Guidelines for Cardiac Rehabilitation Programs

Sixth Edition

American Association of Cardiovascular
and Pulmonary Rehabilitation

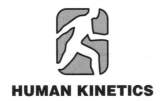

HUMAN KINETICS

Library of Congress Cataloging-in-Publication Data

Names: American Association of Cardiovascular & Pulmonary Rehabilitation, author.
Title: Guidelines for cardiac rehabilitation programs / American Association of Cardiovascular and Pulmonary Rehabilitation.
Other titles: Guidelines for cardiac rehabilitation and secondary prevention programs
Description: Sixth edition. | Champaign, IL : Human Kinetics, [2021] | Preceded by Guidelines for cardiac rehabilitation and secondary prevention programs / American Association of Cardiovascular and Pulmonary Rehabilitation. Fifth edition. 2013. | Includes bibliographical references and index.
Identifiers: LCCN 2019044218 (print) | LCCN 2019044219 (ebook) | ISBN 9781492569695 (paperback) | ISBN 9781492595076 (epub) | ISBN 9781492569701 (pdf)
Subjects: MESH: Cardiac Rehabilitation | Heart Diseases--prevention & control | Guideline
Classification: LCC RC682 (print) | LCC RC682 (ebook) | NLM WG 180 | DDC 616.1/203--dc23
LC record available at https://lccn.loc.gov/2019044218
LC ebook record available at https://lccn.loc.gov/2019044219
ISBN: 978-1-4925-6969-5 (print)

The web addresses cited in this text were current as of October 2019, unless otherwise noted.

Acquisitions Editor: Amy N. Tocco; **Developmental Editor:** Melissa J. Zavala; **Copyeditor:** Joanna Hatzopoulos Portman; **Proofreader:** Leigh Keylock; **Indexer:** Nancy Ball; **Permissions Manager:** Dalene Reeder; **Graphic Designer:** Joe Buck; **Cover Designer:** Keri Evans; **Cover Design Associate:** Susan Rothermel Allen; **Photographs (interior):** ©Human Kinetics, unless otherwise noted; **Photo Production Manager:** Jason Allen; **Senior Art Manager:** Kelly Hendren; **Illustrations:** ©Human Kinetics, unless otherwise noted; **Printer:** Sheridan Books

Printed in the United States of America

10 9 8 7 6 5 4 3 2 1

The paper in this book is certified under a sustainable forestry program.

Human Kinetics
P.O. Box 5076
Champaign, IL 61825-5076
Website: www.HumanKinetics.com

In the United States, email info@hkusa.com or call 800-747-4457.
In Canada, email info@hkcanada.com.
In the United Kingdom/Europe, email hk@hkeurope.com.

For information about Human Kinetics' coverage in other areas of the world, please visit our website: **www.HumanKinetics.com**

Tell us what you think!
Human Kinetics would love to hear what we can do to improve the customer experience. Use this QR code to take our brief survey.

E7357

Contents

Preface..vi

Chapter 1
Cardiac Rehabilitation: An Evolving Model of Care in the Era of Health Care Reform...1

Ana Mola, PhD, ANP-BC

CR and Population Health Management......................................2
CR and Value-Based Care...3
CR and Care Coordination..4
Summary...5

Chapter 2
The Continuum of Care: From Inpatient and Outpatient CR to Long-Term Secondary Prevention......................................7

Cathie Biga, MSN, FACC

CVD Continuum of Care...8
Efforts to Reduce Gaps in the Continuum of Care........................10
The Role of CR in the Continuum of Care................................12
Putting It All Together..12
Summary..13

Chapter 3
CR in Inpatient and Transitional Settings.............................15

Mary Dolansky, PhD, RN, FAAN; Ana Mola, PhD, ANP-BC

Assessment, Mobilization, and Risk Factor Management...................16
Discharge Planning...22
Clinical Pathways..23
Staffing...25
Space and Equipment..26
Transitional Settings..27
Summary..29

Chapter 4
Medical Evaluation and Exercise Testing for Outpatient CR.............33

Sherrie Khadanga, MD

Physical Examination...34
Risk Stratification and Identification of Contraindications for Exercise Training...........36
Summary..47

Chapter 5
Outpatient CR and SP..49

Philip A. Ades, MD, FACC, MAACVPR

Structure of CR and SP...50
Assessment and Management of Risk Factors for CVD Progression..........50
Coaching, Case Management, and Counseling..............................52
Innovation in CR...58
Maintenance CR...59
Future Directions..60
Summary..60

Chapter 6 Physical Activity and Exercise 61

Jonathan Myers, PhD

Cardiorespiratory Endurance Training 62
Exercise Recommendations for Patients Without a Recent Exercise Test 65
PA Outside of CR 65
Resistance Training 66
Flexibility Training 67
Summary 68

Chapter 7 Nutrition Guidelines 69

Ellen Schaaf Aberegg, MA, LD, RD, FAACVPR

Key Nutrition Principles 70
Diet Patterns of Nutrition Intake 74
Evidence-Based Nutrition Guidelines for CVD Risk Factors 76
Nutrition in the CR Care Process 79
Dietitian–CR Professional Partnership 85
Summary 86

Chapter 8 Behavior Modification for Risk Factor Reduction: Guiding
Principles and Practice 87

Diann Galeema, PhD

Overview of Health-Related Behavior Change 88
Summary 96

Chapter 9 Modifiable CVD Risk Factors 97

Sheri R. Colberg, PhD, FACSM; Emma Fletcher, MS, MVB; Carly Goldstein, PhD; Paul M. Gordon, PhD, MPH, FACSM; Joel Hughes, PhD, FAACVPR; Jonathan Myers, PhD; Quinn R. Pack, MD, MsC, FAACVPR; Killian Robinson, MD, FAHA, FACC, FACP

Physical Inactivity 98
Dyslipidemia 103
Diabetes 110
Tobacco Use 119
Hypertension 124
Overweight and Obesity 131
Psychosocial Considerations 136
Environmental Considerations 143
Summary 148

Chapter 10 Cardiac Disease Populations 149

Alison L. Bailey, MD, FACC; Alexis L. Beatty, MD, MAS; Brian Carlin, MD, FCCP, MAACVPR, FAARC; Dennis J. Kerrigan, PhD, FACSM; Steven J. Keteyian, PhD; Kirstine Laerum Sibilitz, MD, PhD; Karen Lui, RN, MS, MAACVPR; Ryan Mays, PhD, MPH; Jonathan Powell, MD; Ray W. Squires, PhD; Diane J. Treat-Jacobson, PhD, RN, FAAN

CR for Patients With CVD (MI, Revascularization, and Stable Angina) 150
Heart Valve Replacement and Repair Surgery 157
Dysrhythmias 160
Heart Failure and Left Ventricular Assist Devices 165
Heart Transplantation 175
Peripheral Artery Disease 186
Chronic Lung Disease 193
Summary 196

Chapter **11** Special Demographic Populations 197

Justin M. Bachmann, MD, MPH, FACC; Daniel Forman, MD; Naomi Gauthier, MD; Alexander Opotowsky, MD, MPH, MMsc; Marta Supervia, MD, MSc, CCRP; Carmen Terzic, MD, PhD

Younger Adults 198
Older Adults 199
Women and Men 209
Race and Culture 214
Socioeconomic Considerations 218
Summary 222

Chapter **12** Program Administration 223

Karen Lui, RN, MS, MAACVPR

Program Priorities 224
Facilities and Equipment 231
Organizational Policies and Procedures 234
Insurance and Reimbursement 235
Documentation 238
Personnel 239
Continuum of Care and Services 242
Summary 242

Chapter **13** Outcomes Assessment and Utilization 243

Sherry L. Grace, PhD, FCCS, FAACVPR, CRFC

Purposes for Measuring Outcomes 244
Outcomes Matrix 244
Measuring, Documenting, Analyzing, and Reporting Program Outcomes 250
Resources 254
Summary 254

Chapter **14** Management of Medical Problems and Emergencies 255

Jason L. Rengo, MS, FAACVPR

Potential Risks in Outpatient CR 256
Intervention Summary 258
Phase 3 CR Programs 262
Alternative Models of SP 263
Summary 264

Appendix A Example of Standing Orders to Initiate Outpatient CR 265
Appendix B Example of Outpatient CR Emergency Standing Orders 266
Appendix C Cardiac Rehabilitation Untoward Event—Physician Notification 270
Appendix D Daily Emergency Cart Checklist 272
Appendix E Monthly Emergency Cart Checklist 274
Appendix F Emergency Equipment Maintenance Log 277

References 278
Index 347
About the AACVPR 356
Contributors 357

AACVPR Membership Application can be found at www.aacvpr.org. Click on the "Join" button and set up an account to begin your application.

Preface

Cardiovascular disease (CVD) is the major cause of death and disability globally. With the advancement in treatment of acute cardiac events, many individuals with chronic CVD are surviving. Additionally, great progress has been made in the treatment and care of patients with valvular heart disease and chronic heart failure. Despite advancement in medical care, there is a high recurrence rate for individuals with CVD, valve disease, and heart failure. Therefore, efforts to prevent secondary events, hasten recovery, and improve physical function and quality of life are essential to the long-term care of patients with cardiac-related chronic disease.

Cardiac rehabilitation (CR) is a medically supervised program that assists with recovery after a cardiac event and with the prevention of disease recurrence and premature death. Cardiac rehabilitation is a complex, multifaceted, and multidisciplinary approach to optimize the health and well-being of individuals with a cardiac-related medical condition. The list of benefits of cardiac rehabilitation participation are lengthy and profound and described in great detail in this sixth edition of *Guidelines for Cardiac Rehabilitation Programs*.

Beginning with the first edition (released in 1991), *Guidelines for Cardiac Rehabilitation Programs* has been an invaluable resource for CR professionals. The diagnoses that qualify a patient for participation in CR continue to expand as we continue to understand the tremendous benefits of exercise training and lifestyle modification. Additionally, with the recent focus on increasing participation, the demographics of participants has become increasingly diverse. Consequently, the interventions employed in CR need to accommodate an evolving patient population and be scientific and evidence based. The sixth edition of the guidelines is an update on the recommendations and guidelines for the treatment and care of this increasingly diverse patient population.

Past editions of the guidelines have used the term *cardiac rehabilitation and secondary prevention (CR/SP)*. The terms *cardiac rehabilitation* and *cardiac rehabilitation and secondary prevention* are often, but not always, interpreted similarly and are used interchangeably. In this edition, for the purpose of consistency, we have defined *cardiac rehabilitation* as including the delivery of secondary prevention services. As described in chapter 1, CR is an integral, cost-effective health care delivery strategy that results in improved patient outcomes. Therefore, in a departure from previous editions, the current edition uses the term *cardiac rehabilitation (CR)* instead of the lengthier *cardiac rehabilitation and secondary prevention (CR/SP)*.

To optimize the care and treatment of patients with cardiac-related disease, CR programs must be connected to the larger continuum of care—from acute hospitalization to transitional medical care facilities to preventive care after the patient has gone home. Chapters 2 and 3 detail the opportunities and challenges of delivering CR and secondary prevention service, beginning with in-hospital care for an acute event and continuing through long-term follow-up.

To optimize health outcomes, it is critical that individuals with a qualifying cardiac-related diagnosis are referred to, enrolled in, and adhere to CR programming. Compared to an otherwise healthy population, individuals eligible for CR are at relatively high risk for recurrent events. Moreover, participants in CR often have the complication of comorbid medical conditions. It is incumbent on CR programs to provide a safe environment that minimizes the risks of adverse events. A key to minimizing risk is to ensure that all patients are properly screened prior to initiating CR. Chapter 4 details the components of the medical evaluation that is needed for any participant prior to enrolling in CR.

A major challenge for all CR programs, which is addressed in chapter 5, is to increase opportunities to provide risk intervention and promote positive health behavior patterns within the limited amount of available resources. Outpatient CR programs must provide patients with low-cost, high-quality programming that moves patients toward taking personal responsibility for disease management and secondary prevention over a lifetime. Disease management involves using efficacious approaches for risk factor intervention, implementing effective education and coaching techniques, increasing physical activity and discouraging sedentary behavior, and recognizing symptoms before an acute episode occurs to decrease cardiovascular disease morbidity and mortality.

A hallmark characteristic of participants in CR has always been low levels of fitness and functional capacity. Not coincidentally, physical inactivity is an independent risk factor for CVD. As a remedy, exercise training is the cornerstone of CR programming. Reflecting this prominent role, this edition includes a new, comprehensive discussion of the topic, with the entirety of chapter 6 dedicated to physical activity and exercise training and prescription.

CR professionals must be diligent in helping people make lifestyle changes that reduce the risk of cardiac-related events. There is perhaps no more important, complex, and challenging topic in lifestyle behavior than nutrition. Chapter 7 is fully revised for the sixth edition and provides CR professionals with information regarding nutritional education and counseling to maximize patient understanding and achieve long-term compliance to dietary advice. Chapter 8, Behavior Modification for Risk Factor Reduction, highlights the critical importance of effectively addressing behavior change in CR. This chapter contains new and updated information that will assist CR professionals with the challenging task of helping patients change behaviors that are associated with the progression of CVD.

Chapter 9 addresses modifiable CVD risk factors. The scientific literature clearly supports the efficacy of participating in CR as a means of CVD risk factor reduction and for the prevention of recurrent cardiovascular events. Many chronic diseases—including coronary artery disease, hypertension, obesity, diabetes, and peripheral vascular disease—have a common underlying pathophysiology. Thus, the preventive and rehabilitative aspects of CR programs can (and should) address six lifestyle-related risk factors: smoking, hypertension, obesity, type 2 diabetes, unhealthy diet, and sedentary lifestyle. The key to effective chronic disease management is adherence to a healthy lifestyle, including high levels of physical activity, no tobacco use, and a healthy dietary pattern. Adherence to existing medical therapy underpins the healthy lifestyle choices.

Chapter 10 is new to this edition and explores the different qualifying diagnoses for which CR is appropriate. The secondary prevention model employed in CR also allows for program transition into the management of other chronic diseases that have similar underlying pathophysiology. Thus, CR programs can be models for other disease management programs. One clear example of expanding opportunities is the treatment of patients with peripheral artery disease. A portion of chapter 10 provides a detailed description of the important aspects of peripheral artery disease programming within the setting of outpatient CR. Chapter 11 focuses on special demographic populations typically seen in CR.

It is a challenge to integrate the many and varied aspects of CR programming together to deliver comprehensive CR services. Changes in (and interpretation of) federal regulations affecting reimbursement and program design continue to influence how CR services are delivered. Chapter 12 addresses the complexity of delivering CR programming in an integral, cost-effective service that results in positive health outcomes for patients. To this end, measuring patient- and service-related outcomes is critical to demonstrating the value that CR delivers directly to the patient and to the overall health care system. The outcomes generated through the care of patients in CR reflect program performance and quality. Chapter 13 details the process of measuring, collecting, and analyzing patient outcomes.

Even when a thorough process for screening patients has been put in place (as explained in chapter 4), adverse events will occur. Consequently, CR professionals need to be ready to respond and deliver emergency care as expeditiously and effectively as possible. Chapter 14 describes the critical elements needed for CR programs to be prepared to respond to emergent situations in CR.

As in the previous editions, it is acknowledged that all programs may not have the personnel or resources to provide specific expertise in each area, but the core components of CR should be part of every program. Changes in program delivery and the professional expertise of CR practitioners may be necessary to make this happen. This edition provides the basis to address the essential components in a manner that is in keeping with the delivery of a comprehensive CR program.

The challenge to CR professionals is to select, develop, and deliver appropriate, state-of-the-art rehabilitative and secondary preventive services to patients and to tailor the method of delivery of these services to the individual needs of each patient. Determination of the best approach in each case should involve both health care provider recommendations and patient preferences. The strategy for success should reflect a desire for progressive patient independence in CR and continued compliance with the necessary lifestyle change.

The information in the sixth edition covers the current scope of practice for CR programs and professionals. Keeping up with change is a professional necessity, while keeping up with the science is a professional responsibility. This text is an essential tool to help CR professionals meet program structure and delivery challenges. By participating in writing *Guidelines for Cardiac Rehabilitation Programs*, more than 50 leaders in the field of CR and secondary prevention, cardiovascular risk reduction, reimbursement, and public policy have provided CR professionals with the latest tools and information to successfully start new programs or update and enhance existing ones.

The AACVPR and this text are critical for keeping our profession (and the services that we provide) recognized and valued by the scientific community, federal agencies, third-party payers, and, most importantly, the patients, families, and communities whose lives we touch. The sixth edition of *Guidelines for Cardiac Rehabilitation Programs* provides significant support to help us achieve our goals of continuing professional development and program excellence.

Web Resource

To complement the text, *Guidelines for Cardiac Rehabilitation Programs, Sixth Edition*, has a companion web resource. This resource includes case studies and questions for select chapters. Reproducible questionnaires, charts, consent forms, protocols, records, checklists, and logs are included for use in creating or assessing programs. The web resource will also serve as a location for AACVPR to post biannual updates to book content, as necessary, keeping the guidelines up to date between editions of the text. The web resource can be purchased at www.HumanKinetics.com/ GuidelinesForCardiacRehabilitationPrograms.

Cardiac Rehabilitation

Ana Mola, PhD, ANP-BC

An Evolving Model of Care in the Era of Health Care Reform

Cardiac rehabilitation (CR) is a medically supervised specialty with a multidisciplinary approach to deliver a comprehensive secondary prevention program. Cardiac rehabilitation optimizes cardiovascular disease (CVD) risk reduction, promotes adherence to healthy lifestyle behaviors, and reduces disabilities.[1] Specific components of CR include medical evaluation, psychosocial assessment, physician-prescribed exercise, cardiac risk factor modification, education, behavioral counseling, and outcomes assessment.

OBJECTIVES

This chapter provides an overview of the following:

- The definition of cardiac rehabilitation (CR)
- The goal of decreasing the cost burden of cardiovascular disease (CVD) to the overall health care system
- The role of CR within the health care economy that prioritizes value over volume with a focus on improved patient outcomes and quality of care
- CR as an integral, cost-effective health care delivery strategy that results in improved patient outcomes

Cardiac rehabilitation has evolved tremendously since the 1970s. Going forward, rather than be viewed as a clearly defined intervention with 3 or 4 distinct phases, CR needs to evolve to maintain its status as a value-based service that coordinates care across a wide continuum of secondary disease prevention.[2] The chronic state of underutilization of CR services needs to be addressed with a collective voice that amplifies innovation, accessibility, and adaptability. U.S. government agencies involved in population health, such as the Centers for Disease Control and Prevention (CDC), are steadfast in reinforcing a collective capacity to improve the nation's health by responding to the epidemic of chronic diseases and promoting community wellness.[3]

The Million Hearts Collaborative 2022 is a national initiative co-led by the CDC and the Centers for Medicare and Medicaid Services with a goal to prevent 1 million heart attacks and strokes. Increasing referral, enrollment, and adherence to CR services are critical to achieving the goals of the Million Hearts Collaborative[4]. To frame this national initiative and emerging national trends, *Guidelines for Cardiac Rehabilitation Programs, Sixth Edition,* provides a blueprint for evidence-based clinical and administrative practices and illustrates the practical and innovative strategies to increase CR participation.

The Patient Protection and Affordable Care Act (ACA) was established in 2010. It includes clear provisions for comprehensive models of care, which in practice deliver interventions that provide safe, efficient, and high-quality care to at-risk populations such as patients with multiple chronic conditions.[5] Historically, CR has delivered clinical services such as team-based and patient-centered care, chronic disease management, prevention strategies, and models of care coordination across a continuum of care that is cost-effective, safe, and high in quality.[2] However, even with long-standing national recommendations encouraging use, CR services are underutilized.[6] *Guidelines for Cardiac Rehabilitation Programs, Sixth Edition,* provides strategies and alternative delivery models of CR services that will assist programs in meeting the challenges of underreferral, enrollment, and adherence.

CR and Population Health Management

By 2035, more than 130 million adults in the U.S. population are projected to have CVD, and total costs of CVD are expected to reach $1.1 trillion.[8] The national agenda to decrease the CVD cost burden and to deliver safe, effective, and efficient care will be imperative to the viability of U.S. health care and of the future of CR services. To attain the American Heart Association's (AHA) 2020 Impact Goals of reducing deaths attributable to CVD and stroke by 20%, innovative delivery of care is needed to prevent and treat CVD events and promote secondary prevention through risk factor reduction strategies.[8] When CR is practiced within the population health approach, emphasizing care coordination and a care continuum model with guideline-based care, it provides a high-yield investment.

The goal of health care reform is to broaden the population that receives health care coverage, improve the access to health care specialists and programs, improve the quality of health care, and decrease the cost of health care. The Institute for Healthcare Improvement (IHI) set forth the Triple Aim framework. According to this framework, new designs must be developed to simultaneously pursue the following three dimensions of optimal care: (1) improving the quality of care, (2) improving the health of the population, and (3) lowering the cost of care.[7] The framework, in context, is operational within a population heath management model. *Population health management* refers to integrated health care for patients in a health system. It applies strategies and interventions across the continuum of care to improve the health care experience and outcomes at competitive costs.[9]

Comprehensive CR services can deliver sustainable improvements in medication adherence, tobacco cessation, weight management, stress management, and increased physical activity. Expansion of innovative outreach models of CR services is feasible utilizing the Triple Aim framework to improve patients' health through prevention and rehabilitation programs across the continuum. The AHA encourages health care providers and clinicians to intervene directly and as members of a multidisciplinary health care team to help patients adopt healthier lifestyles and advocate for health care system and policy improvements to address behavior change needs more effectively.[10]

Analytic frameworks for quality assessment have guided performance measure development by the Institute of Medicine (renamed National Academy of Medicine). One of the most influential frameworks includes the following six domains of a national quality strategy for the health care system.[7,11,12]

1. *Safe:* Avoid harm to patients from the care intended to help them.
2. *Effective:* Provide services based on scientific evidence to all who could benefit and refrain from providing services to those not likely to benefit (avoiding underuse and misuse, respectively).
3. *Patient centered:* Provide care that is respectful of and responsive to the individual patient's preferences and needs, ensuring that the patient's values guide clinical decisions.
4. *Timely:* Reduce wait times and harmful delays for those who receive care.
5. *Efficient:* Avoid wasting equipment, supplies, ideas, and energy.
6. *Equitable:* Provide quality care regardless of gender, ethnicity, geographic location, and socioeconomic status.

The American College of Cardiology and the AHA developed performance measures to evaluate the quality of care provided and to identify opportunities for improvement. The performance measures are aligned with the national agenda of quality of care and "pay-for-performance" initiatives for the delivery of care that is timely, safe, effective, efficient, and patient centered. In 2016, AACVPR revised performance measures for CR. In addition, new measures to benchmark and improve the quality of care for CR patients have been developed. Further insight into the meaning and impact of these CR performance measures in optimizing referral to CR in alternate delivery payment models and the overall contributions of CR to measure outcomes of the care experience are discussed in other chapters in this book.[13,14,15]

CR and Value-Based Care

The U.S. health care system's traditional fee-for-service based payment model offers incentives for providers to increase the volume, but not necessarily quality, of services. Due to concerns about rising costs and poor performance on quality indicators, purchasers of health care are pushing for a transition to value-based payment models. *Value* in health care is a measure of beneficial and significant quality results and outcomes, per dollar spent. With a new health care economy defined by value over volume, payers and providers are collaborating to improve quality of care.

The premise of value-based payments is to align physician and hospital bonuses and penalties with cost, quality, and outcomes measures.[16] Value is conceptualized as the optimization of the Triple Aim framework in clinical practice. The combination of care experience and cost enables measurement of efficiency. Similarly, the combination of population health outcomes and care experience enables measurement of effectiveness of care or the comparative effectiveness to alternative treatments.[17] The 2018 AHA Heart Disease and Stroke Statistics report highlights the large number of patients who could benefit from CR. A systematic review has shown that after a heart attack, CR participants were 53% less likely to die from any cause and 57% less likely to experience cardiac-related mortality than were those who did not use CR.[18] Studies have also found that CR participation is associated with a 20% to 30% reduction in hospital readmission during the year after a postmyocardial infarction.[19] Therefore, CR is an integral, cost-effective service that can produce a positive "return on investment."[20]

BOTTOM LINE

The CR team creates value and return on investment by doing the following:

- Enhancing medication reconciliation as patients transition to the next level of care (e.g., inpatient to skilled nursing facility to outpatient to primary care)
- Decreasing hospital length of stay with early mobilization and self-care education
- Decreasing the need for high-cost post-acute services
- Preventing or reducing 30-day readmissions
- Providing tobacco cessation and relapse prevention services
- Implementing established turnkey strategies for increasing referral, enrollment, and adherence
- Improving the patient (inpatient and outpatient) experience and satisfaction
- Creating lifelong health and wellness

CR and Care Coordination

The ACA specifically identifies care coordination as a main strategy for achieving national quality objectives.[21] Medicare and Medicaid programs now reimburse providers for selected care coordination services. Increasingly, health care insurances companies are offering care coordination as a benefit to their members.[22]

The National Quality Forum (NQF) mission is to advance performance measurements in health care and has endorsed measures for care coordination as a national quality strategy. The NQF defines care coordination as a:[23]

> "...function that helps ensure that the patient's needs and preferences for health services and information sharing across people, functions, and sites are met over time."

Care coordination intertwines the various parts of the system together to ensure that patients and families receive the care in a timely manner. Effective care coordination supports patients as they proceed through various levels of care settings in a synchronized care continuum.

BOTTOM LINE

Care coordination strategies include the following: Prevent gaps in care; communicate important information to patients, providers, and insurers; and orchestrate services to achieve desired health, quality, and cost outcomes.[24]

An example of a care coordination healthcare reform alternate payment model is the *bundled payment care initiative (BPCI)*. *Bundled payment* is a single payment for an episode of care over a specified period for a procedure or condition. It may consist of clinicians receiving a lump sum for services related to a procedure or care episode instead of individual payments for encounters, services, tests, and procedures. Bundled payments aim to reward clinicians who offer efficient, high-quality care across the continuum of care.[25] For example, the Medicare demonstration project of the elective BPCI included voluntary participating providers assuming financial risk for the selected diagnoses of myocardial infarction, heart failure, and cardiovascular surgery (coronary bypass and valvular).[2] The BPCI Advanced

Model, an alternative payment model, continues a value-based care payment program with some modifications from the previous BPCI program. The aim is to align incentives among participating health care providers for reducing expenditures and improving quality of care.[26,27]

The trends of care coordination are naturally entrenched in CR. CR can play a pivotal role in value-based care BPCI and other alternative payment models. CR delivers a comprehensive CVD risk reduction program over a cycle of care, not separate encounters, and aligns performance measures to ensure safe, efficient, and effective care.[2] In practice, value-based payment models address various opportunities for hospitals and their partners to improve quality and reduce spending by reaching out to patients during their hospitalization and after discharge, when patients transition to the next level of care, such as to a postacute care facility or home. To reduce readmissions and increase quality of care, transitional care interventions such as reconciling medications, scheduling timely post-discharge follow-up appointments with primary care physicians or specialists, establishing plans for addressing common health concerns, and coordinating with post-acute care providers have proven beneficial.[28] These established, patient-centric activities and care coordination interventions already occur in CR. For example, the care coordination occurs with the activation of the CR team when the patient presents in the emergency department with an acute myocardial infarction, and is followed through revascularization, to discharge. With established CR liaisons and engagement with postacute care partners, CR activities can continue with ongoing communications to acute rehabilitation, skilled nursing facilities, and a referral to a hybrid model of CR home care or center-based CR rehabilitation.

Going forward, a significant challenge is the prevalent underutilization of CR services. Particular focus needs to be directed to include patients from traditionally underrepresented groups, such as people of lower socioeconomic status, racial and ethnic minorities, women, and the elderly. Mobile and other health-related technology is advancing rapidly and has enormous potential for CVD prevention and management. Also, alternatives to the traditional CR model can be considered. For example, home-based CR programs may provide an effective means to increase accessibility to CR-related services. Some evidence suggests that home- and center-based CR programs are similarly effective in improving clinical and health-related quality of life outcomes. This finding supports the continued expansion of evidence-based, home-based CR programs.[29,30] However, more research is needed in order to help differentiate the relative benefits of nontraditional CR programming. Studies of CR hybrid models of both center-based and home-based programs are needed to advance greater options of care coordination across the continuum.

Summary

CR programs must continue to evolve and provide value to patients and the health care system. Going forward, CR has an opportunity to play a prominent role with the focus of hospitals and payers shifting to quality patient care and meaningful patient outcomes. A major challenge for all CR programs is to increase opportunities to provide services within the finite limit of available resources. CR programs need to continue to evolve in order to provide evidence- and value-based care to patients. Practitioners and payers working collaboratively will be instrumental in the continued growth of CR services with the ultimate goal of enhanced patient outcomes. Conventional fee-for-service payment is becoming less viable, and enrollment in new payment models will be emerging. Therefore, CR programs will need to be innovative, engaging, accessible, and adaptable when developing value-based care that is coordinated across the continuum of care.

The Continuum of Care

Cathie Biga, MSN, FACC

From Inpatient and Outpatient CR to Long-Term Secondary Prevention

In the past, health care focused largely on fee-for-service care; providers were paid according to the number of visits, services, and tests performed. The IHI launched the Triple Aim to help organizations and providers redesign health care delivery.[1] The intention was to adopt new processes that would simultaneously pursue these three goals: (1) improve the patient experience of care (both quality and satisfaction), (2) improve the health of populations, and (3) reduce the per capita cost of health care in the United States. This conceptual shift in health care delivery has become widely accepted, but it has resulted in the unintended consequence of provider burnout. Thus, the Triple Aim evolved into the Quadruple Aim[2]; the fourth aim is to prevent provider burnout. As the health care delivery model evolves, it is imperative to remember that not only is the patient at the center of care, the patient also needs competent and caring providers at every stage of the delivery system.

OBJECTIVES

This chapter provides an overview of the following:
- CR in the continuum of care with the goals of improved patient outcomes, better patient experience, cost reduction, and provider well-being
- Key trends in health care
- How best to implement CR guidelines into the continuum of care
- The operational structure and sequence of CR programming
- Opportunities to redesign existing programs to optimize performance within an evolving continuum of care

The trajectory of comprehensive health care reform continued with the passage of the ACA then the Health Care and Education Reconciliation Act. Every provider needs to look at how, when, where, and why health care is delivered. Management of CVD was among the first disease conditions impacted by these reforms. With the Health and Human Services (HHS) mandate and the passage of the Medicare Access and the Children's Health Insurance Program [CHIP] Reauthorization Act (MACRA),[3] the transition to payment based on the value of care delivered truly ramped up. The HHS-mandated payment reform resulted in alternative payment models (APMs) and not fee-for-service care. By 2018, 90% of payments were tied to quality or value, with 50% being paid through APMs. Some of the more common APMs are Accountable Care Organizations (ACOs) such as Medicare Shares Savings Program (MSSP), Next Generation ACO, and Pioneer ACO models. MACRA created these two payment pathways for physicians: the Merit-based Incentive Payment System (MIPS) and the Advanced Alternative Payment Model (AAPM) track. The MIPS adjusts payment based on performance in these four performance categories: quality, cost, improvement activities, and advancing care information. With the scoring of four categories and resultant penalties and/or bonus payments, MACRA will continue to evolve and become an integral component in the delivery of CVD care.

The changes brought about will continue to drive improvements to the delivery of care by mandating better care at a lower cost with better patient outcomes and satisfaction. These legislative mandates were only the beginning of the path referred to as *payment reform* or *movement from volume to value*. Health care administrators have learned that one size does not fit all. Rather, successful system change requires collaboration and coordination of the entire health care team, including payers, providers, and patients.

What does this massive change in care delivery have to do with CR? With the advent of caring for patients throughout their disease continuum, CR programs have taken on more importance and a sense of urgency. The call to action is louder and more of an imperative than ever before. Health care providers must care for CVD patients beyond their initial diagnosis and treatment.

Changes in health care have accelerated with a focus on the continuum of care, not only during an acute illness but afterward as well.[4-6] There is an increased emphasis on providing patient care along a continuum, particularly in the area of CVD medicine.[7-10] As payment reform continues to evolve, postacute care has become one of the key areas of focus. As new programs were proposed, such as Bundled Payments for Care Improvement (announced in 2013) and Bundled Payments for Care Improvement—Advanced (announced in 2018),[11] as well as the ongoing evolution of APMs, CR services represent a critical component of postacute care. Several factors help explain this growing focus, including the following:

- Survival of patients experiencing an acute myocardial infarction has improved, resulting in more patients with chronic CVD.
- Effective medical and lifestyle secondary prevention (SP) therapies have been developed that improve long-term survival of patients with CVD.
- The majority of patients with chronic CVD do not receive optimal SP care. In fact, only a minority of patients receive appropriate SP treatments and follow-up services.
- Private and governmental organizations have noticed the gaps in the continuum of care and have established policies to bridge important gaps in the continuum of CVD care.

CVD Continuum of Care

While the continuum of care for CVD should begin early in life (before the clinical manifestation of CVD),[12,13] for the purposes of this discussion the continuum of care for the patient with CVD begins at the time of the clinical diagnosis or event. The 2018 release of the CR Performance and Quality measures targeted recognized gaps in the quality of care.[14] This set of guidelines included six performance and three quality measures. Steps in the CVD continuum of care include the following (figure 2.1):

1. *Treatment of acute event.* The initial step in the CVD care continuum occurs with treatment given to address the acute event. For an acute coronary syndrome, prompt provision of antiplatelet therapy, thrombolytic therapy, percutaneous coronary intervention, or some combination of these treatments is critically important for survival and to minimize myocardial damage.[15]

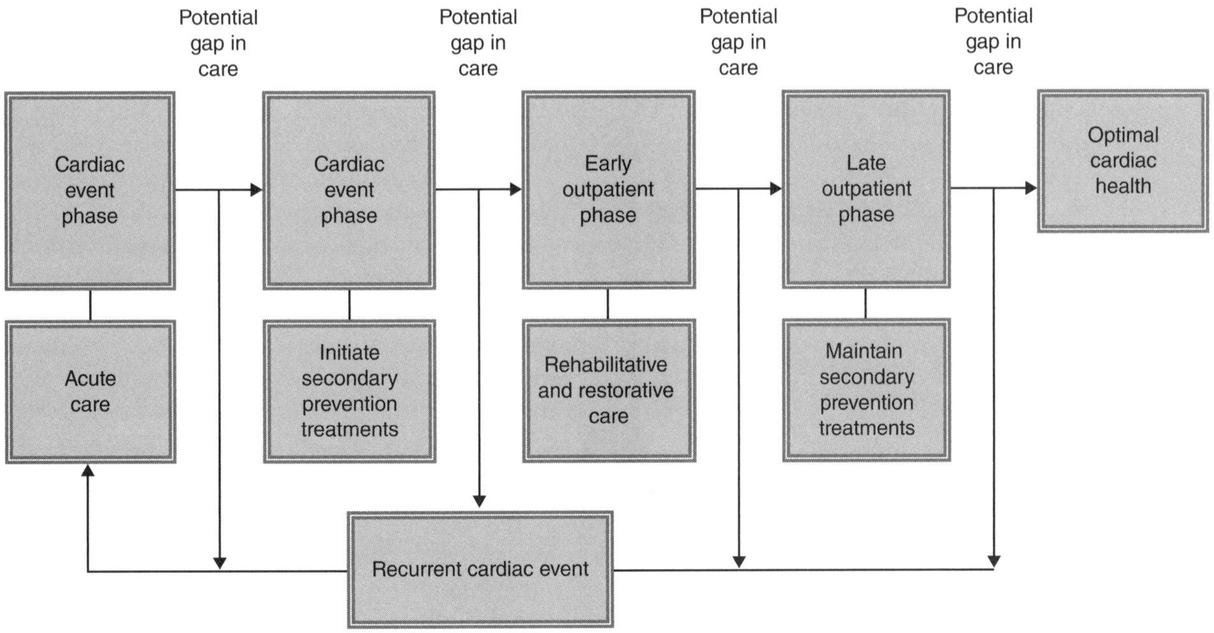

Figure 2.1 Continuum of cardiovascular care following a cardiac event, highlighting potential gaps in the care continuum.

2. *Initiation of SP therapies.* The second step in the care continuum occurs shortly after the acute event has resolved and a longer-term treatment plan is initiated. This long-term plan generally includes lifestyle and medical therapies, and it is optimally started before hospital discharge. In fact, evidence shows that when SP treatments are started in the hospital, patients are more likely to adhere to those treatments in the long term and are more likely to remain free from recurrent CVD events than when those treatments were not started before discharge.[16]

3. *Early outpatient CR.* Typically, this phase includes up to 36 sessions following a CVD event. An important hand-off occurs at the time of patient discharge from the hospital and prior to commencing with CR in the outpatient setting, under the supervision and guidance of health care professionals. Unfortunately, this important step is often a misstep when enrollment in CR is delayed or not undertaken. It is notable that a significant number of referred patients never attended CR. Just under 40% of patients surveyed in the Behavioral Risk Factor Surveillance System, who had a myocardial infarction (MI), participated in CR.[17] Gaps in adherence to the SP plan can occur for a variety of reasons, including

patient, provider, environmental, socioeconomic, and health care system factors.[18-22]

From the patient perspective, the time following hospitalization for a CVD event is filled with concerns, questions, and confusion. Patients diagnosed with CVD are often prescribed an array of new therapies. Concerns about costs and potential side effects, as well as uncertainty about treatment benefits, may lead patients to avoid prescribed treatments.[23,24] In addition, depression and anxiety, which are commonly experienced following a CVD event, make it even more challenging for patients to maneuver through this difficult time.[25] CR services can help bridge the divide between the hospital and outpatient settings. Patient education and counseling services are provided and give needed guidance and resources to help initiate and maintain the SP plan. In addition, outpatient CR programs help promote coordination of care between health care providers.[26, 27]

4. *Long-term CR and SP.* Following the early rehabilitation phase after a CVD event, patients shift into long-term CR, another time where gaps in the CVD care continuum occur. Patients who participate in an early outpatient CR program and continue with long-term maintenance CR are likely to continue to receive effective therapies and the associated morbidity and mortality benefits.[28-35] However, many patients who complete an early outpatient CR program fail to continue with a long-term follow-up program and do not continue with the recommended SP therapies.[24,36] Equally problematic is that patients who do not participate in an early outpatient CR program are unlikely to receive effective SP therapies in the long term as well.[33]

BOTTOM LINE

The care of patients with CVD should be viewed as a continuum that includes the following:

- Initial treatment of an acute event
- Identifying cardiovascular risk factors and initiating SP treatment
- Referral, enrollment, and adherence to early outpatient CR programming
- Long-term maintenance of SP interventions

The American College of Cardiology (ACC)/AHA performance measurements are intended to provide practitioners who deliver CR services with tools to measure the quality of care provided and identify opportunities for improvement.[14] The intention is to accelerate the translation of scientific evidence into clinical practice. With the ongoing evolution of payment reform, this document should serve as the infrastructure for all CR programs. The tools allow programs to measure the quality of care and to facilitate the movement to value and continuous quality improvement. One of the key aspects is clearly differentiating quality measures from performance measures. Program administrators have the opportunity to embed quality measures in their programs to assess outcomes while understanding that they are not publicly reportable. As supporting scientific evidence becomes available, quality measures may be promoted to the status of performance measures.

The six performance measures and three quality measures are summarized in table 2.1. Two of the quality measures that programs should initially focus on are *CR time to enrollment* and *CR adherence*. Designing inpatient and outpatient capture processes is critical to ensure not only the enrollment but also participation in CR.

Efforts to Reduce Gaps in the Continuum of Care

Considerable effort has been made to identify, understand, and reduce the gaps in SP. Gaps in inpatient care, commonly due to systematic barriers and inefficiencies, have been reduced with organized approaches to quality improvement. For instance, critical pathways of care and standing orders have been found to improve the inpatient provision of SP therapies.[16,37,38] Furthermore, the use of automatic referral systems has been found to improve referral to outpatient CR.[21,39,40] Likewise, systematic approaches to enrollment of patients in outpatient CR have been fruitful.[39] However, despite these advances, only a minority of patients receive appropriate CR services. Women, the elderly, underserved minorities, the less educated, and uninsured patients are particularly at risk of not receiving SP services.[41,42]

Various national health care organizations have developed and disseminated clinical practice guidelines with the intent to improve the delivery of care. Prior clinical practice guidelines alone

 Guideline 2.1   Components of the Continuum of Care

To demonstrate its place in the continuum of care, each CR program should have

- an outline of the structure or sequence of cardiovascular care and SP within its operation;
- a written description of the scope of CR services including medical evaluation, psychosocial assessment, physician prescribed exercise, cardiac risk factor modification, education, behavioral counseling, and outcomes assessment; and
- standards of care that outline how each service will be delivered and evaluated.

Table 2.1 ACC/AHA 2018 Clinical Performance and Quality Measures for CR

No.	Measure title	Care setting	Attribution	Measure domain
PERFORMANCE MEASURES				
PM-1	CR patient referral from an inpatient setting	Inpatient	Facility level	Communication and care coordination
PM-2	Exercise training referral for chronic heart failure from inpatient setting	Inpatient	Facility level	Communication and care coordination
PM-3	CR patient referral from an outpatient setting	Outpatient	Facility or provider level	Communication and care coordination
PM-4	Exercise training referral for HF from an outpatient setting	Outpatient	Facility or provider level	Communication and care coordination
PM-5a	CR enrollment—claims based	Outpatient	Provider level	Effective clinical care
PM-5b	CR enrollment—registry/ electronic health records based	Inpatient	Provider level	Effective clinical care
QUALITY MEASURES				
QM-1	CR time to enrollment	Outpatient	Facility or provider level	Effective clinical care
QM-2	CR adherence (≥36 sessions)	Outpatient	Facility or provider level	Effective clinical care
QM-3	CR communication: patient enrollment, adherence, and clinical outcomes	Outpatient	Facility or provider level	Communication and care coordination

have not been sufficient to reduce the gaps in CVD SP, in part because of the variable rates at which clinicians adopt guidelines.[43] However, such guidelines have been important in their influence on establishing standards of care and decisions in health care policy.[44]

Various organizations have made efforts to improve the quality of health care services, including the IOM, Joint Commission, IHI, Physician Consortium for Practice Improvement, and the National Quality Forum (NQF). These organizations have promoted improvements in health care quality by increasing the national focus on transparency and accountability in health care delivery. One quality improvement method that has been promoted by these and other organizations is the use of quality indicators or performance measures. Performance measures are designed to promote high-quality care through (1) measurement of important processes and outcomes of care provided by a health care provider or organization, (2) identification of performance gaps in the processes and outcomes measured, and (3) use of quality improvement methods to revise and

improve the processes of care and thereby reduce gaps in care. A standard approach to developing performance measures has been published by the ACC and the AHA.[45]

The six performance measures of the 2018 ACC/AHA guidelines accelerated this concept. Targeting gaps in care that are Class 1 practice guidelines will accelerate the enrollment and completion of CR. Noting that it is critical to capture patients in both the inpatient and outpatient settings, these performance measures should align both facility and provider care coordination.

Early enthusiasm for the use of performance measures was tempered by evidence suggesting minimal effects on patient outcomes.[46] However, the use of performance measures that are highly correlated with desired outcomes appears to improve the likelihood of success.[47] The CR performance measures were specifically designed to cover these two main aspects of CR: (1) referral of eligible patients to a CR program and (2) delivery of care to eligible patients through multidisciplinary CR programs. The AACVPR has developed specific tools to track patient outcomes and program performance related to evidence-based guidelines for SP. Value-based care and turnkey strategies are available to assist programs to thrive. Value-based care initiatives are resources that will assist CR professionals to do the following:

- Assign accountability.
- Target efficiencies.
- Strategize operational transformation.
- Restructure the care delivery model.
- Implement effective technology solutions in management.
- Ultimately improve the patient and practitioner experience.

Turnkey strategies allow CR programs to use resources to ensure that patients have a path through the continuum of care. As the emphasis for provider and hospital reimbursement shifts to value rather than volume, the time is right for CR programs to become actively involved to assure that appropriate patients are referred for CR services. CR participation clearly impacts many of the outcomes measured within episode-based payment models (such as ACOs or BPCI-A), and inclusion of the referral to CR performance measures in the ACC and AHA registries facilitates benchmarking and tracking. In addition, credentialing bodies and payers are now stressing performance improvement activity by providers, which presents an opportunity for CR programs to work with other providers to develop systems and processes to close the gap in CR referrals. Minimizing the delay between hospital discharge to first appointment is paramount to the success of the program and optimal patient outcome.

The Role of CR in the Continuum of Care

Endorsement of the CR referral performance measures by NQF identified CR as one of the most critically important steps in the continuum of care for patients with CVD. The decision by NQF to endorse the CR referral performance measures is based on several factors, including a growing body of evidence that CR services reduce gaps in the delivery of CR therapies, thereby improving the care and outcomes of patients.[28-35]

The beneficial effects that result from participating in CR are multifactorial. The benefits occur all along the care continuum. Specifically, beneficial effects of CR include the following:

- Positive vascular, metabolic, and rheologic changes related to exercise training[34]
- Improvement in patient adherence to medical and lifestyle therapies for SP[24]
- Improvement in the control of CVD risk factors[33]
- Identification and management of comorbid conditions, including depression and other psychological disorders, resulting in improved quality of life[48-50]
- Coordination of care between a patient's health care providers, helping patients understand, receive, and continue with appropriate SP treaments[26]

Although CR fills an important role in the continuum of CVD care, gaps continue to exist in the utilization of CR due to relatively low referral and enrollment rates.[41,42] The future success of efforts to improve the delivery and impact of CR will depend directly on how well those efforts can extend CR to all eligible patients. As new, effective models are added to current delivery models for CR, and as federal and private health insurance plans provide coverage for those expanded services,[51-55] success is more likely to occur.

Putting It All Together

Several important factors are essential as health care organizations seek to bridge gaps in the continuum of CVD care and provide high-quality SP care to patients. These factors reflect an organizational culture that supports quality improvement efforts through the following common threads[56,57]:

- Organizational values and goals
- Involvement of key leaders
- Staff expertise and participation
- Systems and tools that support collaboration, problem solving, and learning

Professionals in the field of CR can play a valuable role in improving the continuum of SP care that is provided to patients with CVD. Specific steps that can be taken to promote a culture of quality improvement in their practice area include the following:

1. Gain an understanding about and experience with important quality improvement issues and strategies that involve CR.

2. Establish a culture of quality improvement in your CR program, and develop effective delivery models that address the needs of all patients who are eligible for CR, both in the early outpatient phase and over the longer term of CR.

3. Develop collaborative relationships with leaders in the hospitals and practices who care for patients with CVD in the local area.

4. Communicate with local health care leaders and other key partners about the important gaps in CR that exist, using local data if available.

5. Work with local leaders to establish common goals for quality improvement efforts in CR.

6. Work together with leaders and key staff members to develop and carry out quality improvement projects that are in alignment with the goals of the organization.

7. Communicate results of quality improvement efforts, and continually work to improve upon those efforts.

Summary

An increased focus exists on meeting patient needs along the entire continuum of CVD care from inpatient to outpatient settings. CR is recognized as an essential part of the continuum of care for patients with CVD. Gaps exist along that continuum, especially in the provision of CR. These gaps in care ultimately result in suboptimal patient outcomes. Quality improvement strategies, including the use of performance and quality measures for the referral of eligible patients to CR programs, increase the accountability of health care organizations and providers for the referral of patients to CR.

CR programs are ideally positioned to deliver SP services to eligible patients. To do so, CR programs must be actively involved in efforts to implement new strategies that improve the reach and impact of SP services. CR programs will be successful in bridging gaps in the continuum of SP as they develop and implement a variety of delivery models and options to meet individual patient circumstances and needs. Changes must also continue to occur in the arena of health care policy and reimbursement to promote and cover effective models of care that can bridge the current gaps in CR.

CR in Inpatient and Transitional Settings

Mary Dolansky, PhD, RN, FAAN; Ana Mola, PhD, ANP-BC

The initial stage in the CR continuum of care occurs after an acute cardiac event; it begins in the inpatient setting. This chapter provides recommendations regarding the structure and process of inpatient and transitional CR services while recognizing the dynamic and evolving opportunities and trends in health care reform to adapt CR services to innovative clinical practices.

OBJECTIVES

This chapter provides an overview of the following:

- Recommendations regarding the structure and process of delivering rehabilitative services across the continuum of care, from inpatient and transitional care to outpatient CR
- The challenges of delivering rehabilitative services in the inpatient setting
- The process of transitioning patients from one care setting to another
- The process of initiating and progressing early ambulation and physical activity
- The importance of providing patient education regarding CVD risk factor reduction

Emerging hospital patient discharge efficiencies are impacting how and where patients receive treatment. Decreasing patients' length of stay has reduced the overall time for staff to provide care to patients during their hospitalizations. Decreasing length of hospital stay following an acute event needs to be balanced with care teams that focus on delivering expedited quality of care services, particularly in older patients with multiple comorbidities.[1] The mean length of hospital stay is 3.7 days following an uncomplicated cardiac event, including acute coronary syndrome (ACS), ST-elevation myocardial infarction (STEMI) or non-STEMI, and heart surgery (coronary artery bypass grafting [CABG]; or valve repair, replacement, or both).[2,3] The role and function of inpatient health care teams have evolved to adapt to the constraints of the decreasing length of stay while maintaining safe, effective, and efficient quality of care.

A major factor affecting the patient length of stay has been the metric of discharge before noon (DBN). Late afternoon hospital discharges contribute to admission bottlenecks, overcrowding, and increased length of stay. Increasing the DBN rate correlates with admissions arriving earlier in the day and reductions in high-frequency peaks of emergency department admissions.[4] Consequently, the time until discharge has been shortened, so the inpatient CR team needs to be organized to provide timely, focused, meaningful therapy services and appropriate discharge instructions to the patient.

One approach to meet the challenge of shorter length of stay is early progressive mobilization that can begin in the cardiothoracic intensive care unit (CTICU). Benefits of early progressive mobility include patients in the CTICU experiencing shorter time to first physical therapy evaluation and treatment compared to other hospital floor units.[5] Additionally, early rehabilitation programs have led to an earlier discharge from the hospital and improved functional recovery.[6] The early delivery of physical and occupational therapies results in a higher likelihood of achieving independent functional status, less CTICU acquired weakness, and greater unassisted ambulation distance at hospital discharge.[7] Furthermore, early rehabilitation is significantly effective and safe for postoperative recovery in octogenarians after heart valve surgery.[8] Early progressive rehabilitative services can be delivered as a value-based care service to assist in achieving shorter length of stay.

BOTTOM LINE

Instituting early ambulation as part of an inpatient rehabilitation program results in improved patient outcomes, including increased functional capacity at hospital discharge.

A comprehensive patient assessment is a vital component to addressing concerns related to decreasing length of stay, DBN, and the intervention of early rehabilitation in CTICU assessment. A comprehensive assessment ensures patient clinical clearance for the initiation of CR therapy and identification of risk triggers for readmissions, including review of social determinants (living alone, transportation, finances for medication adherence), and planning for a safe discharge to the next transitional setting (skilled nursing facilities, home care services, and referral to outpatient CR). Since the initiation of inpatient CR (IPCR), a variety of postacute or transitional care settings have existed to bridge acute IPCR and discharge to home. These settings have become increasingly important given the shortened length of stay following a cardiac event. This chapter addresses the continuum of care from the acute event to successful discharge to home.

Assessment, Mobilization, and Risk Factor Management

Patient assessment, mobilization, identification of CVD risk factors, and discharge requirements (including basic education regarding self-care and management and facilitating entry into outpatient CR) are cornerstones of CR services in the acute care setting. IPCR commences once a referral is made (guideline 3.1).

Generally, activity progresses from supine through sitting and standing to ambulation. Assessment may include activities of daily living (ADLs), such as grooming, dressing, and bathing (showering). Occasionally, patients may require medical intervention before resuming certain types of physical activity. Abnormal physiologic

Guideline 3.1   Cardiac Rehabilitation Within the Inpatient and Transitional Settings

Following a physician referral or by standing order, patients hospitalized for a cardiac event or procedure and discharged to a transitional setting should receive CR services consisting of (a) initial and daily clinical status assessment; (b) early progressive mobilization; (c) identification of and information regarding modification of cardiovascular risk factors; (d) self-care; and (e) a comprehensive discharge plan including follow-up options for traditional center-based or hybrid outpatient CR.

Assessment of patients referred for CR services is accomplished through a chart review, a patient interview, and a physical examination (guideline 3.2).

Guideline 3.2   Initial Patient Assessment

The initial interview of patients referred to inpatient or transitional CR should consist of the following: assessment for admitting diagnosis, present clinical status, code status and advance care planning, prior level of function, current signs and symptoms, past medical and social history, employment status, risk factors for CVD and other chronic diseases, comorbidities, alcohol or substance abuse, cognitive function, mental health, knowledge and capacity to self-manage, and identification of support systems for future health behavior change and medical issues. The variable trajectory of CVD recovery makes it difficult for patients and families to adequately prepare and direct their future health needs and outcomes; hence, this incertitude makes advance care planning important for patients. Transparency in patient–clinician bidirectional communication about advance care planning, including an exploration of patient values and goals for care in the context of their prognosis, is essential to patient-centered treatment decision making.[9]

The purpose of the chart review and assessment is to

- verify diagnosis, current medical condition, and code status;

- identify CVD risk factors (figure 3.1) in order to begin planning education and interventions; and

- determine the existence of comorbidities or complications that may increase the risk of a recurrent cardiac event, rehospitalization, and emergency room utilization.

To supplement medical information, a patient interview is helpful for gathering information on personal, family, and social history; home self-management needs (diet, physical activity, medication adherence, home and food insecurities); and availability of resources after discharge. Management beyond CVD risk factors is critical to the success of the CR program. However, emphasis during this initial encounter should be on assessing the patient for

- readiness for physical activity (figure 3.2),
- readiness to learn (figure 3.2), and
- discharge requirements to an appropriate transitional setting.

The CR professional should assess whether patient goals are reasonable and realistic (guideline 3.3). Early recognition of unrealistic goals allows staff to determine the need for counseling and education.

Guideline 3.3   Assessment of Patient Goals for Cardiac Rehabilitation

Patient goals for rehabilitation should be assessed to facilitate compliance and ensure adherence and integration into the community. As appropriate, goals should be developed for

- return to activities of daily living,

- risk factor reduction through health behavior change,
- psychological well-being and quality of life, and
- family and social support.

Figure 3.1 CVD Risk Factor Checklist

Smoking	Dyslipidemia	Hypertension
__ Current smoker or quit at time of hospitalization Number of packs per day _____ Years smoked _____ Total pack-years _____ __ Former smoker, quit smoking <6 months before admission Total pack-year history _____ __ Never smoked or quit ≥6 months before admission Total pack-year history _____ __ Uses other tobacco products Identify: _____	__ Abnormal lipid levels diagnosed before admission __ Pt reports compliance with prescribed lipid-lowering medication __ Previous lipid values or lipids drawn within 24 h of admission Chol _____ LDL _____ HDL _____ Trig _____ __ Unknown __ History of normal lipid levels	__ Diagnosed before hospitalization BP _____ __ Pt reports compliance with anti-HTN medication __ Pt reports discontinuing current medication __ Unknown __ History of normal blood pressure
Physical inactivity	**Stress or psychological concerns**	**Body composition**
__ Pt did not exercise 3 or more times per week or ≥150 min per week in 3 months before hospitalization __ Pt reports regular exercise	__ Pt reports history of high stress levels __ History of prior psychological or psychiatric treatment __ No history of perceived high stress or prior problem Appears, acts, or reports being __ angry __ depressed __ hostile __ lonely	Current height _____ Current weight _____ BMI _____ __ Healthy weight, BMI <25 __ Overweight, BMI 25-29.9 __ Obese, BMI 30-40 __ Very obese, BMI >40 __ Waist circumference _____ At risk: __ Males >102 cm (>40 in.) __ Females >88 cm (>35 in.)
Diabetes	**Alcohol or substance abuse**	**Other**
__ Elevated blood glucose levels on admission or diagnosed __ Fasting BS or __ HbA1c __ Normal blood glucose levels __ Metabolic syndrome	__ History of alcohol or substance abuse at time of admission __ Pt denies history but initial presentation suggestive __ No evidence of alcohol or substance abuse	_____ _____ _____

Response is required in each category. Abbreviations: Pt, patient; BP, blood pressure; Chol, cholesterol; LDL, low-density lipoprotein; HDL, high-density lipoprotein; Trig, triglycerides; HTN, hypertension; BMI, body mass index; BS, blood sugar; HbA1c, glycosylated hemoglobin

Figure 3.2 Assessment Parameters for Inpatient and Transitional Settings Education

Is the patient physically able to learn now?	Is the patient psychologically willing to learn now?
Stable physical condition Adequate energy level and alertness (may be limited by fatigue, medication) Absence of brain injury with event (anoxia or hypoxia not present)	Appropriate emotional state (may be limited by anxiety or depression) Awareness of cardiac problem (informed of diagnosis; not in denial)

If assessment indicates that a patient is not ready to learn, *do not proceed with teaching;* document the assessment, and defer teaching due to lack of readiness.

1. **Before proceeding with any teaching encounter,** confirm readiness to learn.
2. **To determine the teaching sequence,** ask the patient to complete a learning assessment tool (see Sample Learning Assessment Tool), then proceed to teach topics that the patient identified as priorities.

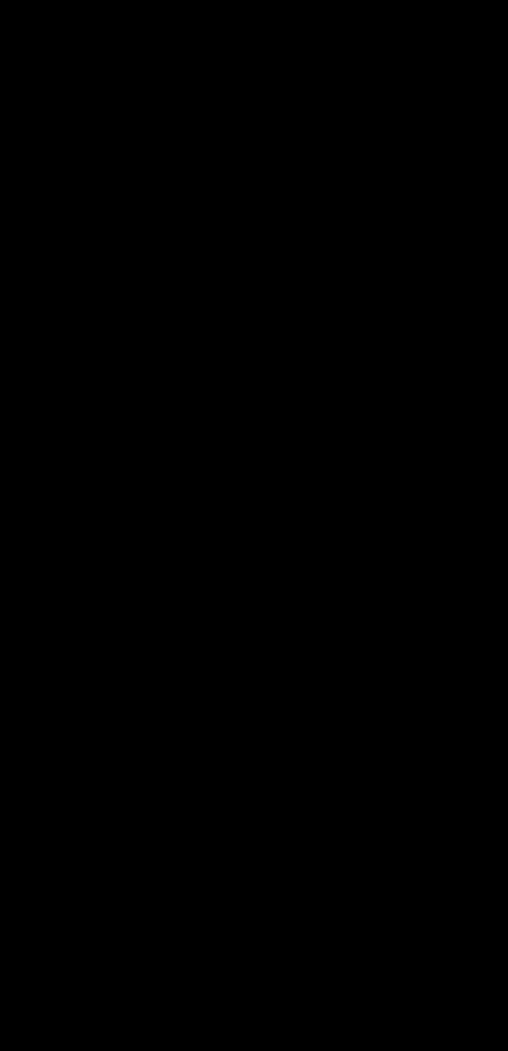

Assessment Parameters for Inpatient CR and Transitional Settings

Advancing Daily Ambulation Safety Criteria of Cardiopulmonary Clinical Parameters

- No new or recurrent chest pain during previous 8 h period
- Stable or declining creatine kinase or troponin levels
- No new signs of decompensated failure (e.g., dyspnea at rest with bibasilar rales)
- No new significant, abnormal rhythm, or electrocardiogram changes during the previous 8 h period[12]

Progression of Activity

Progression of activity depends on the initial daily physical assessment. Progression of activity should be considered when response to activity includes

- appropriate heart rate increase (<30 bpm, absence of chronotropic incompetence)
- appropriate systolic blood pressure (SBP) response to activity (increasing with activity, 10-40 mm Hg from resting SBP);
- no new arrhythmia or ST changes with activity; and
- no new cardiovascular symptoms such as palpitations, dyspnea, excessive fatigue, or chest pain with activity.

Patients experiencing any abnormal physiologic response should be assessed by a physician prior to resumption of activity.

---

responses must be documented and brought to the attention of the physician (see Abnormal Responses to Inpatient Physical Activity). On the other hand, if no contraindications are noted, patients may proceed with ambulation as tolerated.

Early progressive mobility is a series of planned movements in sequence from a patient's current mobility status with a goal of returning to pre-hospital level. Progressive mobility techniques include head of bed elevation, range of motion, continuous lateral rotation therapy, tilt training, leg dangling, chair position, and ambulation on or off a ventilator.[10] Safety criteria for early progressive mobilization can be standardized regarding the following: (a) respiratory conditions, including intubation status, ventilatory parameters, and percutaneous oxygen saturation levels; (b) cardiovascular considerations, including the presence of devices, cardiac arrhythmias, and blood pressure

(BP); (c) neurological considerations, including level of consciousness and sedation; and (d) other considerations, including lines, drains, tubes, and surgical or medical conditions.[11]

Progression of activity depends on the initial and daily assessment. The physician or physician's designate should assess patients on a daily basis before ambulation or activity within IPCR. Daily chart review and assessment by CR professionals before activity should include review of progress notes as well as assessment of heart rate (HR) and BP as they relate to ambulation and physical activity (guideline 3.4).

Progression may vary from a more rapid increase in physical activity in low-risk patients (uncomplicated patients without left ventricular dysfunction) to a slower progression in higher-risk or more debilitated patients. Table 3.1 lists common activities used in IPCR as well as approximate metabolic equivalent (MET) values

---

Abnormal Responses to Inpatient Physical Activity

- Abnormal BP changes including decrease in SBP of ≥10 mm Hg; and increase in SBP of >40 mm Hg
- Significant ventricular or atrial arrhythmias
- Second- or third-degree heart block
- Signs or symptoms of physical activity intolerance, including angina pectoris, marked dyspnea, or electrocardiogram changes suggestive of ischemia

Guideline 3.4   Physical Assessment and Initial Physical Activity Mobilization by Inpatient CR

- Before beginning the activity portion of IPCR, a baseline physical assessment should be made of heart and lung sounds, palpation of peripheral pulses, and self-care skills and ability. Results of the physical assessment along with HR, BP, and cardiac rhythm must be documented.

- Daily assessments must include chart review (after physician or nursing rounds, if possible) and assessment of heart rhythm and HR, BP, and current clinical status.

Table 3.1   Types of Activities Commonly Used in Early Cardiac Rehabilitation

Activity	Method	METs
Toileting	Bedpan Commode Urinal (in bed) Urinal (standing)	1.5-2.5
Bathing	Bed bath Tub bath Shower	1.5-2.0
Walking	Flat surface 2 mph 2.5 mph 3 mph	 2-2.5 2.5-2.9 3-3.3
Upper body exercise (low to moderate effort; no resistance)	While standing Arms Trunk	2.5-3.0
Stair climbing	1 flight = 12 steps Down 1 flight Up 1 or 2 flights	3.0-4.0

Based on Ainsworth et al. (2011).

for those activities. The patient's individual response is always the determining factor when considering progression of physical activity.

Management of risk factors begins with the assessment of patient readiness to learn and capacity to understand the disease process. Providing the patient and family with information and resources for risk factor intervention is critical. However, the reduced length of stay and time constraints often restrict the IPCR staff to addressing only the most important concerns, such as survival skills and smoking cessation (guideline 3.5).

Adult learning theory provides the foundation for effective in-hospital patient education. An understanding of the patient's discharge needs promotes patient-centric education that enhances

self-care management, and decreases postsurgical complication and hospital readmissions.[15] The concept of self-management has its roots in cognitive learning theory and reflects patients' active participation in their own treatment.[15] Evidence supports that multiple, shorter sessions of education are more effective than a single-session intervention; and education interventions designed to enhance self-care management, communication, and problem-solving skills may be more effective in behavioral and clinical outcomes than delivering only knowledge-based education.[15,16]

IPCR education programs are based on individually selected learning priorities, with the exception of the universal need for safety-related information. Materials such as handouts, pamphlets, and videos can be used to supplement the

Guideline 3.5   Tobacco Smoking Cessation Intervention

- The smoking status of each patient must be assessed and documented.
- Everyone who was a current smoker at hospital admission must be offered an intervention.
- Tobacco cessation medication as well as educational and behavioral intervention should assist patients through the period when they are not smoking in the hospital, assess readiness to continue smoking cessation after discharge, and provide information on maintenance of smoking cessation if patients are amenable.
- If a patient is contemplating quitting, refer the patient to the Smoker's Quitline associated with the patient's U.S. state of residence. Smoking cessation counseling intervention that was initiated in hospital and extended as follow-up support for at least one month after discharge increased smoking cessation rates by 65%.[13] The IPCR team should be aware that when counseling patients about electronic cigarettes, the evidence suggests that these products are not harm free but may be viewed as reduced-harm alternatives to conventional cigarettes. The utility of e-cigarettes is still being investigated and not supported by conclusive evidence, especially considering the wide variation between e-cigarette products.[14]

Sample Learning Assessment Tool

Dear Patient:

Like most people with heart problems, you probably have many questions. During the next few days we want to address those concerns that are uppermost in your mind. So, to help plan our discussions, please check all topics for which you would like more information:

___ structure treatments and related equipment

___ heart and function

___ heart arteries, normal/abnormal

___ activity progression during hospital stay

___ what to do for chest pain

___ emergency planning for home*

___ heart attack and healing

___ your risk factors

___ how to take your pulse

___ high blood pressure

___ high blood cholesterol

___ your medications

___ fitness and health

___ eating for a healthy heart

___ sexual activity and your heart

___ emotional changes after heart problems

___ development of heart disease

___ stress and your heart

___ smoking and your heart*

___ alcohol and your heart

___ guidelines for activities at home*

___ activity/exercise precautions*

___ heart catheter procedure

___ bypass graft surgery

___ heart balloon procedure

___ stent placement

___ heart failure

___ internal cardiac defibrillator

___ CR program*

___ treadmill exercise test

___ effects of heart problems on families

___ return to daily activities/work questions*

___ heart rhythms

Other questions you would like to have answered:

*These topics will be discussed by the CR staff before you go home.

learning experience. Staff must choose materials that best reinforce topics of importance, giving special attention to the reading level of selected teaching aids. Materials appropriate for a 6th- to 8th-grade reading level are recommended. Resources for many appropriate IPCR topics are available on the Internet.[17-19]

Management of CVD risk factors requires behavior counseling along with patient education. Chapter 9 discusses risk factor management in detail. Reduced length of stay often precludes interventions for modifying specific risk factors. Consequently, the role of IPCR staff is to identify risk factors and, when possible, inform patients of their implications as well as provide information about how they may obtain additional assistance for risk factor intervention following hospital discharge. In addition, clear, concise documentation about when and with whom the patient should follow up within the first weeks after discharge will ensure the continuum of care (figure 3.3). Early family involvement in the management of risk factors and continued care is critical to the success of the interventions and must be encouraged. In the United States, informal caregivers provide almost $470 billion in unpaid care, with an additional average of $7,000 per year in out-of-pocket costs for home modifications, transportation, reduced work time, unpaid leave, and reduced savings.[20] Assessment of the need for informal caregiving and the capacity for nonprofessional caregivers to meet the patient's needs must be considered in planning for discharge.

Discharge Planning

Discharge planning has taken on greater significance with decreased length of stay. An IPCR can no longer be viewed as a phase that the patient will finish before being discharged; thus, discharge planning should focus on assisting patients and families through the care continuum pathway (i.e., referral to an outpatient CR program *before* hospital discharge). The IPCR team needs to engage in enhanced communications with the interdisciplinary team to direct referrals to outpatient CR. AACVPR performance measures related to referral to outpatient CR indicate that programs consider implementing an automatic referral process in the discharge orders.[21-24] For

Figure 3.3 Sample Discharge Instructions and Intervention Follow-Up Checklist

Item	Provider of service	Responsible for follow-up	Date of appointment
Transitional care or home health			
Physician follow-up: Cardiologist Surgeon Primary care physician			
Outpatient CR/SP program			
Risk-factor follow-up: Smoking cessation program Lipid management Hypertension management Stress management, psychosocial counseling, or both Weight management Diabetes management Medication management			
Insurance and reimbursement issues			
Transportation			
Additional therapies: Physical therapy Occupational therapy			

example, the referral process could include a prescription for CR in the discharge packet, along with a list of programs close to the patient's home (including contact information). The performance measures for referral to outpatient CR stipulate that information about the inpatient course should be sent to the outpatient facility and that the patient should be provided with information about how to enroll. Also included is a sample script for inpatient practitioners to use to endorse the benefits of outpatient CR to patients. Chapter 2 discusses turnkey strategies to increase timely referral and enrollment to CR.

Patients are more likely to enroll in CR if their health care practitioners strongly encourage them to attend. The AHA (endorsed by AACVPR) encourages consistent communication about the importance of CR from all health care professionals who interact with a patient.[25] This advisory also recommends that an inpatient CR director be identified and empowered to direct the IPCR process, including working with administrators and other health care professionals to facilitate enrollment in CR after discharge.

BOTTOM LINE

It is critical that all appropriate and eligible patients are referred to outpatient CR. One of the most important things patients should learn during inpatient rehabilitation is where they can go to participate in early outpatient CR.

Figure 3.3 provides a sample checklist for discharge instructions and follow-up interventions. Health care providers, including the CR staff, should address the following discharge planning issues during the first month after discharge:

- Return to work
- Driving
- Household activity
- Stair climbing
- Lifting
- Sexual activity
- Walking
- Recreational and social activities

Transition to Outpatient CR

All patients hospitalized with an appropriate diagnosis should be referred to an outpatient CR. However, regardless of where (or whether) the patient continues outpatient CR, addressing safety is the highest priority for discharge planning. Survival skills (recognition of signs and symptoms, nitroglycerin use, when to call the doctor, and emergency assistance) and recommendations specifically with respect to ADLs, physical activity, and basic self-care are essential. IPCR professionals should be active participants in the discharge planning, especially by providing the patient assistance in evaluating options for continuation of CR. Formal program options (transitional programs) that precede entrance into a more typical outpatient program are discussed in the next section.

Implementation Strategies

Checkpoints and criteria for discharge readiness assessment[26] include

- physiological and symptom stability,
- functional and cognitive ability,
- cognitive and psychomotor competency to perform adequate self-care,
- perceived self-efficacy,
- availability of social support and services, such as housing and food security, and
- access to health care resources.

A validated and reliable instrument is available to assess core components of discharge readiness in the older adults. Implementing this assessment in discharge protocols could promote identification of patients who do not have adequate physical well-being, self-management capabilities, or social support to handle postdischarge recovery at home.[27]

IPCR staff should document functional level and tolerance for physical activity on a daily basis; this documentation provides data that are useful for home activity guidelines and CR.

Clinical Pathways

Exercise and physical activity, education, and behavior counseling have traditionally been provided to patients within the construct of a structured and sequenced IPCR program. Clinical pathways are structured interdisciplinary care plans used by health services to detail essential steps in the care of patients with a specific clinical problem. The aim is to link evidence to practice and optimize clinical outcomes while maximizing clinical efficiency.[28] The use of a clinical pathway provides a framework for the overall care of patients and integrates IPCR services into a comprehensive care plan.[29]

Clinical pathways provide a description of the typical course of treatment for patients with a cardiac diagnosis. The purpose of a clinical pathway as a case management tool is to standardize care so that length of stay is predictable for the majority of patients in the respective diagnostic groups. As clinical guides, the pathway provides a protocol for progressing patients through the hospital stay. Furthermore, they serve as tools for evaluating both the process and the outcomes of patient care. Clinical pathways are intended to be comprehensive and multidisciplinary and are specific to each facility. Categories of patient care typically mapped out on the path include the following:

- Physical activity
- Consultations
- Diagnostics
- Discharge planning
- Education
- Medications
- Nutrition
- Treatments

Table 3.2 provides a simplified sample of a clinical pathway. Clinical pathways allow visualization of the overall plan of care by outlining the sequence of intended care. Because activity progression and education are core elements of the IPCR program, these services are listed in the Activity and Education rows. Note that this pathway is only an example of the activity progression and that both activity progression and teaching must be individualized. Additionally, special visits by the IPCR staff for the initial assessment or predischarge instructions may be included under the Consults heading. To ensure optimal integration of IPCR services as well as to clarify roles and responsibilities, staff members, including those from IPCR, should participate

Table 3.2 Sample Grid for Clinical Pathway

	Day 1	Day 2	Day 3	Day 4
Consults		CR to assess: • Readiness for activity • Readiness to learn		
Activity	Stay in bed rest until stable, then move OOB in chair. Use bedside commode.	Do routine CCU activities. Do sitting warm-up, walk in room.	Up in room; do standing warm-up. Walk 5 to 10 min in hall 2 or 3 times a day (first time with supervision).	Up in room; do standing warm-up. Walk 5 to 10 min in hall 3 or 4 times a day. Walk down and up flight of stairs with supervision.
Education	Orient to CCU. Give basic explanation of event and treatment plan.	Assess readiness to learn; when patient is ready, teach survival lesson; e.g., signs and symptoms recognition, preventive medications, nitroglycerine use, emergency plan.	Assess readiness to learn. Discuss safety, self-care, precautions for home.	Review survival lesson. Discuss postdischarge plans: • Provide phone number to call with questions. • Discuss CR/SP follow-up: where, when. • Discuss MD and specialist follow-up.
Discharge planning				Provide CR/SP predischarge visit. Evaluate for follow-up CR/SP services: home, transitional, outpatient.

MI length of stay = 4 days. Abbreviations: OOB, out of bed; CCU, coronary care unit; CR/SP, cardiac rehabilitation/secondary prevention.

in the multidisciplinary team that designs each cardiac-related clinical pathway.

Once clinical pathways for cardiac patients are developed and implemented, patients progress accordingly. Variations in a clinical pathway secondary to comorbidities or complications such as those listed in the section titled Variations in the Pathway may occur. Although such problems may disrupt the treatment timeline, they usually do not eliminate the need for IPCR services. The IPCR specialist may make case-by-case adjustments, documenting those adjustments so that other members of the rehabilitation team are aware of the variance and can implement associated changes accordingly. Variance tracking is a part of the data collection requirements of clinical pathways.

Staffing

Considerations for staffing have been previously described, and they include defining responsibility, competency, and productivity (guideline 3.6).[30] CR specialists, including exercise physiologists, physical and occupational therapists, nurses, and other staff, are traditional providers of IPCR services. Table 3.3 provides an example of such role delineations. The particular role assigned depends on the needs, expectations, and resources of each facility.

CR Specialist

Even within the dedicated CR specialist role, variations in practice patterns exist. Responsibilities range from daily delivery of physical activity and education services to a single, focused pre-discharge visit. Figure 3.4 contrasts the various roles. Again, the AACVPR Core Competencies outline and detail these competencies for CR professionals.[30]

Other Health Professionals

Clinical pathways encourage multidisciplinary involvement in the CR process. To optimize results, qualified health care professionals may share responsibility with the CR specialists for activity progression, patient education, and other aspects of the CR process as long as they meet the specific core competency. Once the extent of the involvement of CR specialists and other staff has been clarified, respective job descriptions must be revised to reflect roles and responsibilities. CR specialists are expected to meet the AACVPR Core Competencies and to be working toward appropriate specialty certification.[30]

All professional staff members require ongoing in-service education to maintain CR program excellence. It is recommended that programs combine classroom instruction with supervised clinical practice. Such training not only improves the quality of patient care but also helps fulfill the expectation for specialty training that

Guideline 3.6 Staff Responsibilities

Competencies for each member of the IPCR team should be defined as specified in the AACVPR Core Competencies document.[30]

Variations in the Pathway

Preexisting Conditions	Cardiovascular Complications
General frailty	Postoperative bleeding
Chronic renal insufficiency	Arrhythmia
Cerebrovascular accident	Pulmonary infections
Orthopedic problems	Perioperative myocardial infarction
Cognitive impairment	Reduced left ventricular function
	Cerebrovascular accident
	Postoperative wound infections

Table 3.3 Clinical Pathways and Staff Allocation

Role	Focus	Function
Cardiac or diabetic educator (RN, clinical exercise specialist, PT, dietitian, other allied health staff)	All cardiac patients in hospital	Responsible for teaching preventive strategies for risk factor modification and recovery from medical or surgical interventions
Rehabilitation specialist (RN, clinical exercise specialist, PT, OT, other allied health staff)	Postacute recovery	Responsible for evaluation, ambulation and exercise, and education of patients eligible for IPCR
RN or LPN	Postacute, postsurgery recovery and nursing care	Responsible for assisting with daily care (e.g., getting patients OOB, inspecting incision sites, doing medication teaching, assisting with transfer) as well as exercise and education where appropriate and necessary
Cardiovascular clinical nurse specialist, NP, PA, or case manager	Selected or all cardiac patients	Role defined by institution; may include implementation of teaching, activity progression, and discharge planning, or may include the coordination of the bedside RN staff for purposes of IPCR

Abbreviations: RN, registered nurse; PT, physical therapist; OT, occupational therapist; LPN, licensed practical nurse; IPCR, inpatient cardiac rehabilitation; NP, nurse practitioner; PA, physician assistant; OOB, out of bed.

Figure 3.4   Inpatient CR Specialist Role Variations

Minimum	Moderate	Maximum
Predischarge visit: Education—emergency plan, precautions for home Exercise—activity evaluation (e.g., stair climbing, 6-minute walk test), treadmill demonstration, and home program Discussion of need for CR/SP or transitional follow-up; seek referral to the outpatient program	Shared responsibility with unit nursing staff for daily services: Responsible for education, exercise, or both Responsible for a selected combination of risk factor topics and exercise Discuss need for CR/SP or transitional follow-up; seek referral and provide patient with information to facilitate enrollment	All day-to-day rehabilitation services: Education—daily sessions based on individual priorities Exercise—daily assessment and activity advancement based on protocol or clinical pathways Discuss need for CR/SP or transitional care follow-up; provide referral

Abbreviation: CR/SP, cardiac rehabilitation/secondary prevention

ensures competence.[31] Continuing education modules using conferences and webinars are offered through various organizations, including AACVPR. Productivity and staffing standards must be consistent with the volume of IPCR patients.

Space and Equipment

The most common physical site for the delivery of IPCR services is the patient room and care unit where the patient is housed, usually the intensive care unit, coronary care unit, or intermediate-care unit or nonmonitored medical–surgical bed.

Bedside activity and patient and family education can take place in the room or in another facility, while progressive ambulation can be carried out in adjacent hallways and stairwells.

Ideally, facilities have dedicated space for evaluations, physical activity, or both. A room specially equipped with treadmills and bicycle ergometers to limit hallway traffic and further advance functional capacity before discharge can be useful. Alternatively, patients may be transported to the CR center (time and space permitting) for an introductory visit or even brief activity before discharge. An outpatient center visit may encourage expeditious entry into the CR.

Educational equipment and supplies, including an audiovisual system with a collection of educational programs, along with pamphlets and other handouts are recommended. Office and storage space that serves as a work area and contact point for IPCR staff is also recommended. Access to a conference room or small classroom is useful for group teaching. If an electronic health record is available, customized patient education tailored to the patient's cardiovascular event or procedure can be also pulled into the patient portal system for the patient's review after hospital discharge.

Transitional Settings

Patients must leave the hospital with a clear plan for follow-up. Patients must be advised and instructed about progression of activity that is initiated in the hospital. Unfortunately, shortened length of stay and limitations in patient readiness to learn often reduce opportunities to deliver effective teaching in the hospital; this is particularly true in older more medically complex patients with significant preexisting comorbidities. When patients do not move directly from the inpatient to the outpatient setting, the immediate postdischarge (transition) period may provide an opportunity for participation in a transitional program, depending on the needs and capabilities of the individual patient as well as the options available in the area. Figure 3.5 illustrates admission criteria for three of the most current transitional settings.

Because of cardiac complications, comorbidities, or age-related frailty, some patients are medically ready for discharge from acute-care facilities without the ability to perform ADLs or to ambulate household distances, while others may require physical therapy or other services in addition to CR in order to return to home safely. These types of patients benefit from referral to an alternative level of care such as subacute rehabilitation in a skilled nursing facility (SNF), acute inpatient rehabilitation in a hospital unit, or an inpatient rehabilitation facility (IRF; figure 3.5).

Skilled Nursing Facility

Skilled nursing units may be available within the acute-care hospital or as independent centers. Such facilities have specific admission criteria based on patient ability to carry out ADLs. Patients who require assistance with basic ADLs such as feeding, toileting, dressing, grooming, bathing, transferring, and walking after a cardiac event may qualify for admission to a skilled nursing facility. Approximately 25% of older adults who are discharged from the hospital transition to skilled facilities.[32] Staff in skilled nursing facilities are not necessarily trained in CR competencies and, consequently, there is often a gap in CR care.[33] Clinical guidelines are available to improve care in skilled nursing facilities related to heart failure.[34]

Inpatient Rehabilitation Facility

Inpatient rehabilitation facilities have been developed as a bridge between the acute-care facility and independent home living.[35-36] These programs prepare patients for a safe and independent return to home using a multidisciplinary approach that includes physical, occupational, vocational, and recreational therapy; speech pathology; nutrition; psychology and psychiatry; and continued medical and nursing management. Such a team approach should reduce fragmentation of care; improve patient outcomes; and enhance patient, family, staff, and physician satisfaction.

Figure 3.5 Admission Criteria for Transitional Settings

Skilled nursing facility	Inpatient rehabilitation facility	Home health care
Patients are temporarily unable to carry out some ADLs. They do not need 24 h rehabilitation nursing or evaluation and management by a rehabilitation physician as many as 3 times per week.	Patients require specific rehabilitation therapies; patients should be capable of participating in at least 3 h of combined rehabilitation per day; they should require 24 h rehabilitation nursing and evaluation and management by a physician with expertise in rehabilitation at least 3 times per week.	Patients are limited in their ability to provide for themselves independently at home and are in need of skilled nursing care or home physical or occupational therapy or social work services.

Admission criteria to IPCR programs generally include a greater need for skilled nursing, physician, and rehabilitation care compared to subacute or skilled nursing facilities. This can include management of medical issues such as fluid status; dysrhythmia; tracheotomy care; oxygen and bronchodilator therapy; wound care; intravenous therapy; and adjustments of medications for comorbidities such as depression, postoperative confusion, diabetes, and hypertension. The frequency and intensity of therapy sessions are greater. Sessions include individual and group education; gait retraining; strength, endurance, and range of motion exercise; ADL evaluation and retraining; cognitive evaluation and retraining; and therapy specific to any preexisting or postoperative neurological or musculoskeletal disabilities that may interfere with recovery.

Inpatient rehabilitation services can play a critical role in the recovery of various subgroups of cardiovascular patients. For example, an increasing population of patients is receiving a left ventricular assist device (LVAD). Approximately half of the patients who received LVADs were admitted to inpatient rehabilitation. After the implantation of LVAD and inpatient rehabilitation, significant functional improvements were observed.[37] Additionally, patients with permanent disabilities (e.g., paraplegia, amputation, neuromuscular disorders) also benefit from the multidisciplinary assistance that an inpatient rehabilitation hospital can provide. Cardiac patients who transition to intermediate rehabilitation facilities, compared to those who transition to skilled facilities, are more likely to attend outpatient CR.[38] Inpatient rehabilitation facilities use standardized, objective, and valid tools to measure outcomes. Evaluations such as the Functional Independence Measure, among others, are used to measure improvement from admission to discharge.[36] Longstanding national registries track outcomes for these patients related to functional improvement, discharge destination, and readmissions. Published data demonstrate the efficacy of such programs with respect to functional outcomes.[39-41]

Home Health Care

Home care patients tend to be older, functionally impaired, clinically complex, and drive high cost of medical expenditures.[42] Improving patient care coordination with decreasing length of stay through secondary prevention of CVD posthospitalization has become a reality for patients discharged directly to their home setting. Home care clinicians are often the first line of rehabilitation and support for patients posthospitalization. The immediate postdischarge window is where the most variation in health care spending occurs; home care can mitigate the social and economic barriers to receiving CR. Home-based CR models represent a novel approach to improving care and reducing hospital readmissions among patients with CVD and delivering patient care in a lower cost setting. Cardiac patients with Medicare may qualify for a 60-day episode of home care if deemed homebound (i.e., unable to leave home unassisted). However, skilled home care services do not typically include standardized CR.[43] Pilot studies on innovated integration of CR services into home care demonstrated a positive impact on attending outpatient CR.[44] Home health services and adaptation of a home-based CR model represent a promising approach to improving care and reducing hospital readmissions among patients with CVD.

Cardiac patients may qualify for home care based on physical limitations, lack of mobility, or temporary restrictions imposed by the medical team (e.g., driving restrictions). A patient who is being transported by another person for any reason other than medical appointments is not considered homebound and, therefore, can not receive reimbursed services. The maximum length of time for insurance coverage is determined individually. Payers may cover follow-up home care for a fixed number of visits or weeks as a routine component of total case management.

A patient navigator transitional program has demonstrated promise in bridging the gap between discharge and the start of early outpatient CR. Patient navigators (either lay or health care professionals) collaborate with patients and families to facilitate access to patient-centered care, assist with identifying and overcoming potential barriers, sequence treatments ensuring access to timely treatment, and improve communication between patients and clinicians.[45] Patient navigators increase utilization of recommended treatments and reduce hospital readmission rates among older, higher-risk patients.[46] Additionally, a patient navigator program reduced readmissions for patients with heart failure and myocardial infarction.[47] Use of lay patient navigators has also shown considerable promise for increasing participation in CR.[48] Use of navigators during the transition from hospital to CR is consistent with evidence that early interaction with CR clinicians improves overall participation rates.

Specific Considerations for Transitional Settings

When exploring patient options for transitional settings, the two major considerations to address are (1) who provides care and (2) the level of reimbursement. Nurses, physical therapists, and others who typically staff skilled nursing facilities and home care agencies are trained to provide services designed to meet specific functional and medical goals to enable a patient to return to (or stay at) home. Therefore, staff may not receive specific training regarding CR issues. However, these staff members can develop competencies through in-service training provided by CR professionals; alternatively, CR specialists may staff these programs. Physical assessment skills should include identification of signs and symptoms of worsening medical condition and electrocardiogram monitoring, which is not typically available in skilled nursing facility or home settings. Although transitional settings may provide CR physical activity and education services, CR services alone in these settings are usually not reimbursable by Medicare. Medicare reimburses only for skilled nursing or specific therapies, such as physical or occupational, based on medical necessity. This emphasizes the need for specialized training and experience related to CR for these providers if the delivery of postacute care for cardiac patients in these transitional settings is to be effective.

The clinical pathway can also be a primary tool for service delivery in transitional settings. Transitional clinical pathways can build on the inpatient programming results by gradually increasing ambulation and introducing upper body activities. Performance parameters similar to those used with inpatient programs apply; and the same education assessments, curricula, and teaching aids can be used to address individual priorities.

In an attempt to provide continuity of CR service from one setting to the next, transitional clinical pathways and programs have been established. Two major advantages have been documented with this approach. First, downtime between CR settings is minimized; second, referrals from tertiary treatment centers to community CR programming are maximized.[49]

This continuity of care is as beneficial to the uncomplicated patient who is discharged quickly as it is to the more complicated patient who requires transitional care. Ironically, patients considered uncomplicated may have the fewest options for posthospitalization or transitional care, because it tends to be provided most often to patients at higher levels of acuity and dysfunction. Additionally, because uncomplicated patients often have a shortened length of stay, less time is available for education and physical activity. Unfortunately, some uncomplicated patients may not be able to enter an outpatient CR program immediately. Therefore, traditional outpatient CR program staff should consider developing transitional programs.

Summary

U.S. hospital stays are becoming increasingly brief, and there are now many places where patients go after hospital discharge to receive a continuum of care from inpatient to early outpatient. The innovative transitional settings discussed in this chapter and summarized in Summary of CR Structure Recommendations in Inpatient and Transitional Settings and Summary of CR Process Recommendations in Inpatient and Transitional Settings meet the expectation of a quality continuum of rehabilitation care.

Summary of CR Structure Recommendations in Inpatient and Transitional Settings

Physical Activity

1. Design and implementation of physical activity/exercise plan should be based on physiological principles that can be used by a variety of health professionals within either an inpatient or a transitional setting, and should be integrated into a cooperative clinical pathway.

2. Flexibility in the physical activity plan is critical to individualization; recommendations should be individualized, and advancement should be done as clinically indicated.

3. Specific criteria for beginning and advancing inpatient activities are required.

Education

1. A standardized collection of cardiac teaching plans that outline the content area topics (see figures 3.3 and 3.5) should be available.

2. Appropriate and understandable teaching aids are required in order to reinforce patient education.

3. Patients must be involved in identifying the educational priorities.

4. Patient ability and readiness to learn should be assessed.

5. Each teaching encounter should be evaluated; this evaluation includes patient and family or significant other comprehension.

Discharge Planning

1. At a minimum, one predischarge visit for every CR patient must
   - address survival skills and postdischarge dos and don'ts,
   - evaluate and estimate predischarge functional and cognitive ability, and
   - provide information about outpatient CR programming.

Summary of CR Process Recommendations in Inpatient and Transitional Settings

Mechanism

1. Define the purpose and goals of the inpatient or transitional CR program.
2. Clarify CR expectations between rehabilitation specialists and other health care professionals.

Resources

1. Specify the extent of responsibility each rehabilitation specialist has.
2. Document the time required for delivery of rehabilitation services.
3. Complete the scope of practice statement for all professionals involved in CR service delivery.
4. Develop and present in-service training for health care professionals outside the immediate inpatient team who will assume some rehabilitation responsibilities.
5. Develop standards clarifying the criteria for educational and physical activity within the inpatient and transitional settings.

Continuity

1. CR staff must participate in discharge planning to facilitate CR follow-up.
2. Identify potential transitional resources and respective patient qualifications, including
   - skilled nursing facilities,
   - acute rehabilitation hospitals, and
   - home care follow-up.
3. Advisory and educational assistance should be available to transitional programs.
4. Continuation to CR programming after transition is complete is strongly recommended.

Medical Evaluation and Exercise Testing for Outpatient CR

Sherrie Khadanga, MD

Data gathered from the initial medical evaluation of patients before entry into CR are used to design and implement an effective program in which specific outcomes are defined and targeted. The AHA guidelines for comprehensive secondary prevention provide a useful framework for evaluation and management of prevention guidelines.[1] This information is most useful for stratifying the patient in these two ways:

- It establishes patient risk for progression of atherosclerosis and the likelihood of future cardiac events.
- It establishes patient risk for adverse cardiac events during prescribed exercise training as well as whether exercise is contraindicated and, if not, the level of supervision and monitoring recommended during the initial training period. (Stratification of these factors is discussed separately in chapter 5.)

OBJECTIVES

This chapter discusses the following:
- Components of the patient history and physical examination
- Methods and protocols for exercise tolerance testing
- Interpretation of exercise testing results
- Additional exercise testing imaging modalities
- Alternative methods for evaluating functional status

Information from the medical evaluation and exercise testing may be provided by the primary care physician, cardiologist, or surgeon before initiation of CR or through direct evaluation by the CR medical director during the initial session (guideline 4.1). A medical history, with particular attention to cardiovascular status, and a detailed review of risk factors and their management, are essential components of the initial assessment and will serve to target and individualize the program (see Components of the Medical History). Either the physician or CR staff member should determine whether patients are experiencing symptoms of angina, dyspnea, palpitations, or syncope, and should ask about a previous history of MI, percutaneous coronary intervention, systolic chronic heart failure (EF <35%), peripheral vascular disease, transcatheter valve replacement, and valvular or coronary artery bypass surgery. Ideally, measurements of cardiac function via echocardiography and coronary anatomy should be available and noted. A complete list of prescribed and over-the-counter medications, dosing intervals, and compliance with the drug regimen should be reviewed. Comorbid conditions such as pulmonary, endocrine, and neurological illnesses and behavioral and musculoskeletal conditions should be evaluated.

Detailed social and occupational histories yield valuable information and allow the tailoring of exercise training and goals to meet individual needs. When developing the patient assessment protocol for all patients, CR staff should seek consultation, as needed, from social services and vocational rehabilitation specialists who are familiar with the array of medical, psychological, economic, and legal factors that influence return-to-work issues. Family and community resources that can assist patients with family concerns and returning to work should also be considered.

Physical Examination

The initial physical examination should be performed by a physician or another appropriately trained and qualified health care provider (under the direction of a physician who is actively involved in the routine care of patients with CVD; see guideline 4.2). A resting standard 12-lead ECG is useful in assessing HR, rhythm, conduction abnormalities, and evidence of prior MI. The resting ECG serves as an important reference for future comparison, particularly if the patient develops new signs or symptoms suggestive of ischemia, infarction, or dysrhythmia.

Musculoskeletal complaints and injury are not uncommon, especially when a patient is beginning an exercise program.[2] It is not unusual for patients' comorbid conditions to be more of a barrier to physical activity than their heart condition. The list of possible comorbid conditions is lengthy, but more common examples include arthritis; peripheral vascular disease; orthopedic disorders; neurological disorders; cognitive, hearing, and vision deficits; and pulmonary disease. Therefore, comorbid conditions should be assessed before exercise training begins. Assessment of lower extremity strength, flexibility, and balance should be performed with hopes of preventing injuries related to weight-bearing exercise. CR staff should assess posture and

---

Guideline 4.1   Medical Evaluation and Exercise Testing

- To establish a safe and effective program of comprehensive CVD risk reduction and rehabilitation, each patient should undergo a careful medical evaluation and, ideally, exercise tolerance test before participating in an outpatient CR program.

- The 6-minute walk test (see later subsection on this test) can be used as a surrogate measure of exercise capacity when standard exercise tolerance testing is not available.

- The specific components of the medical evaluation should include a medical history, physical examination, relevant lab work, and resting electrocardiogram (ECG).

- The exercise test should be repeated when symptoms or clinical changes warrant, as well as in the follow-up assessment of the exercise training outcome.

Components of the Medical History

1. **Medical diagnoses:** A variety of diagnoses should be reviewed, including, but not limited to, CVD including existing coronary artery disease; previous MI, percutaneous intervention, chronic systolic heart failure, valvular disease, cardiac surgery, angina, and hypertension; pulmonary disease, including asthma, emphysema, and bronchitis; cerebrovascular disease, including stroke or transient ischemic attack; diabetes mellitus; peripheral vascular disease; anemia, phlebitis, or emboli; cancer; pregnancy; musculoskeletal imbalances and neuromuscular and joint disease; osteoporosis; emotional disorders; and eating disorders

2. **Symptoms:** Angina pectoris; discomfort (pressure, tingling, pain, heaviness, burning, numbness) in the chest, jaw, neck, or arms; atypical angina, such as light-headedness, dizziness, or fainting; shortness of breath; rapid heartbeats or palpitations, especially if associated with physical activity, eating a large meal, emotional distress, or exposure to cold

3. **Risk factors for atherosclerotic disease progression:** Hypertension, diabetes mellitus, obesity, dyslipidemia, metabolic syndrome, smoking status (current or former and use of electronic cigarettes and vaping), chewing tobacco, and physical inactivity

4. **Recent illness, hospitalization, or surgical procedure**

5. **Medication (both prescribed and over-the-counter) dose and schedule, drug allergies**

6. **All supplements** (prescribed or otherwise)

7. **Other habits,** including alcohol or illicit drug use

8. **Physical activity history:** Information on habitual level of physical activity, such as frequency, duration, intensity, and type of activity

9. **Work history:** With an emphasis on current or expected physical and mental demands, noting upper and lower extremity requirements; estimated time to return to work

10. **Psychosocial history:** Living conditions and cohabitants; marital and family status; transportation needs; family needs; domestic and emotional problems; depression, anxiety, or other psychological disorders

Based on Fletcher et al. (2013).

 Guideline 4.2   Physical Examination

At a minimum, the physical examination should focus on the resting HR; BP; and pulmonary, cardiac, vascular, and musculoskeletal areas (see Components of the Physical Examination).

alignment and determine whether the patient has a history of musculoskeletal injury. A pre-CR program evaluation is critical in identifying special considerations for prescribing exercise and physical activity. It is important to refer patients or consult with other professionals to assist with physical activity limitations (e.g., physical and occupational therapy).

In patients who have undergone coronary artery bypass or valvular surgery via median sternotomy, it is important to evaluate for sternal stability by identifying any movement in the sternum, pain, clicking, or popping. Sternal bone healing to attain adequate sternal stability is usually achieved by eight weeks postsurgery.[3] Infection, nonunion, and instability occur in about 2% to 5% of cases and are often predisposed by clinical factors such as diabetes mellitus, obesity, immunosuppression, advanced age, and osteoporosis.[4]

Components of the Physical Examination

1. Body weight, height, body mass index, waist (measured at the midpoint between the lower margin of the last palpable rib and the top of the iliac crest) and hip (measured around the widest portion of the buttocks) circumferences, and waist-to-hip ratio

2. HR and HR regularity

3. Resting BP

4. Auscultation of the lungs, with specific attention to uniformity of breath sounds in all areas (absence of rales, wheezes, and other abnormal breath sounds)

5. Auscultation of the heart, with specific attention to murmurs, gallops, clicks, and rubs

6. Palpation and auscultation of carotid, abdominal, and femoral arteries

7. Palpation and inspection of lower extremities for edema and presence of arterial pulses and skin integrity (particularly in patients with diabetes)

8. Absence or presence of xanthoma and xanthelasma

9. Examination related to orthopedic, neurologic, or other medical conditions that might limit exercise testing or training

10. Examination of the chest and leg wounds and vascular access areas in patients after coronary bypass surgery, valvular surgery, or percutaneous coronary revascularization

Based on Fletcher et al. (2013).

Risk Stratification and Identification of Contraindications for Exercise Training

Recommendations for risk stratifying patients as they enter outpatient CR are outlined in chapter 5. Risk stratification recommendations are presented as a means of classifying patients with respect to the likelihood of an adverse event during exercise and probability of progression of atherosclerosis. The risk stratification recommendations do not consider accompanying comorbidities (e.g., insulin-dependent diabetes mellitus, morbid obesity, severe pulmonary disease, complicated pregnancy, or debilitating neurological or orthopedic conditions) that may constitute a contraindication to exercise or necessitate closer supervision during exercise training sessions. Patients with conditions as outlined in Absolute and Relative Contraindications to Exercise Training should be considered for exclusion from exercise training or delayed until the underlying problem is rectified.

Exercise Testing

An exercise tolerance test is a key component of the initial assessment made before a patient begins an exercise program. Graded exercise tests are used to assess the ability to tolerate increased physical activity; ECG, hemodynamic, and symptomatic responses are monitored for manifestations of myocardial ischemia, dysrhythmias, or other exertion-related abnormalities. The exercise test may be used for diagnostic, prognostic, and therapeutic applications.[5] The exercise test may also bolster a patient's confidence and provide motivation and verification to the family about the patient's readiness to resume physical activities and participate in CR. Various published position statements present additional in-depth information regarding applications of exercise testing, methods of conducting exercise tests, and guidelines for managing exercise testing laboratories.[5-8] Apart from their use as a diagnostic tool, exercise tests are equally useful to staff as a tool to assess functional status. The test is helpful in assessing cardiorespiratory fitness and for developing an exercise prescription.

Absolute and Relative Contraindications to Exercise Training

Absolute

- Recent change in the resting ECG suggesting significant ischemia, recent MI (within two weeks), or other acute cardiac event
- Unstable angina
- Uncontrolled cardiac arrhythmias
- Symptomatic severe aortic stenosis or other valvular disease
- Decompensated symptomatic heart failure
- Acute pulmonary embolus or pulmonary infarction
- Acute noncardiac disorder that may affect exercise performance or may be aggravated by exercise (e.g., infection, thyrotoxicosis)
- Acute myocarditis or pericarditis
- Acute thrombophlebitis
- Physical disability that would preclude safe and adequate exercise performance

Relative*

- Electrolyte abnormalities
- Tachyarrhythmias or bradyarrhythmias
- High-degree atrioventricular block
- Atrial fibrillation with uncontrolled ventricular rate
- Hypertrophic obstructive cardiomyopathy with peak resting left ventricular outflow gradient of >25 mm Hg
- Known aortic dissection
- Severe resting arterial hypertension (SBP >200 mm Hg or diastolic BP [DBP] >110 mm Hg)
- Mental impairment leading to inability to cooperate with testing

*Contraindications can be superseded if benefits outweigh risks of exercise.

Adapted from R.J. Gibbons et al., *ACC/AHA 2002 Guideline Update for Exercise Testing. A Report of the American College of Cardiology/American Heart Association Task Force on Practice Guidelines* (Committee on Exercise Testing), (Bethesda, MD: American College of Cardiology, 2002), 5. Available: http://my.americanheart.org/idc/groups/ahaecc-internal/@wcm/@sop/documents/downloadable/ucm_423807.pdf

It can also be used to measure functional changes over time to assess exercise training outcomes. Exercise tests and simulated work tests also help determine an individual's ability to return to work.[9] Patients should not be denied participation in CR solely on the basis of not having undergone preentry exercise testing. Information regarding exercise prescription for patients without exercise testing is presented in chapter 6. The following section outlines the contraindications to exercise testing.

Safety and Personnel

Exercise is associated with an increased risk for a cardiovascular event. However, the safety of exercise testing is well documented, and the overall risk of adverse events is quite low. Among several large series of subjects with and without known CVD, the rate of major complications (including MI and other events requiring hospitalization) is <1 to as many as 5 per 10,000 tests, and the rate of death is <0.5 per 10,000 tests; however, the incidence of adverse events varies depending on

Absolute and Relative Contraindications to Exercise Testing

Absolute

Acute MI (within 2 days)

High-risk unstable angina

Uncontrolled cardiac dysrhythmias causing symptoms or hemodynamic compromise

Active endocarditis

Severe symptomatic aortic stenosis

Decompensated symptomatic heart failure

Acute pulmonary embolus or pulmonary infarction

Acute noncardiac disorder that may affect exercise performance or be aggravated by exercise (e.g., infection, renal failure, thyrotoxicosis)

Acute myocarditis or pericarditis

Physical disability that would preclude safe and adequate test performance

Inability to obtain consent

Relative*

Untreated left main coronary stenosis or equivalent

Severe stenotic valvular heart disease

Electrolyte abnormalities

Tachyarrhythmias or bradyarrhythmias

Atrial fibrillation with rapid ventricular rate, such as >150 bpm

Hypertrophic cardiomyopathy

Mental impairment leading to inability to cooperate with testing

High-degree atrioventricular block

Severe resting arterial hypertension (SBP >200 mm Hg or DBP >110 mm Hg)

*Contraindications can be superseded if benefits outweigh risks of exercise.

Adapted from R.J. Gibbons et al., *ACC/AHA 2002 Guideline Update for Exercise Testing. A Report of the American College of Cardiology/American Heart Association Task Force on Practice Guidelines* (Committee on Exercise Testing), (Bethesda, MD: American College of Cardiology, 2002), 5. Available: http://my.americanheart.org/idc/groups/ahaecc-internal/@wcm/@sop/documents/downloadable/ucm_423807.pdf

the study population.[10] For the 2,331 patients who completed exercise testing in the HF-ACTION study (Heart Failure: A Controlled Trial Investigating Outcomes of Exercise Training), there were no deaths, and the rate of nonfatal major cardiovascular events was <0.5 per 1,000 tests.[11] Patients with recent MI, reduced left ventricular systolic function, exertion-induced myocardial ischemia, and serious ventricular arrhythmias are at highest risk.[8]

Central to the prevention of exercise-induced complications are appropriate screening and risk stratification of patients before beginning an exercise program. Although the risk of an event is greater in patients with CVD, several clinical characteristics are associated with patients at highest risk. Matching of patient medical history and clinical status to established contraindications to exercise should be incorporated into the assessment protocol before the patient gives informed consent and prepares for testing.[12]

Before the exercise test, the patient must give informed consent. A detailed explanation of the exercise test should be provided to the patient. The patient should have ample time to read the consent form before testing and given an opportunity to ask questions about the consent form or the test procedures. Satisfactory explanations should be provided before proceeding.

Maintenance of appropriate emergency equipment, establishment of a workable emergency plan, and regular practice of the plan (with critiques) are fundamental to ensuring the safety of a CR program. Chapter 14 discusses considerations for managing emergency situations.

The AHA has described the requisite supervision for exercise testing.[6] The level of supervision depends primarily on the clinical characteristics of the patient being tested. For patients who are at higher risk, such as those with recent MI, heart failure, or arrhythmia, the supervising physician should determine the necessity for directly monitoring the test.[6] In other cases, properly trained nonphysician health care professionals may conduct the test and directly monitor patient status throughout testing and recovery, provided that they have been deemed competent by the physician supervisor per established guidelines.[13] In all cases, the supervising physician must be immediately available to respond. For nonphysicians, certification in the clinical track by the American College of Sports Medicine (ACSM) provides evidence of competencies to supervise exercise testing.[7] The CR program medical director is responsible for ensuring the availability of proper equipment and staffing of the exercise testing laboratory, including establishing laboratory policies and procedures. The physician is also responsible for final data interpretation and approval and delivery of emergency care (including advanced cardiovascular life support [ACLS]), according to established standards.[6,13]

Medications

Although diagnostic exercise tests typically are performed with medications withheld to better assess any underlying ischemic response, functional exercise testing performed before entrance into a CR program should occur with the patient taking medications as prescribed. For example, withholding beta-blockers before exercise testing will preclude using HR for the prescription of exercise training intensity. By withholding the beta-blockers, the patient will likely have a higher heart rate and may experience angina. Under ideal conditions, the exercise tolerance test should be administered at a time when the patient normally exercises and following normal medication ingestion time.

BOTTOM LINE

Prior to commencing with CR, all participants should undergo an assessment that includes a review of medical history, physical exam, review of a complete list of prescribed and over-the-counter medications, confirmation of medication use, and assessment of functional capacity.

Exercise Test Modality and Protocol

The testing modality and protocol should be selected after an initial patient assessment. A patient may have exercise limitations due to musculoskeletal, orthopedic, or neurodegenerative disorders that may affect their performance, therefore limiting the usefulness of the exercise test. Exercise tests may be submaximal or maximal with respect to the effort required. In addition to common indications for stopping the exercise test (see Indications for Terminating Exercise Testing), submaximal exercise testing often has a predetermined endpoint, namely, a specific peak HR such as 120 bpm, a percentage of predicted maximum HR such as 70%, an arbitrary MET level such as 5 METs, or a submaximal rating of perceived exertion (RPE) such as 13 to 15. Submaximal tests may be used before hospital discharge at 4 to 6 days after acute MI.[14] A submaximal test can provide sufficient data for evaluating the ability to engage in ADLs or other physical activity, and can serve as a baseline for early ambulatory physical activity recommendations.

Symptom-limited tests are designed to continue until the patient demonstrates signs and symptoms that require termination of exercise.[5] Symptom-limited tests are usually selected when testing is performed more than 14 days after an acute MI. Minimum required physiological and perceptual measurements to be collected before, during, and following exercise testing are listed in Minimum Requirements for Measures Assessed During Exercise Testing.

Although several exercise testing protocols are available for both treadmill and stationary cycle ergometers, it is most important that the protocol be selected according to the individual patient-estimated physical fitness based on age,

Indications for Terminating Exercise Testing

Absolute Indications

- ST elevation (>1.0 mm) in leads without Q waves (other than V1 or aV$_R$)
- Drop in SBP of >10 mm Hg (persistently below baseline) despite an increase in workload, when accompanied by any other evidence of ischemia
- Moderate to severe angina (grade 3 to 4; Frequently Used Angina and Dyspnea Rating Scales presents descriptions and grades for angina scale)
- Central nervous system symptoms (e.g., ataxia, dizziness, or near-syncope)
- Signs of poor perfusion (cyanosis or pallor)
- Sustained ventricular tachycardia
- Technical difficulties monitoring the ECG or SBP
- Patient request to stop
- Development of bundle branch block that cannot be distinguished from ventricular tachycardia

Relative Indications

- ST segment or QRS changes such as excessive ST displacement (horizontal or down sloping of >2 mm), or marked axis shift
- Drop in SBP of >10 mm Hg (persistently below baseline) despite an increase in workload, in the absence of other evidence of ischemia
- Increasing chest pain
- Fatigue, shortness of breath, wheezing, leg cramps, or severe claudication
- Dysrhythmias other than sustained ventricular tachycardia, including frequent multifocal ectopic beats including ventricular pairs, supraventricular tachycardia, heart block, or bradyarrhythmias

Adapted from R.J. Gibbons et al., *ACC/AHA 2002 Guideline Update for Exercise Testing. A Report of the American College of Cardiology/American Heart Association Task Force on Practice Guidelines* (Committee on Exercise Testing), (Bethesda, MD: American College of Cardiology, 2002), 6. Available: http://my.americanheart.org/idc/groups/ahaecc-internal/@wcm/@sop/documents/downloadable/ucm_423807.pdf

underlying disease, and current activity level. Patients who are deemed to be higher risk (e.g., recent history of dysrhythmia or symptoms during low levels of effort) or who are significantly deconditioned should be tested using a less aggressive exercise protocol. Validated questionnaires, which estimate a person's exercise capacity and assist in appropriate protocol selection, are available.[15] ACSM summarizes a wide variety of treadmill and cycle ergometer testing protocols.[7] Treadmill and cycle ergometers may employ staged or continuous ramp protocols. Work rate increments during staged protocols can vary from 1 to 2.5 METs (1 MET = 3.5 mL $O_2 \cdot kg^{-1} \cdot min^{-1}$), whereas those of ramp protocols are designed to use less abrupt increments. Treadmill testing provides a more common form of physiological stress (i.e., walking), with subjects more likely to attain a higher oxygen uptake and HR. Cycling

may be preferable when orthopedic or other specific patient characteristics limit ability to walk or bear weight during exercise. The most frequently used stepped treadmill protocols are the Bruce (table 4.1), the modified Bruce, and the Naughton.[7] Ramp protocols are designed to have stages no longer than 1 min and for the patient to attain peak effort within 8 to 12 min. Thus, ramp protocols must be individualized to patient effort (table 4.2).

The cycle ergometer is smaller, quieter, and less expensive than a treadmill. Because the cycle ergometer requires less movement of the arms and thorax, quality ECG recordings and BP measurements are easier to obtain. Stationary cycling may be unfamiliar to many patients, and its success as a testing tool is highly dependent on patient motivation. Thus, the test may end before the patient reaches a true cardiopulmonary end

Minimum Requirements for Measures Assessed During Exercise Testing

Pretest Procedures and Assessments

- Minimum of 5 min of rest before initial measures are taken
- Informed consent
- Demonstration of equipment use (as required)
- Explanation of maximal effort or desired end point(s)
- Explanation of rating scales (use standardized instructions where available)
- 12-lead ECG in supine and in position of exercise
- Blood pressure in supine and in position of exercise
- Assessment of medications, when last taken
- Current symptom status

Exercise Assessments

- 12-lead ECG during last minute of each completed stage and when exercise is terminated
- Blood pressure and perceived exertion during last minute of each completed stage and when exercise is terminated
- Other rating scales as appropriate

Posttest Procedures and Assessments

- Minimum of 6 min in sitting or supine position, or until near-baseline measures are reached. A period of active cool-down may be included in the 6 min recovery period; for functional (nondiagnostic) exercise tests, a 1 to 3 min cool-down is recommended, depending on the level of exertion (additional time for heavier exertion), to minimize postexercise effects of venous pooling in the lower extremities.
- 12-lead ECG every minute.
- Blood pressure immediately after exercise, then every 1 or 2 min until normotensive or near-baseline measures are reached.
- Rating of symptoms each minute as long as they persist after exercise. Patients should be observed until all symptoms have subsided and the ECG is within acceptable limits as determined by the supervising clinician.

Table 4.1 Bruce Protocol for Treadmill Testing

Stage	Time	Speed (mph)	Grade (%)	METs
Rest	00.00	0.0	0.0	1.0
Modified Bruce Protocol	3.00	1.7	0.0	2.2
	3.00	1.7	5	3.4
1	3.00	1.7	10.0	4.6
2	3.00	2.5	12.0	7.0
3	3.00	3.4	14.0	10.1
4	3.00	4.2	16.0	12.9
5	3.00	5.0	18.0	15.1
6	3.00	5.5	20.0	16.9
7	3.00	6.0	22.0	19.2

Table 4.2 Approximate MET Loads During Cycle Ergometer Assessments

BODY WEIGHT		EXERCISE RATE KG · M · MIN⁻¹/WATTS						
kg	lb	300/50	450/75	600/100	750/125	900/150	1050/175	1200/200
50	110	5.1	6.6	8.2	9.7	11.3	12.8	14.3
60	132	4.6	5.9	7.1	8.4	9.7	11.0	12.3
70	154	4.2	5.3	6.4	7.5	8.6	9.7	10.8
80	176	3.9	4.9	5.9	6.8	7.8	8.8	9.7
90	198	3.7	4.6	5.4	6.3	7.1	8.0	8.9
100	220	3.5	4.3	5.1	5.9	6.6	7.4	8.2

Based on American College of Sports Medicine (2006).

point. However, unlike treadmill testing, which is fully weight bearing, cycle testing protocols are independent of weight because the seat supports the body weight. As shown in table 4.2, the MET level attained varies with patient body weight. The energy requirement (oxygen uptake) of non-weight-bearing activity is inversely proportional to body weight. That is, at the same workload, the higher the body weight, the lower the oxygen uptake.

The following recommendations may assist in selecting an appropriate cycling protocol:

- Select a protocol appropriate to level of fitness.
- When using a mechanically braked ergometer, keep pedal revolutions per minute constant, for example at 50 rpm.
- After a zero-load warm-up of 1 to 2 min, use 25 W or less (150 kilopond-meter [kpm]) increments for patients who are deconditioned or weigh less than 150 lb (68 kg). Use 50 W (300 kpm) increments for more fit or heavier patients.
- Set stages at a minimum of 2 min in duration, increasing the load by 25 W or less as clinical judgment indicates.
- When ramping protocols are used, electronically braked cycle ergometers are preferred because they generally allow programming of incremental workloads at stages <1 min. Similar to treadmill ramp protocols, customized cycle ergometer ramp protocols that accommodate a wide range of fitness levels need to be established by individual exercise testing laboratories.

Once the appropriate test equipment and protocol are selected, the exercise component of a symptom-limited exercise test should last approximately 8 to 12 min.[16] Low-level ramps or protocols that increase metabolic demand by 1 MET per stage are appropriate for high-risk patients with functional capacities less than 7 METs; metabolic demands ≥2 METs per stage may be appropriate for low- to intermediate-risk patients with functional capacities ≥7 METs. Similar considerations are necessary when one is adjusting ramp rates. Smaller increments in MET requirements for each stage permit a more specific determination of the ischemic or anginal threshold and result in a more accurate estimation of oxygen uptake at the corresponding work rate. The widely used Bruce treadmill protocol (2-3 METs per stage) is less accurate in this regard.[17]

During treadmill exercise, encourage patients to walk freely, using the handrails for balance only when necessary. Excessive gripping alters the BP response and decreases the oxygen requirement (METs) for each workload, resulting in an overestimation of exercise capacity and inaccurate HR- and BP-to-workload equivalents. Most patients adapt quickly if instructed to lightly rest a finger or two from one or both hands on the handrail. Exercise capacity can be reasonably estimated for functional purposes from both treadmill and cycle workloads provided that the equipment is calibrated regularly and accurately. When precise determination of oxygen uptake is necessary, as in assessing patients for heart transplant, evaluation by expired gas analysis is preferred.

Symptom Rating Scales

Before exercising, patients should be familiarized with the symptom rating scales. RPE and scales for angina, dyspnea, and claudication are shown in Frequently Used Angina and Dyspnea Rating Scales and Intermittent Claudication Rating Scale.

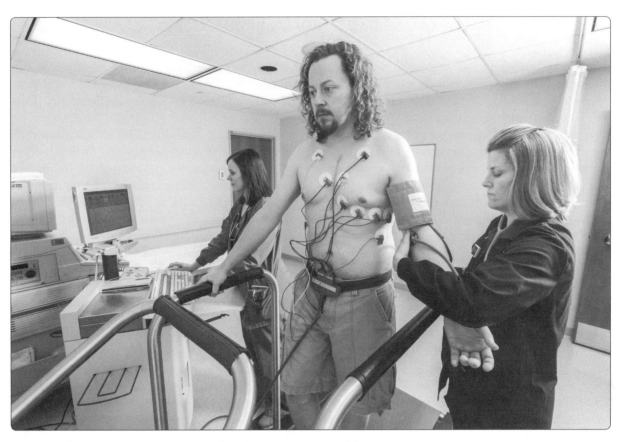

When performing an exercise test, closely monitor HR and BP.

Frequently Used Angina and Dyspnea Rating Scales

Five-Grade Angina Scale

0   No angina
1   Light, barely noticeable
2   Moderate, bothersome
3   Severe, very uncomfortable
4   Most pain ever experienced

Five-Grade Dyspnea Scale

0   No dyspnea
1   Mild, noticeable
2   Mild, some difficulty
3   Moderate difficulty, but can continue
4   Severe difficulty, cannot continue

Intermittent Claudication Rating Scale

0   No claudication pain
1   Initial, minimal pain
2   Moderate, bothersome pain

3   Intense pain
4   Maximal pain, cannot continue

Cardiopulmonary Exercise Testing

Cardiopulmonary exercise testing (CPX) uses ventilatory gas exchange analysis during exercise and is the gold standard for the assessment of exercise capacity.[5] Measures of gas exchange primarily include oxygen uptake ($\dot{V}O_2$), carbon dioxide output ($\dot{V}CO_2$), minute ventilation, and ventilatory threshold. Oxygen uptake at peak exercise is considered the most reliable measure of peak aerobic capacity and cardiorespiratory function. The technical aspects and clinical applications of CPX are discussed in detail elsewhere.[10] CPX is also indicated for

- evaluation of exercise capacity in selected patients with heart failure to assist in the estimation of prognosis and assess the need for cardiac transplantation;
- assistance in the differentiation of cardiac versus pulmonary limitations as a cause of exercise-induced dyspnea or impaired exercise capacity, when the etiology is uncertain;
- evaluation of the patient response to specific therapeutic interventions in which the improvement of exercise tolerance is an important goal or end point; and
- a more precise determination of the appropriate intensity for exercise training through identification of the ventilatory threshold.[18]

Normative values for peak oxygen uptake among patients entering CR[18] and healthy adults are available and serve as a useful reference in the evaluation of exercise capacity.[19] Exercise training intensities to maintain or improve health and fitness among individuals with or without heart disease can be derived from direct measurements of peak oxygen uptake.[16] This information may be most useful when the HR response to exercise is not a reliable indicator of exercise intensity (e.g., in patients with atrial fibrillation or patients who have a change in chronotropic medication).

Contemporary exercise testing systems have simplified techniques of CPX testing. However, these systems require maintenance and calibration for optimal use. Personnel involved with both test administration and interpretation must be trained and proficient in these techniques. Finally, the test requires additional time as well as patient cooperation.[10]

Diagnostic Utility

Exercise tolerance tests are useful in the detection of ischemia for diagnostic and management purposes. Abnormalities in exercise capacity, HR, BP, and exercise ECG are important findings. Cardiac events are more likely to occur in patients with lower exercise capacities and those who exhibit exercise-induced hypotension. Other markers of adverse prognosis are abnormal HR recovery (HR drop of <12 bpm within the first minute of recovery),[24] inability to attain 85% maximal predicted HR (unless on beta-blocker therapy),[25] and frequent ventricular ectopy in recovery (ventricular couplets or runs of ventricular tachycardia).[27]

The most common and useful ECG definition of a positive test for cardiac ischemia is a horizontal or downsloping ST depression that is ≥1 mm for at least 60 to 80 ms after the end of the QRS complex.[5] Stress test ECG findings must be interpreted in the context of clinical information regarding the baseline ECG, the patient's cardiovascular history, and the presence or absence of symptoms. Clearly, exercise testing in patients with documented CVD entering CR is not used for diagnosis, but rather for the detection of inducible ischemia, disease management, and estimation of prognosis. With patients for whom the diagnosis is in question, the description of symptoms can be most helpful. Typical angina can be defined as substernal chest discomfort (it may also begin in, or radiate into, the arms or jaw) that is provoked by exertion or emotional stress and is relieved by rest or nitroglycerin. Typical or definite angina, particularly in men older than 50 years and women older than 60 years, makes the pretest probability of disease so high that the test result does not dramatically change the probability of the presence of CVD. Atypical angina is defined as chest discomfort that lacks one of the earlier-mentioned characteristics. It may also include discomfort other than in the chest, arms, or jaw, and other symptoms such as shortness of breath, all of which serve to complicate the diagnosis. Symptoms of atypical angina generally indicate an intermediate pretest likelihood of CVD, particularly in men older than 30 years and women older than 50 years.[5]

Sensitivity is the percentage of patients with disease (e.g., ≤50% lesion of at least one major coronary artery) who will have an abnormal test.

Specificity is the percentage of patients free of disease who will have a normal test. The sensitivity and specificity of exercise ECG are each approximately 70%. However, those levels are affected based on the subgroup of patients being evaluated.[5] *Positive predictive value* of an abnormal test result is the percentage of people with an abnormal test who have the disease, whereas the *negative predictive value* of a normal test result is the percentage of people with a normal test who do not have the disease. It is important to understand that the positive and negative predictive values of the test are dependent on the prevalence of disease within the population being tested. Thus, evaluation of the pretest likelihood of disease allows for the most appropriate interpretation of the test results. For example, an abnormal test result is more likely to be a true positive (high positive predictive value) in a 60-year-old man with typical angina, and more likely to be a false positive (low positive predictive value) in a 25-year-old woman with atypical symptoms.

Several other factors influence test interpretation. Failure to achieve 85% maximum predicted HR limits the estimation of posttest probability if no abnormalities are detected, because the patient has not reached a diagnostic level of stress from which sensitivity estimates have been derived.[5] Beta-blockers are often prescribed as an antianginal therapy and can affect the sensitivity of the test. Galeema et al. reported that 82.7% of CR participants are on a beta-blocker.[27] Additionally, the presence of left bundle branch block, left ventricular hypertrophy with repolarization abnormalities, or resting ST-segment depression (≥1 mm) and the use of digoxin therapy confound the interpretation of the exercise ECG.[8] In such patients, exercise testing with either nuclear or echocardiographic imaging offers the advantage of greater sensitivity and specificity for the detection of CAD. In severely debilitated patients who are unable to perform an exercise test, pharmacologic testing has been used to evaluate ischemia. Unfortunately, the data from pharmacologic tests are not particularly useful in exercise prescription because hemodynamic and ischemic responses during such tests are not directly related to exercise effort. These tests are discussed later in this section.

Exercise Testing With Imaging Modalities

Cardiac imaging modalities are indicated when potential ECG changes are likely to be nondiagnostic, when it is important to determine the extent and distribution of ischemic myocardium, or to confirm an exercise ECG. Cardiac imaging with echocardiography before and after exercise can diagnose and localize the extent of myocardial ischemia. Radioactive agents are used to obtain nuclear myocardial perfusion scans at rest and with exercise.

Exercise Echocardiography

Echocardiography can be combined with exercise ECG in an attempt to increase the sensitivity and specificity of stress testing, as well as to determine the extent of myocardium at risk for ischemia. Echocardiographic images at rest are compared with those obtained during or immediately after exercise. Images must be obtained within 1 to 2 min after exercise, because abnormal wall motion begins to normalize after this point.

Myocardial contractility normally increases with exercise, whereas ischemia causes hypokinesis, akinesis, or dyskinesis of the affected segments. Therefore, a test is considered positive when wall motion abnormalities develop in previously normal areas with exercise or worsen in an already abnormal segment. Exercise echocardiography has a weighted mean sensitivity of 86%, specificity of 81%, and overall accuracy of 85% for the detection of CAD.[28] Patients with a normal exercise echocardiogram have a low risk of future cardiac events, including revascularization procedures, MI, or cardiac death. Exercise echocardiography has been shown to be highly accurate in diagnosing CAD in patients in whom there may be an increased incidence of false positive exercise ECG (e.g., women).[28,29]

Exercise Nuclear Imaging

Exercise tests with nuclear imaging are also performed with ECG monitoring. Several different imaging protocols use only technetium (Tc)-99m or thallous (thallium) chloride-201. These agents are usually injected about 1 min before the end of exercise, and images are obtained. Rest images are compared to exercise images to determine the areas of myocardial ischemia. Perfusion defects that are present during exercise but not seen at rest suggest ischemia. Perfusion defects that are present during exercise and persist at rest suggest previous MI or scar. In this manner, the extent and distribution of ischemic myocardium can be identified. Exercise nuclear single photon emission computed tomography (SPECT) imaging has a sensitivity of 87% and specificity of 73% for detecting CAD with ≥50% coronary stenosis.[30]

Pharmacologic Stress Testing

Patients unable to undergo exercise stress testing for reasons such as deconditioning, peripheral arterial disease, orthopedic disability, neurological disease, or concomitant illness can often benefit from pharmacologic stress testing. Two of the most common tests are dobutamine stress echocardiography (DSE) and nuclear scintigraphy with dipyridamole, adenosine, or regadenoson. Indications for these tests include establishing a diagnosis of CAD, determining myocardial viability before revascularization, assessing prognosis after MI or in chronic angina, and evaluating cardiac risk preoperatively. Little information can be gained from these tests to aid in the exercise prescription, because the HR and BP response at the ischemic threshold cannot be directly compared to that during exercise. However, pharmacologic studies can provide information regarding ventricular function and the extent of myocardium that may become ischemic; thus they are useful in risk stratification, particularly as it relates to the exercise program.

Dobutamine is a synthetic catecholamine and acts predominantly as a beta-1 agonist but also has some beta-2 and alpha-1 stimulatory effects. At lower doses, it increases cardiac output by causing an increase in contractility and HR. At higher doses, its principal effect is to bring about an increase in HR. Patients who have inadequate HR response to dobutamine may also receive an additional infusion of atropine to further stimulate HR response. As a result of the increased cardiac work, myocardial oxygen demand increases. If significant coronary artery stenoses are present, an oxygen supply-and-demand mismatch may occur, resulting in ischemia and abnormal wall motion.[28]

Dipyridamole, adenosine, and regadenoson cause coronary vasodilation in normal epicardial arteries but not in stenotic segments. As a result, a coronary steal phenomenon occurs, with a relatively increased flow to normal arteries and a relatively decreased flow to stenotic arteries. Nuclear perfusion imaging under resting conditions is then compared with imaging obtained after coronary vasodilation. Interpretation of the test is similar to that for exercise nuclear scans.[30]

Alternative Opportunities for Evaluating Physical Activity Status

Several opportunities exist for the evaluation of physical activity status in addition to symptom-limited exercise testing. These tests include the 6-minute walk test; and estimation of exercise tolerance from the clinician–patient interview, questionnaires, and direct assessment of job simulation and ADLs.

Six-Minute Walk Test

The 6-minute walk test (6MWT) can be used as a surrogate measure of exercise capacity when standard treadmill or cycle testing is not available.[31] However, the 6MWT is not useful in the objective determination of myocardial ischemia and is best used in a serial manner to evaluate changes in functional capacity with training over time. An alternative for assessing functional capacity in CR patients is the North Carolina 6-minute cycle test, a valid and reliable measure of physical performance in cardiac patients.[32]

Clinician–Patient Interview and Questionnaires

Although interviews and surveys are not a substitute for exercise testing, clinicians may obtain rough estimations of exercise tolerance by using MET activity tables and questioning patients about those activities that induce fatigue or symptoms.[33,34] In addition, a number of physical activity surveys have been used to quantify activity.[35] The Duke Activity Status Index and the Specific Activity Scale are examples of such scales.[36,37]

Controlled Job Simulation

Data from an exercise test can be compared to readily available MET tables to assist in making recommendations for safe vocational and avocational activities.[23] However, mechanical efficiency, specific job-task requirements, and environmental and psychological stressors can substantially alter the responses measured in the laboratory. While not usually performed in CR programs, controlled simulation of physical tasks can aid physicians and employers in determining whether a patient can safely return to work.[9]

Integrated assessment tests that attempt to measure a person's capacity to do everyday activities are available.[38] The most common tools have been developed to assess function in geriatric populations. Examples of these tests are the 30-second chair stand, the timed up and go, continuous scale physical functional performance–10, and the short physical performance battery. These tests can provide useful information related to functional mobility in patients with low functional capacity. Because of a ceiling effect, these tests have limited utility in younger, higher-functioning patients.

Summary

A careful evaluation of patient medical and functional status before participation in CR is essential to identifying limitations to exercise participation, describing the patient CVD progression risk factor profile, and facilitating the development of patient and staff goals as they relate to expected outcomes. Recognizing the appropriate methodologies for accomplishing these objectives and understanding potential alternatives to the evaluation of physical activity status are integral to the CR process, and ultimately to the success of the individual patient in CR.

Outpatient CR and SP

Philip A. Ades, MD, FACC, MAACVPR

The importance of comprehensive health behavior change in the prevention and management of CVD is an established component of CR. CR is effective at improving survival, decreasing rehospitalizations, and improving quality of life.[1] Collaboratively, patients and CR professionals must address the prevention of atherosclerotic disease progression and the risk of recurrent cardiac events. Moreover, CR professionals should be cognizant of changing demographics as patients become older, have more comorbid conditions, and more are obese.[2] Simultaneously, eligibility criteria for CR have expanded to included chronic systolic heart failure and heart valve replacement and repair. It is critical not only to expand participating patient populations, but also to implement and deliver effective models for SP through a variety of programming techniques. Integrating the rapidly growing knowledge base of the etiology and progression of atherosclerosis, as well as the efficacy of healthy behaviors as agents for primary and SP in CR, are necessary to positively affect patient outcomes. Primary prevention and SP of CVD have been the subject of epidemiological and experimental research for decades. Many prominent groups have issued practice guidelines for primary prevention and SP (see chapter 5 of the web resource for these statements), including the AACVPR, the ACC, and the AHA. These documents present the basis for the utilization and efficacy of a CR as a multifaceted program for SP of CVD. The notion that SP is not only possible, but also feasible and effective, is well established.[3,4] An aggressive therapeutic regimen, using optimal targets for intervention that addresses all modifiable risk factors, has become the basis for managing patients with CVD.[3] A broad array of assessments and treatment modalities along with follow-up is required for comprehensive SP. Tracking and reporting outcomes to patients, physicians, and payers is essential to the ongoing reimbursement, success, and acceptance of SP programs.

OBJECTIVES

This chapter focuses on the following:

- Assessment and management of risk factors for atherosclerotic CVD progression
- Stratification of risk for adverse events during CR
- Outlining the appropriate amount of monitoring and medical supervision
- Implementation of models for SP of CVD

Case management approach is the most effective method for delivering preventive and rehabilitative services in CR.[5-7] Inclusion of CR in the clinical pathway of cardiac patients beginning in the acute-care phase and continuing through the outpatient phase is absolutely necessary for comprehensive patient care.

Secondary prevention efforts within the health care setting are increasing as health care reform progresses. However, utilization rates of CR during 2007 to 2011 remained relatively unchanged compared to 1997, when studies found that only 11% to 37% of eligible patients were participating in outpatient CR.[8-10] Despite the evidence that outpatient CR confers reductions in mortality and morbidity (21-34%),[1,12,13] vulnerable populations such as minorities, women, the elderly, and people of lower socioeconomic status are the least likely to participate.[11] Thus, despite widespread confirmation of the safety and efficacy of CR, as well as an emphasis aimed at the medical community to aggressively implement this therapy and recommended lifestyle interventions, CR is not optimally utilized. With a goal of increasing participation, AACVPR, AHA, and American College of Cardiology Foundation (ACCF) released a statement on performance measures to include specific referral guidelines.[14] Future efforts to increase participation need to focus on methods to increase referral rates for patients with eligible diagnoses.[15]

Structure of CR and SP

AACVPR/ACCF/AHA statements regarding performance measures, core components, and SP guidelines provide standards that specify structure for CR.[3,14,16] Assessment and management of all established CVD risk factors and associated health behaviors are addressed in both documents. The European Society of Cardiology and Societies on Cardiovascular Disease Prevention in Clinical Practice provide additional preventive strategies for CVD.[17] These guidelines and subsequent statements issued by national organizations can guide CR structure and development and may be useful for maintaining and updating program design concurrent with a rapidly evolving body of literature.

The core components of CR have been formulated with the primary goals of reducing CVD morbidity and mortality, improving physical and psychological function, and enhancing quality of life.[16] These goals can be accomplished through changing health behaviors that lead to disease progression, including tobacco use, medication adherence, dyslipidemia, nutrition, exercise and physical activity, stress, psychological health, and control of metabolic disorders such as type 2 diabetes mellitus, metabolic syndrome, and obesity. Optimal management of lifestyle behaviors and metabolic disorders results in stabilization and regression of the atherosclerotic process.[5,18,19] Less-than-optimal, or *usual* care, is significantly less effective than active and more intensive lifestyle interventions in preventing the progression of CVD and recurring events.[5,18,19] Thus, a paradigm focusing on aggressive health behavior change along with adjunctive guideline-based medical therapy need to be prioritized (guideline 5.1).

Optimal SP requires a team of health care professionals to function in close collaboration with physicians to assist and guide patients toward efficacious preventive therapies. Core competencies for CR professionals are specified in an AACVPR/AHA position statement.[22] It is critical that CR programs foster close partnerships with primary care and specialty physicians to coordinate medical management for patients enrolled in CR.

Assessment and Management of Risk Factors for CVD Progression

The progression and vulnerability of established or newly developed atherosclerotic plaque are mostly dependent on the presence of risk factors, in particular, lipid abnormalities, smoking, insulin resistance, and other pro-inflammatory factors.[23]

Thus, ongoing assessment and management of CVD risk factors through the use of medications and behavior change are the most important spheres of influence of CR on positive patient outcomes.

Risk factor assessment should, at a minimum, be performed at entry into and exit from CR (guideline 5.2). Additionally, reassessing risk factors throughout participation in the program provides educational opportunities that may facilitate the behavior change that is critical to

Guideline 5.1   Structure of CR Programming

- At entry, all CR patients should be assessed for the presence and severity of modifiable CVD risk factors, including smoking, physical inactivity, overweight/obesity, dietary pattern, psychosocial dysfunction including depression, diminished exercise capacity, hypertension, dyslipidemia, impaired glucose tolerance, and type 2 diabetes mellitus.

- Depending on the medical history and physiological and psychological status, the majority of patients should pursue strategies for aggressive SP initiated in the hospital that should continue after discharge.

- Standard practice guidelines for preventive pharmacologic therapy should be followed.

- Strategies for SP that are initiated in hospital need to be verified, reassessed when indicated, and optimized at the CR baseline medical evaluation.

- Outcome assessment should include objective clinical measures of exercise performance and self-reported measures of exertion and behavior as required by the Centers for Medicare and Medicaid Services.[20]

- An in-hospital computerized automatic referral to CR should occur for all eligible patients to increase referral rates.[21] A specific health care professional directly involved in patient care should be identified and act as the liaison to facilitate the transition from IPCR to outpatient CR.[21] The use of referral and transition from IPCR to outpatient CR is a critical point in the enrollment process to early outpatient CR.

Early outpatient CR should begin within one to three weeks (or as soon as possible) of discharge from the hospital. Most patients, including those with uncomplicated percutaneous coronary interventions, should begin CR as soon as one week after hospital discharge. Other patients, such as those who experienced a sternotomy for bypass or heart valve surgery, may enter as soon as two to three weeks after hospital discharge. The evaluation, intervention, and expected outcomes are specified in the AACVPR Performance Measures document.[14]

Guideline 5.2   Screening and Assessments*

At the time of program entrance and exit, all patients should undergo the following assessments:

- Current medical history—medical or surgical procedures, including complications, comorbidities, and other pertinent medical history

- Physical examination—cardiopulmonary systems assessment and musculoskeletal assessment

- Current medications, including dose and frequency

- CVD risk profile, including the following:

  o Identification of age, sex, and menopausal status

  o History of electronic cigarettes, tobacco use, and nicotine containing products

  o History of legal or illicit drug use

  o History and level of control of hypertension

  o History and level of control of dyslipidemia, including lipid profile (total cholesterol, low-density lipoproteins [LDLs], high-density lipoproteins [HDLs], and triglycerides); lipid profile at the time of the index event and four weeks post-event or after initiating lipid lowering therapy

  o Dietary pattern, specifically macronutrient content including dietary fat, saturated fat, and caloric intake along with qualitative factors such as the consumption of processed foods, vegetables and fruit, and likeness to a Mediterranean diet

  o Body composition (weight, height, body mass index, waist circumference)

  o Fasting blood glucose or hemoglobin A1c and history of diabetes mellitus

  o Symptom-limited exercise tolerance testing to assess safety, exercise capacity, HR, BP, arrhythmias, and ECG response

  o Physical activity status, including leisure time physical activity, daily sitting, or sedentary time

  o Psychosocial history, including evidence of depression, anxiety, level of anger, hostility, and social isolation

  o Quality of life questionnaire data

*For a complete discussion of evaluation and assessment, see chapter 4.

improved patient outcomes. This reinforcement is one of the most effective tools that CR professionals can employ. CR professionals should consider prioritizing and implementing all required variables for assessment included in the document on performance measures.[14]

The presence of multiple CVD risk factors increases the risk of recurrent cardiovascular events exponentially.[23] Additionally, the specific combination of risk factors that includes elevated levels of LDL and triglycerides and impaired glucose metabolism (insulin resistance/metabolic syndrome or diabetes) is associated with significantly increased risk in patients with CVD.[24] Assessment and treatment of CVD risk factors are outlined in chapter 9.

After the initial assessment, establishing patient-centered goals according to a patient's readiness to change and self-efficacy should be prioritized. (Chapter 8 includes a detailed discussion of the basic principles of health behavior change.) One of the most effective ways to facilitate positive health behavior change is to work with a CR professional to specifically define patient-established short-term and long-term goals.[25] In addition, documenting agreed upon goals in writing (often in contractual form) can be effective for promoting health behavior change.[26]

Modifying risk factors has been shown to be efficacious for reducing risk of subsequent events and progression of CVD.[5,7,17] The national guidelines, practice standards, and scientific statements available in the chapter 5 section of the web resource provide significant support and documentation for the efficacy of risk factor modification. For more information on treatment recommendations for CVD risk factors, see chapter 9.

Coaching, Case Management, and Counseling

The usual-care therapeutic approach to health behavior change, in which a knowledgeable expert simply prescribes medications and creates goals consistent with national practice standards, is not an effective means to foster behavior change. Individualized case management is an integrated process that provides specific behavioral risk factor intervention strategies for disease management.[5,7] The patient is the center of the process and takes an active role, particularly in goal setting, to accomplish mutually agreed-upon short- and long-term goals and outcomes that reduce CVD risk. Therapeutic approaches should be coordinated with other health care professionals as necessary. Case management techniques are especially efficient in CR using a team approach consisting of these three primary steps:

1. Assess risk factors for disease progression and recurrent CVD events, and subsequently guide patients to make positive changes in health behaviors associated with those risk factors.

2. Establish rapport, and maintain communication with patients through motivational interviewing, electronic communication, and smartphone reminder techniques as appropriate.

3. Provide follow-up care to assess progress, and reset goals as appropriate.

Finally, continued support for health behavior change is essential for addressing lapses and for promoting long-term change. This model allows for both group teaching and individualized therapeutic modalities along with implementation of algorithms for each risk factor with full patient agreement and understanding.

Contemporary CR provides the patient support necessary for successful behavior change. Consistent contact over an extended period of time gives CR staff the opportunity to provide feedback and reinforce positive health behavior changes. Patient and staff interaction can take many forms, including personal discussion during exercise and education sessions, telephone calls, electronic messaging, letters or other written correspondence, or visits to the facility for follow-up counseling and testing.

Stratification of Risk for Events During Exercise

It is prudent to assess for the risk of complications prior to an individual with CVD commencing with an exercise program. The sidebar Stratification of Risk for Cardiac Events During Exercise Participation provides information relative to the level of risk for individual patients. A patient's level of risk will influence the recommended

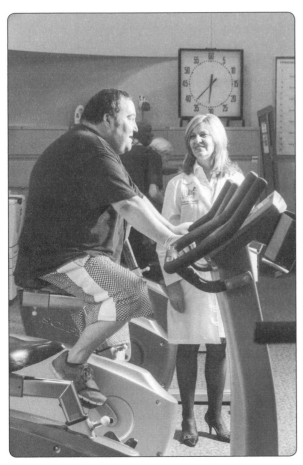

Consistent contact with patients, such as personal discussion during exercise, provides CR staff opportunities to reinforce positive health behavior changes.

intensity of monitoring during exercise and the frequency of behavioral counseling required. Current clinical status and extent of behavior change required must be considered when setting goals with patients. Patient-set goals and goal ownership are significantly related to achieving the desired outcomes.[25]

The goal of an exercise program is to balance safety with the patient's desire to achieve optimal physiological, symptomatic, psychological, and vocational benefits. A key element of safety is stratification of patients according to risk for acute CVD complications during exercise (guideline 5.3).[26] Risk stratification criteria for events during exercise or activity are not absolute nor are they differentiated from risks related to general mortality. Despite these potential limitations,

stratification of patients for risk of an event during exercise is a clinical tool that can help determine the appropriate level of supervision for individual patients.

For patients diagnosed with CVD and properly evaluated, including a symptom-limited stress test, the risk of adverse events during exercise is exceedingly low.[27,28] It has also been reported that the risk of an event for patients with chronic heart failure during exercise is minimal.[29] Physical activity (especially unaccustomed activity) can transiently trigger CVD events, but increased habitual physical activity and higher levels of cardiopulmonary fitness significantly lower risk of events during exercise.[30]

CR can minimize risk through appropriate assessment at program entry, gradual advancement of the exercise prescription, frequent and high-quality training of CR professionals in emergency response, and ongoing clinical and symptomatic assessment of patients prior to and during each exercise session. This fact does not diminish the potential importance of ECG monitoring. However, CR professionals should understand that monitoring, in itself, does not prevent or reduce complications during CR.

The risk stratification model presented in the sidebar Stratification of Risk for Cardiac Events During Exercise Participation uses variables common to established models and allows categorization into a single level of risk. This model is helpful for identifying the lowest-, moderate-, and highest-risk patients. Lowest-risk patients have all of the characteristics listed, whereas the highest-risk patients have any one of the characteristics listed. Those who do not fit either classification are considered to be at moderate risk.

Patients who have not undergone exercise testing before entering CR and those with non-

Guideline 5.3 — Stratification of Risk for Exercise Events

All patients entering CR should be stratified according to risk for the occurrence of adverse events during exercise and for risk of progression of atherosclerotic disease.

Stratification of Risk for Cardiac Events During Exercise Participation

Characteristics of patients at highest risk for exercise participation (any one or combination of these findings places a patient at high risk)

- Presence of complex ventricular arrhythmias during exercise testing or recovery
- Presence of angina or other significant symptoms (shortness of breath, light-headedness, or dizziness at low levels of exertion [<5 METs] or during recovery)
- High level of silent ischemia (ST-segment depression ≥2 mm from baseline) during exercise testing or recovery
- Presence of abnormal hemodynamics with exercise testing (i.e., chronotropic incompetence or flat or decreasing systolic BP with increasing workloads) or recovery (i.e., severe postexercise hypotension)
- Functional capacity ≤3 METs

Nonexercise testing findings

- Left ventricular dysfunction with resting ejection fraction <35%
- History of cardiac arrest
- Complex dysrhythmias at rest
- Complicated myocardial infarction or incomplete revascularization procedure
- Presence of heart failure
- Presence of signs or symptoms of post-event or post-procedure ischemia
- Presence of clinical depression
- Implanted cardiac defibrillator

Characteristics of patients at moderate risk for exercise participation (any one or combination of these findings places a patient at moderate risk)

- Presence of stable angina or other significant symptoms (e.g., unusual shortness of breath, light-headedness, or dizziness occurring only at high levels of exertion [≥7 METs])
- Mild to moderate level of silent ischemia during exercise testing or recovery (ST-segment depression <2 mm from baseline)
- Functional capacity <5 METs

Nonexercise testing findings

- Rest ejection fraction = 35% to 49%

Characteristics of patients at lowest risk for exercise participation (all characteristics listed must be present for patient to remain at lowest risk)

- Absence of complex ventricular dysrhythmia during exercise testing and recovery
- Absence of angina or other significant symptoms (e.g., unusual shortness of breath, light-headedness, or dizziness during exercise testing and recovery)
- Presence of normal hemodynamics during exercise testing and recovery (i.e., appropriate increases and decreases in heart rate and systolic blood pressure with increasing workloads and recovery)
- Functional capacity ≥7 METs

Nonexercise testing findings

- Rest ejection fraction ≥50%
- Uncomplicated myocardial infarction and/or complete revascularization procedure
- Absence of complicated ventricular arrhythmias at rest
- Absence of heart failure
- Absence of signs or symptoms of postevent or postprocedure ischemia
- Absence of clinical depression

Reproduced from *Cardiology Clinics,* Vol. 19, M.A. Williams, "Exercise testing in cardiac rehabilitation: Exercise prescription and beyond," Copyright 2001, with permission from Elsevier.

diagnostic exercise tests may be inadequately categorized using criteria from the sidebar Stratification of Risk for Cardiac Events During Exercise Participation. For such patients, the approach to risk stratification should be more cautious, and the initial exercise prescription should be conservative. Patients with nondiagnostic exercise tests or tests that may not be useful for exercise prescription include patients with abnormal resting ECG, including left bundle branch block, left ventricular hypertrophy with or without resting ST-T wave changes, nonspecific intraventricular conduction delays, Wolff-Parkinson-White syndrome, and ventricular-paced rhythms.

Clinical Supervision During Exercise

Decisions regarding the intensity of clinical supervision, including necessary personnel and the type and duration of the supervision and frequency of ECG monitoring (continuous v. intermittent), should be established by the CR program medical director and staff. An appropriate staff-to-patient ratio to ensure safety will need to account for the increasing age and complexity of contemporary CR patients.[2]

BOTTOM LINE

Important considerations to promote patient safety include the following:

- More intense clinical supervision is required for patients deemed to be at a higher level of risk, who exhibit new or recurring cardiovascular symptoms or potentially deleterious arrhythmias, or who experience a change in health status.

- Enhanced surveillance of patient status during exercise is prudent when the intensity of the exercise prescription is increased. The monitoring of clinical parameters before, during, and following exercise provides further safeguards (see guideline 5.4).

- CR professionals must provide thorough instruction regarding patient self-assessment and reporting responsibilities about symptoms and feelings of well-being to CR staff.

- The safety and efficacy of the exercise program can be maximized through ongoing communication with patients and conducting and implementing frequent clinical and symptomatic assessment for well-being and clinical status, as well as for compliance with the exercise prescription.

Early Outpatient Exercise Program

Early outpatient CR may begin within one to three weeks post-discharge from the hospital if clinical status allows and may last up to 36 sessions (or longer based on medical necessity).[31] Sessions are most commonly scheduled three days per week, although numbers of sessions per week may vary from one to five and may include more than one session per day if greater than 1 hour of intensive counseling or teaching is added to an exercise session. The intensity of clinical supervision is usually highest during early outpatient CR and may include ECG monitoring. The sidebar, Physician Roles in CR, outlines the physician roles in the provision of clinical supervision.[32] There are no specific federal requirements regarding professional designation for CR staffing. Professionally qualified CR staff members include registered

---

Guideline 5.4   Recommended Methods and Tools for Daily Assessment of Risk for Exercise

The pre-exercise assessment should include interviewing the patient about recent signs and symptoms, adherence to the medication schedule, and subjective feelings of well-being. Risk may also be assessed with the following clinical measures:

- Signs or symptoms of effort intolerance

- Continuous or intermittent ECG monitoring
- BP
- HR
- RPE
- Exercise tolerance

Reducing Cardiovascular Disease Complications During Exercise Within Cardiac Rehabilitation

Program Policies

- Ensure that all patients have a physician referral and the appropriate assessment before entry into the program and at periodic follow-up intervals.
- Ensure that all patients receive ongoing assessment before, during, and after each exercise session.
- Maintain an emergency plan for adverse events, and provide for frequent mock emergency practice and critique sessions for all staff members.
- Maintain physician standing orders for potential emergent and nonemergent medical events.
- Ensure on-site medical supervision; monitoring and resuscitation equipment, including a defibrillator (as well as maintenance of such equipment); and appropriate medications.

Patient Education

- Emphasize to patients that they must be knowledgeable about and alert for warning signs and changes in their medical status, both at home and within the CR program, including, but not limited to, angina-like symptoms, light-headedness or dizziness, irregular heart rate, abrupt weight gain, and shortness of breath.
- Instruct patients about the appropriate responses to such changes in their medical condition.
- Emphasize the importance of adhering to the exercise prescription (including target HR or RPE, exercise workloads, duration of effort, and choices of exercise equipment).
- Emphasize the importance of warm-up and cool-down as they relate to the safety of exercise.
- Remind patients to adjust exercise levels according to various environmental conditions such as heat, humidity, cold, and altitude.

Expectations During the Exercise Session

- Evaluate each patient before exercise for recent changes in medical status, body weight, BP, medication adherence, and ECG.
- Use ECG monitoring as appropriate. It is important to note that there are no specific mandates regarding ECG monitoring in CR. Most programs employ ECG monitoring for the initial three to six sessions of CR for the majority of patients after a thorough baseline medical evaluation.
- Adjust the intensity and duration of the exercise prescription based on the clinical status before and in response to exercise.
- Maintain supervision during and following exercise, including periodic checks of shower or locker room facilities, until all patients have vacated the facility.
- Modify recreational physical activities as appropriate, and minimize high-intensity competition.

nurses, clinical exercise physiologists, physical therapists, and exercise specialists.

ECG Monitoring in Early Outpatient CR

Continuous ECG monitoring does not ensure safety or efficacy of CR. Rather, ECG monitoring is one of several methods and techniques that can be used for clinical supervision of patients. The duration of ECG monitoring for a given patient should depend on the level of risk of an individual patient. ECG monitoring during exercise sessions may be required for insurance reimbursement. ECG monitoring is most useful for the detection of exercise-induced arrhythmias whereas it is less

Physician Roles in CR

- *The supervising physician* is immediately available and accessible for medical consultations and medical emergencies at all times during which services are being provided to patients within CR programs.

- *Standards for supervising physicians.* Supervising physician must possess all of the following:

  1. Expertise in the management of individuals with cardiac pathophysiology

  2. Training in basic life support or advanced cardiac life support

  3. A license to practice medicine in the state in which the CR program is offered

- CR services are initially prescribed and supervised by a physician pursuant to a written Individualized Treatment Plan established, reviewed, and signed by a physician every 30 days (in consultation with appropriate staff participating in the program). The plan sets forth the diagnoses; the type, amount, frequency, and duration of the items and services provided under the plan; and the goals under the plan.

- *The medical director* is the physician who medically supervises a CR program at a particular site.

- The medical director, in consultation with staff, is involved in directing the progress of individuals in the program and must possess all of the following:

  1. Expertise in the management of individuals with cardiac pathophysiology

  2. Training in basic life support or advanced cardiac life support

  3. Expertise in CR, exercise physiology, and the principles of exercise training in cardiac patients

  4. A license to practice medicine

- The medical director and the supervising physician are not necessarily the same person.

Reprinted from U.S. Code of Federal Regulations, 2019. http://edocket.access.gpo.gov/cfr_2010/octqtr/pdf/42cfr410.49.pdf

useful, in the clinical setting, for the detection of coronary ischemia and as a predictor of coronary events.[33,34] Ideally, the ECG monitoring and the length of supervised CR should be determined on an individual basis according to attainment of outcomes and individual needs. Further recommendations for the use of ECG monitoring and duration of CR based on risk of exercise events are presented in the sidebar, Recommendations for Intensity of Supervision and Monitoring Related to Risk of Exercise Participation.

The use of ECG monitoring seems to be linked with a lower risk, but no firm predictors exist to help identify patients for whom it may not be necessary. Continuous ECG monitoring is intended to

- detect potentially deleterious arrhythmias,

- monitor compliance with the exercise prescription, especially with respect to HR, and

- increase patient self-confidence for independent activity.

Given the variable occurrence of dysrhythmias, however, and given that the safety of exercise regimens has been determined only by means of aggregate data, the use of continuous versus intermittent ECG monitoring remains a matter of clinical judgment. The type and frequency of ECG monitoring depend on the overall clinical status of the patient and the response to the exercise session. Intermittent ECG monitoring enables observation when indicated, such as at the time of a suspected change in clinical status as assessed by observation, measurement, or symptomatology, but does not afford detection of silent or sudden-onset dysrhythmias and thus should be used judiciously. Accordingly, the optimal approach balances patient benefit with safety. Clinicians may request monitoring in specific clinical situations, such as when a patient is symptomatic or when a concern exists for paroxysmal atrial fibrillation.

Recommendations for Intensity of Supervision and Monitoring Related to Risk of Exercise Participation

Patients at Lowest Risk for Exercise-Related Event

- Direct medical supervision of exercise should optimally occur until a safe and appropriate exercise response during exercise sessions has been demonstrated. This often begins with continuous electrocardiogram (ECG) monitoring and decreasing as appropriate (e.g., after 3-6 sessions).

- For the patient to remain at lowest risk, the hemodynamic findings must remain normal; there should be no development or progression of abnormal signs and symptoms or intolerance to exercise within or outside the supervised program. Progression of the exercise regimen is appropriate.

Patients at Moderate Risk for Exercise-Related Event

- Direct staff supervision should occur until a safe exercise response has been demonstrated. This begins with continuous ECG monitoring and decreased to intermittent or no ECG monitoring as appropriate (e.g., after 3-6 sessions).

- To move the patient to the lowest risk category, hemodynamic findings during exercise must be normal; there should be no development or progression of abnormal signs and symptoms or intolerance to exercise within or outside the supervised program. Progression of the exercise regimen is appropriate.

- Abnormal ECG or hemodynamic findings or the development or progression of abnormal signs and symptoms or intolerance to exercise within or outside the supervised program, or the need to dramatically decrease exercise levels, may result in the patient remaining in the moderate risk category or even moving to the high-risk category.

Patients at Highest Risk for Exercise-Related Event

- Direct staff supervision of exercise should occur for a minimum of 18 to 36 sessions beginning with continuous ECG monitoring and decreasing to intermittent ECG monitoring as deemed appropriate for the patient by clinical criteria.

- For a patient to move to the moderate risk category, ECG and hemodynamic findings during exercise should be normal; there should be no development or progression of abnormal signs and symptoms or intolerance to exercise within or outside the supervised program. Progression of the exercise regimen is appropriate.

- Findings of the development or progression of ischemic symptoms such as angina or abnormal ECG or hemodynamic findings during exercise, including intolerance to exercise within or outside the supervised program, should be evaluated immediately. Significant limitations in the ability to participate may result in discontinuation of the exercise program until appropriate medical evaluation and intervention, when indicated, can take place.

Innovation in CR

The traditional structure of CR needs to be reconsidered. Barriers to program participation need to be addressed. Programs need to alter and adapt program structure to accommodate a greater number of patients that will result from efforts to enhance patient referral, participation, adherence, and completion. Innovations in CR can take the form of altered exercise programming or delivery of SP services.

Examples

- It has been demonstrated that an exercise format using increased duration and frequency of exercise with a goal of maximizing caloric expenditure can significantly increase weight loss in CR and effectively modify several CVD risk factors and the risk for metabolic syndrome.[35]

- Whereas most group teaching sessions on risk factor treatments are currently given on-site, programs have been experimenting with smartphone technologies to deliver equivalent risk factor teaching in the home setting.[36]

- Hybrid CR programs have combined on-site exercise and teaching sessions (currently reimbursed) with home sessions (currently not reimbursed), sometimes with smartphone ECG monitoring capability.[36] The Veterans Administration health care system has expanded its use of home-based CR by combining on-site with home sessions along with an educational program.[37]

The traditional structure of CR needs to be reconsidered. Programs will need to alter and adapt program structure to accommodate a greater number of patients that will result from efforts to enhance patient referral, participation, adherence, and completion.

Maintenance CR

Maintenance CR is a term that is often used to describe programs that are less medically super-vised than early outpatient CR. Typically, maintenance CR programs utilize the same physical space as early outpatient CR. Participants usually pay an out-of-pocket fee to participate. Patients who have completed early outpatient CR or who have CVD risk factors can benefit from attending maintenance CR to facilitate ongoing exercise and health behavior change associated with disease prevention and reductions in recurrent CVD events.[38] Indeed, maintenance CR and the accompanying healthy lifestyle behaviors encouraged through continued secondary prevention are integral to decreasing morbidity and mortality and enhancing health-related quality of life in patients with CVD.[39,40]

Maintenance CR can take many forms and is often structured around an individualized exercise prescription tailored to clinical status and comorbidities, orthopedic considerations, and cardiorespiratory fitness. Patients are monitored less intensively than in early outpatient CR, and physicians may not be on-site. CR staff are

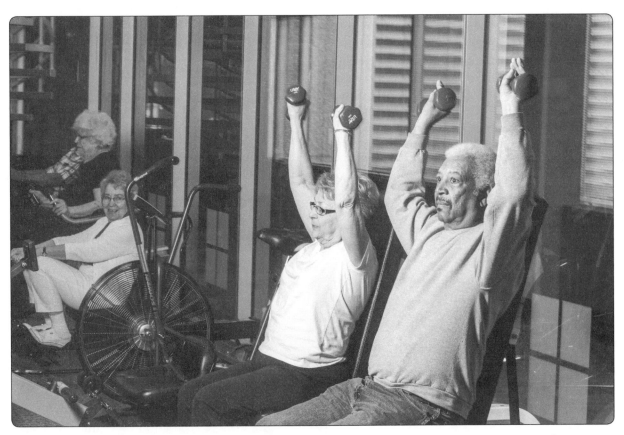

Beyond basic exercise sessions using standard equipment, supplementary programming such as group resistance training sessions may increase program adherence.

always available, and avenues for obtaining urgent medical care when needed have been established. Patients may receive periodic HR and BP assessment; intermittent or quick-look ECG monitoring; and counseling and support regarding health behavior change and risk factors, cardiovascular symptoms, and exercise prescription. Qualified staff (e.g., registered nurse, ACSM Registered Clinical Exercise Physiologist, ACSM Certified Clinical Exercise Specialist, and other certified clinical professionals) should be immediately available and properly trained to administer emergency support. Exercise progression and cardiovascular indicators should be monitored for changes in clinical status. Moreover, professional staff can determine whether ancillary programming, such as diabetes education, psychosocial evaluation, or weight loss or nutrition counseling, may be beneficial to patients and make referrals as indicated. Annual reviews that include assessment of CVD risk factor status and symptom—limited exercise tolerance are appropriate and can be performed by either CR staff or by an individual patient's health care provider.

In addition to exercise instruction and monitoring, maintenance CR provides a setting for continued risk factor modification and behavior change. Education can take many forms, including group lectures, individualized chart reviews, and newsletters or other written material, as well as verbal interaction during exercise sessions. A group education format also provides opportunities for social interaction among patients.

Finally, identifying barriers to participating in maintenance CR such as financial considerations, transportation issues, time constraints, and orthopedic limitations allows patients and staff to work cohesively toward developing an action plan to circumvent factors limiting compliance.

Future Directions

For many reasons, attendance at on-site CR will never reach all eligible patients. Efforts to expand the reach of CR by establishing hybrid and home CR programs should be implemented with use of modern technologies.[15] Innovative efforts should also be made to reach patients who do not attend CR, including the provision of various SP programs designed to ensure that patients are taking evidence-based preventive medications, maintaining a tobacco- and nicotine-free personal environment, and engaging in adequate physical activity profiles. Case managers who are knowledgeable in CR and SP, assigned in the hospital for patients unlikely to attend CR, would be optimal personnel to manage such an effort.

Summary

Given that CR has been shown to reduce CVD morbidity and mortality as well as to improve physical function and quality of life,[15] implementation of comprehensive CR needs to be greatly expanded. The treatment of risk factors associated with the progression of CVD requires a multifactorial effort by a multidisciplinary CR staff. Entry assessments for patient safety and CVD risk factors assist program staff to establish priorities for therapeutic modalities, help patients to recognize those health behaviors that require change, and identify the most efficacious therapies. The level of clinical supervision and patient monitoring depend on individual patient characteristics and level of risk. Hybrid and home programming for patients, with or without supervised CR, is an excellent adjunct to a patient-centered program of CVD risk reduction.

Physical Activity and Exercise

Jonathan Myers, PhD

CR should provide patients with knowledge and skills needed to enhance the adoption or resumption of an optimal level of physical activity (PA). This part of the CR process is important not only for the period following a cardiac event but also for gaining knowledge, skills, and confidence to maintain a more active lifestyle in the long term. To this end, programs should give patients recommendations for both structured exercise training and leisure-time PA. The overall goal should be to increase habitual PA to a level that promotes health, improves CRF, and reduces chronic disease risk. This chapter reviews the general recommendations for exercise during CR participation. For more specific recommendations with respect to specific patient conditions during CR participation, see chapters 9, 10, and 11.

OBJECTIVES

This chapter discusses the following:

- General recommendations for developing and implementing exercise to patients participating in CR
- Recommendations for aerobic-based exercise
- Recommendations for resistance-based exercise
- Recommendations for range of motion–based exercise
- Specific safety information for beginning and progressing exercise training in a CR program

Guideline 6.1   Considerations for the Prescription of Exercise and Physical Activity

When developing an exercise prescription, consider the following factors:

Safety Factors

- Clinical history
- Risks associated with CVD progression or instability
- Ischemic and angina thresholds
- Cognitive or psychological impairment

Associated Factors

- Vocational or avocational requirements
- Orthopedic limitations
- Previous and current activities
- Personal health and fitness goals

An important initial consideration in exercise planning is safety. Safety considerations apply to both structured exercise training and leisure-time PA. While most patients can engage in exercise without incurring undue risks, appropriate risk stratification should be performed. Guideline 6.1 provides key variables to consider when developing an exercise prescription. Safety and risk stratification are discussed in detail in chapters 4 and 5. Recommendations for supervision and ECG monitoring can be found in chapter 5. Later in this chapter, tables 6.1 and 6.2 present basic principles of exercise prescription. A model for risk stratification for cardiovascular events is outlined in the sidebar Stratification of Risk for Cardiac Events During Exercise Participation in chapter 5. After risk stratification, recommendations for supervision, ECG, monitoring and prescribed intensity and duration of exercise training can be made.

Comprehensive, evidence-based recommendations for structured exercise training in CR are available from several prominent organizations[1,3,8] and are only summarized here. A comprehensive exercise program includes cardiorespiratory, musculoskeletal, and flexibility components. Specific elements for each component are summarized in the tables in this chapter and include guidelines for intensity, duration, frequency, and type of exercise for training. Each of the elements should be prescribed relative to one another and in a way that effectively addresses predefined training goals (e.g., increased aerobic or musculoskeletal fitness, weight reduction, control of blood glucose, or resumption of occupation).

Cardiorespiratory Endurance Training

Cardiorespiratory endurance training should be the foundation of most exercise routines for adults with or at risk for CVD. This type of exercise training is the most effective way to increase CRF. Elements of an exercise prescription for increasing CRF are presented in table 6.1. The relative training intensity may vary between 40% and 80% of maximal heart rate reserve (HRR) or metabolic reserve ($\dot{V}O_2R$). Initially, programs should focus on the lower part of the intensity range, with progression to higher intensities as patients adapt to the program.[7] RPE (e.g., Borg Scale of Perceived Exertion 6-20; Borg CR10 Scale; Omni Picture System of Perceived Exertion) are considered adjunctive to HR monitoring, but they may become more important as a subjective intensity guide as patients gain experience with exercise training and learn how to use the scale. Exercise training duration varies as a function of the overall energy expenditure goals of the patient. A *minimum* of 20 continuous minutes of exercise per session is commonly recommended within structured programs, although some patients may follow an intermittent (i.e., interval) exercise regimen. Some patients may need to accumulate shorter bouts (e.g., multiple 10 min bouts) throughout the day due to comorbidities, symptoms such as claudication or musculoskeletal discomfort, or lifestyle factors. Ideally, patients should be active most days of the week,[1-7,9] but structured programs are often designed with a frequency of two to four sessions per week.

Once the initial exercise prescription is established, patients should progress gradually toward predefined or redefined program goals. There is no set format with respect to progression because many factors, including fitness level, motivation, and orthopedic limitations, influence the rate at which a patient may progress. In general, it is prudent to change one component and provide some time (a minimum of one exercise session) to assess the adaptation to the new level before progressing further. When time permits, increases in duration and frequency should precede increases in intensity. Modest increases in intensity, when appropriate, are likely to be tolerated and should be based on the observations of the staff and subjective responses of the patient, provided that the changes remain within the limits specified in the most recent evaluation.

A guiding principle should be progression of the total volume or dose of exercise such that the patient achieves desired energy expenditure thresholds within a three- to six-month period. Therefore, given that most patients' participation in CR lasts no longer than three months, it is important to educate and encourage patients to continue exercising even after CR participation has ended. The most appropriate volume of exercise depends on the individual CVD risk profile, training goals, and comorbidities (i.e., diabetes, hypertension, obesity, arthritis). An accumulating body of evidence has affirmed a dose–response relationship between the volume of PA and health outcomes.[1,3,6-8] Whether exercise has a role in reversing coronary artery disease is an issue that remains controversial; however, thresholds of approximately 1,500 and 2,200 kcal/week are associated with stability and regression of coronary artery lesions, respectively.[18] Notably, multiple studies document that energy expenditure

Table 6.1 Exercise Prescription for Cardiorespiratory Endurance Training of Cardiac Patients Cleared for Participation

Component	Recommendation

Intensity	• 40%-80% of HRR or $\dot{V}O_2R$ or $\dot{V}O_2$ peak if maximal exercise data are available (See table 6.2 when exercise test data are not available.)
	• RPE of 12-16 on a 6-20 scale as adjunct to objective measure of HR
	• 10 bpm below HR associated with any of the following criteria:
	  • Onset of angina or other symptoms of cardiovascular insufficiency
	  • Plateau or decrease in SBP; SBP >240 mm Hg; DBP >110 mm Hg
	  • >1 mm ST-depression, horizontal or downsloping
	  • Radionuclide evidence of reversible myocardial ischemia or echocardiographic evidence of moderate to severe wall motion abnormalities during exertion
	  • Increased frequency of ventricular dysrhythmias
	  • Other significant ECG disturbances (e.g., second- or third-degree AVB, atrial fibrillation, SVT, complex ventricular ectopy)
	  • Other signs or symptoms of exertional intolerance

Duration	• 20-60 min per session • Longer durations or multiple sessions accumulated throughout the day are recommended to enhance total energy expenditure for weight reduction. Daily goal can be accumulated in single or multiple shorter sessions
Frequency	Ideally, most days of the week (i.e., CR 2-4 days/week and supplemented with 2-4 days of home-based exercise)
Type	Rhythmic, larger muscle group activities (i.e., walking, cycling, stair climbing, elliptical trainers, and other arm or leg ergometers that allow controlled movement and consistent intensity)

Abbreviations: HR, heart rate; HRR, heart rate reserve; $\dot{V}O_2R$, maximal oxygen uptake metabolic reserve; RPE, rating of perceived exertion; SBP, systolic blood pressure; DBP, diastolic blood pressure; ECG, electrocardiogram; AVB, atrioventricular block; SVT, supraventricular tachycardia.

Based on ACSM (2018).

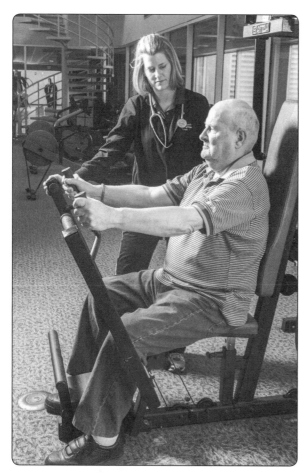

Once a patient has been cleared for participation in a resistance training program, a measure of baseline muscular strength helps to establish a safe initial routine and monitor adaptations over time.

in structured CR does not typically meet either of these thresholds.[11-14] Therefore, patients will likely need to engage in PA outside of the structured program to achieve the optimal levels of energy expenditure.

Few studies have supported the efficacy of structured exercise training as a singular strategy to normalize body weight and body composition in patients with CVD. This underscores the importance of multiple behavioral strategies in weight reduction programming for overweight patients. Studies show that achieving weight loss goals requires a simultaneous change in dietary habits in addition to greater physical activity patterns. The volume or dose of exercise associated with the typical CR training session may be a limiting factor, and there is only a 1 to 2 kg weight

loss during CR participation. It is likely part of the explanation for a low amount of weight loss during CR is due to a lack of focus on helping patients lose weight. As mentioned previously, numerous studies have shown the weekly dose to be inadequate for weight or fat reduction. As an example, a typical exercise session for an outpatient with a peak functional capacity of 7 METs might be 30 min at a heart rate that would equate with about 4 METs. The following formula provides a method to estimate the caloric costs of the exercise session:

$$\text{Calories/min} = [\text{METs} \times \text{body weight in kg} \times 3.5] / 200$$

It should be noted that the 4 MET value in this example includes the resting energy expenditure component (1 MET). Therefore, the *net* caloric cost of the exercise would be based on only 3 METs. If the hypothetical patient in this example weighed 100 kg (220 lb) and exercised 3 days per week for 30 min, the net caloric expenditure would be approximately 480 kcal/week (5.3 kcal/min × 30 min × 3 days/week). Although patients can clearly improve exercise tolerance with this regimen, the estimated caloric expenditure falls well short of contemporary recommendations for PA and in most cases would not be effective for weight or fat loss.[15] For example, 40 min sessions, five times per week, would result in an expenditure of approximately 1,060 kcal per week. Again, this calculation highlights the importance of increasing PA outside of the structured or in-hospital program. Thus, adjustments must be made about frequency and duration of exercise to allow patients to achieve greater energy expenditures to enhance program outcomes. However, these adjustments must be with the caveat that although it is prudent to increase exercise volume progressively, staff must carefully consider the risk that a higher-volume program may lead to higher dropout rates. Therefore, overweight patients must be educated about the need to develop and maintain fitness as the core of their exercise regimen, with the additional volume of PA facilitating weight loss and other goals. Finally, as CRF improves, patients are able to exercise at a higher metabolic rate (more kcal/min) at a given relative intensity (% maximal HRR). This adjustment allows patients to accumulate a greater caloric deficit over time.

Exercise Recommendations for Patients Without a Recent Exercise Test

While a maximal exercise test is the foundation of an appropriate exercise prescription, the test is not always available. For patients entering a CR program without an entry exercise test, staff should implement exercise programs conservatively with close patient surveillance. The program director and referring clinician should advise on the upper limit of training intensity. Initial exercise intensities can be determined according to the length of time from cardiac event, hospital discharge, and patient assessment (including ADLs). At a minimum, monitoring should include signs and symptoms, RPE, HR, and signs of overexertion. While ECG monitoring is not needed for most patients, it is often advisable to use ECG monitoring for at least a few initial sessions in patients who have not had an exercise test. This is particularly true in patients with an ischemic etiology, especially if they have not been revascularized and are being medically managed (although these patients are ideal for an exercise test to assess for indications of ischemia). A submaximal exercise evaluation, such as a 6-minute walk test with conservative termination criteria, can be helpful to determine exercise session parameters. Table 6.2 outlines initial recommendations for patients entering a program without a recent exercise test.[16] A patient who responds normally to three to six exercise sessions as outlined in table 6.2 may gradually be progressed to an exercise prescription more consistent with that presented in the table. Progression should be individualized and based on a normal response to exercise along with the absence of abnormal signs or symptoms during and following exercise sessions.

One way to establish an initial exercise intensity is to begin with 2 to 3 METs and observe HR, BP, and other physiological responses, including fatigue, at this workload. The RPE scale (Borg 6-20) is helpful for determining how the patient tolerates the exercise load, with a suggested range of 11 to 13. Another starting point often used is resting HR + 20 to 30 beats/min. However, such levels (METs, HR, or RPE) should be used with caution; interindividual variation likely exists within each of the approaches.[9] Progression of the components in table 6.2 should be based on the patient's signs and symptoms, monitored response, and RPE. If the patient remains asymptomatic, exercise staff under the direction of the program director or referring clinician may gradually increase exercise intensity. Over time, stable patients typically progress to exercise plans such as those presented in table 6.1. Comparisons of training outcomes between patients with and without a program entry exercise test have reported similar physiological improvements.[16]

PA Outside of CR

As noted earlier, many patients involved in CR do not achieve desired energy expenditure levels, especially when they attend only two or three

Table 6.2 Components of Initial Cardiorespiratory Endurance Exercise Prescription for Patients Without a Recent Symptom-Limited Exercise Tolerance Test

Component	Initial recommendation
Warm-up	Stretching and low-level calisthenics followed by 5-10 min of very low-level cardiorespiratory exercise types
Cardiorespiratory fitness	Intensity (guides) • HR + 20-30 bpm over resting HR • 2 METs • RPE 11 to 14 Duration: 20-30 min, possibly in 2-3 bouts Frequency: 3 days/week Type: Simplest modes such as a treadmill, leg or arm ergometer, or a recumbent device
Cool-down	5-10 min

Abbreviations: METs, metabolic equivalents; RPE, rating of perceived exertion; HR, heart rate.

Data from ACSM (2018).

sessions a week, typically expending <300 kcal per session.[11-14] Additionally, most patients with CVD perform even less PA on days they do not participate in CR.[17-20] Moreover, it is important to recognize that most patients who enroll in CR have previously been insufficiently active. Thus, they face the challenge of changing another aspect of their lifestyle (along with possibly quitting smoking, changing their dietary habits to support weight loss, or making changes to their medication regimen for control of risk factors such as lipids, glucose, or BP) in addition to becoming regularly physically active. Although patients should be routinely instructed to achieve more than 30 min of moderate-intensity PA on days they do not attend CR, many patients may need more support or alternative approaches in order to be more active. Having patients track and record their PA outside of CR is helpful in increasing PA.[21] PA assessment instruments are described in chapter 9 in the Physical Inactivity section. Principles of behavior modification that apply to changing behavior, including physical activity, are covered in chapter 8.

Resistance Training

For appropriately screened patients with CVD, resistance training should be incorporated into the exercise program when time permits following cardiorespiratory training. Because many forms of resistance training exist and many CVD patients may not be familiar with resistance exercise, instruction on technique is often necessary. The perception that resistance exercise is harmful to CVD patients, or at the least is not beneficial, is not supported by the scientific literature.[22] Lower myocardial demand, attenuation of ischemic responses, and higher subendocardial perfusion have all been observed in studies of resistance exercise training compared to that with dynamic exercise in patients with CVD. In addition, although the caloric expenditure during resistance exercise is less than with endurance exercise, increased muscle mass has been associated with an increased basal metabolic rate and may therefore be an important training adaptation contributing to attainment and maintenance of healthy body weight. Finally, improving and maintaining strength and endurance may

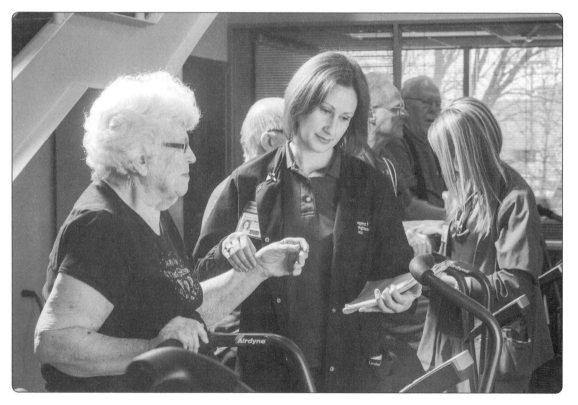

Cardiorespiratory endurance training should be the foundation of most exercise programs for adults with or at risk for CVD.

hasten return to vocational and recreational activities and may prolong functional independence for older patients.

Although ample evidence supports the safety and efficacy of resistance exercise, careful selection of patients is prudent. Patient criteria for clearance for safe participation are identified in guideline 6.2. Patient clearance should be a staff decision with approval of the medical director, surgeon, or other primary provider as appropriate. See chapter 10 for information on sternotomy precautions. Once a patient has been cleared for participation, a measure of baseline muscular strength will help establish a safe initial routine and monitor adaptations over time. Patients should be monitored for HR, RPE, ECG, and responses throughout the baseline evaluation, and proper breathing techniques (e.g., no breath holding or straining) should be emphasized. BP can be measured before the repetitions begin and then again immediately after completion of the final repetition. Methods for baseline assessment of muscular strength include the following:

- One-repetition maximum (1RM)—Determines the maximal amount of weight that a patient can lift once, but not twice, while maintaining correct technique without straining.
- Multiple RM (6RM to 15RM)—Determines the maximal amount of weight that a patient

can lift 6 to 15 times, maintaining correct technique and without straining.

- Experienced CR staff can also use a trial-and-error technique when performing the baseline assessment. It typically involves a verbal assessment of a patient's general strength, followed by the loading of resistance and allowing the patient to try and perform the resistance movement. Depending on the observed response, loading is either increased or decreased as appropriate.

While the 1RM assessment is commonly used in healthy people, the multiple RM assessment is less stressful and can provide a reasonable baseline level of musculoskeletal fitness for most patients with CVD. The elements of a safe and effective resistance training routine are identified in table 6.3. As with cardiorespiratory endurance training, the prescriptive elements within the table must be individualized to the needs and goals of the patient.

Flexibility Training

Optimal musculoskeletal function requires that a patient maintain an adequate range of motion (ROM) in all joints. It is particularly important to maintain flexibility in the lower back and posterior thigh regions. Lack of flexibility in these

Guideline 6.2   Patient Selection Criteria for Participation in a Resistance Training Program

A resistance training program is defined here as one in which patients lift weights >50% of their 1RM. Elastic bands, 1 to 3 lb (0.45-1.3 kg) hand weights, and light free weights may be used in a progressive fashion starting at outpatient program entry provided that no other contraindications exist.[19,22] When determining whether a patient is eligible to begin resistance training, CR staff should consider the following:

- Minimum of 6 to 10 weeks after date of MI or cardiac surgery, including 4 weeks of consistent participation in a supervised CR endurance training program
- Minimum of 3 weeks following transcatheter procedures (PCI, other), including 2 weeks of con-

sistent participation in a supervised CR endurance training program

No evidence of the following conditions:

- Acute congestive heart failure
- Uncontrolled dysrhythmias
- Severe valvular disease
- Uncontrolled hypertension; patients with moderate hypertension (SBP >160 or DBP >100 mm Hg) should be referred for appropriate management, although these values are not absolute contraindications for participation in a resistance training program.
- Unstable symptoms

Table 6.3 Components of an Exercise Prescription for Muscular Strength and Endurance for Cardiac Patients Cleared for Participation

Component	Recommendation
Intensity	• Use resistance that allows ~10-15 repetitions without significant fatigue (RPE of 11-13 on Borg 6-20 scale). • Complete movement through as full a ROM as possible, avoiding breath holding and straining (Valsalva maneuver) by exhaling during the exertion phase of the motion and inhaling during the recovery phase. • Maintain a secure but not overly tight grip on the weight handles or bar to prevent an excessive BP response. • RPP should not exceed that identified as threshold for CRF exercise.
Volume	• Perform a minimum of one and maximum of three sets per exercise, avoiding significant fatigue. • May increase to two or three sets once accustomed to the regimen and, if greater gains are desired, ~8-10 different exercises using all major muscle groups of the upper and lower body: e.g., chest press, shoulder press, triceps extension, biceps curl, lat pull-down, lower back extension, abdominal crunch or curl-up, quadriceps extension, leg curl (hamstrings), and calf raise
Frequency	2 or 3 nonconsecutive days/week
Type	• Variable: Use free weights, weight machines, resistance bands, pulley weights, dumbbells, light wrist or ankle weights. • Select equipment that is safe, comfortable, effective, and accessible.
Progression	Training loads may be increased ~5% when the patient can comfortably achieve the upper limit of the prescribed repetition range.

Abbreviations: RPE, rating of perceived exertion; BP, blood pressure; RPP, heart rate × systolic rate–pressure product; CRF, cardiorespiratory fitness; ROM, range of motion.

Based on data from ACSM (2018); Williams et al. (2007).

Table 6.4 Components of an Exercise Prescription for Musculoskeletal Flexibility

Component	Recommendation
Intensity	Hold to a position of tightness or slight/mild discomfort (not pain). Exercises should be performed in a slow, controlled manner, with a gradual progression to greater ROM.
Duration	Gradually increase to 15-30 s, then as tolerable to 90 s for each stretch, breathing normally. Do 3-5 repetitions for each exercise.
Frequency	≥2-3 days/week; ideally daily
Type	Static, with a major emphasis on the lower back and thigh regions

Data from ACSM (2018); Williams et al. (2007).

areas may be associated with an increased risk for the development of chronic lower back pain. Therefore, preventive and rehabilitative exercise programs should include activities that promote the maintenance of flexibility.[23] Lack of flexibility is prevalent in the elderly and contributes to a reduced ability to perform ADLs. Accordingly, exercise programs for the elderly should emphasize proper stretching, especially for the upper and lower trunk, neck, and hip regions. The elements of a musculoskeletal flexibility training routine are identified in table 6.4. As with CRF endurance exercise and musculoskeletal resistance training, the prescriptive elements within the table should be individualized to the needs and goals of the patient.

Summary

The physical activity and exercise recommendations in this chapter are meant to provide a general base from which to develop personalized exercise prescriptions for the variety of patients enrolled in CR programs. For more definitive exercise prescription recommendations, refer to chapters 9, 10, and 11 containing specific information about these patients.

Nutrition Guidelines

Ellen Schaaf Aberegg, MA, LD, RD, FAACVPR

There is clear evidence demonstrating that a Western (i.e., standard American) diet is inextricably linked to the development and progression of CVD. A large amount of dietary related information is available, but much of the information can be confusing, especially to the general public. The information provided in this chapter derives primarily from the 2015 USDA Dietary Guidelines for Americans (DGA)[1]; AHA/ACC 2013 Guidelines for Lifestyle,[2] Lipids,[3] Obesity,[4] or Heart Failure[5]; National Lipid Association Recommendations for Patient-Centered Management of Dyslipidemia[6]; and the 2017 ACC/AHA/AAPA/ABC/ACPM/AGS/-APhA/ASH/ASPC/NMA/PCNA Guideline for the Prevention, Detection, Evaluation, and Management of High Blood Pressure in Adults.[7] Further, the 2016 Recommended Dietary Pattern to Achieve Adherence to the AHA/ACC Guidelines reflect updates to the 2013 guidelines based on the DGA.[8]

OBJECTIVES

This chapter provides an overview of the following:

- CVD-related nutritional information regarding micro- and macronutrients, specific food categories, and dietary patterns
- Nutrition recommendations for the prevention and treatment of CVD
- How to incorporate dietary recommendations into standards of care and education of the CR participant
- Prioritizing the multitude of recommendations into achievable goals and behavioral objectives on the individual treatment plan (ITP)

Key Nutrition Principles

Understanding diet is not solely possessing knowledge of nutrients. Diet choices that lower CVD risk are complex. Figure 7.1 illustrates that food choices are not solely based on what is considered healthy but also by numerous internal and external influences. For example, internal influences such as taste preference may overwhelm a patient's decision to eat healthfully. Taste and preference have genetic and environmental origins. Food is consumed for sustenance, emotional comfort, entertainment, as a coping strategy, and as a means to mediate social dynamics. Further, external influences such as environment and historical context affect food choices; how cultures season food, celebrate life events, and frame a food's meaning or religious significance strongly influence diet choices. Firmly held belief systems, such as those formed by parental influences on food type, timing, and volume as reward or punishment, can last a lifetime. Moreover, the inadequate availability of healthier foods in poorer U.S. neighborhoods limits food choices, and patients of lower socioeconomic status have less healthful eating behaviors.[9] Understanding these concepts allows the CR professional to recognize potential obstacles to change and aid in recommendations that are most helpful in lowering a patient's CVD risk.

Macronutrients

The primary macronutrients are carbohydrate (CHO), fat, and protein. Macronutrients are chemical compounds that provide energy. While water does make up a large proportion of a diet, it does not provide any nutritional value. Alcohol is a calorically dense compound that can provide large amounts of calories although it is not a necessary dietary component.

Carbohydrate

The four types of CHO are (1) mono-, (2) di-, (3) oglio-, and (4) polysaccharides. Carbohydrates provide approximately 4 kcal/g. Recommendations suggest 45% to 65% of total energy should come from CHO consumption.[1] Mono- and disaccharides are simple CHOs that are quickly absorbed in the gastrointestinal tract and may increase BP, cause weight gain, raise low-density lipoprotein (LDL) and triglyceride (TG) levels, and decrease high-density lipoprotein (HDL) levels. Consumption of excess sugar (e.g., sucrose, a disaccharide) may increase insulin resistance, promote fat accumulation in the liver,[10] decrease HDL levels, profoundly increase TG levels, and

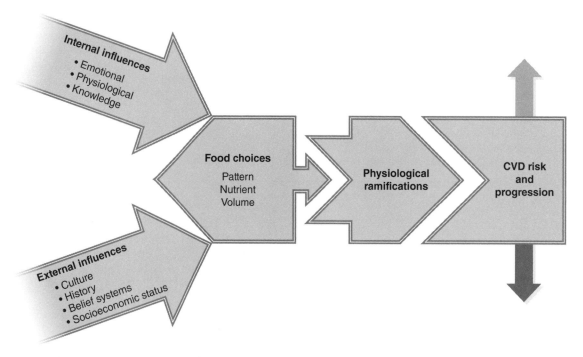

Figure 7.1 CVD prevention: nutrients, food, and dietary patterns.

worsen type 2 diabetes mellitus (T2DM) control.[11] Conversely, these negative associations are not seen with the consumption of naturally occurring mono- or disaccharides found in fruit, whole grains, or milk.[12]

The term *complex CHOs* refers to oglio- and polysaccharides, which are found in foods such as peas, beans, and white and whole grains. Complex CHOs provide vitamins, minerals, and fiber that are important to good health. The majority of a person's diet should consist of complex CHOs and naturally occurring rather than processed or refined sugars. Consuming complex CHOs improves glucose/insulin homeostasis and endothelial function, and it reduces inflammation.[13]

Dietary fiber is indigestible CHO and provides minimal caloric content. Fiber is a beneficial component of fruits and vegetables, legumes, whole grains, nuts/seeds, and soluble fiber supplements. Many studies have found that the highest intakes of fiber were associated with reduced risk of CVD and cardiac morbidity and mortality.[14,15] The two primary forms of fiber are soluble and insoluble. Insoluble fiber adds nondigestible plant components to the diet accompanied by many micronutrients. Soluble fiber (glycan, psyllium gums, and pectin) lowers LDL[16] by forming a gel when combined with water. This gel binds to and can increase elimination of bile acids, thus stimulating hepatic conversion of CHO to create bile acids, increasing hepatic uptake of LDL and reducing serum LDL.[17] Consumption of whole-grain sources of fiber lowers LDL without lowering HDL.[18]

The term *glycemic index* refers to the serum glucose raising capability of a food compared to pure glucose. Although a helpful descriptor, a specific glycemic index score loses significance when foods of varying macronutrient content are consumed at a single meal. Yet diets composed primarily of low, rather that high glycemic index foods have been associated with lower risk of CVD and T2DM.[19]

Fat

Dietary fats are either saturated (with hydrogen) or unsaturated (mono- or polyunsaturated). All dietary fats provide 9 kcal/g. The type, rather than the quantity, of fats consumed is particularly relevant for CVD risk reduction.[20, 21] The total fat content of a healthful diet can range from 20% to 35%.

Saturated fatty acids (SFAs) negatively increase blood coagulation, inflammation, adiposity, and insulin resistance.[20,21,22] SFAs are found in meat from animals, dairy products, and tropical oils (e.g., palm, coconut). The favorable relationship between reduced consumption of SFAs and lowered risk and incidence of CVD is clear.[6,8,23] A concern is what nutrients or food items replace the SFA (i.e., polyunsaturated fatty acid [PUFA] and monounsaturated fatty acid [MUFA], or simple or complex whole-grain CHO). Replacement of SFA with PUFA, and to a lesser extent MUFA, has the most beneficial effect on lipid profile and lower CVD event rates.[23] Conversely, the replacement of SFA with simple or unrefined CHO raises LDL levels.[2,23]

Most PUFAs and MUFAs come from plant sources, although some MUFAs are found in animal products. Some PUFAs are not synthesized by humans and thus are considered essential; they include alpha-linolenic acid (an omega-3 fatty acid) and linoleic acid (an omega-6 fatty acid). Supplemented omega-3 fatty acids are associated with an approximately 10% decrease in CVD mortality.[24] MUFA intake has a favorable effect on the lipid profile.[23] Although the current evidence for the cardiometabolic benefits of total MUFA consumption is not as strong as that of PUFA consumption,[1] the other nutrients in MUFA-rich foods may alter these health effects.[25]

Trans fats result during the manufacturing of partially hydrogenated oil from liquid oils. Trans fats retain the deleterious characteristics of SFAs and, furthermore, lower HDL cholesterol. Trans fats have the strongest adverse relationship with CVD risk factors and are unhealthful to consume. By U.S. federal mandate, food manufacturers are not permitted to use trans fats.

Protein

Proteins are polymers composed of varying combinations of 20 different amino acids. Dietary proteins/amino acids are used to replace muscle mass lost in cell turnover and catabolism. Proteins provide 4 kcal/g. Recommended protein intake is 10% to 35% of total calorie intake.[26] The Recommended Dietary Allowance (RDA) for protein is 0.8g/kg body weight per day.[27] In older or malnourished adults, modestly higher intakes of high-quality protein (1.0-1.5 g/kg per day) evenly distributed throughout the day, may maximally stimulate muscle protein synthesis. Increased protein consumption has little effect on cardio-metabolic risk factors[28,29] but may be beneficial in weight reduction, maximizing protein synthesis, minimizing sarcopenia, and maintaining muscle mass in older adults.[30,31]

Alcohol

Ethyl is the predominant form of alcohol found in beverages. Alcohol provides 7 kcal/g. Consumption of 1 or 2 drink equivalents (1 drink = 4-5 oz wine, 12 oz beer, or 1.5 oz 80-proof spirits) has been associated with an approximately 35% lower relative risk for CVD mortality, fatal and non-fatal MI,[32] and increases in HDL and TG.[33] The "drier" the wine or beverage is (i.e., lower sugar content), the less likely it is to raise TG. Red wine has a cardioprotective effect by providing polyphenols (resveratrol) and by reducing LDL, raising HDL, and inhibiting clotting mechanisms. Conversely, the negative consequences of long-term alcohol consumption in excess of 30 g/day include hypertension, cardiomyopathy, arrhythmias, and stroke.[34] Furthermore, alcohol supplies calories but few nutrients (i.e., high in calories and low in nutrient density). Consumption of alcoholic beverages may contribute to weight gain or impede efforts to lose weight.

Micronutrients: Vitamins and Minerals

Micronutrients are dietary components that are essential and required by organisms in small quantities. Micronutrients are referred to as vitamins and minerals. They sustain metabolism, maintain tissue function, and decrease inflammation.

Foods high in vitamins and mineral content have a beneficial effect on lipid profiles, T2DM, CVD incidence, and mortality. Vitamins function as coenzymes, antioxidants, and hormone-like regulators. Nutritive minerals are required in trace quantities to fulfill structural and functional roles. Phytochemicals include carotenoids (plant precursors of vitamin A) and polyphenols (phenolic acids, flavonoids, and stilbenes/ligans) and are active in the homeostatic response to inflammation. Serum levels of micronutrients generally reflect diet intake but may be confounded by age, sex, smoking, alcohol intake, and race.[34]

The micronutrients found in food are accompanied by other beneficial nutrients. Antioxidants naturally found in foods such as fruit, vegetables, and legumes may produce synergistic interactions and have more positive physiological effects on CVD than when consumed alone.[35] Supplementation of vitamins and minerals does not have any specific benefit on CVD outcomes unless the individual is otherwise deficient.

The mineral sodium is ubiquitous in the modern Western diet. Sodium is 40% of the salt (sodium chloride) molecule. One teaspoon of salt contains 2,300 mg sodium. Salt is a preservative and enhances the flavor of food. Commercially prepared meals, convenience foods, snacks, and bakery items account for the majority of sodium consumption, while additional quantities are ingested from salt added at meals. Fresh, non-processed fruit, vegetables, lean meat, dairy, and whole grains have minimal sodium. Average sodium intake in the United States is estimated to be at least 3,400 mg/day.[14] The consumption of fewer high-sodium foods and more foods high in potassium and calcium results in lower BP in hypertensive and normo-tensive individuals.[36,37] The DGA recommend limiting sodium to 2,300 mg/day.[1] Label reading skills aid in reduction of quantity of sodium consumed.[38] Fortunately, once a person adheres to a low sodium consumption habit, taste preferences adapt, ultimately providing a negative feedback mechanism to reinforce dietary change.

Polyphenols are plant metabolites that contribute to color, flavor, odor, and oxidative stability.[39] Polyphenols are potent inhibitors of LDL oxidation and antiplatelet and anti-inflammatory effects. Polyphenols increase HDL, improve endothelial function, and may contribute to stabilization of the atheroma plaque.[40] Flavonoids are the most abundant polyphenols in people's diets.

Phytosterols (plant sterols and stanols) are chemically related and structurally similar to cholesterol. Consumption of phytosterols is associated with decreased levels of total cholesterol (TC) and LDL.[41] Sterols have been added to foods such as milk, margarine, orange juice, olive oil, cheese, snacks, and breads,[42] which are examples of functional foods (in which the health benefit is derived from the addition of a specific nutrient). Plant sterols/stanols interfere with fat-soluble vitamin absorption. Therefore, if phytosterols are consumed in increasing quantities, eating foods rich in fat-soluble vitamins (vitamins A, D, E, and K) is recommended.[43]

Role of Specific Categories of Food

A key component to a heart-healthy diet is to consume nutritious foods from various categories of food. Food categories consist of different foods that contain similar nutrients. To meet nutritional requirements, it is necessary to eat a variety of foods from within the various categories, or food groups.

Vegetables and Fruits

Diet patterns that are plentiful in vegetables and fruits show substantial improvement in lipid profiles, inflammatory biomarkers, and endothelial function. Brightly colored vegetables and fruits are more likely to have a higher antioxidant content. All guidelines cite evidence demonstrating the benefits of vegetables and fruit.[44] A 12% to 15% CVD risk reduction is observed in otherwise healthy individuals with increasing intake of vegetables (up to about 5 servings/day) and fruits (up to about 2.5 servings/day).[45] The benefits of vegetables and fruit stem from their content of micronutrients, fiber, phytochemicals, antioxidants, polyphenols,[48,46] enhanced nutrient bioavailability,[47] and their potential replacement of less healthful diet components.[45]

Nuts

Most nuts have moderate protein content.[40] The PUFA and MUFA, amino acid, fiber, and micronutrient content of nuts are the beneficial components in the reduction of CVD risk.[48] Nut consumption reduces TC, LDL, and apolipoprotein. Numerous studies have shown that nuts are not associated with higher body weight or weight gain despite relatively higher caloric content. The risk of CVD decreased by approximately 21% with increasing intake of up to 7 to 10 nuts/day.[46]

Whole Grains

Whole grains consist of bran, germ, and endosperm components. Although original versions of the Dietary Approaches to Stop Hypertension (DASH) and Mediterranean (MEDIT) diets did not designate whole-grain versions of the starches/bread group, the *whole grain* designation is included in all current dietary guidelines. Consumption of whole grains is associated with improvements in glucose homeostasis, lipid profile, and endothelial function.[12] The risk of CVD is decreased by 17% with increasing intake of whole grains up to about 6 servings/day.[46]

Fish

Fish contains high quality protein and poly- and monounsaturated fats. Fatty fish such as anchovies, sardines, trout, white tuna, and salmon contain the highest amounts of omega-3 fatty acids. The AHA recommends 1 or 2 servings of omega-3 containing seafood per week.[49] Fish intake is associated with lower TG, reduced inflammation, improved endothelial function, and reduced platelet aggregation.[50] In the general population, increasing fish intake decreased the risk of CVD by approximately 15%.[46]

Meats: Red, White, and Processed

The effects of red meat consumption on CVD are inconsistent.[51] Although red meat consumption is associated with a higher CVD and mortality risk,[46,52] in many studies neither the SFA content nor the fresh/preserved/processed status was standardized.[52] Respectively, unprocessed and processed meats have been associated with a 19% and 40% higher risk of CVD.[53] The higher CVD risk associated with processed meats (e.g., ground meats, smoked or deli meats, bacon, sausage) is facilitated by the higher sodium and SFA content and the presence of preservatives, nitrites, and other processing agents.[54,55] Differences between red (beef, some pork, lamb) and white (chicken, some pork) meat is difficult to ascertain and may be due to SFA, cholesterol content, or heme iron.[56] Replacing red meat with fish, poultry, nuts, legumes, low-fat dairy products, and whole grains lowers CVD risk.[57]

Eggs

Cholesterol is an organic molecule found in cell membranes and serves as a precursor to biosynthesis of some hormones and vitamin D. Eighty-five percent of blood cholesterol is created endogenously, and 15% comes from food intake. Previously, recommendations restricted egg consumption to fewer than twice a week due to eggs' high cholesterol and moderate fat content. However, little evidence exists that dietary cholesterol consumption is associated with CVD. Eggs contain high-quality protein, antioxidants, and choline (an essential nutrient important in neurotransmitters and cell membranes). Removal of specific dietary cholesterol limitations allows for less restrictive egg consumption recommendations.

Dairy Foods

Dairy foods contain calcium and other minerals, high-quality protein, linoleic acid, vitamins, SFA, MUFA, and PUFA. Milk, cheese, and yogurt consumption has been inversely associated with CVD risk.[19] Studies have shown that the potential harm from eating high-fat dairy products is mitigated by the addition of calcium.[58] Further research is needed to elucidate the role of nonfat rather than full-fat dairy products and to scrutinize the unique type of SFA found in dairy foods that may be less harmful.

Diet Patterns of Nutrition Intake

Current dietary guidelines focus on food patterns as opposed to individual foods or nutrients, with qualifiers regarding specific nutrient content. Focusing on patterns facilitates flexibility and individuality in behavioral counseling.[1,59] Making recommendations based more on dietary patterns and less on specific nutrients is likely to encourage greater dietary variety, compliance, and nutrient density. In addition, a focus on dietary patterns reduces consumer confusion and demonization of certain foods.[60]

Dietary patterns should be adapted to meet individual energy requirements and relevant nutrition therapy goals. The three most studied and referenced healthful diet patterns are the Dietary Approaches to Stop Hypertension

(DASH) plan,[61] Mediterranean (MEDIT) diet,[62] and 2015-2020 DGA.[1] Vegetarian plans that include a range of patterns (vegan, lacto-ovo, plant-based, etc.) that eliminate some or all animal products are associated with lower CVD risk and incidence.[63] In general, the diet patterns that emphasize fruits, vegetables, legumes, and whole grains demonstrated lowest risk of CVD and morbidity/mortality, and lowest inflammation indices.[64] The food plans differ on meat, dairy, and alcohol recommendations, and the relative emphasis on olive oil. Table 7.1 highlights the similarities between the food plan recommendations.

Dietary Approaches to Stop Hypertension Plan

The Dietary Approaches to Stop Hypertension (DASH) plan encourages intake of fruit, vegetables, whole grains, poultry, low-fat dairy products, nuts, and fish. It inherently has low levels of sodium by relying on fresh, minimally processed foods. The recommendations of the DASH plan[2,65,67,69] take into consideration the rich content of other beneficial nutrients such as potassium, calcium, magnesium, protein, and fiber. The plan is beneficial in lowering BP in individuals with hypertension (HTN). The DASH plan also demonstrates significant reductions in CVD risk[65] and mortality,[1] and improvements in blood lipids.[66] Adherence to the DASH plan is inversely associated with T2DM incidence.[67]

 Guideline 7.1   Dietary Recommendations for CVD Risk Reduction

The overarching goal of dietary guidance is to reduce the risk and incidence of CVD while encouraging a dietary pattern that accommodates personal, cultural, ethnic, and economic factors.[8] Any favorable dietary pattern includes the following:

- Vegetables and fruits
- Whole grains
- Low-fat dairy products
- High quality protein sources (from plants or animals, with saturated or trans fats removed and limited processing)
- Nuts and legumes
- Monounsaturated and polyunsaturated fats
- Limited saturated fat, sodium, red meat, sweets, and sugar-sweetened beverages
- Elimination of trans fats and tropical oils
- Avoiding high-calorie, low-nutrient-dense foods

Table 7.1 Similarities Between Food Plan Recommendations

Food	2015 DGA[1] (amounts determined by calorie needs)	2016 AHA/ACC pattern recommendations[8]	DASH plan	MEDIT diet	Vegetarian diet
Grains	Whole grain	Whole grain	Whole grain	Whole grain	Whole grain
High quality protein	Variety plus eggs, legumes, nuts, and soy Limit red meat	Variety plus eggs, legumes, nuts, and soy Limit red and processed meats.	Poultry, fish Reduce red meat to <0.5 servings/day	Fatty fish emphasis Includes limited meat	Variety of legumes, nuts, soy, +/– eggs and whey products
Vegetables	Variety of colorful vegetables Include legumes	4-5 servings/day	4-5 servings/day	High intake	High intake
Fruit	4-5 servings/day	4-5 servings/day	4-5 servings/day	High intake	High intake
Dairy products	Variety; not whole fat	Variety, not whole fat	2-3 servings low fat	1-2 servings Fat content often not specified	+/– inclusion
Fats and oils	<10% calories from SF replaced with PUFA or MUFA	Vegetable nontropical oils <7% calories from SF (<6% if CVD) replaced with PUFA or MUFA	2-3 servings PUFA or MUFA	Olive oil (with added polyphenols[66]) emphasis plus other PUFA and MUFA	Vegetable, nontropical recommended
Sodium	<2,300 mg and <1,500 mg High risk: at least 1,000 mg less	<2,300 mg and <1,500 mg High risk: at least 1,000 mg less	<2,300 mg and <1,500 mg High risk: at least 1,000 mg less	Fresh emphasis, not commercially prepared	Not specified
Nuts, seeds, dry beans, and peas	Included with protein foods	Same as DGA	4-5 servings weekly	Walnuts, almonds, hazelnuts, and other nuts encouraged daily[66]	Encouraged
Sweets	<10% calories from added sugars	Women: up to 100 kcal (6 tsp)/day Men: up to 150 kcal (9 tsp)/day Children: up to 100 kcal (6 tsp)/day	<5 weekly Replace sugar with protein or unsaturated fat	Not specified	Not specified
Alcohol	Moderation: 1 drink for female, 2 for male	Moderation: 1 drink for female, 2 for male	Not specified	Red wine, low to moderate intake	Not specified

Mediterranean Diet

The MEDIT diet includes fruit, vegetables, grains, fatty fish, wine, and relatively high amounts of olive oil. Research has demonstrated that the lowest CVD mortality rates occur in countries that consume the MEDIT diet.[11,68,69,70,71] The MEDIT diet, although emphasizing similar foods as the DASH plan, is generally described as relatively higher in total fat (32%-35% of total calories) and in MUFA (due to emphasis on olive oil), it includes alcohol in modest amounts, and it may include high-fat dairy; whereas the DASH plan emphasizes the inclusion of low-fat dairy. Recent iterations of the MEDIT diet emphasize less meat and dairy and more whole grains.

2015-2020 Dietary Guidelines for Americans

Previous editions of the Dietary Guidelines for Americans (DGA) focused primarily on individual dietary components. The newer version emphasizes inclusion of a variety of vegetables and fruits, whole grains, low-fat dairy, lean meats, moderation in caffeine intake, and minimal added sugars and sugar-sweetened beverages,[11] SFA and trans fats, and sodium (<2,300 mg/day).[1,72] Further, there is more of an emphasis on the type and quality of fat versus on a low-fat diet, per se.

Vegetarian and Vegan Diets

Vegetarianism (avoidance of flesh foods but possible inclusion of dairy products and/or eggs) has beneficial effects on LDL-C, BP, and body weight and is associated with reduced risk of CVD.[11,73,74,75,76,77] If vegetarian versions of the DASH or MEDIT diet are advocated, then the intake of adequate high-quality protein and vitamin B_{12} needs to be assured. Dietary patterns that are plant based, but not exclusively vegetarian (plant-centric, flexitarian), may be less intimidating yet still contain larger quantities of vegetables, fruits, and whole grains.

BOTTOM LINE

While there is much controversy surrounding the optimal diet for cardiovascular health, the emphasis of dietary counseling should be on the inclusion of healthful dietary choices rather than restricting or limiting specific foods. Thus, the focus of nutritional counseling for participants in CR should be on dietary patterns rather than specific components of the diet.

Evidence-Based Nutrition Guidelines for CVD Risk Factors

The development and progression of a number of CVD risk factors are directly linked to nutritional factors. The following section describes the nutritional recommendations to address specific CVD risk factors.

Hypertension

The 2017 ACC/AHA Guidelines for Hypertension[7] state that of the six nongenetic causes of HTN, four are related to nutrition: weight management, sodium, potassium, and alcohol. Similarly, five of the six most effective nonpharmacologic therapies address these four nutrition concerns in addition to DASH diet recommendations.[7] The nonpharmacological interventions plus exercise may be sufficient to meet BP reduction goals in patients with mild to moderate (stage 1) HTN, and are an integral part of the management of persons with more severe (stage 2) HTN.

The BP-lowering effect of weight loss in overweight patients with HTN has an apparent dose–response relationship of about 1 mm Hg per kg of weight loss.[7] A weight loss of 4.5 kg reduces BP or prevents HTN in a large proportion of overweight people.[78]

Reduced sodium intake lowers BP in HTN, normotensive, and medication-treated individuals.[79] The higher the initial BP, the greater benefit. There is a clear dose–response relationship between sodium intake and BP, with progressively lower levels of sodium intake associated with lower levels of BP.[80] The threshold of benefit and how much reduction that should be recommended, however, has been debated.[81,82] Major health benefits are associated with reductions in sodium from the current 3,000-4,000 mg sodium/day[82] down to 1,500-2,300 mg/day[1,7,8,83,84] and with the less specific recommendation of decreasing sodium intake by 1,000 mg/day.[27] The focus on a 1,000 mg reduction may allow the CR professional the flexibility to individualize recommendations based on patient assessment and personal preferences.

The sodium/potassium ratio appears to be more strongly associated with BP outcomes than either sodium or potassium alone.[85] Insufficient dietary intakes of potassium, calcium, and magnesium have been implicated in HTN. Intakes of 3,500 to 4,700 mg potassium/day is suggested,[86] although the DRI is 2,600-3,400 mg/day[87] (4-5 servings of fruits and vegetables will usually provide 1,500-3,000 mg of potassium).

The AHA/ACC Lifestyle[2] and Hypertension[7] Guidelines recommend a diet plan that emphasizes vegetables, fruits, whole grains, low-fat dairy products, poultry, fish, legumes, nontropical vegetable oils, and nuts. Limits on sweets, sugar-sweetened beverages, and red meat are recommended. The American Heart Association/American College of Cardiology (AHA/ACC) Guidelines[8] endorses the DASH plan, which encourages fresh versus processed foods and emphasizes a variety of fruit, vegetables, and whole grains to increase dietary intake of beneficial nutrients such as potassium, calcium, magnesium, protein, and fiber. A small positive association between the MEDIT diet and BP exists,[88] yet the sodium decrease may be what exerts the mediating effect.[7,89]

The benefit or harm of alcohol ingestion is related to the quantity consumed. An immediate effect of alcohol ingestion is vasodilation. It is likely that the hypotensive effect of alcohol is mediated by neural, hormonal, or other reversible physiologic changes. Alcohol intakes of ≤2 drinks a day for men and 1 drink per day for women may reduce BP by 2 to 4 mm Hg.[7,90] However, sustained high blood alcohol levels result in elevation of BP.[91,92] The World Health Organization (WHO) attributes 16% of all HTN disease to excess alcohol intake.[93] Therefore, recommendations to moderate the quantity of alcohol should be prioritized.

Caffeine intake is often scrutinized in patients with HTN. Single doses of caffeine up to 200 mg (2-4 8 oz cups of coffee) are unlikely to induce clinically relevant increases in BP.[94] The caffeine related pressor effect is due to the elevation of peripheral vascular resistance rather than enhancement of cardiac output. Progressively larger BP responses to caffeine are observed in persons with increasing risk of HTN.[81] The DGA recommend no more than 400 mg/day.[1] Individual variability in physiological response to a caffeine dose also confounds guidelines for "safe" levels; they should be individually determined.

Diabetes Mellitus

Lifestyle interventions including nutrition therapy, exercise, weight loss, and glucose lowering medications are the foundation of T2DM prevention, treatment, and management. Patient education and self-care practices are essential.[95] A dietitian should initiate medical nutrition therapy (MNT) as early as possible.[96] Lifestyle interventions need to be sustained throughout the patient's life. The CR professional is instrumental in supporting these lifestyle changes. Healthful choices and portion control are most important in food selection.[97]

Patients who participated in intensive MNT showed greater improvements in BP control, glycated hemoglobin (HbA1c), weight loss, fitness, and lipid profile than those in normal care. Education in T2DM self-management skills yields improvement in glycemic control and improved quality of food intake[98] and weight control. The CR professional can support the MNT/self-care effort by assisting the patient in CHO monitoring; CHO record keeping; and emphasizing the need for weight loss, exercise, and medication compliance.[99]

The goal of glycemic control is to maintain optimal blood glucose levels. Macronutrient proportions of each meal should be individualized and balanced to meet metabolic goals and individual preferences.[98] High intakes of refined grains, sugar-sweetened soft drinks, and processed meat were all significantly associated with T2DM risk.[98] The MEDIT diet and DASH plan each have a strong potential for preventing T2DM.[100]

Monitoring CHO intake remains a key strategy in achieving glycemic control.[101] Monitoring practices include specifically counting CHO consumed, following a defined diet plan, or experience-based estimation. There is no absolute recommended mix of CHO, protein, and fat that applies to the diet for the treatment and prevention of T2DM.[102] Lower ranges of CHO intake are associated with tighter glycemic control, lower TG, and higher HDL levels. However, higher CHO vegan plans are associated with lower LDL levels.[103] Glycemic control at individual meals depends on the absolute amount and type of CHO consumed and other meal components. The consumption of other foods (protein or fat) temper rates of glucose absorption and may confound the specific prescription of CHO proportions. If the patient is on insulin, consideration of the amount of CHO in the meal should match the dose of insulin accordingly. Foods containing a high percentage of soluble fiber decrease glycemia.[104] Protein has no effect on blood glucose levels and should not be used to treat hypoglycemia. Protein increases insulin response and is an important component of every meal.

Heart Failure

In heart failure (HF), the heart compensates for the loss of cardiac output by increasing the force and rate of contraction by stimulating the angiotensin system, and by retaining sodium and fluid.[105] Excess sodium intake influences blood volume expansion, and extra- and intracellular fluid shifts. Despite being the most widely recommended self-care measure for patients with HF, evidence remains scarce and mostly observational for dietary sodium restriction.[106] The level of sodium intake that achieves optimal outcomes for patients with HF is unknown; and although the evidence suggests that high-sodium intake worsens outcomes, evidence also shows that sodium restriction is associated with increased risk of untoward events.[107] Because of unintentional negative nutritional consequences that may occur with significant sodium restriction and the risk of malnutrition in an ill HF patient, the quality of the whole diet—not just restrictions—should be considered.[108] The <2,300 mg sodium DASH diet[109,110] or low-sodium MEDIT diet[111] have been shown to have beneficial outcomes in HF. The AHA/ACC 2013 Guidelines for HF recommend that early stages (A and B) of HF warrant sodium restriction (1,300–3,000 mg sodium per day in conjunction with fluid restriction) and later stages (C and D) of HF may benefit from less rigid restriction.[4]

ACC/AHA Guidelines[5] for HF cite fluid restriction (1.5-2.0 L/day) as being reasonable in stage D HF. If a CR patient has a fluid restriction and sweats profusely during exercise sessions, the CR professional should ask the physician if an increase in fluid allowance is appropriate. Weighing the patient pre- and postexercise and using the factor 1 L H_2O/kg body weight lost during the exercise session may be helpful in avoiding symptomatic hypotension.

Despite conventional thought that obesity would aggravate peripheral resistance and worsen HF, some studies have shown that morbidity and mortality are lower in HF patients who have a BMI >30 and slightly higher in patients with a BMI >35.[112] Paradoxical evidence suggesting favorable outcomes with higher BMI values is merely observational. The relation between survival and quality of life may be different.[113] Because concern exists that intentional weight loss may mask cardiac cachexia and result in subsequent worse outcomes, weight loss is not prioritized in the 2013 ACC/AHA Guidelines for HF.[5] Recommendations by the patient's physician would best guide the CR professional regarding the benefit of weight loss in each patient.

Obesity

Obesity is a major risk factor for CVD and impacts nearly all the other risk factors. Consequently, the topic is addressed separately in the Overweight and Obesity section of chapter 9.

The majority of diet plans prescribed for weight loss focus on the number of servings of different food types. A desirable macronutrient composition can range from 30% to 50% of calories from CHO, 15% to 30% of calories from protein, and 30% to 40% of calories from healthful fats. Essentially, any mix of macronutrient will result in weight loss as long as a calorie deficit is elicited.

Gradual weight loss is the goal for most overweight CR participants. Caloric intake goals should include a daily deficit of 250 to 750 kcal. The goal is to target an average of 0.25 to 1 kg weight loss per week. Very low-calorie plans need close supervision and are generally not recommended. The most important consideration is the number of calories consumed relative to the number of calories expended; hence, an energy deficit can be created by more expenditure and/or less intake.

Initial weight loss may be rapid due to changes in fluid balance. If the caloric intake is too restrictive and the diet is intolerable or unsustainable, adjusting calorie intake up may be helpful in accomplishing long-term success.[4,45] The timing of protein consumption may affect satiety. For example, the consumption of protein at breakfast has been associated with greater satiety throughout the day.[114] The consumption of low energy density foods (e.g., vegetables, fruits, whole grains, low-fat dairy products) is associated with weight loss magnitude and weight loss maintenance.[115]

Numerous studies demonstrate that weight loss during the initial six-month period is often not sustained[116] and 30% to 50% of weight is regained even with intensive lifestyle therapy.[117] Therefore, the issue of weight loss recidivism needs to be addressed early in the care process. Studies have shown that maintaining high levels of physical activity is the most critical factor in preventing weight regain.[118] Addressing the patient's non-nutritive concerns for food (e.g., emotional eating and eating in response to stress, coping strategies, self-awareness, and self-monitoring) is essential. Not doing so will likely lead to lack of success and weight regain.[119,120,121]

BOTTOM LINE

Many of the risk factors for CVD are profoundly affected, both in a positive and negative manner, by dietary factors. It is incumbent on CR professionals to understand and be able to communicate to patients the potential impact that dietary components have on specific CVD risk factors.

Nutrition in the CR Care Process

Knowing the recommended diet guidance is the first step in the provision of nutritional care in CR. Motivating participants to eat in a healthful manner can be challenging. Research has shown that eating habits are difficult to modify because of their multifactorial nature.[122] Merely recommending and providing a standard diet or plan will not result in long-term changed behavior nor provide care that is individualized. Nutritional care of CR participants includes assessment, identification of relevant target eating behaviors, goal setting, nutrition education, evaluation, goal modification, and reevaluation until discharge.

Objectives include identifying the following:

- Eating behaviors that contribute to the CVD process
- Participants who are at nutritional risk
- Individuals who would benefit from or require follow-up with a dietitian
- Participants' level of readiness to change eating behavior

Nutrition Assessment in CR

In order to evaluate diet, a variety of assessment tools have been developed. Advantages and disadvantages vary and depend on the patient (literacy, stage of illness, and readiness for change), what diet component is targeted for measurement, and the ability of the assessor to interpret findings.

Unfortunately, there is no single ideal tool. Diet history, dietary records, and 24-hour recalls rely on self-report and may yield an accurate analysis of nutrient content. These methods may be used in clinical care, to provide counseling and education, or as a means to determine the necessity to refer a participant to a dietitian. However, because they are impossible to standardize, these tools cannot be used in CR pre- and post-assessments or in outcomes reporting. The accuracy of the data collected depends on patient motivation, training in food volume assessment, and ease of use.[123]

Food frequency questionnaires (FFQs) are checklists of foods and beverages with a frequency response section for patients to report how often each item was consumed over a specified time period. FFQs yield a single score that can be compared to clinical indicators of risk. Brief FFQs are screeners that assess consumption of targeted nutrients or patterns. For example, tools can measure fruit and vegetable intake or focus on only fat intake. Screeners are helpful as a means to evaluate need for further diet counseling or for referral to a dietitian. Brief FFQs may have only 12 to 22 targeted questions and take less time to administer, but yield only information regarding high, medium, or low ranges of food groupings. Extended FFQs can have at least 100 questions, and they are able to address subcategories of food as well as quantities of macro- and micronutrients. Computerized versions of FFQs may improve reliability of the measure by using photographs to estimate portion sizes and increase questionnaire completion and accuracy.[124]

The availability and suitability of particular FFQs or indices for use in CR is under review.[125, 126,127.]

Table 7.2 lists the parameters obtained at program entry and used to evaluate need for education and intervention.

Nutrition Care Plan in CR

A concrete, behaviorally focused nutrition care plan should result from clinical and diet assessments. As with other aspects of care in CR, the nutrition care plan needs to be individualized. The objective of the plan should be to result in behavioral changes that reflect adherence, not compliance. A prescribed one-size-fits-all "diet" external to the patient leads to reliance

Table 7.2 Summary of Relevant Clinical Parameters in Nutrition Assessment in CR

	Clinical parameter	Evaluation criteria
Anthropometric	Height, weight, BMI, unintentional weight loss >5% in the past 6 months	All CR participants If >5% unintentional weight loss in the past 6 months, then referral to dietitian may be warranted. If BMI <15 or BMI >35, consider referral to dietitian.
	WC	Elevated risk if WC men ≥ 40 in.; women ≥ 35 in.
BP	BP at rest and exercise	All CR participants
Serum blood values	Fasting lipid profile	All CR participants
Serum blood values	Glucose, glycated hemoglobin	All CR participants with DM
	BNP	All CR participants with HF
	Iron status (hemoglobin, hematocrit), protein (pre-albumin, creatinine), dehydration, chronic (creatinine)	Abnormal values, if available, may indicate need for physician referral to dietitian.

Abbreviations: BMI, body mass index; BP, blood pressure; WC, waist circumference; BNP, B-type natriuretic peptide; HF, heart failure.

on preprinted menus, charts, and restrictions; resulting behavioral changes conform to imposed structures and thus are temporary. Patients may request a formal, structured strategy (e.g., "Just tell me what to eat"). The resulting behavioral changes, however, merely conform to the imposed external structure. The participant does not internalize the principles guiding the "diet." Thus, the behavioral changes are temporary and do not lead to diminished long-term CVD risk. Obtaining adherence involves shared goal setting aimed at diet pattern targets, utilizing strategies that promote self-efficacy and empowerment.

Diet Pattern Behavioral Targets

Dietary recommendations that focus on diet patterns and not on specific nutrients or energy component ratios are preferred. Various individual aspects of each plan may appeal to patients. Focusing on key behavioral targets that are common to all the recommended plans allows for specific guidance in goal setting (table 7.3).

Guideline 7.2   Nutritional Evaluation

Assessing eating habits and determining target areas for nutritional intervention should be identified in all CR participants.

Strategies for Behavioral Change

CR professionals should employ psychological models shown to be successful at stimulating behavior change. Behavioral change strategies are discussed in detail in chapter 8. Motivational interviewing is an individually directed counseling style for affecting behavior change to support better health. The goal is to help patients identify and resolve ambivalence with targeted eating behaviors. Motivational interviewing centers on the processes that facilitate a positive change and can influence fruit and vegetable consumption.[128]

Principles of mindful eating (ME) include consciously being aware of each bite taken, eating slowly with intention, consuming high-nutrient and lower-calorie-dense foods, finding comfort and soothing without food, and eating without distraction.[123] A corollary of ME is increased awareness of mind*less* eating and how environment and cues shape eating behavior.[129]

Intuitive eating (IE) involves being aware of hunger, fullness, and satiety cues; recognizing that no foods are bad; and encouraging food consumption only when hunger is perceived.[130] The primary principles of IE are to reject the diet mentality, respect hunger, make peace with food, respect fullness and satisfaction, and acknowledge feelings without using food.

Table 7.3   Key Behavioral Targets and Sample Goals

Key behavioral targets	Provisos (List is suggestive, not exhaustive.)	Sample behavioral goal (To be SMART, each behavioral goal needs a time frame.)
Increase servings of fruits and vegetables.	Select variety in type and texture.	Select 3 different greens for salad.
	Include colorful orange, red, and green options.	Add 1/2 cup strawberries and blueberries at breakfast.
	Use fruit to replace sweets.	Eat an apple after dinner instead of dessert.
	Keep portions of 100% juice to 1/2 cup.	Drink orange juice from a small 4 oz glass.
	Use non-starchy vegetables to fill up.	Eat a salad with vinaigrette prior to evening meal.
Select a variety of fish, lean and unprocessed meats and poultry, and low-fat dairy in order to decrease saturated fat. Choose MUFAs and PUFAs.	Prepare lean meats at home, and package leftovers in freezer.	Replace processed deli meat with homemade roasted options.
	Purchase only lean meat and poultry.	Select lean ground meat (93%) or poultry to make meatloaf.
	Select low-fat dairy foods.	Select low-fat yogurt as dessert instead of whole milk for dinner.
	Replace butter or hard spreads with soft spreads made with olive oil, canola oil, or yogurt.	Try olive oil spread on vegetables.
	Decrease portion size of high-fat meats.	Eat 1/2 instead of a whole grilled chicken breast.
Increase whole grains, nuts, and seeds.	Substitute refined with whole grain. Eat whole grains containing ≥3 g fiber/serving.	Select whole-grain bread for sandwiches.
	Try new grains.	Try a side dish recipe that includes quinoa.
	Replace former snacks with whole grains.	Make homemade instead of store-bought popcorn during a football game.
	Replace sugary cereals with whole-grain options.	Make oatmeal with nuts for breakfast.
	Read labels to see which brand has more fiber and verify whole grains first in ingredient list.	Spend 10 min reading food labels at the bread section of the grocery store.
Decrease sodium intake by 1,000 mg or to <2,300 mg daily.	Use unsalted nuts.	Add 2 tbsp walnuts to a salad.
	Eat home-cooked meals more often.	Make date night a home-prepped meal with candlelight.
	Remove the saltshaker from the meal table.	Keep the saltshaker on the top shelf of the cabinet.
	Read food labels and select lower sodium snack foods.	Read the labels of 5 products, and select snacks made with 50% less salt.
	Use more fresh or dried herbs, singular or blends.	Make the herb blend recommended at class today, and use on grilled chicken breast.
Lose weight if BMI >25 (consider age and comorbidities).	Eat smaller portions.	Use MyPlate guide to gauge portions.[140]
	Adjust meal timing and frequency to fit hunger patterns.	Eat breakfast to avoid midmorning hunger. Decrease lunch portion to accommodate.
	Eliminate calories by reducing consumption of high-sugar content foods.	Select low-fat mayonnaise for chicken salad.
	Address emotional issues with food.	Document how often I eat when stressed.
	Keep food intake records.	Use an app to track foods eaten.
Decrease intake of sugar-sweetened beverages.	Use fruit to flavor water.	Add a lemon slice to water at my desk.
	Replace regular pop with diet pop or flavorings.	Select diet root beer instead of regular cola.
	Add other flavorings instead of sugar to coffee or tea.	Add vanilla extract to brewed coffee.
	Try a new sugarless beverage such as sparkling or herb/vegetable infused waters.	Infuse water with cucumber, kiwi, or mint.
	Select smaller serve ware.	Use 4 oz glass of beer instead of 12 oz during social event; alternate with water or calorie-free beverage.

Abbreviation: BMI, body mass index.

Goal Setting Goal setting provides clarity regarding the proposed behaviors' structure, specificity, and expected outcomes. Diet goals are most effective when made collaboratively between CR professional and participants using motivational interviewing techniques. Diet goals should be specific, measurable, achievable, relevant, and time-bound (S.M.A.R.T.).[131] The CR professional can help identify and address barriers to change that are unique to food and eating behaviors (e.g., financial/food insecurity, hunger, taste, habituation of food intake, holiday/religious practices, work-related policy and hours, and lack of accessibility to purchase healthful food).[125]

Problem-Solving Strategies Problem-solving strategies aid the participant in identifying antecedents to behaviors and then setting goals or strategies to cope with those antecedents. For example, the patient identifies that afternoon candy snacking at work is a problem. The patient identifies behaviors or decisions they made prior to eating a candy bar at their work desk. (The patient experiences work stress and hunger, places money in their pocket, walks to a vending machine, then returns to the desk and quickly eats the candy bar.) Then the patient and CR professional develop strategies to intervene. (The patient uses stress coping strategies, replaces the candy with sugarless gum, places the pocket change in a jar, and walks to the courtyard instead of the vending machine.)

Self-Monitoring Self-monitoring is the most important component of successful behavioral change strategies.[117,132,133] The value of self-monitoring accentuates awareness or cues for healthful decisions. Self-awareness aids the transition to mindfulness. The record-keeping process provides immediate stimuli to modify food choices, therefore participants have more success in maintaining a specific behavior change. Effective means of monitoring include food records, behavior records, and journaling in all their variant forms—paper or electronic, structured or formless.

Individual Treatment Plan Assessment, Reassessment, and Discharge

Documentation on the individual treatment plan (ITP) should be brief but specific to the individual patient. Figure 7.2 provides examples of possible charting styles; they are not meant to be proscriptive.

Education

The goal of dietary education in CR is to assist patients to make healthful eating choices and to support nutrition-related behaviors. Limiting dietary education solely to the communication of information on what constitutes a nutritious diet is not necessarily the most effective strategy for helping CR participants to make the necessary dietary changes. Effective dietary education should incorporate a combination of educational strategies designed to facilitate adopting healthful food choices and other food and nutrition-related behaviors conducive to overall health. Effective dietary education can be delivered in multiple ways. The following section addresses providing dietary education in the CR setting.

Topics

CR programming should include the following topics.

Food Plans

- Provide descriptions of the DASH plan, MEDIT diet, and vegetarian diet emphasizing commonality and what *can* be consumed rather than focus on restriction.

- Use the USDA MyPlate guidelines as a graphic means of describing optimal food choices with an emphasis upon portion sizes. The MyPlate presentation emphasizes the larger portions of vegetables, fruit, whole grains, modest portions of lean meat, and the inclusion of low-fat dairy. Less specificity of included foods allows for regional differences. Details are available on the ChooseMyPlate website.[134]

Guideline 7.3   Dietary Interventions

Providing patient education is just one aspect of the provision of nutritional care in CR. Motivating participants to eat in a healthful manner can be challenging. Nutritional care of CR participants includes assessment, identification of relevant target eating behaviors, goal setting, nutrition education, evaluation, goal modification, and reevaluation. Incorporating behavioral change models and compliance strategies into dietary counseling sessions is critical to helping patients achieve long-term compliance with dietary recommendations.

Figure 7.2 Sample ITP Documentation

Nutrition Assessment

Document the results of clinical and diet assessment.

Example 1—Clinical: BMI = 30, overweight, hypertensive

Diet assessment: Scores low on vegetable and fruit intake.

Summary: Overweight, hypertensive, low fruit/vegetable intake.

Example 2—Clinical: BMI = 18, 20 lb weight loss since surgery (9% over 5 months)

Diet assessment: Eats infrequently, scores low on all diet components.

Summary: At risk for malnutrition; refer to RD.

Example 3—Clinical: BMI = 23, TC = 300, HDL = 32, LDL = 222, TG = 420, glucose = 122

Diet assessment: Limited food selection. Scores low on all plant-based food components.

Summary: Borderline high glucose, abnormal lipids, normal weight.

Nutrition Plan

Establish SMART goals designed in collaboration with participant.

Example 1—Weight reduction: Substitute sugar-free iced tea for cola.

Example 2—Target increased daily caloric intake: Add a healthful snack 3 times/day.

Example 3—Elevated lipids and glucose, normal weight: Substitute butter with olive and canola oil.

Interventions

Example 1—Keep food records using phone app daily for one week and discuss results.

Example 2—Keep food and appetite records daily. Appointment with dietitian on 5/15/20.

Example 3—Keep food records in notebook daily. Plans to talk to dietitian after class on 5/15/20.

Education

Example 1—Provided weight reduction strategies. Plan: Attend weight reduction class on 5/15/20.

Example 2—List of healthful snack options was provided, and patient stated plan to add a high-protein breakfast shake daily in addition to current caloric intake.

Example 3—Patient enthusiastically attended all nutrition classes provided. Patient was able to state plans for changing grocery selection.

Nutrition Reassessment

Example 1—Gained 2 lb. Iced tea had sugar. Keeping food records. Will have single sandwich at lunch and single portion at dinner.

Example 2—Appetite still poor. Weight stable. Has added daily breakfast shake. Will add a can of nutritional supplement at night.

Example 3—Food records revealed that meat portions are fried and large. Will bake or grill chicken/fish 3 times this week. Will continue food records.

Nutrition Discharge/Follow-Up

Example 1—Total diet score improved as did fruit and vegetable components. Portion sizes decreased. Has lost a total of 5 lb while in program. Enjoys using phone app and will continue to keep daily. Will weigh two times/week at home. Will bring in lunch to work and only eat out on Fridays.

Example 2—Appetite continues to be poor but has regained 5 lb. Will continue to add 3 healthful snacks along with moderate meals daily. Will see dietitian in one month.

Example 3—Total diet score did not increase significantly. Patient stopped food records. States is frying foods again, but with canola oil. Skipped dietitian appointment. Reviewed obstacles to change; states spouse is resistant and unsupportive of change. Discussed negotiating skills plan. New dietitian appointment made.

Target Lipids

- Identify link between food sources of fat and cholesterol and resultant blood levels.
- Identify foods high in SFA. Replace SFA with olive, canola, or other PUFAs.
- Refer the participant to a weight management session.

Diet and HTN

- Emphasize the importance of lowering sodium intake by 1,000 mg or to <2,300 mg/day.
- Use label reading to identify food and beverages with high sodium content.
- Explain how to increase potassium and calcium in the diet.
- Offer alternative means to season foods, including herbs, spices, citrus juice or zest, vinegar, low-sodium spicy sauces, salsa, and healthful commercial products.
- Provide the DASH diet plan.
- Refer the participant to a behavioral weight loss program.

Weight Management

- Key concepts of energy balance (calories consumed v. calories expended)
- Portion control
- Self-monitoring via food records or journaling
- Recognition of emotional relationships with food
- Emphasizing choice rather than restriction
- Identifying and managing antecedent behaviors that may stimulate a specific response

T2DM

- Key concepts and coping with high and low blood glucose readings
- CHO control versus restriction, including portion size and/or CHO counting
- Sources of simple CHOs and high-fiber foods
- Refer participant to behavioral weight loss program.
- Meal composition

HF

- Signs and symptoms
- Sodium and fluid guidance based on risk or physician prescription
- Weight maintenance versus weight loss

Education Methodologies

Given that participants have varying time availability, learning styles, capacity for learning, prior experience, and knowledge, CR programs should provide a variety of means to educate each participant. Educational interventions are associated with positively related improvements in dietary habits.[135]

Classroom: Experiential Versus Didactic   Traditionally, the most common methodology to promote diet change is education. Although having an intellectual foundation is a component in behavior change, the patient may have no buy-in; thus, behavior change is unlikely. Educational materials may be more important when providing tools for the patient who is ready to make a change, and content must fit the audience. The temptation to provide as much information as possible must be constrained to avoid overwhelming or distracting the patient with unneeded or unwelcome information. Providing health information in the iPEEP format (outlined next) is helpful.

iPEEP Format

- *Interesting.* The more senses a learner engages, the more likely the ability retain facts in memory (e.g., food models, imitation muscle/fat, or sensory input with food demonstration or sampling).
- *Prioritize* the topics by how they will impact the health of CR patient. (E.g., methods of weight loss may be a higher priority topic than a detailed description of fatty acids, due to positive impact on CVD risk factors.)
- *Engaging.* Ask questions frequently (every 3-5 min) or use polling technology.
- *Essential.* Identify what knowledge the CR participant must have in order to make behavioral change. Any additional information may be distracting and hinder learning.
- *Practical.* Fun facts such as how to identify saturated fats or how to season foods in a healthful manner retain the interest of the CR participant.

Education on Exercise Floor   The CR professional should use the time during the exercise session to ask questions and stimulate conversations among participants. Videos of healthful diet content and food demonstrations can be shown on the exercise floor and will stimulate conversation among participants. The CR professional may provide more intensive or focused counseling for those who want a discrete interaction.

Games, Challenges, and Contests Healthy competition among participants discourages complacency and raises consciousness of certain behaviors. Competition embodies play, is pleasurable, and enhances knowledge acquisition. Competition among individual participants or groups (e.g., by session) or among participants and the CR staff incentivizes behaviors or outcomes targeted. Examples of competition include weight loss challenge, number of servings of vegetables, grains, and fruit consumed in a day, and guessing or nutritional trivia contests.

Written Materials Educational material must match the audience for content, cultural bias, literacy, social impact, and readability (format). The CR professional must resist including as much information on the page as possible and employ readability assessments to ensure that main points are understandable.[136] Written materials supplement the behavioral change process; they do not replace it.

Dietitian–CR Professional Partnership

Engagement of a dietitian in the CR program is a necessity, not a luxury. Minimally, a dietitian should evaluate policy and procedures regarding nutritional evaluation and should be engaged in nutrition competency evaluation and continuing nutrition education of CR staff. Although budgets may be tight, dietitian engagement enhances quality of care and outcomes.[137] Therefore, creative means of funding dietitian engagement with CR participants may be required.

Role of Dietitian

The dietitian brings a unique skill set in providing nutrition education that is practical and efficacious. Other health care professionals can learn nutrition-related facts, but dietitians are the only group with standardized education, clinical training, continuing education, and national credentials in place specifically for nutrition.[138] Patients counseled by dietitians demonstrate greater improvements in clinical outcomes than when instructed by other clinical staff.[139,140,141]

Criteria for Referral of CR Patient for Nutritional Consult

CR programs should establish referral policies based on their program needs. Awareness of local insurance and Medicare coverage should inform policy. Medicare covers MNT for diagnoses of kidney failure and T2DM, and private payers have varying policies regarding coverage for dietitian services. Suggested optional criteria for a referral to a dietitian could include the following: previous or extended failure at diet modification in high-risk individuals, newly diagnosed or uncontrolled T2DM, unintended weight loss or gain, clinical evidence of malnutrition, patient request, newly diagnosed HF, and early onset of CVD.

Reimbursement for Dietitian Services

Although the details of reimbursement are determined by local coverage determinations (LCD), the code 93797 can be used for nutrition educational sessions, either in group format or in individual sessions. Dietitian services are available by a variety of means: direct dietitian

---

Guideline 7.4 Nutritional Education and Counseling

Nutritional education and counseling are critical components of CR programming. Nutritional education delivered in CR should be multifaceted. Effective dietary education should incorporate a combination of educational strategies designed to facilitate the adoption of healthful food choices and other food and nutrition-related behaviors conducive to overall health. Ultimately, the goal of nutritional education and counseling is to maximize patient understanding and achieve long-term compliance to dietary advice.

employment by the CR program either by hiring or by consultation, transfer of hours between CR program and nutrition department, shared service agreements, and employment of persons with dual specialty degrees and certifications.[142]

Summary

Nutrition is an essential component of the CR patient's plan of care and reduction of CVD risk. Clearly, a poor-quality diet is a contributing factor to the development and progression of CVD. Professionals in CR need to creatively advocate increasing the consumption of healthful foods and diminishing unhealthful choices. Encouragement of the DASH plan, MEDIT diet, or plant-based diets is a positive message that patients can comprehend and follow. Nutrition education can be delivered in group or individual settings or using a variety of interactive or written means. Each CR team member is responsible for establishing specific behavior goals at entry and practicing regular follow-up and reinforcement with patients.

Behavior Modification for Risk Factor Reduction

Diann Galeema, PhD

Guiding Principles and Practice

The aim of this chapter is to provide health professionals with guidance on promoting health-related behavior change within the context of CR.

OBJECTIVES

This chapter provides an overview of the following:

- The complexity of behavior change
- Assessing patient needs
- The necessity of an individualized approach to behavior change
- Steps for implementing a behavior change plan

Overview of Health-Related Behavior Change

Patients entering CR will most likely need to change at least one health-related behavior for risk factor control. Promoting behavior change can be challenging. This chapter outlines the steps a health care provider can take to best support patients in making changes in their behavior. The described methodologies are adapted from various fields within behavioral psychology, including theories of reinforcement,[1] cognitive psychology, and the transtheoretical model.[2] The interventions draw from methods that take into account various aspects of the patient's social and physical environment as well as their physical and psychosocial characteristics.[3,4]

It is not sufficient to merely target education as a means to bring about a sustained change in behavior. A patient's ability to systematically process information and successfully implement a behavior change program is influenced by emotions that are associated with surviving a cardiac event (depression, anxiety, anger, fear).[5,6] CR professionals must design risk factor modification programs that take into account the specific characteristics of each patient involved, including an understanding of how each patient views their own behavior as a part of their overall recovery and their role as active participant in the behavior change process. Thus, overall, the process of supporting behavior change requires learning about an individual patient's knowledge, needs, and environment; identifying the behaviors needed for risk factor control; making a plan of action in collaboration with the patient; monitoring and rewarding progress; and making changes to the plan as needed. Crucial throughout this process is to remember that successful behavior change is a collaborative and iterative process.

It is also important to consider that behavior change cannot be supported in a patient who does not enter CR. It is incumbent to maximize participation through proven approaches such as automatic referral and rapid entry following hospital discharge.[7] Programs are encouraged to devote efforts to actively recruit and retain patient populations who are underrepresented in CR, such as women, patients of low socioeconomic status, racial and ethnic minorities, current smokers, young patients, and elderly patients.[5,8-12]

Many of the principles outlined in this chapter include behavior change support, which requires health professionals to have effective counseling skills to assist patients with lifestyle modification. Professionals are encouraged to pursue techniques that have demonstrated effectiveness, such as acceptance and commitment therapy (ACT) and motivational interviewing.[4,13]

Programs should support their staff by providing training in behavior change strategies. To optimize success, CR programs should address the points in guideline 8.1.

 Guideline 8.1   Program Resources to Support Health-Promoting Behavior Change

To support behavior modification, programs should address the following points:

- Address behaviors in hospital that may interfere with attendance at cardiac rehabilitation (e.g., smoking, depression, lack of social or financial support).
- Allocate resources for *all* modifiable risk factors.
- Provide patient education on disease processes, management of cardiac emergencies, and maintenance of psychosocial health.
- Develop plans for risk factor modification using current clinical practice methodologies.
- Train staff in health behavior counseling skills.

- Employ a variety of strategies and materials that take into account the individual patient and family needs and preferences.
- Foster patient–provider collaboration.
- Provide resources for objective measurement of progress toward goals (logs, pedometers, etc.).
- Create and provide resources for plans for returning to work and the need for job retraining, where appropriate.
- Allocate resources to facilitate patient transition to as full a level of independence postdischarge as possible.

Step 1: Performing the Initial Assessment

To maximize the chances of successful behavior change, CR professionals need detailed information about the patient. Initial assessments should include information about risk factors, environment, and the patient's thoughts and feelings surrounding the behaviors that require changing.

First, identify the behaviors that need changing. AHA/AACVPR guidelines[14] outline the targets for risk factor reduction in detail. The patient should be assessed on their specific risk factors and the behaviors associated with control of that risk factor. Are they smoking? Are they struggling with depression or other psychosocial issues? Is their physical fitness compromised? Are they adherent with taking medications as prescribed? Risk factors should be listed and ranked in importance and behaviors associated with each identified.

Second, what are the individual characteristics of the patient? The approach taken to behavior change should be done in consideration of relevant characteristics. These characteristics include the following:

- *Demographics.* Be aware of the influence of age, gender, education and literacy level, race-ethnicity, culture, and linguistic differences.
- *Cognitive function.* Consider existing knowledge of the disease process, ability to learn (attend to, process, retain, and apply new knowledge), and the presence of distractions to cognitive processing (e.g., fear, anxiety, hostility, and depressive symptoms).

Third, query the patient about their environment (both physical and social). Where do they live? Whom do they live with? With whom do they associate? By asking questions, you can identify potential positive aspects of a person's environment (e.g., they live in a walkable neighborhood or next to the pharmacy) or potential challenges (e.g., they live in an area with no sidewalks or the nearest grocery store is a 30-minute drive away). Questions about their social environment will yield useful information about people who

may help (e.g., a spouse very concerned about the patient's health and committed to providing a supportive environment) or hinder (e.g., friends who are smokers with no intent to quit) attempts at behavior change. Both physical and social environments can have significant effects on behavior. For example, living in an area with a large number of fast food restaurants is associated with weight gain in adults while community walkability is associated with weight loss.[15] On the social level, researchers have described health-related behaviors as "contagious;" people become more like those they associate with (e.g., losing or gaining weight) even when those associations are not in the person's control (e.g., which military base someone is assigned to).[16] Accordingly, both the physical and social environment are important considerations when supporting behavior change.

Fourth, engage with the patient to find out their thoughts on their recovery. Ask about prior experiences with the behavior and related successes or failures. Such questions can provide information about a patient's self-confidence in being able to change as well as methods that may or may not have worked for them in the past. A solid foundation based on where the patients are starting from will help inform how to help them succeed in changing their health-related behaviors.

Promoting change is a collaborative effort. The patient must be an active participant in executing any plans for change. Accordingly, it can be helpful to know what they value and how that value relates to their recovery. By identifying particularly important aspects of a person's life (e.g., getting to play with grandkids, returning to work, freeing their spouse from having to care for them) allows behavior change (e.g., improving fitness, medication adherence, etc.) to be couched in terms that relate to specific goals and values. For example, explain to an elderly woman that strength training is useful for improving her ability to climb stairs and carry groceries, outcomes she values because she wants to remain independent. Several proven behavior change techniques, including motivational interviewing and ACT, tap into the values of the patients to help motivate positive behavior change.

BOTTOM LINE

Sample steps in supporting behavior change include the following:

1. What is the problem, and what are the modifiable (behavior related) causes of the problem?
   - List behavior(s) that must be modified for risk reduction and management.
   - Rank in order of importance for health improvements.

2. For each behavior, discuss the following with the patient:
   - What does the patient know about the connection between the behavior and the risk factor? Educate as necessary.
   - What are the patient's values around this behavior?
   - Does the patient believe they can change? Is the patient ready to change?
   - What are the barriers to performing the behavior (e.g., physical, social, financial, cognitive)?

3. Prioritize behaviors in order of importance and changeability. Select behavior(s) that will be the target for short-term goals.

4. Develop specific goals (short-term and long-term) and the strategies to achieve them.
   - Use SMART guidelines to outline goals. (For a definition of SMART goals, see Goal Setting in chapter 7.)
   - Recruit support from the patient's family and friends.
   - Discuss how to modify the environment (physical and social) to support the change.

5. Create a specific monitoring and feedback plan.
   - How will the patient objectively measure behavior?
   - How will that information be relayed to the health care professional?
   - Discuss with the patient potential challenges and possibility of lapse or relapse.

6. Reward progress.
   - What can the clinic or the patient provide as a reward for meeting goals?

7. Reevaluate and adjust the plan.
   - Expect that repeated attempts will be necessary.
   - Be prepared to provide a variety of approaches to help support the patient.

Step 2: Educating the Patient

When supporting behavior change, appropriate information is necessary but often not sufficient. Once the provider has established what the patient's risk factors are, the patient needs to understand why control of these risk factors is important. Patients must have sufficient knowledge of health risks and benefits, understanding what positive and adverse consequences can be expected from success as well as failure. These consequences can include the following:

- The physical effects that a behavior is likely to produce (e.g., weight loss, functional improvements, muscle soreness due to exertion)
- Social effects (approval or disapproval of others in their social circle)
- Cognitive effects (improvements or decrements in depressive level or self-esteem)

Selecting and developing materials to promote knowledge among patients requires careful consideration. The average reading level in the United States is between the 8th and 9th grade level, and almost two of five older Americans (65 and over) read below the 5th grade level.[17] Literacy on health-related topics is similarly limited.[18] Due to strong social stigma, most people with a reading problem do not tell a health professional. Educational attainment may also not be a good indicator of literacy level, because adults tend to read three to five grade levels lower than the years of education completed. Research has demonstrated that many patient education materials are written at or above the college reading level.[19] If print materials are used, they should be reviewed with patients to improve comprehension.

Elderly patients generally find materials with large print on nonglossy paper more readable. Also, many patients do not speak or read English or English is a second language. It is helpful to have materials available in multiple languages that are appropriate to the community served. The AHA has translated many of their brochures into Spanish,[20] and other publishers and pharmaceutical companies can supply educational materials in other languages. For health care professionals interested in developing new health education materials rather than using existing products, a step-by-step tool to guide the development of effective communication products, called Making Health Communication Programs Work, can be obtained at no cost from the National Cancer Institute.[21]

After providing information in a manner best suited to each person, it is also important to test comprehension. One way to do so is to have the patient explain back to the provider the risks and benefits of various behaviors. By having to echo the information back, the patient will (1) demonstrate comprehension and (2) further process the information. Requisite knowledge of behavioral factors that increase their risk of a secondary event or procedure and ways to effectively prevent or reduce that risk is critical, so comprehension should also be assured.

However, although knowledge gain is necessary, it is not sufficient by itself to ensure behavior change. Well-informed people may have low motivation or lack the skills and personal resources necessary to bring about a positive behavior change. As pointed out previously, it is important for health care providers to perform baseline assessments and provide tailored interventions to appropriately address the unique needs, capabilities, and values of each patient.

Step 3: Assessing Patient Willingness to Change

After identifying risk factors, it is important to assess the patient's willingness to change. One way to do so is to work through the list of risk factors and assess the patient's stage of change for each behavior. The *stages of change* are five ordered categories of readiness to change behavior that have been identified to describe the process of modifying health behaviors. Assessing stage of change helps to match a patient to the fol-lowing stage-appropriate behavior modification strategies:[2]

• *Precontemplation stage.* There is no intention to change the behavior in the near future (usually defined as within the next 6 months). Patients in this stage may believe that they do not have a problem or that the behavior is not serious enough to warrant attention. They may lack understanding of the potential consequences of not changing. It also is possible that patients in this stage recognize the need to change their behavior but have no serious intention of trying to do so. They may lack self-efficacy about their ability to be successful due to past unsuccessful attempts to change. People in this stage believe that the costs of change significantly outweigh the benefits. At the precontemplation stage, patients may have little or no interest in changing; therefore, repeated, gentle confrontation may be helpful.

Polite and respectful confrontation helps patients see discrepancies in their beliefs and actions. Confronting patients does not imply that health professionals take an adversarial role. Rather, it means that a statement such as "I see you've missed several sessions" allows for honest feedback, giving the patient an opportunity to respond. Confrontation should not take the form of a question like "Why are you missing appointments?" Such a question could put the patient on the defensive. Strategies that might help patients progress to the next stage include the use of brochures, books, newsletters, videos, newspaper articles, and guest speakers who are positive role models of success.

• *Contemplation stage.* Patients in this stage are giving serious consideration to changing the health behavior within the next 6 months. They are thinking but are indecisive and lack commitment to make a plan of action. In the contemplation stage, interventions should be aimed at providing information in the form of written materials, videos, and persuasive role models (such as graduates of the program, ideally of similar gender and age) that can demonstrate the benefits of change (outweighing the costs).

Discussions with the patient regarding the particular behavior should include an appeal to what seems to be a motivating force for that person. Common examples include a desire to engage in a favorite recreational activity or to return to work, family, or social activities. In addition, at this stage a cost–benefit analysis is often quite useful. Help the patient write down all the costs (negative consequences, such as fear of failure, giving up favorite foods, or time required to attend the program) and benefits (positive consequences, such as improved fitness and functioning) of making a particular change. Professional staff should be aware that most patients need help listing immediate benefits and may need counseling to minimize the influence of costs. However, it is probably time well spent. A patient may conclude that the behavior is not worth changing unless it is apparent that the short- and long-term benefits truly outweigh the costs. Once this cost–benefit list is developed, it is useful to have the patient keep the list for reference during difficult times.

• *Preparation stage.* People in this stage tend to act on the health behavior change in the immediate future, usually within the next 30 days. Patients in this stage may make a plan of action and take small steps toward action, such as talking to health professionals and seeking advice and trying out the new behavior (e.g., acquiring low-fat diet recipes, joining a health club, quitting smoking for a day). The combination of intending to change and having enacted recent attempts to change is the hallmark characteristic of the preparation stage.

• *Action stage.* Patients in this stage have a plan and are in the act of changing the health behavior or have made specific changes within the last 6 months. In order to qualify as action, the behavior must occur at a level that is acceptable for optimal health benefits according to current knowledge and standards. For example, only the time period in which total abstinence from smoking was achieved is counted as within the action stage. The period of time in which the number of cigarettes was reduced, but abstinence was not total, falls within the preparation phase.

Most interventions are designed for the preparation and action stages. They are the skill-building stages, when staff and patients begin to set goals and to solve problems of barriers to continuous success (preparation), then implement plans (action) and make adjustments as required. The action stage includes implementation of the new behavior and requires strategies to provide environmental support, feedback, and reinforcement.

• *Maintenance stage.* At this stage, the health behavior has been successfully maintained continuously for more than 6 months. For some behaviors (e.g., smoking cessation), the maintenance stage is a lifelong task and not a discrete period of time. The focus for health professionals who support patients at this stage of change is to assist with relapse prevention by promoting problem-solving and coping skills to overcome challenging situations that may trigger relapse. Most people who relapse at a later stage do not return to precontemplation.

Querying Patient Readiness Using Stages of Change: Example With Exercise Behavior

Question to a Patient From a Health Professional[22,23]

"Do you exercise regularly? By regular exercise, I mean any planned physical activity (e.g., brisk walking, aerobics, jogging, bicycling, swimming, rowing) performed at a level that increases your breathing rate and causes you to sweat. Such activity, if performed regularly, is done three to five times per week for 20 to 60 min per session. According to this definition, do you exercise regularly?"

Response Options

1. "Yes, I have been for more than 6 months." (Patient is in maintenance.)
2. "Yes, I have been for less than 6 months." (Patient is in action.)
3. "No, but I intend to in the next 30 days." (Patient is in preparation.)
4. "No, but I intend to in the next 6 months." (Patient is in contemplation.)
5. "No, and I do not intend to in the next 6 months." (Patient is in precontemplation.)

Once determined, the stage can guide the professional in choosing appropriate strategies. Program staff should be aware that patients can move quickly and unexpectedly forward or backward in the change process due to influences within and outside the rehabilitation program; therefore ongoing monitoring of progress and adjustments are required in order to optimize effectiveness.

Step 4: Identifying Barriers to Engagement

After establishing target behaviors, it is important to identify potential barriers to change. Many aspects of a patient's life can contain barriers that will hinder their efforts at change. Barriers can be the following:

- *Environmental.* A patient may be limited by their physical environment. The patient may live in a neighborhood with no sidewalks, or in a place where walking around is not easy or safe. They might also be far away from the nearest grocery store, making obtaining fresh, nutritious food challenging. Limitations may also occur in resources. For example, a patient may not have access to reliable transportation, or may not be able to afford co-pays to attend CR sessions or to obtain their medications.

- *Social.* A patient may be surrounded by people who are not invested in engaging in health-promoting behaviors. For example, the main socializing that takes place in their family may be at meals, where large helpings of unhealthful food are encouraged. Their friends may generally gather to socialize in an environment where drinking and smoking are the norm. They might have no one in their friend or family group who would be interested in scheduling daily walks together.

- *Physical.* The patient's physical status may also be a barrier. A patient who is extremely deconditioned or has mobility-reducing comorbidities (e.g., severe arthritis) may be limited in the physical activity they can engage in.

- *Psychological.* The psychological characteristics of a patient may also provide barriers to behavior change. For example, a patient who has a psychological disorder (e.g., depression) that is not being sufficiently treated will likely struggle.[24] For such patients, getting them into appropriate treatment is vital.

When you identify barriers in advance, you can work with the patient to figure out potential ways to overcome those barriers.

Step 5: Making a Plan

Once the behaviors have been identified, it is time to establish a concrete plan of action. Staff should encourage patients to set both short-term and long-term SMART goals.[25] Change should begin with goals of high priority and also goals that a patient knows are more easily achievable. Behavior change targets should reflect the most current clinical practice recommendations. As a part of this principle, it is important to assist patients to prioritize which behaviors they are willing to change. As a part of developing a plan, patients require counseling to identify potential obstacles and figure out how they will cope with temptations or make adjustments to promote the likelihood of success. Patients should be encouraged to develop both short-term and long-term goals. Short-term goals focus on small incremental changes in behaviors that will build mastery for taking actions needed for achieving the overall long-term goal. The ultimate goal is improvement in personal health through sustained risk factor modification and management. An example of a long-term goal is *I will walk five days a week for 30 min each day, within six months.* An example of a short-term goal is *This week I will walk three days a week for 10 min a day.* The short-term goals should be achievable so that the patient can experience success. By setting achievable short-term goals in small, gradually increasing steps, the patient can eventually attain the long-term goal. If the short-term goals are not achieved, the patient and professional staff should reappraise and alter as needed.

One way to counsel a patient to set realistic goals and create an action plan to achieve those goals is to ask the patient, "On a scale of 0% (not at all confident) to 100% (completely confident), how do you rate your confidence in achieving the goal?"[26] If the patient is less than completely confident, discuss with the patient what actions can help increase confidence (e.g., figuring out ways to reduce barriers that must be overcome as a part of the program plan). If despite achieving behavioral goals (e.g., improvement in intensity or duration of regular physical activity) a patient continues to be unable to reach health outcomes (e.g., control of hypertension, achievement of weight loss goal), the clinical team should work collaboratively to discuss a potential change in approach.

When designing change plans, the following tips can help increase chances of success:

1. *Make the plan in close collaboration with the patient.* The patient is more likely to implement the plan if the provider understands the patient's motivations for change and the patient is closely involved in setting the goals.

2. *Make the plan formal.* Type it up, print it out, have clear steps listed, have the patient sign the bottom of it, and have them share the plan with friends and family. These actions will help reinforce the patient's commitment to the plan of action, which will help improve outcomes.[1]

3. *Remember to make the steps small and achievable.* Early success bolsters further effort, while failure punishes effort. Even if that step is only reducing from drinking six sodas a day to five, or forgoing 1 of the 20 cigarettes a day a person smokes, that change is a positive one that can snowball over time.[27]

Step 6: Setting the Stage

One of the most effective ways to engender change is to reduce the barriers to performing the wanted behavior (identified in step 4) and increase the barriers to performing the unwanted behavior. Work with patients to help them shape their environment so that it is supportive of the changes they want to make. This modification can take many forms. For example, if a patient is trying to improve their diet, you can increase barriers to unhealthful eating by having them remove the unhealthful food from the house. Removing barriers to the targeted behaviors could include grocery shopping while not hungry (to reduce temptation buying) or ordering groceries online to be picked up at the store so that food choices can be made further in time and distance from the food (which will increase healthy choices).[28] Similar efforts can support any behavior. For example, CR professionals can support medication adherence by setting up automatic refills to be mailed to the patient, support walking by having the patient schedule walks with a friend in advance, and support smoking cessation by having the

patient declare (widely) that their home is now smoke free. Patients may also need support to avoid challenging social situations, such as areas at work or other gathering places where smoking is permitted, or gatherings where unhealthful food is the only option. In addition, they may need help to identify and seek out alternative environments that provide support for health-promoting behaviors, such as participating in activities that require physical activity or are held in areas that don't permit smoking. The patient may lack a supportive social environment. Providers should endeavor to connect the patient with supportive peers, whether through creating support groups of current patients or recent graduates or by connecting patients with appropriate online groups.

Patients can set up cues in their environment that will remind them of the behaviors they want to perform and remove cues that lead to undesired behaviors. Setting up cues that occur in the time and place the behavior should be happening will help to set the stage for the occurrence of that behavior.[29] Examples of positive cues include reminder calls the day before a CR session or programmed reminders on personal devices, food logs on or next to the refrigerator to prompt dietary intake tracking, or reminders of the underlying motives for behavior change such as an inspirational photograph of a loved one or of the patient engaging in a favored activity. In addition to helpful cues to prompt desired behaviors, it is important to remove cues for undesired behaviors from the environment (e.g., remove takeout menus, throw out all tobacco products).

It is also important to use knowledge gained about the patient's social environment when setting the stage for change. People in the patient's life may be barriers or facilitators to change. Recruit the facilitators, and make them part of the change plan. For example, a supportive spouse can agree to buy and cook appropriate food or set up times to go for walks together. Also, work with the patient to identify who may be a barrier to change and figure out ways to minimize negative influences. For example, if a patient enjoys socializing with a friend who is still smoking, maybe they can agree to socialize in environments where smoking is not allowed. Overall, in-depth knowledge of their social and physical environment will be key in helping patients shape their environment to best support their attempts.

Step 7: Monitoring and Feedback

When working on behavior change, behaviors require careful monitoring so that the patient has feedback and objective evidence of progress toward goals. In addition, the mere act of tracking a behavior can cause it to change (e.g., tracking smoking or meals can significantly change intake).[30] Patients should be encouraged to self-monitor health behaviors. People can self-monitor using a wide range of tracking mechanisms, from low-tech ones (paper and pen) to high-tech ones (wearables, mobile devices, etc.). Records to monitor progress should be simple to use and readily accessible. Ideally, behavior should be recorded as it is occurring, or immediately following; it will result in higher accuracy than trying to recall behavior a week or even a day later. Work with the patient to find a way to monitor behavior progress. For example, to measure physical activity, consider the following: Do they have a smartphone or activity tracker that they can use to monitor step counts? Can they be given a simple pedometer? Would they be more comfortable making a paper log of their exercise minutes? Identify a monitoring plan, and use it to have the patient log their activity. Similarly, a smoker should keep track of the number of cigarettes smoked per day. This tracking can be as simple as having an index card that is marked every time a cigarette is smoked. For a patient who is a current smoker, measuring their carbon monoxide (CO) level during each visit provides an objective measurement of progress. Objective monitoring allows patients to see their progress, and it allows the health care provider to monitor progress, provide feedback, and adjust goals as necessary.

Monitoring provides important information for the patient. For example, consider a patient who experiences muscle soreness after an exercise session. The patient should be counseled that it is not unusual or deleterious and that it is a positive indication of effort. Soreness can be tracked, so you can use further reduction of soreness after exercising as a measure of progress. Additionally, records of exercise efforts can be affirming. For example, a patient can see how they started with only being able to do 5 minutes on the treadmill and can now do 20. Similarly, a patient who is attempting to quit smoking should be counseled and supported through the initial withdrawal, but they will be able to see from CO measurements how their exposure to heart-harming substances is decreasing while also marking their progress through decreased shortness of breath. It is the responsibility of the health care provider to educate the patient on the short- and long-term effects of the behavior changes. Patients will require support to get through the initial, potentially negative outcomes to be successful long enough to encounter the positive, longer-term outcomes. Informing patients about the potential short- and long-term effects will bolster success.

Step 8: Rewarding Effort and Progress

Supporting initial attempts at change is crucial to patient success. Often initial changes come with negative consequences. Medications may come with side effects that need to be addressed, starting physical activity can come with pain and fatigue, and smoking cessation creates distressing symptoms of withdrawal. Concepts from behavioral economics can help explain the challenge of new changes as well as possible ways to assuage the negatives. For example, the concept of delay discounting (or temporal discounting) says that people weigh current outcomes (the discomfort of these new behaviors) more heavily than more distant outcomes (e.g., more energy, less shortness of breath, more stamina, etc.).[31] The pain of the current attempt weighs much more heavily than the positive outcomes that are off in the future. Accordingly, it is imperative that initial behavior changes be paired with something positive in order to overcome this discounting.

One can increase the likelihood of a behavior occurring in many ways. Many more resources on behavioral economics and operant reinforcement are available,[29,32] but a few examples are listed here:

• *Premack principle.* If you follow a behavior you want the patient to increase with an activity the patient likes to engage in, the occurrence of the wanted behavior will increase. First, find a behavior the patient enjoys (e.g., reading a book). Have them agree not to engage in that behavior until they have completed the wanted behavior (e.g., going for their 20-minute walk).

• *Temptation bundling.* You can also combine the wanted behavior with a positive behavior. For example, the patient can agree not to watch their favorite TV show unless they are doing exercises at the same time, or have the patient only listen to their favorite audiobooks or podcasts if they are walking. One way to increase the effectiveness of these approaches is to have the patient make these decisions public to friends and family.

Additionally, rewards (self-rewards as well as rewards by program staff) for achieving short- or long-term goals are key in reinforcing adherence to health behavior change. Rewards need not be expensive; they need to be connected with specific milestone achievements such as completing the exercise goal for the week or having gone three days without smoking. Provision of rewards from programs has been tested specially for supporting the goal of CR attendance. Both provisions of small rewards (t-shirts, water bottles) in a general CR population, as well as larger financial incentives in high-risk patients, have been successful at increasing completion of CR sessions.[33,34] Regardless of any external source of reinforcement used, patients need to be aware of the personal rewards inherent in improved health and quality of life. Behavior change will likely be easier to sustain when supported by intrinsic reinforcement (e.g., ability to play with a grandchild or perform a desired recreational physical activity).

Step 9: Making Adjustments as Necessary

Remember that lapse (a temporary slip, such as a discontinuation of a behavior) and relapse (a long-term discontinuation of the behavior) are highly likely in behavior change, and patients should be counseled to this effect. Patients should be encouraged to view lapse or relapse not as a failure but rather as an opportunity to learn and try new strategies. Support patients by telling them that change is challenging and so-called failure is very common. Reframe failure as a learning opportunity; each time a patient fails, they are actually learning something about what doesn't work for them, that success often takes multiple tries and approaches to achieve, and that each try is getting them closer to their goal. For example, it may take an established smoker on average 30 tries to quit, but additional attempts are predictive of eventual success.[35]

Regardless of the reasons for difficulties with change, these difficulties must be used as cues to reassure the patient that they are not failing or doing anything wrong and work with them to adjust the plan or find new strategies. As necessary, the provider should go through the previous eight steps with the patient to identify where the plan needs modification. The patient is attempting to change behaviors they spent a lifetime obtaining, so it is expected that multiple attempts and different approaches will be required.

BOTTOM LINE

Supporting positive behavior change requires a multistep approach, including the following:

- Performing a baseline patient assessment regarding behavior change
- Providing patient education regarding the importance of changing deleterious behaviors
- Assessing the patient's willingness to change
- Identifying barriers to behavior change
- Establishing a plan for implementing changes in behavior
- Setting the stage for change by reducing or removing barriers
- Monitoring and providing feedback regarding progress toward achieving behavior change goals
- Establishing a reward system for achieving progress toward behavior change
- Making adjustments based on progress toward achieving behavioral change goals

Summary

Behavior change is challenging. However, following the steps in this chapter will help the health care provider work with the patient to increase the likelihood of success. Overall, the behavior change process is collaborative and iterative; it will necessitate effort by both the health care provider and the patient, and it will require monitoring and modification to maximize the chances for long-term success.

Modifiable CVD Risk Factors

Sheri R. Colberg, PhD, FACSM; Emma Fletcher, MS, MVB; Carly Goldstein, PhD; Paul M. Gordon, PhD, MPH, FACSM; Joel Hughes, PhD, FAACVPR; Jonathan Myers, PhD; Quinn R. Pack, MD, MsC, FAACVPR; Killian Robinson, MD, FAHA, FACC, FACP

A hallmark of SP for CVD is risk factor modification. Since the previous edition of these guidelines, much has been learned and published regarding control of modifiable risk factors. In fact, the AHA/ACC guidelines for HTN have been updated during that time period. In addition, the dyslipidemia guidelines have been updated twice. In 2013, AACVPR published and endorsed the ACC/AHA Guideline on the Assessment of Cardiovascular Risks.[46] Within this publication, a 10-year CVD risk calculator was published and is available for download on smart devices.

OBJECTIVES

This chapter provides an overview of the following:

- The modifiable risk factors that contribute to the development of cardiovascular disease
- Contemporary guidance on controlling modifiable risk factors based on published professional organization guidelines when available
- Suggestions for the implementation of methods to affect modifiable risk factors in the CR setting

As stated in the previous edition of these guidelines, CR programs are primarily risk factor modification programs. It is vital to identify individual risk factors on which patients are prepared to intervene at CR program entrance. Providing information and skills for patients to intervene should be emphasized both individually (e.g., discussions during exercise class) and in small group settings either before or immediately after the exercise portion of CR. Specific individual risk factor interventions may be informed by, as well as enhance, the level of patient awareness by using the 10-year risk calculator.

This chapter reviews the following risk factors:

- Physical inactivity
- HTN
- Dyslipidemia
- Diabetes
- Tobacco use
- Obesity/overweight
- Psychosocial concerns
- Environmental concerns

Physical Inactivity

Physical inactivity is one of the five primary risk factors for CVD,[1] but it is frequently overlooked clinically in favor treating the more traditional risk factors such as smoking, HTN, and lipid abnormalities.[2-4] One of the major challenges for secondary prevention programs is the recognition that physical inactivity not only leads to a higher incidence of CVD but is also associated with higher mortality and rates of reinfarction, stroke, and other cardiovascular conditions after an initial cardiac event.[3,5,6] Thus, it is critical that CR practitioners encourage patients to remain physically active beyond the period of rehabilitation. Indeed, because CR generally provides only a short window in which to intervene (about 12 weeks), a critical function of the CR practitioner is to provide patients with the education, motivation, and resources necessary to maintain a lifestyle of regular PA in the long term.

U.S. national statistics suggest that the majority of adults do not meet the minimal PA recommendations widely publicized by the federal government and other prominent health organizations.[1,7-13] This fact presents another challenge for CR programs, because patients with known CVD tend to be even more sedentary than the broader U.S. population.[14,15] In addition, both low CRF[16-19] and accumulated sedentary or sitting time[20-24] are associated with increased risks for CVD and all-cause mortality. A robust body of evidence suggests that the relationships between CVD risk and levels of PA and CRF are inverse, graded, and most importantly, modifiable.[16-19,25,26] This growing body of evidence regarding the strength of the association between CRF and CVD risk provided the impetus for a recent AHA scientific statement supporting CRF as a risk factor.[19] In fact, many studies have shown that low CRF is a more powerful predictor of risk than the traditional risk factors for CVD (HTN, smoking, lipid abnormalities), and this is true among individuals both with and without CVD.[16-19,24,26] Therefore, allied health professionals should view increasing PA and CRF, as well as reducing overall sitting time, as important goals in SP programs. The following sections provide information related to definitions, risks, assessment, and recommendations for PA and CRF.

There are numerous national and international public health statements related to physical activity. These documents are consistent in terms of defining a PA threshold below which one would be considered habitually *inactive*.[7-10,12,13,27] The concept that accumulating <150 min/week of moderate-intensity PA (or <75 min of vigorous-intensity PA) is widely used to identify an insufficiently active lifestyle. In addition, a growing number of studies[20-24,28] focused on physical inactivity from a different perspective, that is, time spent seated each day (termed *sitting time* or *sedentary time*). These studies suggest that daily sitting time, independent of leisure-time PA, is strongly related to all-cause and CVD mortality. Operational definitions for physical *inactivity* will continue to evolve as better assessments of leisure-time PA become available and are deployed within population-based studies of CVD risk (see Assessment of PA, later in this chapter).

Unlike PA, which is a *behavior*, CRF is an attribute. CRF is typically directly measured or predicted from the results of an exercise tolerance test. The most common definition of CRF is the capacity of the body to consume oxygen, often referred to as peak oxygen uptake (peak $\dot{V}O_2$) or $\dot{V}O_2$max. PA is the most important behavioral factor that affects CRF, therefore PA and CRF are interrelated. A chronic increase (or decrease) in PA often leads to a similar change in CRF. However, an increase in PA does not lead to an increase in CRF in all individuals, and some may respond more favorably to higher-intensity PA. CRF is influenced by a genetic component; that is, some people are inherently more fit than others regardless of their PA patterns.

Relative Risk of Physical Inactivity

Prospective observational studies have typically shown that the relative risk for CVD is approximately 2 to 4 times greater when the least active individuals are compared to the most physically active within a study cohort.[3,18,21,29] This relative risk is similar to that reported for many of the other risk factors reviewed in this chapter. In addition, among studies that analyzed disease risk across multiple ordinal categories of reported PA (e.g., low, moderate, high), the risk is graded, indicating that CVD risk decreases progressively across categories of PA from low through moderate to high. An example is shown in figure 9.1. It is often referred to as a *dose–response* relationship and has been summarized in public health messages in the following way[13]:

- Important health benefits (CVD risk reduction) can be obtained by including a moderate amount of PA on most, if not all, days of the week.

- Additional health benefits (further CVD risk reduction) result from greater amounts of PA.

Given the combination of high prevalence of inactivity in much of the Western world (> 50%) and the two- to fourfold relative risk for CVD, interventions that target inactive lifestyles have significant potential to lower the overall CVD risk burden. Moreover, inactivity is a unique risk trait in that it has both a direct and an indirect impact on CVD risk. While numerous studies have shown that the CVD risk associated with inactivity is independent of other CVD risk factors such as smoking, HTN, obesity, T2DM, and lipid abnormalities, well-controlled clinical trials of exercise training have consistently shown that habitual PA has a modulating effect on these CVD risk factors.[3,10,18,19,25,26] Therefore, the importance of targeting physical inactivity in risk reduction programs, such as CR, goes beyond the independent influence that a more active lifestyle has on lowering CVD risk.

As mentioned, observational reports have also focused on inactive time. A growing number of studies have reported that greater amounts of time spent sitting are associated with adverse health outcomes. Katzmarzyk and colleagues[22] reported a progressively higher risk of CVD mortality across increasing hours of sitting time among 17,013 Canadians aged 18 to 90 years.

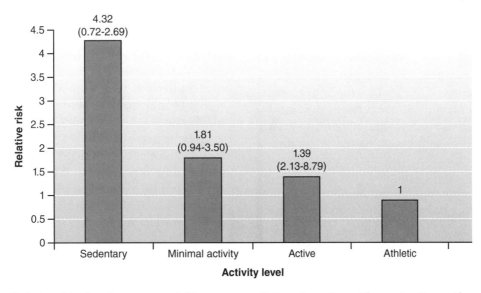

Figure 9.1 Relative risks for all-cause mortality among activity categories, with most active as the reference group (p for trend <.001; relative risks and 95% CIs above each bar). Subjects in the active category were considered to meet the minimal guidelines for PA.

Reprinted by permission from J. Myers et al., "Improved Reclassification of Mortality Risk by Assessment of Physical Activity in Patients Referred for Exercise Testing," *American Journal of Medicine* 128 (2015): 396-402.

Their findings were also independent of self-reported leisure-time PA. Stamatakis and coauthors[23] followed 4,512 Scottish men for about five years and quantified the amount of moderate- to vigorous-intensity PA at baseline as well as screen viewing time per day. After adjustment for traditional CVD risk factors, including leisure-time PA, incidence of CVD was twice as likely among men who reported ≥4 hours of screen time per day compared to those reporting <2 hours/day. In a recent meta-analysis including 14 studies, prolonged sedentary time was independently associated with deleterious health outcomes regardless of PA status.[28] Greater sedentary time was associated with higher risks for all-cause and CVD mortality, CVD incidence, cancer mortality, cancer incidence, and incidence of T2DM. Moreover, incorporating a higher number of breaks in sedentary time is associated with better health outcomes. While these recent reports confirm the lower CVD risk associated with moderate to vigorous PA, they extend the understanding of the unique risks associated with significant amounts of sedentary time. In other words, even people who adopt a more active lifestyle can likely reduce their risk further by limiting the amount of time they spend watching television or engaging in other screen-based activities that typically coincide with sitting for prolonged periods.

Relative Risk of Low Cardiorespiratory Fitness

Numerous prospective, observational studies show that lower CRF predicts all-cause and CVD morbidity and mortality independent of other CVD risk factors.[13,16-19,25,26] This finding is consistent for both primary and secondary prevention, as well as across studies that employed varying measures of CRF (i.e., measured v. predicted $\dot{V}O_2$max, treadmill v. cycle ergometer modalities, and maximal v. submaximal tests). Large, prospective cohorts including the Aerobics Center Longitudinal Study,[30,31] the Veterans Exercise Testing Study,[16,32,33] and the Henry Ford Exercise Testing (FIT) project[34-36] report that each 1 MET increase in CRF is associated with a 10% to 20% reduction in mortality. In addition, a consistent observation in these studies is the fact that the greatest reductions in risk occur at the low end of the fitness spectrum. Stated differently, the greatest benefits occur between the least fit (typically

<5.0 METs) and the next least fit group, while more modest benefits are observed among people who are moderately or highly fit. Given that a large proportion of patients begin a program with relatively low CRF levels, this information is encouraging. Moreover, studies have shown that even small improvements in CRF through CR are associated with considerable improvements in short and long-term health outcomes.[37-38]

Assessment of PA

An accurate assessment of the presence of all CVD risk factors includes assessing physical inactivity. As stated earlier, a person is considered to be physically inactive without *sufficient PA*, which is defined as not meeting the recommendations from the 2018 Physical Activity Guidelines for Americans.[8] As with smoking status, the length of time (months, years) a patient has been inactive should also be assessed. Although a standard has not been established, a pattern of inactivity ≥3 months is often the measure indicating a sedentary lifestyle.

Physical activity is multidimensional and is a complex behavior to measure.[39] To determine whether a person is achieving sufficient PA, the components of PA (duration, frequency, and intensity) need to be assessed. One challenge in PA assessment involves determining the intensity of PA, which can be classified as either relative to the individual (i.e., % of maximal capacity) or absolute (moderate and vigorous intensity are operationally defined as 3-5.9 METs and ≥6 METs, respectively).[39] Expressions of PA patterns that combine both intensity and duration such as MET-h/week (the MET level of a given activity times the number of hours per week) or MET-min/week, are widely used in epidemiologic studies and are useful for CR programs.[8,21,37] Meeting the recommended minimal threshold of 150 min of moderate PA/week[8] is generally considered the equivalent of 9-10 MET-h/week. Inappropriate or crude measures of PA are likely to yield misleading results.[39] Thus, it is important for CR staff to carefully consider the methods they use to assess PA.

The two most common methods used to assess PA status are self-report questionnaires (subjective) and use of PA monitors (objective). The advantage of questionnaires is that they are inexpensive and require little time to administer. However, subjective methods are limited by the ability of the respondent to accurately remember PA behaviors and to accurately classify the intensity of PA. Technology related to wearable PA monitors has advanced considerably in recent years. Many of these instruments are inexpensive and are useful for objectively estimating ambulatory movement, including exercise intensity. An increasing number of wearable monitors have been designed to track HR and energy expenditure in CR programs or other clinical populations,[40] and some can be used to monitor other health behaviors such as dietary and sleep patterns.

A low-cost option for helping people increase their PA is using a pedometer.[39-42] Pedometer features range from simple daily step counts that need to be manually recorded to weekly or longer storage that can be downloaded to a computer. Many wearable monitors today include both a pedometer and an accelerometer, which allows patients to monitor steps as well as time spent in moderate- or vigorous-intensity PA and time spent inactive. Wearable devices that include an accelerometer can have a great deal of utility in CR programs; they capture PA duration, frequency, and intensity, and they can also quantify duration of inactivity. Patients usually require standardized instructions for use of these devices. A typical assessment period might be seven days, but many devices can be used intermittently or throughout the duration of CR. Criteria for acceptable data from a PA monitor include that it be worn a minimum of 12 h/day and that a minimum of four complete days are recorded. Accelerometer data can often be stored on a computer and processed by device-specific software, which can generate various types of reports. CR staff can review this information from patients to provide feedback and support to help them achieve their PA goals.

Examples of data reports from accelerometers that can be used to determine PA behavior are shown in figures 9.2 and 9.3. These examples show patient data from the first week of maintenance CR and then again following 12 weeks of participation. This patient significantly increased PA measured as steps per day and moderate- to vigorous-activity minutes per day. Limitations of wearable monitors have been studied extensively and described[39]; they include the fact that non-ambulatory PA is not captured, purchasing the monitors and replacing lost or damaged devices entail an expense, and some monitors require a degree of technical skill that some patients do not have.

BOTTOM LINE

- Knowledge of a patient's PA pattern helps to optimize the exercise prescription, optimize adherence by providing insight into normal activity preferences, and to set individualized goals for activity.
- Many questionnaires have been validated for assessing PA patterns.
- Following baseline activity assessment, an accelerometer may be worn to provide an objective measure of activity.
- To get a valid estimate of activity, the accelerometer should be worn for a minimum of 12 h/day and a minimum of four days.
- The wearable device may be used intermittently during the CR program to provide objective estimates of activity while exercising at home.

While numerous questionnaires are available to assess PA, the International Physical Activity Questionnaire (IPAQ) that follows (available on the IPAQ website) is one example of a widely used tool for standardizing PA assessment in CR (figure 9.4). This instrument quantifies PA duration, frequency, and intensity. Moreover, the types of activities can be customized to those most common in the population being assessed. The IPAQ also provides information on sitting time which, as previously mentioned, may be useful in determining an overall CVD risk profile.[21-24,28] It is easy to compare time and frequency reported for moderate and vigorous PA on the IPAQ to the recommended standards of >150 min/week (moderate) or >75 min/week (vigorous). The IPAQ can also provide a classification into one of three levels (see IPAQ Classification Categories) and

 Guideline 9.1   PA Assessment in CR

All CR participants should have an initial PA assessment.

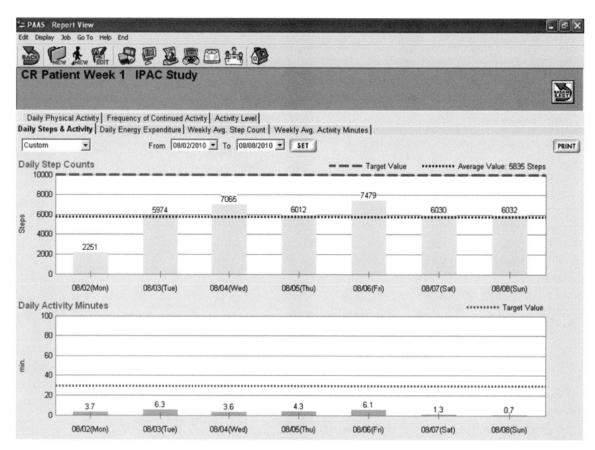

Figure 9.2 An accelerometer report from a baseline PA assessment at the beginning of a maintenance CR/SP. The results show that the patient is insufficiently active (averaging only 5,835 steps/day and accumulating only 26 min/week of moderate to vigorous PA).

Courtesy of Ball State University Clinical Exercise Physiology Program.

uses the MET · min^{-1} variable mentioned in the 2018 Physical Activity Guidelines for Americans to help quantify the total volume of PA.[8]

An alternative, time-tested, and inexpensive alternative to wearable devices is for patients to complete a weekly log of their daily PA or use a weekly recall questionnaire. Daily activity logs or weekly recall questionnaires can also serve as an adjunct to wearable devices to help ascertain that the device is providing accurate information. Patients can complete them with online support, in person, or as part of weekly phone calls by CR staff. Patients can be given clear goals (e.g., minimum of 150 min/week of moderate-intensity PA outside of CR), and the patient's ability to comply with activity recommendations can be reviewed on a weekly basis.

Patients may also consider using the Internet to obtain resources and support for making lifestyle changes and monitoring PA patterns. These online resources vary. For example, some are specific platforms that have a monthly or yearly fee and support access to materials and/or staff in assisting the user; some are free and require patients to enter their PA data; and some are free with the purchase of a wearable device or smartphone or accelerometers, allowing for downloading data directly from the PA monitor.

Providing patients with an assessment of their PA habits can be invaluable. These assessments allow for clear feedback regarding whether patients are meeting the thresholds of >150 min/week (moderate) or >75 min/week (vigorous) PA that are recommended for health benefits. Similarly, these assessments can inform patients and their clinicians of inactivity (sitting time). Although currently no clear standards for sitting time exist, it is becoming increasingly clear that

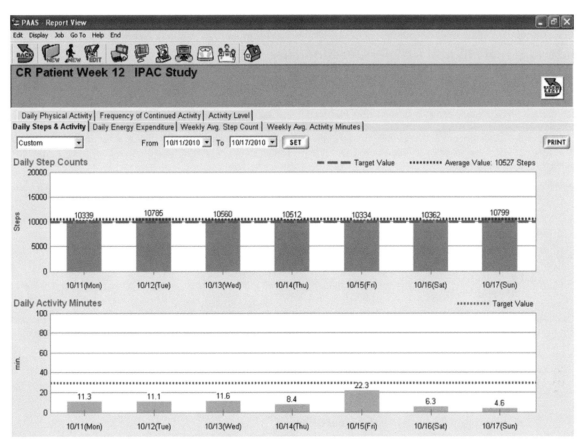

Figure 9.3 An accelerometer report from a PA assessment at the 12th week of a maintenance CR/SP. The results show that the patient has significantly increased her PA level (now averaging 10,527 steps a day and now accumulating about 75 min/week of moderate to vigorous PA).

Courtesy of Ball State University Clinical Exercise Physiology Program.

prolonged sitting or time spent sedentary is deleterious to health, and participants in CR programs should be encouraged to reduce sitting time.[20-24,28]

Assessment of CRF

As mentioned previously, CRF is typically assessed using a maximal exercise test. Because exercise therapy is a cornerstone of CR, it is important to get a baseline assessment in order to most effectively dose the exercise prescription as well as to identify contraindications or potential limitations to exercise training.[1] (See chapter 4, Risk Stratifications and Identification of Contraindications for Exercise Training.) In addition, assessment of CRF with sign- or symptom-limited exercise testing before and after an exercise intervention can yield important objective information related to safety, the appropriate exercise dose, and changes in CRF. However, an exercise test

may not always be possible or recommended, thus the need for assessing functional status of patients using tools described previously. For example, nonexercise test estimates of exercise capacity have been developed,[19] although they generally are not validated in patients with CVD and therefore should be interpreted with caution in the CR setting. Recommendations for the optimal use of exercise testing are available from the ACSM, AHA, and other professional organizations.[1,44,45]

Dyslipidemia

Atherosclerosis begins when cholesterol and other fatty substances deposit in arterial walls and cause arterial inflammation, hardening, and dysfunction. Indeed, when broken down to its Latin roots, the word *athero* describes a substance that is soft, fatty, and pastelike while *sclerosis* describes a hardening. While many risk factors are associated with

Figure 9.4 International Physical Activity Questionnaire

International Physical Activity Questionnaire

We are interested in finding out about the kinds of physical activities that people do as part of their everyday lives. The questions will ask you about the time you spent being physically active in the **last 7 days**. Please answer each question even if you do not consider yourself to be an active person. Please think about the activities you do at work, as part of your house and yard work, to get from place to place, and in your spare time for recreation, exercise, or sport.

Think about all the **vigorous** activities that you did in the **last 7 days**. **Vigorous** physical activities refer to activities that take hard physical effort and make you breathe much harder than normal. Think *only* about those physical activities that you did for at least 10 minutes at a time.

    1. During the **last 7 days**, on how many days did you do **vigorous** physical activities like heavy lifting, digging, aerobics, or fast bicycling?

        _____ **days per week**

        ☐ No vigorous physical activities → *skip to question 3*

    2. How much time did you usually spend doing **vigorous** physical activities on one of those days?

        _____ **hours per day**
        _____ **minutes per day**

Think about all the **moderate** activities that you did in the **last 7 days**. **Moderate** activities refer to activities that take moderate physical effort and make you breathe somewhat harder than normal. Think only about those physical activities that you did for at least 10 minutes at a time.

    3. During the **last 7 days**, on how many days did you do **moderate** physical activities like carrying light loads, bicycling at a regular pace, or doubles tennis? Do not include walking.

        _____ **days per week**

        ☐ No moderate physical activities → *Skip to question 5*

    4. How much time did you usually spend doing **moderate** physical activities on one of those days?

        _____ **hours per day**
        _____ **minutes per day**

Think about the time you spent **walking** in the **last 7 days.** This includes at work and at home, walking to travel from place to place, and any other walking that you might do solely for recreation, sport, exercise, or leisure.

    5. During the **last 7 days,** on how many days did you **walk** for at least 10 minutes at a time?

        _____ **days per week**

        ☐ No walking → *Skip to question 7*

    6. How much time did you usually spend **walking** on one of those days?

        _____ **hours per day**
        _____ **minutes per day**

The last question is about the time you spent **sitting** on weekdays during the **last 7 days.** Include time spent at work, at home, while doing course work and during leisure time. This may include time spent sitting at a desk, visiting friends, reading, or sitting or lying down to watch television.

    7. During the **last 7 days,** how much time did you spend **sitting** on a **week day**?

        _____ **hours per day**
        _____ **minutes per day**

More Information

More detailed information on the IPAQ process and the research used in the development of IPAQ instruments is available on the IPAQ website and in ML Booth, Assessment of Physical Activity: An International Perspective, *Research Quarterly for Exercise and Sport,* 2000;71:s114-120. Other scientific publications and presentations on the use of IPAQ are summarized on the website.

IPAQ Classification Categories

Low (Category 1)

- Not active enough to meet criteria for Categories 2 or 3

Moderate (Category 2)

- ≥3 days of vigorous activity of ≥20 min/day OR
- ≥5 days of moderate activity or walking of ≥30 min/day OR
- ≥5 days of any combination of walking, moderate, or vigorous activity achieving a minimum of 600 MET-min/week

High (Category 3)

- Vigorous activity >3 days/week achieving at least 1,500 MET-min/week OR
- ≥7 days of any combination of walking, moderate, or vigorous activity achieving a minimum of 3,000 MET-min/week

Abbreviations: IPAQ, International Physical Activity Questionnaire; MET, metabolic equivalent

---

Reprinted from U.S. National Institute of Health. Available: www.ipaq.ki.se. LONG LAST 7 DAYS SELF-ADMINISTERED version of the IPAQ. Revised October 2002.

Guideline 9.2 Assessment of CRF

CRF should be assessed when a patient begins a CR program. CRF is optimally obtained from a maximal exercise test using a metabolic system that determines maximal oxygen uptake ($\dot{V}O_2$max or peak $\dot{V}O_2$). Because exercise testing is often performed clinically without a metabolic system, CRF is frequently estimated from the work rate achieved (peak speed/grade on a treadmill or peak watts on a cycle ergometer). CRF can be expressed as a MET (metabolic equivalent of task) level achieved; this term is convenient for making activity recommendations because most activities have an approximate MET level ascribed to them.

When a maximal exercise test is not available, many other methods are available to estimate CRF, including submaximal estimates of CRF. Questionnaires, such as the Duke Activity Status Index or the Veterans Specific Activity Questionnaire, which assess a patient's functional capabilities or symptoms during daily activities, can also be used to assist the practitioner to develop an appropriate exercise prescription. Nonexercise test estimates of CRF that correlate reasonably well with measured CRF have also been used.

The 6-minute walk test (maximum distance walked in meters during 6 minutes) is generally not considered a measure of CRF. However, this widely used assessment provides an estimate of a patient's functional status, is a reflection of the capacity to perform daily activities, and has prognostic value.

---

atherosclerotic cardiovascular disease (ASCVD), elevated blood lipids are essential to the development of atherosclerosis. In fact, increased lipid levels appear to be so fundamental to the disease process of atherosclerosis that ASCVD is rare in people with lifelong very low lipid levels, even in the presence of other risk factors.[1] As a result, all CR clinicians should be very familiar with the management of abnormal lipid levels and be able to counsel their patients about how to reduce their risk in accordance with the 2018 ACC/AHA Guidelines for the Treatment of Blood Cholesterol and other recent publications.[2,3] These guidelines serve as the primary reference for patients attending CR and SP programs and supersede all other prior guidelines.

Although the evaluation and pharmacologic treatment of hyperlipidemia is beyond the scope of practice for most CR personnel, staff members should be familiar with the causes and treatments of hyperlipidemia. This knowledge helps ensure that education and advice are tailored to the individual patient. CR professionals can also work with physicians and patients to encourage medication adherence and answer questions about indications and side effects of common medications. In this way, CR staff members are an integral part of the treatment team by enhancing the evaluation of hyperlipidemia and amplify its impact.

Cholesterol and Lipoproteins

Blood cholesterol is a fatlike substance (lipid) that is present in cell membranes and is a precursor of bile acids and steroid hormones. Cholesterol travels in the blood in distinct particles that contain both lipids and proteins, called lipoproteins. Blood cholesterol level is determined by genetics, environmental factors, and health behaviors such as diet, caloric balance, and level of PA. The three major classes of lipoproteins found in the blood are low-density lipoprotein cholesterol (LDL-C), high-density lipoprotein cholesterol (HDL-C), and very low-density lipoprotein cholesterol (VLDL-C). VLDL-C is a precursor of LDL-C; and some forms of VLDL-C, particularly VLDL-C remnants, appear to be atherogenic.[4]

LDL-C is typically calculated from measurements of total cholesterol, total fasting TG, and HDL-C. If the triglyceride value is below 400 mg/dL, then its value can be divided by 5 to estimate the VLDL-C level. Because the level of total cholesterol is the sum of LDL-C, HDL-C, and VLDL-C, LDL-C can be calculated as follows (all quantities are in mg/dL):

$$LDL\text{-}C = Total\ cholesterol - HDL\text{-}C - (TG/5)$$

Because the LDL-C value is estimated from measurements that include TG, blood samples should be collected from patients who have fasted for 9 to 12 h, having taken nothing by mouth except water and medications. For patients with TG values over 400 mg/dL, estimation of LDL-C as just described is not accurate. In such cases, direct measurement of LDL by ultracentrifugation in a specialized laboratory is recommended. Cholesterol values can be affected by an acute CVD event. Therefore, it is recommended that the measurement of cholesterol occur within 24 h following the event. Almost all patients who are diagnosed with an acute coronary event or coronary revascularization will be started on a high-intensity statin while in hospital. As a result, blood cholesterol levels should be measured again 4 to 6 weeks later to establish an accurate postevent baseline and to evaluate the efficacy of prescribed medication(s).[3]

Normal Cholesterol Levels

Most analytic laboratories define cholesterol levels by using the population distribution of LDL-C levels. Using this method, most laboratories define a normal LDL-C as any level less than the 1980s population mean (SD) of 130 ± 30 mg/dL. However, because of public health efforts and increased use of medications, the past two decades have witnessed a steady decline in lipid levels, such that the 2010 U.S. population mean LDL-C level was ~115 mg/dL.[5] Even at LDL-C levels of 115 mg/dL, most adults will develop some degree of atherosclerosis by the time they are 80 years old,[6] and lower levels of LDL-C are likely needed to prevent ASCVD across the entire population.

The most important alternative definition of hyperlipidemia is the "physiologic normal," which is the cholesterol level at which atherosclerosis does not occur. Based on the LDL-C levels of healthy newborn babies, hunter-gatherer human populations, and primates, this level appears to fall in the 50 mg/dL range, a range in which atherosclerosis is rarely seen.[7] Moreover, an LDL-C of about 60 mg/dL is the level at which the progression of atherosclerosis no longer occurs and regression is possible.[8] Using this alternative definition of hyperlipidemia, the vast majority of U.S. adults have hyperlipidemia and are at risk for developing atherosclerosis and clinical ASCVD. This definition explains why patients with so-called normal cholesterol levels (using laboratory population norms) still experience myocardial infarction and why they benefit from cholesterol-lowering therapies. These studies, in combination with evidence conclusively demonstrating that LDL-C causes atherosclerosis,[9] create a compelling case for the aggressive treatment of hyperlipidemia for almost all patients to lower LDL.[10] It is particularly true in CR where most patients have experienced a clinical ASCVD event.

Assessment of Hyperlipidemia

Because hyperlipidemia is such an important and treatable risk factor, all patients in CR should have a recent assessment of fasting lipids, preferably performed within the 6 months prior to CR program entry. Typically, lipid measures are obtained during a hospital admission but could be obtained in an outpatient setting or at the time of enrollment in CR. Ideally, a lipid profile is determined prior to the institution of lipid lowering therapies, but it is not required.

In conjunction with the patient's treating physician, clinical evaluation of patients with abnormal lipids should include a detailed history to determine potential contributors to elevated lipid levels such as various disease states, contributing dietary factors, or, in some instances, medications. Secondary causes of abnormal lipids include the following:

- Diabetes mellitus
- Hypothyroidism
- Nephrotic syndrome
- Obstructive liver disease

Drugs that may raise LDL-C levels or lower HDL-C levels, particularly progestins, anabolic steroids, corticosteroids; and certain antihypertensive agents, thiazide diuretics, and loop diuretics, can cause an elevation of total cholesterol, LDL-C, and triglycerides.

Although limited in their impact, beta-blockers without intrinsic sympathomimetic activity or alpha-blocking properties increase serum TG and lower HDL-C. However, these drugs are not contraindicated in the presence of abnormal lipids. The use of beta-blockers must be considered in the context of their benefit in treating other disorders versus their potential adverse effect on the lipid profile.

Because abnormal lipids sometimes are the result of familial genetic disorders, a careful family history can help to determine the etiology and management of LDL-C elevations in affected patients, as well as potentially identify family members who need therapy for high cholesterol levels. Increasing evidence shows that additional factors, such as lipoprotein(a), fibrinogen levels, and immune responses, interact with lipids in

ways that can also increase ASCVD risk.[11] Homocysteine is no longer considered an additional factor to measure or treat for CVD.[12] Therefore, population-wide screening for elevated homocysteine levels is not recommended.

Specific areas of the physical examination relevant to abnormal lipids include a careful examination of the eyes to document corneal arcus, a funduscopic examination to detect retinal changes due to abnormal lipids, and an examination of the skin to detect xanthoma or xanthelasma. Specific laboratory assessment in the hyperlipidemic patient might include thyroid-stimulating hormone (TSH), HbA1c, serum creatinine, and liver function tests at baseline.

Therapeutic Lifestyle Changes

Treatment of dyslipidemia must include therapeutic lifestyle changes, including dietary intervention, physical activity, and weight loss, as a part of any risk reduction program. A full separate lifestyle guideline was published in 2013.[13] The main nutrition recommendation for patients with high LDL-C levels is to "consume a dietary pattern that emphasizes intake of vegetables, fruits, and whole grains; includes low-fat dairy products, poultry, fish, legumes, nontropical vegetable oils, and nuts; and limits intake of sweets, sugar-sweetened beverages, and red meats."[13] Eliminating trans fat and limiting intake of saturated fat to only 5% to 6% of daily calories should be priorities. A dietary pattern that closely resembles the MEDIT diet is associated with improved patient outcomes.[14] In obese patients, significant weight loss (including bariatric surgery) greatly reduces LDL-C levels.[15] This dietary pattern is adaptable to personal and cultural food preferences, and a patient can accomplish it with the help and guidance of a registered dietician. Detailed information regarding dietary recommendations are provided in chapter 7.

Pharmacologic Treatment of Hyperlipidemia

The 2013 ACC/AHA guidelines identified four major groups of patients likely to benefit from statin medication; these four groups are presented in the sidebar.[16] They classified statins into three groups (low, moderate, and high intensity) by the estimated percent reduction in LDL-C observed in clinical trials, with high-intensity statin doses

Guideline 9.3   Evaluation of Lipids

All patients with established ASCVD should have a fasting lipoprotein analysis for LDL-C determination at baseline and again 4 to 8 weeks after medication prescription.

expected to reduce LDL-C by an average of >50% (table 9.1).

Patients with established CVD and those with familial hyperlipidemia (LDL >190 mg/dL) should be started on a high-intensity statin as tolerated.[16] (See guideline 9.4.) Patients with diabetes should be started on moderate-intensity statin medications unless their estimated 10-year CVD risk is ≥7.5%, in which case a high-intensity statin is appropriate. Finally, patients with an estimated 10-year CVD risk of ≥7.5% can be started on either a high- or moderate-intensity statin.

Safety and side-effect profile of statin medications (as a class) are generally excellent. However, up to 10% of patients develop side effects; the most common is mild muscle pain.[17] *Myalgias* are diffuse aches of the large muscles of the legs, buttocks, and back, and they are reversible with discontinuation of the statin medication. Notably, these are rarely associated with joint pain and frequently start within 12 weeks from the first statin dose.[17] In patients negatively affected by lipid lowering therapy, lower intensity statin medication or intermittent dosing schedules should be employed, but these approaches are only recommended when higher intensity medications are not tolerated.[18]

Previously, routine monitoring of liver function was recommended after initiation of statin therapy. However, since 2012, the FDA has recommended liver function tests only when a clinical suspicion for hepatotoxicity exists, because true liver injury from statins is extremely rare.[19] As a result, routine testing of lipids (on an annual basis or other similar time frame) is no longer required unless a change occurs in the patient's clinical status, the patient experiences a side effect, or a medication toxicity results in a change of prescription medication.

In CR, the two groups who do not necessarily need high-intensity statin are patients with heart valve surgery and nonischemic heart failure without concomitant ASCVD. CR patients without CVD may still be prescribed a statin, but they need to have a 10-year risk of ASCVD of ≥7.5%, similar to patients without ASCVD who are taking a statin for primary prevention. This 10-year risk can be calculated using an online tool available at the ACC website; search for the ASCVD Risk Calculator. This calculator estimates a patient's risk and includes age, sex, race, smoking status, BP, total and HDL-C, the presence of diabetes, and the use of anti-hypertensive, statin, and aspirin medications. The calculator uses the 2013 pooled cohort equations to estimate the risk of death from CVD, nonfatal MI, or fatal or nonfatal stroke.[11] This risk tool has been validated in several populations and is improved compared to the Framingham Risk Score, because it includes race and diabetes as risk factors.[20] It also includes the risk of stroke as a key outcome and was developed from recent cohort studies, so it is the preferred risk calculator. If the calculated risk is <5%, a statin medication is generally not recommended. Patients with a risk between 5% and 7.5% may be prescribed statins, but they are recommended only after a discussion of patient preferences.[3]

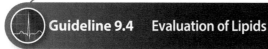

Guideline 9.4   Evaluation of Lipids

All patients with established ASCVD should be prescribed a high-intensity statin as tolerated unless they are age >75, in which case moderate-intensity statin is recommended.

Four Patient Groups With Major Benefit From Statins

1. Patients with clinical ASCVD, which includes patients with prior MI, angina, percutaneous coronary intervention, coronary artery bypass surgery, stroke, transient ischemic attack, peripheral arterial disease, cerebrovascular arterial disease, and abdominal aortic aneurysm

2. Patients with primary elevation of LDL-C >190 ml/dL (familial hyperlipidemia)

3. Patients with diabetes mellitus (either type 1 or type 2), age 40-75, with or without atherosclerotic disease

4. Patients with estimated 10-year CVD risk >7.5% among patients without any prior history of cardiovascular disease, as calculated by the ACC/AHA pooled cohort equation

Table 9.1 Statin Intensity by Drug and Dose

High-intensity statins Daily dose lowers LDL-C on average by ≥50%.	Moderate-intensity statins Daily dose lowers LDL-C on average by 30% to <50%.	Low-intensity statins Daily dose lowers LDL-C on average by <30%.
Atorvastatin 40, 80 mg Rosuvastatin 20, 40 mg	Atorvastatin 10, 20 mg Rosuvastatin 5, 10 mg Simvastatin 20, 40 mg Pravastatin 40, 80 mg Lovastatin 40 mg Fluvastatin 80 mg XL Fluvastatin 40 mg BID Pitavastatin 2, 4 mg	Simvastatin 10 mg Pravastatin 10, 20 mg Lovastatin 20 mg Fluvastatin 20-40 mg Pitavastatin 1 mg

Abbreviation: LDL-C, low-density lipoprotein cholesterol; XL, extended release; BID, twice daily

Reprinted with permission Circulation.2013;128:873-934 ©2013 American Heart Association, Inc.

Use of Non-Statin Medications to Lower LDL-C

The 2018 ACC/AHA guidelines continued to emphasize the essential role of statin medications as the first-line treatment for hyperlipidemia.[3] In all of these decisions, the guidelines strongly recommend regular monitoring of cholesterol levels with the goal of achieving an LDL-C level of <70 mg/dL if possible. While many patients achieve an LDL-C <70 mg/dL with high-intensity statin alone, some patients continue to have elevated LDL-C levels and may benefit from the addition of non-statin medications to further lower LDL-C concentrations to <70 mg/dL. These medications include ezetimibe and proprotein convertase subtilisin/kexin-9 (PCSK-9) inhibitors.

Ezetimibe (10 mg daily) blocks cholesterol absorption in the intestine and reduces LDL-C by 15% to 20%. It is generally well tolerated, although a few patients report upper respiratory symptoms and gastrointestinal upset. When added to simvastatin (40 mg), ezetimibe further lowered LDL-C from 70 to 54 mg/dL and resulted in a small but significant 2% absolute (6.4% relative) reduction in morbidity and mortality.[21] Consequently, ezetimibe is generally recommended in patients with ASCVD with an LDL-C >100 mg/dL, and it is reasonable to use in patients who are at high risk of recurrent events and have an LDL-C between 70 and 100 mg/dL. If possible, ezetimibe should always be used in combination with statins and added before the use of a PCSK-9 inhibitor.

PCSK-9 inhibitors work by preventing the degradation of PCSK-9, a protein involved in regulating hepatic LDL receptors. Inhibiting this protein increases hepatic LDL receptors and further reduces serum LDL-C levels even when used in combination with a statin. Two medications are approved for use in the United States (evolucumab and alirocumab) and are injected subcutaneously every two to four weeks. Injection site reactions are common, allergic reactions occur with some frequency, but otherwise these medications are generally well tolerated.[22] When added to a statin, they further reduce LDL-C levels by 50% to 70% and often achieve unprecedented LDL-C levels between 10 and 30 mg/dL.[23] In two outcome trials in patients with ASCVD, these medications significantly reduced the risk of recurrent heart attack and death by 15% to 20%.[24, 25] However, the impact was smaller than expected based on the degree of LDL-C lowering.[10] Additionally, because these medications are very expensive, use is highly restricted by insurance companies due to poor cost effectiveness.[26] As a result, the 2018 guidelines recommend these medications only as third-line medications (after high-intensity statin and ezetimibe). They should only be used in patients who are deemed to be at very high risk of recurrent events and only after a patient–clinician discussion about value and patient preferences. Based on these guidelines, it is likely the PCSK-9 inhibitors will be used only infrequently and primarily among patients with either familial hypercholesterolemia (very high residual LDL-C levels) or among patients who do not tolerate statins and continue to experience recurrent events.

Medications for HDL

While trials of LDL-C lowering therapies generally improve patient outcomes, the same is not true of therapies that modify other components of the cholesterol panel. Specifically, several recent interventions to increase HDL-C (niacin and cholesterol-esterase inhibitors) have failed to show any differences in outcomes, despite sizable changes in HDL-C levels.[27-29] These trials significantly tempered enthusiasm about the potential effects of modulating HDL-C, and these medications are not currently recommended for routine use.[2]

Medications for TGs

When added to statins, most prior studies show only small differences in cardiovascular outcomes for TG altering medications such as fish oil and fibrates.[30,31] As a result, these medications have been primarily used to prevent pancreatitis in patients with TG levels >500 mg/dL.[32,33]

Most of these studies used mixed omega-3 fatty acids (docosahexaenoic acid [DHA] and eicosapentaenoic acid (EPA)], and subjects were generally dosed at 1 g daily. A recent trial tested subjects using 2 g twice daily (4 g total dose) of purified icosapent ethyl (an ethylated form of EPA without any DHA) who were already taking a statin medication.[34] Most (70%) of the population had established ASCVD, and all participants had elevated triglycerides. This medication reduced risk of subsequent cardiac events by 25% but slightly increased atrial fibrillation and bleeding risk.[34] Given these results, it seems likely that many patients in CR will begin using this medication, but no official guideline statements exist at the time of this writing.

Long-Term Follow-Up

Achieving long-term control of dyslipidemia requires application of the same interest and attention on the part of both the patient and the CR staff to long-term management issues as to initial evaluation and treatment. The effective use of adherence-enhancing techniques combined with the effort and participation of a variety of skilled health care professionals, as found in the CR team, has the greatest potential for helping the patient achieve an optimal lipid profile. Specific strategies include the following:

- Teaching patients how adhere to the treatment regimen
- Helping patients identify ways to remember the dose of medication

- Teaching patients to identify, anticipate, and manage side effects
- Providing updates on the effectiveness of treatment and the importance of long-term adherence
- Ensuring mechanisms for patients to contact the health care professionals who supervise the lipid management

Because not all patients have equal response to statin medications, patients should undergo at least one lipid panel within 4 to 12 weeks after the initiation of statin medications to ensure medication effectiveness.[2,3,35] Test results will provide valuable feedback to patients and improve medication adherence. If the medication is effective, additional testing may not be needed as long as the patient remains adherent to treatment.

Diabetes

Diabetes mellitus is a complex metabolic disorder characterized by impaired glucose uptake caused by insufficient pancreatic insulin production or loss of peripheral insulin sensitivity. In 2017, the Centers for Disease Control and Prevention (CDC) estimated that 30.3 million Americans (9.4% of the U.S. population) have diagnosed or undiagnosed diabetes.[1] Of those estimated 30.3 million, approximately 90% to 95% have type 2 diabetes mellitus (T2DM), whereas most of the remainder have type 1 diabetes mellitus (T1DM). Another 84.1 million Americans (33.9% of adults ages 20 or older) have prediabetes, a condition in which blood glucose (BG) levels are elevated, raising their risk for T2DM.

Diabetes Types and Comorbid Health Conditions

T2DM more frequently has its onset in adulthood and is associated with an insulin-resistant state, accompanied by some loss of beta cell production of insulin. T1DM, typically diagnosed at a younger age than T2DM, involves an autoimmune process targeting the beta cells of the pancreas; all with T1DM must take exogenous insulin. Common comorbid health conditions for either type of diabetes include overweight or obesity, HTN, abnormal blood lipids, and low-level systemic inflammation. Diabetes is a significant contributor to premature mortality and morbidity related to CVD, blindness, kidney disease, nerve disease, and amputation.[1] Heart disease, stroke, HTN, and peripheral arterial disease are major causes of morbidity and mortality,[2] and many of these macrovascular health conditions are more prevalent in adults with diabetes.

Weight loss, dietary changes, and regular physical activity have been shown to lessen insulin resistance in people with T2DM and in those with T1DM who have higher levels of resistance, although comprehensive treatment of diabetes of either type frequently involves antihyperglycemic, antihypertensive, and lipid-lowering medications, especially in patients at risk for or with cardiovascular problems. The most important challenge that patients with diabetes face is how to comply with complex treatment regimens, many of which include management of CVD risks along with BG. CR professionals are in a key position to help monitor and motivate compliance with medications as well as with diet and exercise programs. CR staff must work closely with the primary care physician or endocrinologist to help optimize the lifestyle management of diabetes.

Role of Exercise in Diabetes Management

Anyone with diabetes who engages in regular physical activity can gain health benefits. In particular, the benefits of exercise for a patient with T2DM are even more substantial than for their peers without diabetes.[3] Regular exercise improves BG management, reduces the risk for CVD and its complications, and improves overall health and wellness in these patients, most of whom have comorbid health issues. Exercise can prevent or delay the onset of T2DM in high-risk patients with prediabetes.[4]

BOTTOM LINE

Patients with diabetes are at an increased risk of developing CVD. Patients with CVD and diabetes are at an increased risk of future cardiac events. These patients would benefit from SP and CR programs; when appropriate, they should be referred to these programs.

Most of the benefits of exercise and PA with respect to diabetes management are the result of enhancements in insulin sensitivity, accomplished through both cardiovascular endurance and resistance training. Increased CRF is also key. For each MET increase in aerobic capacity, mortality is apparently decreased by 19% and 14% for Caucasian and African American men, respectively, who are diagnosed with T2DM.[5] Enhanced fitness likely results from regular participation in PA, and insulin sensitivity typically remains elevated for hours to days after each exercise training session.[6,7] The following list outlines the role of exercise in patients with T2DM.

Exercise Impact on T2DM Management

- Improved sensitivity to insulin
- Better BG management
- Decrease in required doses of insulin or other hypoglycemic agents
- Reduced levels of plasma insulin
- Improved glucose tolerance
- Lower levels of A1c

While many of these same benefits of exercise are experienced by patients with T1DM, management of BG during and after exercise can be more problematic than for those with T2DM. Exercise increases glucose disposal and insulin sensitivity, but it can make maintaining glycemic balance a challenge when insulin is an additional variable. Adjustment of the therapeutic regimen (insulin and medical nutrition therapy) to allow safe and effective participation is an important management strategy in these patients, including self-monitoring BG levels associated with PA.[3,8,9] Hypoglycemia can occur during, immediately after, or many hours after activity. Hyperglycemia can also result from PA under certain circumstances. Knowledge of the activity-related metabolic responses, as well as sign and symptom awareness and self-management, can minimize these episodes. Tailored insulin therapy provides patients with the flexibility to make appropriate insulin dose adjustments for various levels of exertion rather than solely focusing on carbohydrate or other food supplementation to compensate.

Risks of Exercise in Patients With Diabetes

Most patients with diabetes can exercise safely. However, PA is not without risks for these patients.

Guideline 9.5   Certified Diabetes Educator

CR programs should consider having at least one CDE on staff whenever possible.

CR professionals should be aware of these risks.[3,8] It may be advisable for CR programs to consider having at least one Certified Diabetes Educator (CDE) on staff whenever possible. Many CR professionals may become a CDE, including clinical exercise physiologists and nurses.

Risks Associated with Exercise in Patients with Diabetes

Cardiovascular Risks

- Cardiac dysfunction and dysrhythmias caused by subclinical or diagnosed ischemic heart disease (silent ischemia)
- MI or stroke during PA
- Excessive increases or decreases in BP or HR caused by autonomic neuropathy
- Postexercise and orthostatic hypotension due to autonomic neuropathy

Metabolic Risks

- Hypoglycemia in patients taking insulin or select oral hypoglycemic agents (insulin secretagogues)
- Exacerbation of hyperglycemia
- Dehydration and potential electrolyte imbalances

Musculoskeletal and Traumatic Risks

- Overuse and acute injuries
- Foot ulcers (especially in the presence of peripheral neuropathy)
- Orthopedic injuries related to peripheral neuropathy

Microvascular Risks

- *Retinopathy:* Exercise that involves straining, jarring, or Valsalva-like maneuvers, as well as all vigorous exercise is contraindicated in patients with unstable proliferative diabetic retinopathy.

- *Diabetic kidney disease:* Low- to moderate-intensity activities are safe (even during dialysis), but high-intensity exercise may not be sustainable due to low fitness levels.
- *Peripheral neuropathy:* Comprehensive foot care and daily monitoring are required.

Preexercise Assessment and Testing of Patients With Diabetes

To maximize the benefits and minimize the risks of exercise in this patient population, it may be necessary to provide appropriate screening of patients, emphasize adherence to program design guidelines, and offer education and tools to improve glucose monitoring and overall CVD risk factor modification. It is essential to determine each patient's knowledge and understanding of diabetes and its management, including medication use, dietary considerations, and exercise regimen. This discussion should also specifically include

- insulin and other hypoglycemic agents,
- all other medications taken, including side effects and potential drug interactions,
- self-monitoring of BG levels, and
- current level of regular PA.

A patient's age and prior PA level should be considered when deciding on the necessity and extent of preexercise evaluation. In addition, the presence of diabetes-related health complications (e.g., peripheral neuropathy, severe autonomic neuropathy, and proliferative retinopathy) or other comorbid conditions may necessitate a more thorough evaluation prior to participation.[3,8] Patients should be assessed for conditions that might contraindicate certain types of exercise or predispose to injury, such as uncontrolled HTN, unstable proliferative retinopathy, autonomic neuropathy, peripheral neuropathy, and a history of foot ulcers or Charcot foot. Preexercise evaluation should also include other important assessments, such as a review of current medications and any physical limitations and symptoms suggestive of health complications (see chapter 2).

Due to an increased incidence of asymptomatic coronary artery disease in patients with diabetes, obtaining medical clearance is advisable if previously sedentary persons are to undertake an exercise program. However, in those who are planning to participate in low-intensity modes of exercise such as walking, the physician or health care professional should use clinical judgment in deciding whether to recommend further testing, such as a graded exercise stress test. This testing is not routinely recommended; however, providers should perform a careful history, assess cardiovascular risk factors, and be aware of the atypical presentation of coronary artery disease in patients with diabetes. High-risk patients (based on AACVPR risk categories) should be encouraged to start with short periods of low-intensity exercise and slowly increase the intensity and duration. Patients intending to begin a more vigorous exercise program (i.e., more vigorous than ADLs) should be assessed more fully before starting the program, especially if they are sedentary to start or in the presence of health complications.

General Indications for Exercise Stress Testing in Patients With Diabetes

- Age >40 years
- Age >30 years and any of the following:

  ○ T1DM or T2DM >10 years in duration
  ○ HTN
  ○ Cigarette smoking
  ○ Dyslipidemia
  ○ Proliferative or preproliferative retinopathy
  ○ Nephropathy including microalbuminuria

- Any of the following, regardless of age:

  ○ Known or suspected coronary artery disease (CAD), cerebrovascular disease, or peripheral artery disease (PAD)
  ○ Autonomic neuropathy
  ○ Advanced nephropathy with renal failure

Adapted from Colberg et al. (2010).

Guideline 9.6   Exercise Training

Exercise should be prescribed carefully when health complications (besides CVD complications) are present in patients with diabetes. Use caution to allow patients to exercise safely and effectively and to remain engaged in being physically active.

Exercise stress testing may be performed with intention of evaluating the presence of ischemia, dysrhythmia, and abnormal BP responses to exercise and recovery. Test results also provide more accurate information for the prescription of initial levels of exercise, along with corresponding training heart rates for specific activities, and identify any patient-specific precautions regarding exercise and PA.

Exercise Prescription for Patients With Diabetes

Exercise prescription for people with diabetes must be individualized according to a medication schedule, presence and severity of comorbid health complications, and goals and expected benefits of the exercise program.[3,8] Food intake must be considered with respect to the timing of exercise, particularly for anyone who takes insulin.[9] The primary goals for patients participating in a CR program may include the following:

- Improved management of BG levels, including during and following exercise
- Minimizing health complications of diabetes
- Increased self-management of CVD risk factors
- Increased aerobic capacity, muscular strength and endurance, flexibility, and/or balance
- Enhanced energy levels and well-being

The development and components of an exercise prescription for a patient with diabetes are similar to the standard methods for all individuals, with a few key exceptions (see the following sections: General Exercise Precautions for Patients With Diabetes and Instructions for Foot Care for Patients With Diabetes). Similar to guidelines for most adults,[10] it is recommended that adults with either type of diabetes engage in the following PA[3,8,9]:

- Moderate aerobic activities such as walking for 150 min weekly, 75 min of vigorous PA, or a combination thereof, with no more than two consecutive days without any activity
- Resistance training at least two, but preferably three, nonconsecutive days per week
- Flexibility exercises at least two days per week
- Balance training two or more days per week (especially for all patients over 40 or with neuropathy of any type)

- More daily movement, including frequently breaking up sedentary time with PA

During CR participation, much of the PA recommendation can take place in the program. Patients should be counseled to prepare to perform these exercise recommendations for the rest of their lives.

Education, Monitoring, and Management of Patients With Diabetes

A number of precautions and special instructions for exercise undertaken by persons with diabetes are listed in General Exercise Precautions for Patients With Diabetes. Complications involving the feet are common; therefore, routine foot care is an important consideration. Problems most often develop in patients with peripheral neuropathy or peripheral vascular disease (PVD; compromised blood flow) in the lower extremities. Such problems can include extremely dry skin that may peel or crack; calluses that may ulcerate; and foot ulcers, particularly on the ball of the foot or at the base of the big toe. Patients should be routinely taught to inspect their feet and report any sores, infections, or inflammation to their health care provider. In addition to regular inquiry by the health care staff regarding foot health, initial assessment for peripheral neuropathies and pulses should be performed. CR staff should instruct patients on routine foot care.[11] CR staff should teach the following exercise precautions to their patients with diabetes.

General Exercise Precautions for Patients with Diabetes[8,9]

- Know the signs, symptoms, and management of hypoglycemia and hyperglycemia.
- Avoid vigorous exercise if BG is not adequately managed (particularly if elevated).
- Hydrate adequately before, during, and after exercise.
- Use caution when exercising in the heat, where temperature regulation may be impaired.

- At all times, carry personal identification specifying diabetes along with emergency contacts.
- Carry a mobile phone or have other means of easily reaching others in case of emergency.
- Take these appropriate precautions to avoid hypoglycemia during PA participation, especially when using insulin or oral insulin secretagogues:
  - Check blood glucose frequently as responses may vary with each individual and activity session
  - Always carry a CHO source for rapid treatment of hypoglycemia.
  - Avoid exercise at the time of peak insulin effect by scheduling PA 2 h or longer after meals for which insulin is taken.
  - If exercising while insulin is peaking, consider consuming a CHO snack before or during exercise or decreasing the insulin or oral hypoglycemic dose of select medications before exercise.
  - Be aware that exercise later in the day may increase risk of nocturnal hypoglycemia, mostly in insulin users.
  - Understand that some non-diabetes medications may mask or exacerbate exercise-related hypoglycemia, including beta-blockers, diuretics, calcium channel blockers, and warfarin.
- Patients with central or peripheral neuropathy
  - may require alternatives to palpating pulse for controlling intensity (e.g., commercial heart rate monitor or use of RPE),
  - may have abnormal HR and BP responses to exercise,
  - may have an increased risk of orthostatic hypotension, and
  - should routinely monitor and care for their feet and hands.

Instructions for Foot Care for Patients With Diabetes

Foot Hygiene

- Inspect feet daily for blisters, cuts, and scratches; report any issues to the health care provider immediately.

- If appropriate, a family member may assist with foot inspection, or patients can place a mirror on the floor to view the bottoms of their feet.
- Inspect the interior and the soles of shoes on a daily basis for roughness or inconsistent wear.
- Wash and dry the feet carefully every day, giving special attention to areas between the toes.
- After bathing and drying feet and hands, apply baby oil or other mineral oil to relieve dry skin.
- Do not soak the feet, and avoid bathing in extreme temperatures.
- When trimming toenails, cut straight across.
- Do not cut or trim corns or treat corns and calluses with chemical agents.
- Do not use adhesive tape on the feet.

Note: The health care provider or physician should examine the feet at each visit.

Footwear

- Wear properly fitted socks that keep the feet dry; avoid all-cotton socks.
- Avoid wearing mended socks or stockings with seams that may irritate the feet.
- Change socks and stockings daily.
- Wear warm socks with protective footwear in the winter.
- Wear socks if the feet are cold at night.
- Wear comfortable shoes with a broad and square toe box, laces with three or four eyes per side, and a padded tongue.[12]
- Choose shoes made of high-quality lightweight materials large enough to accommodate a cushioned insole.[12]
- Replace athletic shoes frequently before they become unduly worn.
- Use custom therapeutic footwear to reduce the risk of foot ulcers in high-risk patients.
- Do not wear sandals with thongs between the toes.
- Do not walk barefoot, especially on hot surfaces.

Guideline 9.7   Monitoring BG in CR

When patients with diabetes begin an exercise program, BG responses to exercise should be monitored each session at least until the CR staff is comfortable that the risk of postexercise hypoglycemia is low.[13] It is advisable to check BG prior to and after an exercise session, at least for the first few sessions, to ensure adequate starting values and postexercise values. Patients should continue to be monitored more frequently whenever they are symptomatic or have experienced recent high or low BG levels prior to participation on any given day.

Monitoring and Recording BG Levels

Monitoring and recording BG levels before and after exercise is important because it may

- allow for early detection and prevention of hypoglycemia or hyperglycemia,
- help determine appropriate preexercise BG levels to lower risk of hypoglycemia or hyperglycemia,
- identify patients who can benefit from monitoring BG during exercise,
- provide information for modifying the exercise prescription,
- allow for better adjustment of diabetes regimens to manage all PA, and
- motivate patients to remain more active to better manage BG levels.

Table 9.2 Preexercise Hypoglycemia Management

Preexercise	Plan of care	Intervention
Patients using insulin or select oral agents (insulin secretagogues) may have an increased risk of developing hypoglycemia during exercise.	Assess patient for individual risks for low BG: • Medication use • Time and content of last meal or snack • Planned duration and intensity of PA	Increase or maintain appropriate BG levels during exercise. Patients using insulin or oral agents that increase the risk of hypoglycemia may need to ingest some added CHO if pre-exercise BG is <100 mg/dL, depending on whether they are able to lower insulin doses during the workout (such as with an insulin pump or reduced preexercise insulin dosage), the time of day exercise is done, and the intensity and duration of the activity.[14]
Patients with the need for and access to BG monitoring	BG should be taken immediately before exercise; establish strategies for BG values; encourage patients to look for patterns in their BG response.	Individual BG targets should be set.
Patients with a history of hypoglycemia unawareness or frequent symptomatic hypoglycemia	Assess patient level of understanding about unawareness, and discuss any remaining signs and symptoms of low BG (if any) and treatment if needed.	Patient may require a higher preexercise BG target, increased monitoring, or both during the exercise session; treat appropriately.
Patients using insulin pumps	Consult with endocrinologist or CDE for instructions on insulin dose adjustment (basal and/or bolus) related to exercise.	Every effort should be made to set appropriate BG targets to prevent hypoglycemia from interfering with the exercise session and performance.

Abbreviations: BG, blood glucose; CDE, certified diabetes educator; CHO, carbohydrate.

Adapted by permission from F. Lopez-Jimenez et al., "Recommendations for Managing Patients With Diabetes Mellitus in Cardiopulmonary Rehabilitation. An American Association of Cardiovascular and Pulmonary Rehabilitation Statement," *Journal of Cardiopulmonary Rehabilitation and Prevention* 32 (2012): 101-112.

Table 9.3 Postexercise Hypoglycemia Management

Postexercise	Plan of care	Intervention
Glycemic goal postexercise should be individualized.	BG should be taken within 15 min after exercise and possibly again 1-2 h afterward.	Encourage patients to test BG frequently after exercise to be aware of the potential for a hypoglycemic response that can last 24-48 h after exercise session.
An individualized postexercise BG goal can be used to discharge an asymptomatic patient until a BG pattern and response have been established.	Use clinical discretion regarding the discharge of patients on oral hypoglycemic medication if BG is lower than 100 mg/dL and the patient is asymptomatic; caution should be used in discharging patients on insulin if BG is <100 mg/dL.	Snacks to prevent hypoglycemia after exercise may contain some CHO, protein, and/or fat; CHO should be used to treat hypoglycemia because they are more rapidly digested and absorbed. To prevent hypoglycemia during extended activity, a snack of 15-30 g CHO may be needed every 30-60 min of PA in insulin users or others on insulin secretagogues.
Patients using insulin pumps	Patients using pumps should consult with their endocrinologist or CDE for instructions on insulin dose adjustment (basal and/or bolus) related to exercise and BG targets.	Discuss with patient's physician whether insulin or other medication needs to be reduced before the exercise session; obtain specific goals for exercise BG.

Abbreviations: BG, blood glucose; CDE, certified diabetes educator; CHO, carbohydrate.

Adapted by permission from F. Lopez-Jimenez et al., "Recommendations for Managing Patients With Diabetes Mellitus in Cardiopulmonary Rehabilitation. An American Association of Cardiovascular and Pulmonary Rehabilitation Statement," *Journal of Cardiopulmonary Rehabilitation and Prevention* 32 (2012): 101-112.

Table 9.4 Hypoglycemia Recommendations

Points for consideration	• Treatment of hypoglycemia (BG <70 mg/dL) requires ingestion of glucose- or CHO-containing foods; rapid glycemic response correlates better with the glucose content than with the CHO content. • Ongoing activity of insulin or insulin secretagogues may lead to recurrence of hypoglycemia unless more food is ingested afterward. • People on an alpha glucosidase inhibitor (Precose [acarbose] or Glyset [miglitol]) must use dextrose only (such as glucose tablets) for treatment of hypoglycemia. • Giving 15-20 g of a rapidly digested CHO is the preferred treatment for the conscious patient with hypoglycemia, although any form of glucose containing CHO may be used. • If BG 15 min after treatment shows continued hypoglycemia, the treatment should be repeated; once BG returns to normal, the patient may need an additional meal or snack to prevent recurrence.
Examples of foods and drinks containing ~15 g glucose	• 1-2 bags of candy-coated chocolates (6 g glucose each) • 1-2 pieces of hard or sugary candy (not chocolate) • 4 oz of regular soda • 8 oz of juice • 8 oz of sports drink • 8 oz of skim milk • 2-3 graham crackers or 6 saltine crackers • 3-4 glucose tablets • 1 glucose gel
Intervention	• Help patient determine amount of food or drink or number of glucose tablets that equal 15 g CHO. • Differentiate CHO used to treat a hypoglycemic episode from appropriate CHO intake to prevent hypoglycemia; added fat may retard and then prolong acute hypoglycemic episode. • Explain to patient that overtreating low BG can lead to hyperglycemia and weight gain. • Calibrate patient glucose meter using a control solution or compare against institution-calibrated glucometer. (Note that this does not validate the patient's glucometer but may indicate if an issue occurs with its readings.) • In unresponsive people with diabetes experiencing a hypoglycemic event, follow institution policy regarding glucagon injection or intravenous administration of dextrose.

Adapted by permission from F. Lopez-Jimenez et al., "Recommendations for Managing Patients With Diabetes Mellitus in Cardiopulmonary Rehabilitation. An American Association of Cardiovascular and Pulmonary Rehabilitation Statement," *Journal of Cardiopulmonary Rehabilitation and Prevention* 32 (2012): 101-112.

Table 9.5 Preexercise Hyperglycemia Care for Patients With T1DM

Preexercise	Plan of care	Intervention
• Avoid exercise if fasting BG ≥250 mg/dL and ketosis is present; use caution if >300 mg/dL without ketosis. • A person with T1DM who is deprived of insulin for 12-48 h can develop ketosis with hyperglycemia; exercise can aggravate the hyperglycemia. • It is not necessary to postpone exercise based simply on hyperglycemia if urine, blood ketones, or both are normal.	1. With repeated BG levels of ≥300 mg/dL, obtain BG goals and medication adjustments from the physician for planning treatment, interventions needed for an exercise session, or both. 2. Help patient determine possible causes of increased BG: • Medication compliance • Overconsumption of CHO • Missed insulin dosing • Insulin pump malfunction • Signs or symptoms of an infection • Dehydration	• Obtain individualized BG range for patient if warranted. • If fasting BG or postprandial BG continues to be elevated, consider an adjustment in insulin dosing; refer patient to physician, CDE, or both for further intervention. • Assess patient knowledge and proficiency in following prescribed dosing. • Check medication and test strip expiration dates. • Follow instructions given for checking pump operation. • Patient should postpone exercise and follow up with physician.

Abbreviations: BG, blood glucose; CDE, certified diabetes educator; CHO, carbohydrate; T1DM, type 1 diabetes mellitus.

Adapted by permission from F. Lopez-Jimenez et al., "Recommendations for Managing Patients With Diabetes Mellitus in Cardiopulmonary Rehabilitation. An American Association of Cardiovascular and Pulmonary Rehabilitation Statement," *Journal of Cardiopulmonary Rehabilitation and Prevention* 32 (2012): 101-112.

Table 9.6 Preexercise Hyperglycemia Care for Patients With T2DM

Preexercise	Plan of care	Intervention

• Patients with T2DM should exercise with caution if BG ≥300 mg/dL.
• Routinely testing ketones is not indicated in patients with T2DM unless they are instructed to do so by their physician.
	1. With repeated BG levels of ≥300 mg/dL, obtain BG goals from the physician for planning treatment, interventions, or both for an exercise session.
	2. Help patient determine possible contributors to increased BG:
	  • Medication compliance
	  • Overconsumption of CHO
	  • Signs or symptoms of an infection
	  • Dehydration
		• Obtain individualized BG range for patient if warranted.
		• If fasting BG or postprandial BG continues to be elevated, consider an adjustment in medications; refer patient to physician, CDE, or both for further intervention.
		• Assess patient knowledge and proficiency in following prescribed dosing.
		• Check medication and test strip expiration dates.
		• Patient should postpone exercise and follow up with physician.
		• If elevated BG is caused by timing of meal and patient is asymptomatic, advise exercise with caution; in the absence of very severe insulin deficiency, exercise may decrease the BG level.
		• BG can be evaluated during exercise to make sure it is not increasing; if BG increases, exercise may need to be stopped until patient is within goal range.
		• If hyperglycemic hyperosmolar state is suspected, contact physician immediately.

Abbreviations: BG, blood glucose; CDE, certified diabetes educator; CHO, carbohydrate; T2DM, type 2 diabetes mellitus.

Adapted by permission from F. Lopez-Jimenez et al., "Recommendations for Managing Patients With Diabetes Mellitus in Cardiopulmonary Rehabilitation. An American Association of Cardiovascular and Pulmonary Rehabilitation Statement," *Journal of Cardiopulmonary Rehabilitation and Prevention* 32 (2012): 101-112.

Table 9.7 Postexercise Hyperglycemia Management

Postexercise	Plan of care	Intervention
Patients with diabetes may experience an increase in BG values after exercise if undertreated or PA is performed at intense levels due to an increased catecholamine response (and BG release) to this level of exertion. Hyperglycemia may last for several hours before BG returns to desired levels (or in some cases where meal-time insulin is taken, a dose of such insulin may be needed to lower it). This response does not erase other fitness benefits, but the patient may feel discouraged or have concerns about doing harm.	Assess patient and extenuating circumstances (e.g., consuming a meal just before exercise or timing of PA).	Instruct the patient to continue monitoring, and follow usual treatment guidelines for high BG. Timing or intensity of PA may be modified to prevent a rise in BG from activity. If significant hyperglycemia remains or if the patient is symptomatic, contact the physician.

Abbreviation: BG, blood glucose.

Adapted by permission from F. Lopez-Jimenez et al., "Recommendations for Managing Patients With Diabetes Mellitus in Cardiopulmonary Rehabilitation. An American Association of Cardiovascular and Pulmonary Rehabilitation Statement," *Journal of Cardiopulmonary Rehabilitation and Prevention* 32 (2012): 101-112.

Table 9.8 Signs and Symptoms of Hypoglycemia and Hyperglycemia

Hypoglycemia	Hyperglycemia
Rapid heart rate	Frequent urination
Sweating	Extreme thirst
Anxiety	Extremely dry skin
Shakiness	Drowsiness
Dizziness	Nausea
Weakness and fatigue	Slow-healing cuts or wounds
Headache	Hunger
Irritability	Blurred or impaired vision
Hunger	
Impaired vision or visual spots	

Data P.K. Welton et al., "2017 ACC/AHA Guideline for the Prevention, Detection, Evaluation, and Management of High Blood Pressure in Adults," *Hypertension* 7, no. 6 (2018): e13-e115.

Tables 9.2 through 9.8 describe the procedures for monitoring BG in a CR setting.

Monitoring BG levels is vital for the long-term maintenance of glycemic management and is especially important during exercise given that beta-blocker therapy can mask the onset of hypoglycemia. Done during exercise, such monitoring may also provide positive feedback regarding the regulation or progression of the exercise prescription, which may result in greater subsequent long-term adherence to exercise. Adherence to exercise is particularly important, because exercise is a cornerstone of treatment for diabetes.

Tobacco Use

The treatment of tobacco use should be a major focus for CR staff members. It is a leading cause of death in the United States and is also a performance measure for CR programs.[1] However, the AACVPR does not have specific or distinct guidelines for treating tobacco use in CR programs beyond those found in national guidelines for the identification and treatment of this important risk factor. The most current comprehensive guidelines are in the 2008 U.S. Public Health Service (PHS) Clinical Practice Guideline on Treating Tobacco Use and Dependence.[2] This section summarizes the PHS guideline, which serves as the primary reference for the treatment of tobacco for CR clinicians, although several additional recent reviews may be of interest to readers.[3-5] Additionally, this section discusses some of the unique features of applying smoking cessation to the CR setting.

"Starting today, every doctor, nurse, health plan purchaser, and medical school in the United States should make treating tobacco dependence a top priority."

David Satcher, MD, PhD. Former U.S. Surgeon General. Director of National Center for Primary Care, Morehouse School of Medicine

Epidemiology and Pathophysiology

Tobacco continues to be the single greatest preventable cause of disease and premature death in America today.[6] In 2018, more than 450,000 people in the United States will die prematurely due to tobacco use, and the typical smoker loses 11 years of life to their addiction.[7] Smoking is associated with an increased risk of CVD events in patients with and without established disease, including recurrent MI, sudden death, and restenosis after percutaneous coronary intervention (PCI). In individuals with coronary heart disease (CHD), smoking cessation is associated with a 36% reduction in the risk of all-cause mortality, making it an important SP intervention.[8] Unfortunately, very few smokers are able to quit each year, and even an acute hospitalization for a heart attack or heart procedure results in only 30% to 40% one-year smoking cessation rates.[9] Because of the highly addictive nature of tobacco use, persistent smokers are a group in need of extra attention, and the PHS guideline recommends considering tobacco dependence a chronic disease that requires multiple interventions.[2,10]

Smoking contributes to multiple vascular diseases including CHD, peripheral arterial disease, abdominal aortic aneurysm, and stroke. Smoking injures the vasculature through catecholamine release, which increases HR and BP and thus increases myocardial oxygen demand.[11] In addition, smoking constricts peripheral arteries, interfering with blood flow to tissues; lowers the threshold for ventricular fibrillation; and increases platelet activation. Finally, smoking has adverse effects on the lipoprotein panel, decreasing HDL cholesterol (HDL-C) and increasing the oxygenation of LDL-C, which in turn promotes atherogenesis. Carbon monoxide, another byproduct of smoking, injures vascular endothelium and interferes with the ability of red blood cells to carry oxygen, thus reducing the amount of oxygen delivered to the heart muscle. Many other constituents in tobacco smoke augment platelet aggregability, promoting adherence of platelets to damaged endothelium.[11]

As a result of these pathophysiologic changes, it is not surprising that smoking is a potent risk factor for acute MI and is present in nearly 50% of cases of ST-segment elevation MI; the largest impact is among patients <50 years old.[12] However, the short-term physiologic changes associated with smoking also mean that the beneficial effects of smoking cessation are apparent soon after quitting and in people of all age groups, including the elderly. For example, the risk of MI decreases by 50% within two years of cessation, and the rate of restenosis following PCI and deaths following bypass surgery are decreased after cessation.[13]

Tobacco Use in CR

In 2017, 15.5% of U.S. adults smoked as part of a 20-year downward trend.[14] Thus, because smoking increases the chances for CVD, one should expect that at least 15% (and more likely 20%-25%) of patients in CR should be recent or active smokers. Unfortunately, despite a higher referral rate, smokers are much less likely to attend CR programs and are more likely to drop out prior to program completion.[15] Based on unofficial data from the AACVPR registry in 2017, about 5% of patients who completed CR were current smokers at the time of enrollment. This gap is particularly problematic because attendance at CR has been associated with strong beneficial impact on long-term smoking cessation rates,[16] perhaps even as strong as a formal smoking cessation intervention.[17] Although smokers appear to respond to messages about reducing stress and anxiety through the use of CR and exercise,[18] much greater efforts are needed to seek out and encourage these patients to attend CR.

Assessment of Tobacco Use

Health care professionals should take every opportunity to identify and treat tobacco use in all practice settings.[6] For the purposes of the AACVPR performance measure and most guidelines, *active tobacco use* is defined as someone who used any form of tobacco within 30 days of enrollment into a CR program.[1] *Recent tobacco use* is defined as someone who used any form of tobacco within the past 6 months. This identification and intervention should generally follow the five A's of a tobacco intervention, listed here:

- *Ask.* Identify and document tobacco use status for every patient at every visit.
- *Advise.* In a clear, strong, and personalized manner, urge every tobacco user to quit.
- *Assess.* Is the tobacco user willing to make a quit attempt at this time?
- *Assist.* For the patient willing to make a quit attempt, use counseling and pharmacotherapy to help them quit.
- *Arrange.* Schedule follow-up contact, in person or by telephone, preferably within the first week after the quit attempt.

As noted, the key first step is to assess tobacco use and advise all smokers to quit. To assure that all patients are screened, guidelines suggest considering tobacco use as a vital sign to be assessed at the same time as BP and HR.

Although most CR professionals routinely assess tobacco use and advise patients to quit, many fewer professionals take the additional steps of *assisting* or *arranging* an intervention to actually help patients quit smoking.[19] This tendency is unfortunate given that most cardiac patients are highly motivated to quit smoking[20] but fail to quit because of the highly addictive nature of nicotine. Fortunately, effective treatments are available, and the CR professional is

---

Guideline 9.8   Assessment of Smoking Status

Assess each patient at CR program entry for current smoking status.

optimally situated to offer substantial assistance to tobacco users so that they can quit permanently.

For patients who are ready to make an attempt to quit smoking, additional information about their smoking status is helpful and allows individualized counseling. A smoking history may be useful to ensure a comprehensive assessment of the patient and to plan an intervention. Documenting whether other household members smoke may help determine the patient level of support and whether family members may also benefit from counseling. Determining past experience with serious attempts to quit and length of cessation, success with previous smoking interventions, and previous use of pharmacologic therapies can be helpful in planning an appropriate intervention.

Patients who are unwilling to make an attempt to quit smoking should be offered a brief intervention designed to enhance their motivation. Ways to enhance motivation include

- encouraging patients to indicate why quitting smoking is personally relevant to them and their disease process, being as specific as possible;
- helping patients to identify the short- and long-term risks associated with continued smoking;
- helping patients determine potential benefits of quitting by identifying personal rewards;
- identifying barriers to quitting; and
- repeating the intervention (motivational interview) every time an unmotivated patient visits a clinic setting (see Motivational Interview sidebar).

A key to remembering the structure of such an intervention is to focus on the five Rs, listed here:

- Relevance
- Risks
- Rewards
- Roadblocks
- Repetition

Assessment of Alcohol Use

Alcohol use is strongly associated with smoking relapse and nearly doubles the risk for failure to abstain from smoking, even for moderate drinkers.[21] As a result, smoking cessation guidelines strongly recommend that all smokers attempting to quit also completely abstain from alcohol for at least 1 month and possibly longer. Moreover, recent research has challenged the long-held association that light to moderate alcohol consumption decreases CV events.[22,23] Thus, until more definitive information is available, it seems reasonable that all patients who smoke should be assessed for alcohol use and advised to completely eliminate their consumption for at least one month and perhaps indefinitely.

Additionally, because heavy alcohol use is consistently and strongly associated with worse CV outcomes,[22] all patients should be screened for alcohol abuse. The CAGE Questionnaire is the most common screening tool used for this purpose.[24] A "yes" response to any of the questions may indicate potential alcohol abuse, and two or more positive responses generally requires further evaluation and intervention by a qualified mental health professional.

Intervention

The best time to begin a smoking cessation intervention is during the patient's hospitaliza-

---

Motivational Interview

- Relevance: Personalize why quitting is relevant (e.g., wishes of family members, health) and how the patient's disease process is directly related to their smoking habit.
- Risks: Ask the patient to identify negative consequences of tobacco use.
  - Acute risks: Shortness of breath, chest discomfort, poor taste and smell
  - Long-term risks: MI, stroke, chronic obstructive pulmonary disease (COPD)
  - Environmental: Respiratory infections in children, heart disease in spouses
- Rewards: Ask the patient to identify benefits of stopping smoking (e.g., improving symptoms, saving money, setting a good example for children).
- Roadblocks: Ask the patient to identify barriers to quitting (e.g., weight gain, depression, withdrawal symptoms).
- Repetition: Repeat this intervention at every clinic visit or within any other setting.

tion for treatment of their heart disease. During the hospitalization, patient motivation is usually high and patients are eager to make a fresh attempt at quitting smoking. Moreover, hospitals in the United States are uniformly 100% smoke free, which typically provides two to five days free from smoking; this time can serve as the patient's quit date and first few days of abstinence. Family members can be involved, and any other smokers in the patient's home strongly advised to quit or at the very least begin smoking outside. Hospitalization provides a critical opportunity to counsel patients and prescribe pharmacotherapy in preparation for discharge. These interventions are best provided by a multidisciplinary team, including a smoking cessation treatment specialist, a physician, a nurse, and/or a member of the CR program staff.

Because smoking relapse often occurs very quickly after hospital discharge (as many as 30% of smokers relapse within 1 week),[9,25] it is particularly important that the tobacco intervention be started while the patient is hospitalized. Delaying an intervention to the outpatient CR program or deferring to the primary care physician or cardiologist could potentially leave the patient unsupported during the period of greatest withdrawal symptoms (one to two weeks) and cause them to relapse and lose motivation to make further behavior changes. However, an inpatient smoking cessation intervention is, by itself, insufficient and must be coupled with long-term outpatient follow-up.[26] CR programs are ideally situated to provide such long-term support, which is another critical reason that smokers should be strongly encouraged to attend CR after hospital discharge[18] and hopefully enroll within a week.[27]

At the time of enrollment in CR, if a patient has successfully abstained from tobacco use since their hospital discharge, they should be encouraged and praised for their efforts but should not be treated as nonsmokers. Relapses occur frequently up to one year, and current performance measures recommend that all patients who used tobacco within six months should receive a relapse prevention intervention.[1] Clinicians should inquire about withdrawal symptoms and cravings and identify potential obstacles to long-term smoking cessation success. These obstacles may include frequent contact with friends, family, or coworkers who smoke; high-stress situations at work or at home; concurrent alcohol use; and uncontrolled anxiety or depression. Clinicians should attempt to address any concerns raised and encourage patients to remain 100% abstinent. They can promise anxious or stressed patients that smoking cessation consistently reduces stress and anxiety while improving mental health and quality of life.[28] Clinicians should also emphasize the valuable role of CR and exercise in preventing relapse and dealing with cravings. Finally, after the initial enrollment in CR, staff members should continue

---

Guideline 9.9 Intervention for Tobacco Cessation

Patients who are active tobacco users at the time of enrollment into CR should receive a tobacco cessation intervention, as set forth in the performance measure.[1] This includes any of the following items:

- *Brief tobacco cessation counseling at program entry.* If the patient is not willing to make a quit attempt, intervention should be aimed at helping the patient improve their readiness for an eventual quit attempt.

- *Tobacco cessation pharmacotherapy.* Medication may be provided to patients who are not yet ready to quit but who are ready to reduce to quit.

- *Referral to a tobacco treatment program or specialist.*

Ideally, all three of these interventions would be provided with sustained support throughout the course of CR.

- For those who do not wish to quit smoking, provide consistent education to attempt to move them from the precontemplation to contemplation or preparation stage of change.

- For those who are not ready to quit but willing to reduce smoking, refer to physician for tobacco cessation pharmacotherapy.

- For those desiring to quit, refer to a tobacco treatment program or specialist.

to regularly inquire about tobacco use, offer support and encouragement, and continue to assess tobacco use in individual treatment plans for the entire duration of CR.

Patients should set a quit date within one to two weeks of the tobacco intervention so that their commitment to cessation does not wane. Health care professionals can use this opportunity to review the smoking history, highlighting the most relevant items, such as success with previous attempts, availability of social support, use of alcohol, and problems that may have hindered past success. In addition, CR specialists should prepare patients for their quit day by asking them to remove all ashtrays and tobacco products, inform family members of their intent to quit, and obtain pharmacologic therapies if they have not done so already. After the patient sets a quit date, CR specialists should provide behavioral counseling and monitor the effects of pharmacologic therapies for patients interested in quitting.

Exercise through CR also helps patients as they quit smoking by improving psychological well-being and minimizing weight gain and withdrawal symptoms. Thus, CR professionals should encourage active participation in the exercise component of CR programs. Self-help materials such as pamphlets, text-to-quit services, and online video resources have been developed by the AHA, the American Lung Association, and the American Cancer Society to supplement counseling and to reinforce information provided by program specialists. An abundance of reputable websites and smartphone applications offer resources to help smokers through the early stages of quitting to complement in-person counseling. Individuals may also want to avail themselves of a state-sponsored quitline or the national quitline (1-800-QUIT-NOW). One of the advantages of using the quitlines is the lack of cost associated with this type of intervention and ready access to well-trained smoking cessation counselors. Unfortunately, only about 1% of all smokers avail themselves of these services.[29]

Finally, the clinical practice guideline highlights evidence from randomized controlled trials suggesting these key findings that are important when intervening with smokers:

- The more intense the treatment, the greater the rate of cessation. Intensive interventions are more effective and should be used whenever possible.
- Treatment can be maximized by increasing the length of individual sessions to greater than 10 min and the number of treatment sessions to four or more sessions (≥30 min contact time).
- Use of multiple types of providers (e.g., physicians, nurses, pharmacists) enhances cessation rates.
- Proactive telephone calls and individual and group counseling are effective cessation formats. State quitlines and the national quitline (1-800-QUIT-NOW) are effective compared to little or no intervention.
- Practical counseling (problem-solving and skills training) and use of social support significantly improve cessation outcomes.
- Pharmacologic therapies increase cessation rates and should be encouraged for all smokers, except where contraindications exist. In some cases, combination therapies have been shown to be more effective than single drugs.
- The combination of counseling and medications is more effective for smoking cessation than either one alone; both should be provided.[3]

Many of these recommendations have been applied in helping cardiac patients to quit smoking.[30] In particular, case management with more intensive interventions has been shown to improve cessation rates in those with established CHD.[29,30]

Pharmacologic Therapy

The clinical practice guideline indicates that all patients should be encouraged to use pharmacologic therapies for smoking cessation except in special circumstances.[2] Presently, seven first-line medications are indicated to help smokers in their attempts to quit. They include buproprion SR, varenicline, and these five nicotine replacement therapies: nicotine gum, nicotine inhaler, nicotine lozenge, nicotine nasal spray, and the nicotine patch. Personal preference and previous use can often guide the choice of an agent, although varenicline has the strongest evidence for smoking cessation in patients with CVD.[25] Additionally, because nicotine patches, gum, and lozenges are available without a prescription, all CR programs should be able to confidently recommend and prescribe these medications for their patients without the need for physician involvement.

Although there were initially some concerns about the use of nicotine replacement therapy (NRT) in patients with CVD, numerous studies now clearly indicate a lack of association between the use of nicotine replacement products and acute cardiovascular events.[31-33] Similarly, initially some safety concerns about the use of varenicline existed, but recent studies have shown no association between use of varenicline and either suicidal behavior or increased CVD risk.[34,35]

The following items should be considered when prescribing pharmacotherapy:

- *Smoking while on a nicotine patch is no longer prohibited. The FDA removed this restriction in 2013.* This modification helped create a new reduce-to-quit approach, where complete abstinence may not be the initial treatment goal but is attempted only after the patient has significantly reduced tobacco use.[36]

- *Treatment with pharmacotherapy for at least three months, and more preferably for six months, improves quit rates.*[37] Short-term use of these medications is discouraged.

- *Combination therapy of any of the FDA approved smoking cessation therapies is allowed and in many cases has been shown to be superior to single-agent quit attempts.*[3] Examples include combining the patch and lozenge; or varenicline and gum; or bupropion and inhaler.

- *The AHA does not consider e-cigarettes a treatment agent for smoking cessation and are considered tobacco products.* Their use should be discouraged and has been associated with lower long-term quit rates.[38]

Hypertension

The identification and treatment of hypertension (HTN) is of major importance for clinicians because it is one of the most prevalent and treatable conditions in cardiac rehabilitation (CR) programs. While the AACVPR does not have separate or distinct guidelines for the management of HTN in CR, the AACVPR instituted a performance measure for Optimal Blood Pressure Control in 2017.[1] This performance measure follows 2017 American College of Cardiology/American Heart Association (ACC/AHA) guideline for the Prevention, Evaluation, and Management of High Blood Pressure in Adults which serves as the primary guideline for CR prevention programs.[2]

Diagnosis

For years, the standard diagnostic threshold for the diagnosis of HTN was 140/90 mm Hg. However, based on results of several recent studies, including the landmark 2015 SPRINT trial,[3] the 2017 ACC/AHA guideline changed the definition of HTN.[2] Stage 1 HTN is now diagnosed at a threshold of >130/80 mm Hg; stage 2 HTN is diagnosed at >140/90 mm Hg. Normal BP is now <120/80 mm Hg. (See table 9.9 for all categories of BP.) Based on this new diagnostic threshold, it is estimated that 46% of adults in the United States have HTN, with a greater prevalence among men than women. In CR programs, the prevalence is estimated to be between 75% and 80% (based on 2017 AACVPR registry data) but may further increase as this new cut point becomes more widely applied.

Table 9.9 Categories of Resting BP in Adults*

BP category	Systolic		Diastolic
Normal	<120 mm Hg	and	<80 mm Hg
Elevated	120-129 mm Hg	and	<80 mm Hg
HTN			
Stage 1	130-139 mm Hg	or	80-89 mm Hg
Stage 2	≥140 mm Hg	or	≥90 mm Hg

Abbreviations: BP, blood pressure; HTN, hypertension.

*Patients with SBP and DBP in 2 categories should be designated to the higher BP category.

Adapted by permission from P.K. Welton et al., "2017 ACC/AHA Guideline for the Prevention, Detection, Evaluation, and Management of High Blood Pressure in Adults," *Hypertension* 71, no, 6 (2018): e13-e115.

Measurement

Obtaining an accurate BP measurement is essential to the correct management of HTN, but it is frequently done incorrectly.[4] The AHA has established 11 recommendations in measurement technique,[5] and they were reemphasized in the 2017 ACC/AHA guidelines. Recommendations include properly preparing the patient, using calibrated equipment, using proper technique, and accurately documenting and averaging the readings;[2] see table 9.10 for instructions corresponding to these steps. Although many clinicians fail to follow them, these specific instructions are essential to confidently and accurately establish-ing a diagnosis of HTN. Using proper measurement technique is especially important when the diagnosis of HTN is uncertain or when a change in antihypertensive therapy is being considered.

Although the pace of a typical CR program does not usually allow for the 5 min rest period and 5 min measurement period required for multiple repeated measurements that are then averaged for each patient for every exercise session, a high-quality BP measurement should be done at least intermittently. It should include program entry and exit, because these measurements are the primary data points used in the AACVPR performance measure.[1] It could also include every

Table 9.10 Checklist for Accurate BP Measurement

Key steps for proper BP measurement	Specific instructions
Step 1: Properly prepare the patient.	The patient should avoid caffeine, exercise, and smoking for at least 30 minutes before measurement. Ensure that the patient has emptied their bladder. Ask the patient to remove all clothing covering the location of cuff placement. Have the patient relax in a chair with the feet on the floor with both arms and back supported for 5 minutes. Do not have patients sit or lay on an exam table; measurements made while the patient is sitting or lying on an exam table are less reliable. Neither the patient nor the observer should talk during the rest period or during the measurement.
Step 2: Use proper equipment for BP measurements.	1. Use a BP measurement device that has been validated, and ensure that the device is calibrated periodically. 2. Support the patient's arm (e.g., resting on a desk). 3. Position the middle of the cuff on the patient's upper arm at the level of the right atrium (the middle of the sternum). 4. Use the correct cuff size, such that the bladder encircles 80% of the arm, and note if a larger or smaller-than-normal cuff size is used. 5. You may use either the stethoscope diaphragm or the bell for auscultatory readings.
Step 3: Use proper technique for BP measurements.	1. At the first visit, record BP in both arms. Use the arm that gives the higher reading for subsequent readings. 2. Separate repeated measurements by 1-2 min. 3. For auscultatory determinations, use a palpated estimate of radial pulse obliteration pressure to estimate systolic BP. Inflate the cuff 20-30 mm Hg above this level for an auscultatory determination of the BP level. 4. For auscultatory reading, deflate the cuff pressure 2 mm Hg/s, and listen for Korotkov sounds.
Step 4: Document and average the BP readings.	1. Record systolic and diastolic BP. If using the auscultatory technique, record systolic BP and diastolic BP at onset of the first Korotkov sound and disappearance of all Korotkov sounds, respectively, using the nearest even number. 2. Note the time of the most recent BP medication taken before measurement. 3. Use an average of ≥2 readings obtained on ≥2 occasions to estimate the patient's BP. 4. Provide the patient with the BP reading both verbally and in writing.

Abbreviation: BP, blood pressure.

Data from P.K. Welton et al., "2017 ACC/AHA Guideline for the Prevention, Detection, Evaluation, and Management of High Blood Pressure in Adults," *Hypertension* 7, no. 6 (2018): e13-e115.

6th or 12th session of CR, or at the time of a 30-day individual treatment plan, or more often if the patient is consistently hypertensive. However, at this time, no guideline exists on the exact frequency of high-quality BP measurements, and it is not understood how this factor might improve patient care. Individual programs must make these decisions based on program resources and patient needs. It is important to ensure accurate measurements for the performance measure and to provide feedback to treating clinicians.

Many current CR programs perform a BP measurement before and after each exercise training session. Additionally, some may also measure a BP during exercise. However, no current recommendation exists on the frequency of these measurements; it is unknown whether these assessments improve patient care. However, these measurements might be considered screening readings that can alert CR staff to values that are considered high or low for an individual patient. This information might be used to question the patient about their symptoms, medications, or other factors that may have affected their BP (e.g., smoking, dehydration, high sodium intake).

Because BP can sometimes be markedly different in clinical settings when compared to home or work settings, a new diagnosis of HTN requires confirmation of elevated BP readings on more than one occasion and usually in at least one other setting, unless severe BP elevations (such as >180 mm Hg) are present[6] (see guideline 9.10). At least 3 measurements should be made to confirm the diagnosis; 10 or more measurements

over one to two weeks would be ideal. Similarly, when possible, multiple measurements should be made before making changes in medication. The best time to measure BP is within 2 h of waking, because morning measurements are most closely associated with long-term prognosis.[7] Because the proper management of HTN requires frequent BP measurements, most patients with HTN should purchase a high-quality home BP cuff and be instructed in proper measurement technique.[2] When possible, patients can be encouraged to bring their home system to a CR visit for instruction on its use and to compare to a clinical reading. Home BP measurement can be confidently recommended to all patients with HTN, because it has been associated with greater patient awareness of, engagement in, and active participation in monitoring and controlling their disease. It has also led to improved medication adherence and fewer long-term events.[8]

White Coat Effect and Masked HTN

In clinical settings, such as a physician's office or the emergency department, many patients exhibit an alerting reaction in which BP is temporarily but significantly increased over usual baseline for the period of the clinical interaction.[9] It is termed *white coat effect* because of the association with the laboratory white coats that physicians sometimes wear, although the color and type of clothing do not matter. Importantly, white coat effect can be present in patients both with and without HTN and should not be confused with *white coat HTN*, which only occurs in patients with normal BP at home and elevated BP in a physician's office.

Analogous but much less recognized by clinicians, some patients have HTN at home but exhibit normal BP in clinical settings. This form of HTN is termed *masked HTN* and is more difficult to detect, but CR members should not

Guideline 9.10   Diagnosis of HTN

- HTN should not be diagnosed on the basis of a single measurement and should be done using high-quality measurement techniques. (See table 9.10.)

- Initial elevated readings should be confirmed on at least two subsequent visits over a period of 1 to 2 weeks (unless systolic BP is >180 mm Hg or diastolic BP is >110 mm Hg). Average levels of systolic BP ≥130 mm Hg or diastolic BP ≥80 mm Hg are required for diagnosis.

Guideline 9.11   Home BP Monitoring

The use of home BP measurements should be encouraged and incorporated into the diagnosis and management of HTN in cardiac rehabilitation.

dismiss it as a spurious finding.[10] Masked HTN is most commonly seen in people who have high-stress employment or difficult domestic situations. Such situations can lead to high BP at home and work but normal BP when visiting a physician. Masked HTN should also be suspected when end organ damage (e.g., left ventricular hypertrophy, chronic kidney disease, retinopathy) is out of proportion with the measured clinical BP.

Both white coat HTN and masked HTN have nearly equal prevalence of about 10% to 15%, and both conditions are associated with worse outcomes compared to consistently normal BP.[11,12] Although they do not always require treatment, these patients should be monitored more frequently because they are both risk factors for the development of sustained HTN. All CR staff should be aware of these conditions and teach patients of their potential deleterious impacts.

BP With Exercise

The ACC/AHA guidelines do not give recommendations about the diagnosis or management of HTN during an exercise session. Similarly, they do not stipulate a specific threshold for resting BP where initiating or continuing exercise is contraindicated. They also do not provide a recommendation about the frequency or even the necessity of measuring BP during exercise. As a result, currently no clear standard exists on these issues. Programs are encouraged to consult with their medical director to establish specific guidelines about when exercise is contraindicated, how often to measure exercise BP, and what threshold of exercise BP should prompt an intervention. However, some general considerations may be of use to programs as they develop individual policies.

First, although a resting BP higher than 180/120 mm Hg is necessary for making a diagnosis of hypertensive emergency in the ACC/AHA guidelines, this diagnosis can be made only if the patient also has signs and symptoms consistent with severe HTN (e.g., chest pain, dyspnea, heart failure, blurry vision) and evidence of target organ damage (e.g., hematuria, MI, pulmonary edema, retinal hemorrhage). As a result, the threshold of 180/120 mm Hg specified in these guideline does not apply to patients who are asymptomatic and

who are attending cardiac rehabilitation for an exercise session.

Second, the ACSM uses a threshold of 200/110 mm Hg as a relative contraindication for starting a maximal stress test. ACSM also recommends that an exercise test be stopped when BP >250/115 mm Hg, and it also recommends stopping an exercise test if systolic BP drops by >10 mm Hg. While these guidelines are well accepted for stress testing, it is unclear how they should be applied to routine exercise training in CR.

Third, there is an ongoing clinical trial (TRIUMPH) to test the impact of aerobic exercise training and lifestyle intervention on BP among patients with resistant HTN in cardiac rehabilitation who have usual SBP in the 150 to 170 mm Hg range.[13] Similar to the recommendations from the ACSM, this trial uses a threshold of >200/110 mm Hg to preclude beginning an exercise session and a threshold of >250/115 mm Hg to immediately stop exercise. While the efficacy and safety of this approach are unknown at this time, results from TRIUMPH will likely provide important insights into the management of exercise in patients with significant HTN.

Assessment of Patients With HTN

A pertinent medical history includes many items recommended for the initial evaluation of patients entering the CR program (see chapter 4), with a particular focus on dietary sodium intake, excessive alcohol and caloric consumption, and low levels of PA. The goals of this

> ### Guideline 9.12   Exercise in HTN
>
> - Patients who have symptoms attributable to either high or low BP should not be allowed to exercise and should be referred for rapid additional evaluation by a medical professional.
> - Exercise is contraindicated in all patients with a resting BP >200 and/or 110 mm Hg (systolic and diastolic, respectively).
> - Exercise training is contraindicated in all patients if BP rises above 250 and/or 115 mm Hg (systolic and diastolic, respectively).

evaluation are to determine cardiovascular risk status and the presence (and extent) of target organ damage. The following are additional important aspects of the physical examination related to the evaluation of HTN that an appropriately trained health care professional should perform and document.

- Examination of the eye, including fundoscopy, for presence of retinopathy or hemorrhage
- Examination of the neck for carotid bruits, distended jugular veins, or an enlarged thyroid gland
- Examination of the heart for increased rate or size, precordial heave, clicks, murmurs, arrhythmias, and third (S3) and fourth (S4) heart sounds
- Examination of the abdomen for bruits, enlarged kidneys, masses, and abnormal aortic pulsation
- Examination of the extremities for diminished or absent peripheral arterial pulsations or the presence of bruits or edema
- A complete neurologic assessment

Initial laboratory evaluation should be performed routinely before HTN therapy is started. This includes urinalysis; a complete blood count; a fasting BG, if possible; potassium, calcium, creatinine, and uric acid; and lipid profile. A 12-lead ECG should be used to identify the presence of left ventricular hypertrophy. Based on this evaluation, appropriate and tailored therapy can be started.

BP Therapeutic Goals

Unlike prior guidelines, the 2017 ACC/AHA guidelines recommend that patients be risk stratified prior to beginning pharmacologic therapy to avoid overtreatment of low-risk patients and inducing adverse events in patients unlikely to benefit.[2] To do this risk stratification, the guidelines state that all patients with a BP >130/80 mm Hg should be treated with diet and lifestyle intervention but apply pharmacologic therapy only when the benefits outweigh the risks. Low-risk patients (<10% for 10-year risk of myocardial infarction, stroke, or death according to the ACC/AHA pooled cohort risk calculator) should only

Guideline 9.13   Intervention for HTN

- CR staff should initiate a lifestyle intervention in all patients with BP ≥130 mm Hg systolic or ≥80 mm Hg diastolic. They can intervene with a documented program of weight management, PA, alcohol moderation, and moderate sodium restriction.
- For most patients in CR, antihypertensive medications should be added if BP is ≥130 mm Hg systolic or ≥80 mm Hg diastolic.

be started on pharmacologic therapy when BP >140/90 mm Hg. However, among patients with established vascular disease, diabetes, chronic kidney disease, heart failure, or stroke, pharmacologic therapy should be prescribed when BP >130/80 mm Hg. Given that the vast majority of patients in CR have established vascular disease and are, by definition, not at low risk, most patients in CR should be treated with pharmacologic therapy when BP >130/80 mm Hg (see guideline 9.13).[3]

Individual circumstances (significant orthostasis, neurologic disease, or recurrent syncope or falls) may necessitate a BP goal higher than 130/80 mm Hg. Because the elderly (age 80+) are at higher risk of fall, orthostasis, syncope, and injury with falls, caution is often needed and low dose medications should be tried first in this age group.[14] Additionally, if patients report dizziness with standing, BP should be measured in both the seated and standing positions, with the standing BP occurring ideally during reported symptoms. If significant orthostasis is detected (BP drop of >20 mm Hg with standing) the standing BP should be used to guide therapeutic decisions. However, the vast majority of patients in CR are able to achieve and tolerate a BP of <130/80 mm Hg, so setting a higher BP goal should only be done in careful consultation with the patient's physician.

Lifestyle Intervention

Lifestyle modifications are the foundation for treatment of HTN. Lifestyle modifications are effective in lowering BP for many people who follow them (see table 9.11), and they can often be more effective than a full-dose antihypertensive medication. If properly used, lifestyle modifications offer multiple benefits at little cost and with minimal risk. Even when not adequate in themselves to control HTN, they may reduce the number and doses of antihypertensive medications needed to manage the condition. Additionally, because exercise is an effective therapy for resistant HTN,[15] patients with sustained HTN should generally still be allowed to exercise in CR, even though exercise BPs may be significantly elevated.[13]

As definitive or adjunctive therapy for HTN, the ACC/AHA guideline underscores the foundational importance of lifestyle modifications for all patients, which include weight reduction (when indicated), increased PA, and moderation of diet.[2] Dietary modifications should include these components: (1) Individualize the diet to achieve and maintain a healthy body weight (see Overweight and Obesity section later in the chapter); (2) limit alcohol intake to <1 oz ethanol a day; (3) limit sodium intake; (4) emphasize intake of fruits, vegetables, and low-fat dairy products, particularly ones that are high in potassium; and (5) reduce saturated fat and trans fat in general (see chapter 7). Table 9.11 also outlines lifestyle treatment strategies appropriate for individual risk factors. Initial monotherapy is usually successful in patients with stage 1 HTN.

The DASH diet is the single most important and effective lifestyle intervention for patients with HTN.[16,17] Specifics regarding the DASH diet are discussed in chapter 7. The DASH diet reduces BP in both hypertensive and nonhypertensive people, and particularly in African Americans.[18] It is as potent as maximally dosed antihypertensive medication and reduces BP by 8 to 14 mm Hg. Specifically, the DASH diet emphasizes five to nine servings of fruits and vegetables a day and two to four servings of low-fat dairy products a day. Comparatively, this plan includes substantially more fruits and vegetables than the one or two servings of fruits and vegetables consumed by the average U.S. adult.[19] Additionally, it includes whole grains, fish, poultry, and raw nuts with limits of saturated fat, red meat, sweets, and sugar-containing beverages, which is consistent with current ACC/AHA guidelines and the MEDIT dietary pattern.[20]

The AHA also recommends that all American adults limit their sodium intake; the optimal goal is <1,500 mg/day.[2] This recommendation is particularly important for populations known to be salt sensitive, such as African Americans, adults over the age of 50, and people with existing HTN, diabetes mellitus, or chronic kidney

Table 9.11 Strategies to Promote Lifestyle Modification

Modification	Recommendation	Approximate SBP reduction, range
Weight reduction	Maintain normal body weight (BMI = 18.5-24.9).	5mm Hg/5 kg weight loss
Adoption of DASH diet	Consume a diet rich in fruits, vegetables, and low-fat dairy products with a reduced content of saturated and total fat.	8-14 mm Hg
Dietary sodium reduction	Optimal goal is <1,500 mg/day, but aim for at least a 1,000 mg/day reduction in most adults.	5-6 mm Hg
Enhancing dietary potassium	Aim for 3,500-5,000 mg/day, preferably by consumption of a potassium-rich diet.	4-5 mm Hg
Physical activity	Engage in regular aerobic PA such as brisk walking (at least 30 min/day, most days of the week).	4-9 mm Hg
Moderation of alcohol consumption	Limit consumption to ≤2 drinks/day (1 oz or 30 mL ethanol; e.g., 24 oz beer, 10 oz wine, or 3 oz 80-proof whiskey) in most men and ≤1 drink/day in women and lightweight persons.	2-4 mm Hg

For overall cardiovascular risk reduction, stop smoking. The effects of implementing these modifications are dose and time dependent and could be higher for some individuals.

Abbreviations: SBP, systolic blood pressure; BMI, body mass index calculated as weight in kg divided by the square of height in m (kg/m²); DASH = dietary approaches to stop hypertension.

Data from P.K. Welton et al., "2017 ACC/AHA Guideline for the Prevention, Detection, Evaluation, and Management of High Blood Pressure in Adults," *Hypertension* 7, no. 6 (2018): e13-e115.

disease. If obtaining a sodium intake of <1,500 mg/day is not possible, the guidelines recommend a reduction of sodium intake of at least 1,000 mg from any baseline level, because this number has been associated with improvement in BP control.

Although commonly perceived by patients as a low-sodium diet, the DASH diet is primarily a healthy eating pattern that is rich in potassium, magnesium, and calcium.[16] These minerals appear to be important mediators of the DASH diet's antihypertensive effects.[21] Additionally, increasing dietary potassium intake is now recommended as a strategy to reduce BP and appears to be important to counteracting the impact of high dietary sodium intake.[2] It is still important to counsel patients to reduce their sodium intake, but this reduction is an additive effect rather than the core impact of the DASH diet.[17] This fact should be emphasized when counseling patients about the antihypertensive effect of the DASH diet, because most of the impact of the DASH diet will be lost if the patients only attempt to reduce their sodium intake.

Pharmacologic Treatment

Although prescription of antihypertensive medications is usually beyond the scope of practice of most CR clinicians, staff members can greatly assist the primary care physician and cardiologist in treatment of patients with HTN. The most important role is to identify and diagnose patients with uncontrolled HTN. In addition to this role, CR staff members can encourage consistent medication adherence, educate patients about important factors that impact HTN control, and assess therapeutic responses to medication changes. Unlike physicians who have only episodic and infrequent contact with patients, CR staff members generally have multiple contacts per week over several months where BPs can be measured and the importance of adherence and lifestyle can be reinforced. Thus, CR staff members should play a key role in assuring that BP targets and AACVPR performance measures are met.

If a patient remains hypertensive despite a few weeks of lifestyle and medication therapy, pharmacologic therapy is indicated. In this case, the CR staff should alert the patient and engage their physicians in actively addressing the problem. Communication can include phone calls, messages, and appointments with the patient's physicians. Staff members may find that involving the CR medical director in these communications may be particularly helpful in overcoming clinical inertia and inaction.

Regarding medication prescription, the 2017 ACC/AHA guidelines recommend thiazide-like diuretics, calcium channel blockers (CCBs), and angiotensin-converting enzyme (ACE) inhibitors as first-line medications for the treatment of HTN.[2] These medications can be used as monotherapy or combined, at either low or high doses. When used together at maximally tolerated doses, most patients are able to achieve their goal BP with minimal side effects. In patients who cannot tolerate ACE inhibitors, angiotensin receptor blockers (ARBs) are the preferred agents. In the patient whose BP readings are greater than 20/10 mm Hg over goal, a single drug will likely be ineffective, and combination therapy is indicated.

Patients who remain hypertensive despite taking high doses of an ACE inhibitor, thiazide diuretic, and a CCB are diagnosed with resistant HTN.[22] This diagnosis should prompt physician evaluation for secondary causes of HTN and possible referral to a HTN specialist. Causes of resistant HTN can include obstructive sleep apnea, hyperaldosteronism, renal artery stenosis, pheochromocytoma, and Cushing's disease, although a clear cause for the elevated HTN is never found in most patients.[22] In these cases, the most commonly used medication class is an aldosterone antagonist (e.g., spironolactone); it is a particularly effective medication in resistant HTN.[23] Other medications used in resistant HTN include loop diuretics, alpha antagonists, and direct vasodilators; they should be used only when all other standard therapies have been considered or tried.

Although useful in many circumstances, beta-blockers are notably no longer considered a first-line treatment for HTN.[2] Thus, all three classes of first-line therapies should generally be used before starting a beta-blocker specifically for control of HTN. However, most patients in CR are taking beta-blockers for their cardiac conditions, which is certainly appropriate and should contribute to BP control. Common indications for beta-blockers are the presence of ischemic heart disease, stable angina, systolic heart failure, or for the treatment of arrhythmias such as atrial fibrillation. Combined alpha- and beta-blockers (e.g., carvedilol or labetalol) are commonly used in patients with both ischemic heart disease and HTN, because the addition of the alpha antagonist further reduces BP.

The most important factor that contributes to resistant HTN is poor adherence to long-term treatment, encompassing both lifestyle modifications and pharmacologic therapy. CR programs can be particularly effective in providing education and support aimed at improving patient understanding of specific therapies and treatment goals, correcting misconceptions, adjusting the therapeutic interventions to patient lifestyles, and enhancing family or other social support. These efforts should help patients achieve long-term adherence to treatment schedules and BP control.

Performance Measure

Given the wide range of available medications, the effective impact of lifestyle changes, and the strong beneficial impacts of treating HTN, the AACVPR considers the control of BP at the completion of CR to be the standard of care for all patients who complete the program. This performance measure has been validated and should be a useful tool for programs looking to improve the care of their patients with HTN.[1] This performance measure is available free in the resources section on the AACVPR website. This site is regularly updated. It includes answers to frequently asked questions and an algorithm for determining inclusions, exclusions, and the proportion of patients meeting the measure.

Overweight and Obesity

Obesity continues to be a major public health problem in the United States and elsewhere in the world.[1-3] In the United States in 2014, the reported prevalence of obesity was 35%, and in 2015 and 2016 the National Health and Nutrition Survey reported an overall prevalence of 39.8% among U.S. adults across all ethnic groups (see figure 9.5).[4] Obesity is not only an independent risk factor for CHD,[5] it is also associated with the major risk factors of diabetes, HTN, and hyperlipidemia. Overweight (BMI ≥25-29.9 kg/m²) and obesity (BMI ≥ 30 kg/m²) are also associated with excess cardiovascular deaths.[6]

The mechanisms by which obesity predisposes a person to vascular disease are many, and they include insulin resistance and dyslipidemia. Many accompanying metabolic changes, including altered cytokine production, contribute to a possible proinflammatory state.[7,8]

Excess adiposity predisposes people to other

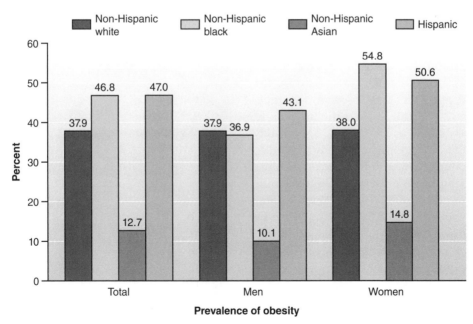

Figure 9.5 Age-adjusted prevalence of obesity among adults aged 20 and over, by sex and race and Hispanic origin: United States, 2015-2016.

Based on Center for Disease Control and Prevention. https://www.cdc.gov/nchs/products/databriefs/db288.htm3

risk factors for CHD such as hypertension, dyslipidemia, and diabetes mellitus.[9] Historically, many authors have reported a high prevalence of overweight in patients undergoing CR.[10,11] Unfortunately, this trend continues. In data recently reported from North Carolina, 1,000 of approximately 1,300 patients (about 75%) were either overweight or obese.[12]

Despite the prevalence and strong link to risk factors and excess mortality, overweight and obesity have not been a primary focus of intervention for many CR programs. Most CR programs focus mainly on exercise. Indeed, while nutritional counseling is also standard of care, it is often directed toward a heart-healthy rather than a weightloss diet.

Physicians caring for patients with CHD frequently treat the consequences of overweight pharmacologically (e.g., diabetes, hypertension, and hyperlipidemia) without a major emphasis on lifestyle changes and dietary intervention. Less than half of CR programs self-report providing a weight management lecture, and very few a weight loss program.[13] These statistics may explain why the amount of weight loss among patients undergoing CR is reported as minimal at only 2.2 to 4.4 lb (1-2 kg).[10,11,14] However, the outcomes in relation to weight loss may not be so bleak and may depend on how it is calculated, because some patients may lose nothing and others may in fact gain weight.[12] In one recent study, very obese patients had the greatest weight loss during CR participation.[12] In addition, the authors suggested that a better metric for CR programs might be the prevalence of a greater than 3% weight change. For individual patients, a significant weight loss might be defined as more than 3% of body weight; this percentage is most likely to lead to clinically meaningful health benefits.[15] Absolute weight loss should be interpreted individually and related to baseline. A loss of 10 lb (4.5 kg) in a patient weighing 200 lb (90.7 kg) may be clinically meaningful (>3%); but in a patient of 400 lb (181.4 kg), though laudable, it may be clinically insignificant (<3%).

Metabolic Syndrome

While the average weight loss is much less than what is required to optimize CVD risk reduction, participation in CR is associated with significant reductions in the prevalence of metabolic syndrome characteristics.[16,17] It also reduces the incidence of new cases of CVD in otherwise healthy individuals with risk factors,[18] and it is associated with a reduced rate of cardiac events.[19] This outcome is anticipated, because weight loss in patients with CVD is associated with improvements in abdominal obesity, insulin resistance, lipid profile, BP,[20] endothelial function,[21] platelet aggregation,[22] and self-reported quality of life.[23] Given that an overall goal of CR is to favorably alter lifestyle-related markers of CHD, programs should concentrate efforts on the careful evaluation and treatment of overweight patients and integrate programs to yield meaningful and long-lasting weight reduction.

Identifying Overweight Patients

The first step in a treatment strategy is to identify overweight patients (guideline 9.14). At a minimum, all patients entering CR should have height and weight measured and recorded and BMI calculated (kg/m²; see table 9.12). Weight can then be measured on a weekly basis and serve as an index to evaluate program effectiveness.[24] Similar to BMI, waist circumference measurement is an effective means of identifying patients who would benefit from a weight loss intervention.[24]

BMI is frequently used as a surrogate measure of body composition. For adults, overweight is defined as a BMI of 25.0 to 29.9 kg/m²; obesity is defined as a BMI ≥30.0 kg/m². Both overweight and obesity are considered risk factors for developing metabolic syndrome. Thus, metabolic syndrome is an overweight-related medical disorder

---

Guideline 9.14 Weight Management

- Weight management interventions should be targeted to those patients enrolled in CR whose weight and body composition place them at increased risk for, or exacerbation of, cardiometabolic disease, including CHD, diabetes mellitus, hypertension, and dyslipidemia.

- Patients generally at risk include those with a BMI ≥25 kg/m² and/or a waist circumference >40 in. (102 cm) in males and >35 in. (88 cm) in females (see table 7.2).

Table 9.12 Classification of Overweight and Obesity

Weight class	BMI (kg/m²)
Normal	18.5-24.9
Overweight	25.0-29.9
Class 1 obesity	30.0-34.9
Class 2 obesity	35.0-39.9
Class 3 obesity	≥40

that increases an individual's risk of developing CVD.[25] Metabolic syndrome is defined by the presence of three of the following five risk factors: large waist circumference, high BP, elevated fasting glucose and TG levels, and reduced HDL-C (see table 9.13).[26] Metabolic syndrome and associated insulin resistance are particularly prevalent among CR patients.[25] The incidence of metabolic syndrome among patients in CR is more than 50%,[27] twice that of the general population.[28] Excess adiposity associated with metabolic syndrome predicts an increased risk of death and recurrent events following a MI.[29-34] Thus, overweight and obesity should be viewed as a highly prevalent and serious medical condition.

Although BMI is often used to indicate adiposity and to define obesity, it has limitations. It may fail to correctly distinguish lean body weight from adipose body weight and therefore underestimate risk leading to an apparent absent or inverse relationship between obesity and death in patients with CVD sometimes called the obesity paradox.[35] In turn, this may be a limitation in its use in predicting outcomes. In one study of patients undergoing CR after coronary artery

disease events, major adverse cardiac events including acute coronary syndromes, coronary revascularization, and stroke were not associated with BMI but with body fat percentage.[36] Nonetheless, BMI has the advantage of simplicity and familiarity and can be useful in measuring obesity in the short term.

The Energy Balance–Weight Loss Equation

Overweight is a heterogeneous problem stemming from genetic, biologic, and behavioral factors that affect the balance between energy intake (calorie content of food consumed) and total energy expenditure. Total energy expenditure is partitioned into three components: (1) resting metabolic rate (~60%-75% of total); (2) thermic effect of food (~10% of total); and (3) physical activity, the most variable of the three components and the one that can be voluntarily modified (~15%-30% of total) through lifestyle changes.[37] To accomplish weight loss, a net caloric deficit (achieved through increased energy expenditure or dietary restriction or both) needs to occur. A caloric deficit of ~3,500 kcal equates with a weight loss of about 1 lb (~0.45 kg) of fat.[38]

Program Components of Weight Loss

Effective behavior change is integral to the success of any weight loss program and must address reductions in energy intake and increases in energy expenditure through physical activity. Initially practitioners should assess motivation and patient readiness for change to ensure that the patient is at least contemplating making a

Table 9.13 Clinical Identification of Metabolic Syndrome

Risk factor	Defining level
Abdominal obesity (waist circumference)	
• Men	>102 cm (>40 in.)
• Women	>88 cm (>35 in.)
Triglycerides	>150 mg/dL
High-density lipoprotein cholesterol	
• Men	<40 mg/dL
• Women	<50 mg/dL
Blood pressure	≥130 / ≥85 mm Hg
Fasting glucose	≥100 mg/dL

Reprinted by permission from National Cholesterol Education Program (NCEP), "Executive Summary of the Third Report of the Expert Panel on Detection, Evaluation and Treatment of High Blood Cholesterol in Adults (Adult Treatment Panel III)," *JAMA* 289, no 19 (2003): 2560-2572.

change.[39] The three standard components of behavioral weight control programs are behavioral modification, dietary patterns, and exercise and physical activity.[40-42]

Behavioral Modification

Behavioral modification principles focus on changing factors that control behavior. Attention is directed toward identifying environmental antecedents or cues that set the stage for behavior or reinforcers that lead to its reoccurrence. Common program components for weight reduction are shown in table 9.14.

Often treatment sessions in a group setting for approximately 60 min are provided by a trained facilitator (registered dietitian, behavioral psychologist, nurse, clinical exercise physiologist, or related health care professional). Evidence suggests that group therapy is more effective than individual treatment.[38] However, patients should be able to choose their treatment option of a group or individual visit setting. Treatment visits often use a structured curriculum and sessions that are focused on reviewing patient progress, reinforcing a provided plan, and problem solving related to barriers to changes in behavior.

Weight loss is of major importance in improving the risk factor profile in patients both with and without coronary artery disease. A major limitation for CR is that most programs last only 12 weeks or less. Therefore, the challenge is to affect the most long-lasting change in a relatively short period of time or to find novel ways to extend CR in content or duration. The AHA has developed practical tips, including educational information such as knowledge of caloric needs to achieve a healthy weight and understanding the calorie contents of food.[43] In addition, important lifestyle changes, such as food choices and preparation as well as portion control,[43] might be emphasized and discussed frequently on both an individual and group basis during CR. Adapting the curriculum so that requisite information is provided in fewer sessions will help to accommodate participants who cannot complete a 12-week program.

Although many CR programs are of short duration, a very low-calorie diet using high-protein meal replacements has been used very successfully and safely to achieve significant weight loss (more than 20% of excess weight).[44] This approach might be applicable to selected patients in CR programs. One novel method to achieve weight loss used at the Mayo Clinic is a digital health intervention combined with standard CR using a smartphone or web-based portal to individually guide patients through CR.[45,46] This method was successful in achieving a greater weight loss than in standard CR and can also be extended to beyond 90 days.[46] Such an approach may help to individualize CR programs, address the problem of limited resources, and promote a long-term commitment to weight loss and other health-promoting habits. Other alternatives include referring patients to community-based weight loss programs, as well as allowing them to attend classes even if they are not formally enrolled in CR, perhaps by developing and using other digital technology. Partnering with employers and financial incentives may also be successful in achieving weight loss and prolong the effect of a CR program in the long term.[47]

Dietary Pattern

Long-term weight loss should be managed by an allied health professional such as registered dietitian, clinical exercise physiologist, or nurse. A registered dietitian should always be the one who provides meal planning and diet instruc-

Table 9.14 Behavior Modification Techniques

Self-monitoring	Systematic observation and recording of eating behaviors
Stimulus control	Altering the environment associated with eating and exercise
Problem solving	Proposing strategies to control factors that may precipitate excessive caloric intake
Assertiveness training	Teaching assertiveness regarding social situations involving eating and exercise
Goal setting	Establishing realistic short- and long-term weight loss and exercise training goals
Relapse prevention	Developing strategies to prevent or recover from relapse into behaviors associated with weight gain
Positive reinforcement	Emphasizing positive behaviors while avoiding negative thoughts

Adapted by permission from K.D. Brownell, *LEARN Program for Weight Control* (Dallas, TX: American Health Publishing Co, 2000).

tion. In general, patients should have a caloric reduction goal approximately equivalent to 500 to 1,000 kcal less than their estimated daily maintenance energy requirements. To estimate the maintenance energy requirement, multiply baseline body weight by 12.[40] For example, for a 220 lb (100 kg) person, the daily maintenance caloric requirement would be 2,400 kcal, and a targeted daily caloric intake would be between 1,400 and 1,900 kcal. The health care provider should consider an initial goal of reducing body weight by approximately 10% from baseline, but the time frame to accomplish this goal must be individualized.

Diet is critically important in patients with coronary artery disease. Also, strong evidence shows that a heart-healthy diet may not only lead to regression of coronary disease[48] but also improve outcomes.[49] In a controlled trial, patients were assigned a low-fat vegetarian diet combined with smoking cessation, stress management, and exercise. Coronary lesions regressed in the treatment group but progressed in the controls.[48] Unfortunately, adherence to this diet is often poor, even in the short term.[50] This fact underscores the need for individualized recommendations for dietary modification, as well as consideration of reasonable goals and likelihood of compliance. The MEDIT diet, which includes legumes, unrefined cereals and vegetables, fish, low amounts of meat and meat products, olive oil, fermented dairy products, and wine,[51] may achieve greater compliance.[49] The Lyon Diet Heart Study, a randomized secondary prevention trial after a first MI, showed a striking protective effect using this diet after an extended follow-up. Cardiac death and nonfatal MI were reduced (14 events v. 44 in the control prudent Western-type diet group), a protective effect of the MEDIT diet being maintained up to four years after a first infarction. Combining this approach with the overall goal of a reduction of caloric intake is shown to be successful in achieving weight loss in high-risk U.S. populations.[52]

Food journaling (if done correctly) is an effective tool for recognizing current eating habits and documenting caloric intake. Diets with different macronutrient compositions have proven to be compatible with weight loss and CHD risk reduction.[53-56] For weight loss to be maintained, foods consumed must be compatible with long-term adherence focusing on a variety of food choices that ensure adequate nutrients and essential vitamins.

Exercise and PA

The primary objective of an exercise and PA program designed for optimal weight loss is to increase daily caloric expenditure. Standard CR exercise alone is of limited benefit in inducing significant weight loss over a three- to four-month time frame.[10,11,14] Increased caloric expenditure using exercise alone,[57,58] or combined with a comprehensive behavioral weight loss strategy,[20] results in significantly more weight loss than standard CR. Moreover, high calorie expenditure exercise training is well tolerated, is perceived to be as enjoyable as standard CR exercise,[23] and is similar in volume to training that supports long-term weight loss maintenance.[59] Formal exercise sessions should focus on exercises that use large muscle groups—thus maximizing caloric expenditure—performed in a continuous fashion. Patients must be counseled on ways to increase their overall daily activity in addition to the formal exercise training.

Intensity Initially, exercise intensity should be approximately 60% to 70% of heart rate reserve, which for most people equates to a fairly light to moderate intensity (RPE of 11 or 12). This exercise intensity is safe, is well tolerated, provides an adequate stimulus to improve cardiovascular fitness,[60,61] and can usually be performed in a continuous fashion for a prolonged duration. With regard to progression, the focus should be on increasing duration first, followed by increases in exercise intensity, which can rise to 80% of heart rate reserve as an upper limit.

Frequency Initially during CR participation, an every-other-day exercise schedule is recommended. After a few weeks, frequency of training should be increased to five to seven days/week. It is helpful to encourage appropriate patients to perform exercise at home on days when they are not participating in CR. Thus, exercise therapy should be viewed as a medicine that is dosed nearly every day for weight control. It will maximize caloric expenditure and reinforce exercise as a consistent part of the daily routine. In addition, the importance of increasing overall daily PA must be reinforced. Adults desiring to lose and control their body weight should increase their aerobic activity to exceed the minimum and move toward 300 min/week. At least two days/week of strength training exercise should also be included.[62]

Modality Barring musculoskeletal limitations, weight-bearing activities provide the greatest caloric expenditure and should be recommended whenever possible.[63] Activities such as free walking, as well as machines such as treadmills or elliptical exercisers, are generally associated with greater caloric expenditure than arm or leg ergometers. If weight-bearing exercises are difficult, modalities that employ large muscle groups should be selected, such as upright or recumbent cycles that use both upper and lower extremities. Caution is warranted with the use of modalities that may be biomechanically difficult for overweight patients. Most equipment has manufacturer recommended body weight limits for safety.

Duration Gradual increases in duration from 30 to over 45 to 60 min are recommended for overweight patients. Intermittent exercise may be necessary for those who are limited in duration or intensity. Patients should be closely monitored and questioned regarding signs of overuse.

In suitable patients, high-calorie-expenditure exercise (3,000-3,500-kcal/week exercise-related energy expenditure) may be used. In one study, when compared with standard CR exercise (700-800 kcal/week), high-calorie-expenditure exercise resulted in double the weight loss (8.2 ± 4 kg v. 3.7 ± 5 kg), as well as greater fat mass loss and waist reduction (–7 ± 5 cm v. –5 ± –5 cm) at 5 months. High-calorie-expenditure exercise is of longer duration and greater frequency but, in fact, lower-intensity (50-60% v. 65-70% peak $\dot{V}O_2$) thus employing a *walk often and walk far* strategy.[20] As one might expect, there were beneficial effects on the risk factor profile. Notably, significant weight loss was maintained at one year.[20]

Lifestyle Activity Increasing PA levels separate from formal, prescribed exercise can lead to additional significant benefit.[64] The amount of PA required for acquiring weight loss or for sustaining weight loss may be greater than the recommendations for general public health. Therefore, overweight and obese adults may need to be gradually progressed from initial recommendations of 150 min/week (1,000 kcal/week) to 250 to 300 min/week (>2,000 kcal/week).[65,66] Another potentially effective recommendation includes simply decreasing the amount of time spent in sedentary activities.[64] Traditionally, bouts of exercise have been recommended. The 2008 Physical Activity Guidelines for Americans recommended that adults accumulate moderate-to-vigorous physical activity (MVPA) in bouts of 10 or more min.[62] However, data from the National Health and Nutrition Examination Survey 2003-2006 and death records available in a follow-up period of over six years suggests that MVPA may reduce mortality independent of how activity is accumulated (i.e., continuous v. various duration bouts).[64] Simple strategies for incorporating an increased amount of overall PA in daily life, reducing dependence on energy-saving devices, and increasing energy expenditure include taking stairs instead of elevators, parking at the outer perimeter of parking lots, exiting public (bus, subway) or private (taxi) transportation several blocks before desired destination, and walking or biking as alternative modes of transportation. Patients should be taught that many home activities, such as lawn mowing, yard work, and housework, all increase overall caloric expenditure. For weight loss and eventual weight maintenance, patients should be advised and instructed about ways to increase their levels of lifestyle PA on all days of the week and to decrease their sedentary time.

Psychosocial Considerations

Many patients with heart disease present to CR with significant psychosocial concerns, including depression, anxiety, social isolation, cognitive impairment, problematic personality characteristics (e.g., type D hostility, narcissism), sexual dysfunction, substance use or abuse (e.g., tobacco, alcohol), and poor adherence. Clearly, heart disease occurs in the context of psychosocial considerations common to all members of society. However, patients with heart disease often have psychosocial risk factors for the development of CVD, such as depression, anxiety, or poor social support. Psychosocial considerations can precede heart disease and the cardiac event or condition that makes someone eligible for CR. Acute events or the stress of managing a chronic condition can also bring these issues to the forefront.

Furthermore, psychosocial considerations often emerge after an acute cardiac event or in the course of a chronic health condition, and it is clear that recovering from cardiac events, managing chronic heart disease, and adjusting to subsequent life changes is a challenge for most cardiac patients and their families.[1]

In this complex interplay of psychosocial factors and chronic disease, CR professionals also recognize that the patients who enroll in CR are likely to be a select subset of those who are eligible. Given the underutilization of CR,[2,3] the rates of various psychosocial considerations within a CR program population can vary widely. For example, poor social support or depression could be barriers to both enrolling in and completing CR, resulting in lower rates of depression in CR patients than would be expected. However, some programs achieve high enrollment for the communities they serve, in which case depression levels in CR may be similar to those observed in the local population of patients with heart disease.

Clinicians in secondary prevention settings such as phase 2 CR should address the psychosocial needs of patients.[4] These needs can be addressed using assessment, feedback, intervention delivered in CR, and referrals as appropriate for evaluation and treatment by mental health professionals outside CR.

Addressing psychosocial considerations improves quality of life regardless of potential impact on cardiovascular mortality, which calls into question whether or not psychosocial considerations are somehow less important if they are not modifiable risk factors for heart disease. In the era of patient-centered care, it is appropriate to address psychosocial contributors to quality of life whenever possible.

Also, psychiatric diagnoses have evolved from the fourth edition of the *Diagnostic and Statistical Manual of Mental Disorders (DSM-4)*[15] to the fifth edition *(DSM-5)*,[16] which is reflected in this updated edition of the AACVPR guidelines. Eligibility for participation in CR or in the CR setting has expanded to include new diagnostic categories (e.g., heart failure, peripheral artery disease), in which the effectiveness of typical interventions may vary. For example, antidepressants do not appear effective for comorbid depression and heart failure.[10-12] Also, AACVPR has issued several new documents such as the Certified CR Professional (CCRP) competencies blueprint, a candidate handbook, and a study guide for CR professionals seeking certification through the certification exam. The mental health infrastructure available to CR professionals for referrals varies and remains inadequate in many areas. Moreover, the literature on psychosocial considerations and heart disease has continued to grow. If CR professionals find the domain of addressing psychosocial considerations in CR to be broad with fuzzy boundaries, it is understandable.

Therefore, this section is limited to a focused and practical overview, aligned with other documents (e.g., CCRP materials), and targeted to outpatient CR professionals. Many worthy topics cannot be covered adequately (e.g., spiritual needs, sexual function), and these guidelines should not be considered as a comprehensive description of the psychosocial concerns that some CR programs may address. For example, addressing sexual concerns in education classes is highly encouraged. Finally, some of the opinions expressed here are those of the contributors and not necessarily those of AACVPR. Therefore, some variability will exist between programs in how psychosocial considerations are addressed.

Key Psychosocial Considerations

The most recent version of the core competencies for CR identifies psychological distress and other psychosocial indicators as key considerations. Psychological distress includes clinically significant depression, anxiety, sexual dysfunction, and marital or family distress. Other psychosocial indicators may or may not be distressing, but they are relevant to treatment. These indicators include social isolation, anger or hostility, and substance abuse. Although tobacco use is considered substance abuse, it is covered by other core competencies and sections of these guidelines.

Depression

Depression is a leading cause of disability and is often comorbid with heart disease. Depression both increases the risk of developing heart disease and increases the risk of a poor outcome (e.g., mortality) in patients with heart disease.[17-20] Furthermore, heart disease may contribute to depression symptoms through physiological (e.g., inflammation, medication side effects) and psychosocial mechanisms (e.g., stress, loss of preferred activities, role changes). Depression is also a barrier to adherence (including exercise),[21] lowering smoking cessation success, impairing medication adherence,[22] and generally reducing the benefit received from treatments involving patient behavior.[23] Depression presents a risk of failing to complete CR.[24,25] Thus, the AHA issued a scientific advisory, endorsed by the American Psychiatric Association, that recommended screening for depression in all patients with heart disease.[26]

A formal diagnosis of a depressive disorder such as major depressive disorder is based on the diagnostic criteria from the *DSM-5* or the *World Health Organization's International Classification of Diseases (ICD-11)*. The symptoms from the *DSM-5* are as follows:

- Depressed or sad mood
- Loss of interest in activities that were previously pleasurable
- Changes in appetite or unintended weight loss
- Changes in sleep (too much or too little)
- Markedly reduced psychomotor activity or agitation that is observable by others
- Fatigue or loss of energy
- Guilty or worthless feelings that are more than guilt about being ill
- Concentration or thinking problems
- Suicidal thoughts or behaviors

Some of these symptoms overlap with those that are common in heart disease. Qualified health professionals, including physicians and psychologists, can formally diagnose depressive disorders. However, all CR professionals should be able to recognize symptoms of clinically significant depression whether or not the threshold for major depression is met.

Anxiety

Many patients with heart disease exhibit symptoms of anxiety. As with depression, anxiety may be involved in the development of CVD and appears to be a risk factor for poorer outcomes. A number of anxiety disorders are listed in the *DSM-5*,[16] including the following:

- Agoraphobia
- Generalized anxiety disorder
- Panic disorder
- Social anxiety disorder
- Specific phobias

Also, the *DSM-5* now lists these categories of disorders that were previously conceptualized as anxiety disorders:

- Obsessive-compulsive and related disorders
- Trauma- and stressor-related disorders (including posttraumatic stress disorder)

As with depression, patients may have clinically significant anxiety that may not meet the threshold of a psychiatric diagnosis. Common symptoms of anxiety include the following:

- Cognitive symptoms such as worry, especially worry that is difficult to stop or control, feeling unable to cope, and feeling that things are not real
- Emotional symptoms such as fear, dread, uneasy anticipation, and irritability
- Physical symptoms such as weakness, numbness, fatigue, headache, muscle tension or ache, stomach churning, shortness of breath, blurred vision, dizziness, heart palpitations, trembling and shaking, feelings of paralysis, sweating, and pressure in the head or chest

Social Isolation and Social Support

Many older Americans experience considerable loneliness, which is often caused by social isolation. A related factor, perceived social support, is also an important psychosocial consideration relevant to CR. Together, social support and social isolation have important implications for prognosis in CVD. For example, a classic study reported that patients who were socially isolated or who lacked a close confidant were more likely to die after a heart attack than those with adequate social support.[27,28] Inadequate emotional or practical social support can be a barrier to participation in CR. Conversely, many patients report that the interaction with staff and other patients is one of the most valued experiences in CR. However, patients with significant levels of loneliness may not receive enough benefit from increased exposure to social interaction, in which case professional mental health services would be necessary.[29]

Addressing Key Psychosocial Considerations

CR programs should have clear procedures in place for assessing psychosocial considerations, providing interventions that fall within the scope of practice for CR, referring patients to qualified mental health professionals for further evaluation and treatment when necessary, and documenting psychosocial outcomes.

Psychosocial Assessment

Assessing psychosocial factors includes both screening for the presence of specific psychosocial considerations using reliable and valid instruments, and a broader evaluation of the patient's psychosocial concerns. That is, the psychosocial evaluation should start with the intake interview, which often provides the most complete information. The most current statement of core competencies advises that staff should be able to provide a comprehensive evaluation that includes assessment of psychosocial concerns related to heart disease, such as depression, anxiety, social isolation, and anger or hostility.[4] The interview represents an opportunity to go beyond the minimum screening requirements. Areas not covered by screening instruments could include sexual functioning, difficulty with adherence to medical recommendations, history of mental health treatment, and spiritual needs. Some level of distress is common; many patients are grieving the loss of health, youth, employment, and role functioning. This topic can be explored during the interview.

Key psychosocial concerns should be documented quantitatively using screening instruments. The areas covered by screening instruments can rise to the level of diagnosable mental disorders or serious impediments to recovery, participation in CR, and the management of heart disease. For example, concerning depression, the 2007 AACVPR/ACC/AHA performance measures[30] included a sample data collection tool to document that this performance measure for the presence or absence of depression is being met. The guidelines specify that the target goal is an assessment of the presence or absence of depression using a valid and reliable screening tool, including formal documentation of the following:

- Patient is assessed for of presence or absence of depression using a valid and reliable screening tool.
- The patient is screened for depression.
- If the patient is depressed, results are discussed with the patient and the health care provider is notified.
- The patient is re-screened for depression prior to completion of the program.
- If the patient is depressed, results are discussed with the patient and the health care provider is notified.

In addition to interview procedures, screening instruments should be administered at the beginning and end of CR for key psychosocial considerations such as depression, anxiety, social isolation, and quality of life. For example, Medicare requires an evaluation of "aspects of family/home situation" that affect treatment (i.e., social support), although the guidelines do not specify screening procedures.[31] In addition to the intake interview, a variety of screening instruments could be employed for social support, such as the ENRICHD Social Support Inventory,[32] which is a 7-item self-report inventory.

Many CR programs also include screening instruments for other considerations such as sexual functioning, anger or hostility, and medication adherence. The results of the screening administered should be documented at the onset

---

Guideline 9.15   Assessment of Psychosocial Factors

Staff should identify clinically significant levels of psychosocial distress using a combination of clinical interview and psychosocial screening instruments at program entry, exit, and periodic follow-up.

- The clinical interview can be broad and cover multiple areas.
- Reliable and valid screening instruments should be administered and the results recorded for key

psychosocial considerations, which would typically include depression, anxiety, social support, and health-related quality of life.

- In particular, the presence or absence of depression should be documented, as well as what action was taken for cases identified (e.g., referral).

and conclusion of participation in CR. The specific tools used vary widely, and the AACVPR website is a great resource for selecting specific instruments. The website content continues to evolve. For example, turnkey enrollment and adherence strategy documents have recently been developed, and toolkits and templates for CR professionals may be available.

Often sex, ethnic, and age differences exist in the expression of psychological symptoms. For example, some people are less likely to admit feelings of depression for cultural or psychological reasons (e.g., not being very self-aware or expressive regarding psychological issues). Women are about twice as likely as men to have clinically significant depression and anxiety. It is also important to repeat screening assessments at the end of CR. Many patients who qualify for a depression diagnosis were already depressed before their cardiac event, and about half of the cases of depression in patients with heart disease emerge in the year following an acute cardiac event.

Providing Interventions in CR

Interventions targeting psychosocial considerations common in patients with heart disease include these three options:

1. Behavioral interventions, such as psychotherapy or counseling

2. Pharmacological interventions, such as medications used to treat anxiety, depression, or sexual dysfunction

3. Behavioral interventions that can be incorporated into the CR program

Most behavioral interventions for psychosocial concerns are beyond the scope of practice for CR, in the sense that a full course of behavioral treatment may not be practical given the other demands of CR programming. Thus, although CR professionals are expected to be familiar with effective behavior change techniques, they are not expected to be trained to provide formal cognitive behavioral therapy for anxiety or depression. Although it would be ideal, there is no requirement (e.g., for program certification) that a psychologist or other mental health provider be housed within a CR program, or even readily available in the health care system for consultation. As is discussed later, many CR programs will need to be innovative and proactive in cultivating referral options.

Pharmacological approaches for depression and anxiety include selective serotonin reuptake inhibitors (SSRI), which are generally safe, affordable, and potentially associated with improved prognosis in heart disease.[14,33] However, their effectiveness for reducing depression relative to placebo varies. For example, in a study of patients with depression who had experienced a heart attack, sertraline only improved symptoms of depression for patients with a prior history of depression.[13] In another study, citalopram was found to reduce depression symptoms in patients with heart disease.[34] In some patients eligible for CR, such as those with heart failure, little evidence shows that antidepressants are more effective than placebos for reducing depression symptoms.[10-12]

Pharmacological treatments are most commonly provided by primary care physicians, although in some cases a psychiatrist may be consulted. Thus, most behavioral interventions and pharmacological treatments for psychosocial considerations require a referral.

Some effective interventions for psychosocial concerns can be provided as part of CR. For example, CR programs have long provided limited individual or small group counseling and education related to a variety of psychosocial concerns such as stress, anxiety, and depression. Education provided in CR is an appropriate way to raise awareness of the high levels of psychological distress among patients with heart disease. Normalizing distress encourages patients to seek help when necessary, even if the CR program isn't equipped to fully diagnose or treat their mental health concerns.

The activities of exercise-based CR are inherently therapeutic. Outpatient CR improves psychosocial comorbidities, improves quality of life, reduces risk factors, and reduces the risk of mortality.[17,35,36] For example, a small body of literature suggested that PA is as effective for depression as SSRIs in healthy older adults.[37-40] Monitored exercise is also an exposure treatment, which is the foundation of most behavioral interventions for anxiety. That is, patients learn in a controlled and safe environment that they can tolerate exercise and expand their physical activity behaviors in ways that they may not have anticipated. This explanation may not address every symptom of anxiety (e.g., worry), but some of the physiological manifestations of anxiety are similar to the effects of exercise (e.g., elevated heart rate, rapid breathing), which can help patients to reframe these symptoms as expected sensations of vigorous exertion and not signs of danger.

Given that psychotherapy and pharmacological treatments for depression do not improve prognosis in patients with heart disease, it could be argued that high-quality CR is an essential treatment for comorbid depression and heart disease. One hypothesis, albeit untested, is that CR targets some of the mechanisms by which depression may confer risk of premature mortality (e.g., physical fitness, autonomic nervous system functioning, adherence, stress, risk factor reduction), while simultaneously reducing depression symptoms. Of course, severe depression cases and those that do not improve during the course of CR would necessitate a referral for additional evaluation and treatment.[26] Most guidelines list first-line treatments for depression and anxiety as being cognitive behavioral therapy and pharmacological treatment, in part because performing randomized clinical trials of CR for comorbid psychosocial distress and heart disease is unethical (all eligible patients should be offered CR). In the absence of such studies, it is unlikely that professional association guidelines will fully recognize the value of CR for psychosocial distress comorbid with heart disease. Nevertheless, CR professionals should feel confident that CR is beneficial for psychosocial considerations, and they have some options for incorporating limited interventions into the program beyond structured exercise.

Support, Education, and Guidance

Support for the patient and family begins at the first contact, and a structured program of education and psychosocial support tailored to the needs identified in the initial evaluation should be developed. Early interactions should emphasize active listening to patient and family concerns and the development of rapport. Patients should be assured that their questions and fears are normal and should receive practical suggestions for the management of stressors that accompany hospitalization and recovery. The CR professional should provide multiple, brief interventions consisting of education and anticipatory guidance.[41] Conceptualization of the illness as an opportunity for growth in multiple domains including physical, mental, and spiritual can lead to more optimistic thoughts, which ought to increase the likelihood of successful outcomes. Proactive coping with stressors should be encouraged, and patients may be empowered through recall of previous success they may have had in dealing with other life challenges.

Stress Management and Relaxation Training

A variety of brief interventions geared toward teaching the patient to relax can be incorporated into routine care. It is common for the education sessions in CR to include time devoted to stress management and relaxation training. Examples of stress management and relaxation training include instruction in abdominal breathing, moderate-intensity progressive muscle relaxation, mindfulness meditation exercises, and similar techniques. Where applicable, patients can be encouraged to recall and use previously learned relaxation strategies, such as the breathing techniques used in Lamaze training. Patients can also be instructed to focus attention on soothing stimuli or visual imagery. The value of stress

---

 Guideline 9.16 Interventions for Psychosocial Factors

CR staff should provide a therapeutic experience in the program, recognizing that a positive and encouraging atmosphere capitalizes on the psychosocial benefits of a comprehensive exercise-based secondary prevention program. CR staff should provide limited behavioral interventions in the course of CR, including individual counseling as necessary and small-group education covering topics such as the following:

- Stress management
- Coping with depression, anger, and anxiety
- Maximizing social support
- Effective principles of health behavior change
- Regular exercise and physical activity

management and relaxation should not be underestimated. A small but important study showed that 12 weeks of stress management incorporated into CR reduced clinical events compared to comprehensive CR alone at up to 5 years post-CR.[8] Where feasible, incorporating more intensive structured stress management training into CR may improve prognosis, although more research is necessary.

Referral to Other Providers

Referring a patient who screens positive for depression, anxiety, or other key psychosocial considerations to a mental health professional is a common decision in CR. Programs should have clear guidelines about what warrants a referral, the process for referring patients for additional evaluation and treatment, and what mental health infrastructure is available.

When to Refer Patients should be referred for further evaluation and treatment for any psychosocial consideration that is outside the scope of practice of CR professionals, including both psychological distress and other psychosocial indicators. Common reasons for referral include severe anxiety or depression, as well as a wide variety of issues for which additional consultation may be helpful. The kinds of psychosocial concerns that may merit a referral will depend on what CR professionals have assessed. For example, some programs may assess sexual dysfunction and marital distress and may have access to specialists that can address these concerns beyond the typical patient education provided by CR. All patients should be referred if they show any indication of suicide risk or self-harm. Certainly, patients should be referred for distress that has not resolved during CR, reinforcing the need for repeated screening and careful discharge planning.

Available Health Infrastructure Patients who are referred for further evaluation may need medications, psychotherapy, spiritual counseling, or social work assistance. If a referral for specialized counseling is necessary, the CR professional should initiate and maintain communication with the counselor whenever possible. For example, where alcohol abuse counseling is indicated, the CR professional should, within the limits of confidentiality, inform the counselor of any observed changes in tolerance, symptoms of withdrawal, or odor of alcohol on the breath.

Effective referral and consultation require a robust local mental health infrastructure. Academic medical centers may be well-resourced with departments of psychiatry and behavioral health housing mental health professionals such as psychiatrists, psychologists, social workers, and counselors. Alternatively, CR programs in some areas may not have access to coordinated mental health services at their location. For example, affiliation with a mental health care provider in the community can improve access to resources that can assist patients with addressing identified needs. Thus, programs are encouraged to identify local behavioral health resources, even when they are outside the hospital system, and cultivate relationships with them.[42]

In practice, an elevated score on a screening instrument (e.g., depression) often results in a referral back to and notification of the primary care physician. An ongoing conversation in CR can reveal whether or not any action was taken and whether or not additional referrals are needed. Finally, some patients with chronic mental health conditions can readily report the services they receive. For example, severely depressed patients will list the medications they are taking for depression during the intake process and can explain

Guideline 9.17 Measuring Outcomes of Psychosocial Factors

For each patient, outcomes of psychosocial considerations should be documented. They include the following:

- The results of screening instruments
- Any follow-up actions taken based on screening instruments (e.g., referral, reevaluate in 30 days)

- Improvement in depression, anxiety, social support, and health-related quality of life
- Attainment of individual treatment goals related to psychosocial outcomes

Performance measures and outcomes should be entered into the registry as appropriate.

whether or not "it's working," including their preference for intensified treatment or desire for a referral. As a caveat, patients typically do not request a behavioral health services referral, so professionals in CR should take the initiative to ask.

Measuring Outcomes

Patients completing CR are evaluated for all their individual treatment goals, including psychosocial considerations. That is, the screening instruments administered at enrollment should be repeated, and the results documented. At minimum, this evaluation would include depression, anxiety, social isolation, and quality of life. These domains are in keeping with Medicare requirements specific to CR[31] and performance measures.[30] Measuring outcomes provides valuable information for thoughtful discharge planning to ensure continuity of care. In addition, documenting outcomes also provides evidence for the value of CR that can be shared with hospital administrators as the occasion arises.

Environmental Considerations

The effects of traditional cardiorespiratory risk factors on disease onset, progression, and mortality are well established. However, despite substantial improvements in prevention, diagnosis, and treatment, the prevalence of disease continues to escalate.[1-3] Therefore, in an attempt to maximize risk reduction, some of the focus has shifted over the last two decades to the identification of other potential causes of disease and disease outcomes, with the environment being a prime target.[3-7]

The cardiorespiratory system is affected by numerous environmental factors. Those most extensively studied include air pollution; the heavy metals arsenic, lead, and cadmium; and extremes in noise and temperature.[1] Because approximately 91% of the world's population is exposed to outdoor air pollution levels that exceed the air quality guidelines of the World Health Organization (WHO),[8] the most extensive environmental threat to public health comes from air pollution.[9-13]

Recent statistics from the Global Burden of Disease Study[14] suggest that exposure to ambient air pollution is the sixth most important risk factor for all-cause mortality worldwide, accounting for approximately 4.1 million deaths annually and 105.7 million disability-adjusted life years (DALYs). Of these air-pollution-related deaths, the vast majority (58%) are due to ischemic heart disease and stroke, followed by chronic obstructive pulmonary disease (COPD) (18%), lower respiratory tract infections (18%), and lung cancer (6%).[8] Furthermore, the disability burden associated with the annual daily exposure to outdoor air pollution is higher than other well-recognized modifiable disease risk factors such as elevated cholesterol levels, excess dietary sodium, and a sedentary lifestyle. In women, the negative ramifications of air pollution on health appear to even outweigh smoking status.[14] If these trends continue, the contribution of outdoor air pollution to premature mortality is projected to double by 2050.[11]

Exposure to air pollution is not just restricted to time spent outdoors. Even though most people remain indoors for approximately 85% of their daily life,[15] significant amounts of outdoor pollution can infiltrate buildings,[16-19] accounting for the majority of risk associated with air pollution.[17,18] Other sources of indoor pollution include smoke from domestic cooking and tobacco.[16,17] Additionally, recent studies have raised concerns about the negative effects of synthetic nanoparticles, which are prevalent indoors.[19]

Regardless of whether the pollutants are present indoors or outdoors, pollution is a complex mixture of many different components.[2,9,19] Of particular concern are the six pollutants, termed *criteria air pollutants*, for which air quality standards are set by the Environmental Protection Agency.[20,21] These are airborne particulate matter (PM), ozone (O_3), sulfur dioxide (SO_2), carbon monoxide (CO), nitrogen dioxide (NO_2), and lead (Pb).[9,19-22] Of these pollutants, PM is considered especially damaging to health, and the terms *particulate matter* and *air pollution* are often used interchangeably.[8-10,19,20] Therefore, PM will be the primary focus of this discussion, and occasional reference to other pollutants will be made if pertinent. This section will examine the acute and chronic effects of environmental pollution on the cardiorespiratory system, explore which individuals have heightened susceptibility, and discuss potential recommendations to help mitigate the risk. Although smoking contributes to air pollution, tobacco smoke is already established as a traditional risk factor for cardiorespiratory disease and thus is beyond the scope of this discussion.

Particulate matter consists of both solid and liquid particles suspended in air. The predominant sources are domestic fuels, vehicle emissions, soil and road dust generated by wind, moving vehicles and construction work, industrial combustion, metal processing, agriculture and the incineration of agricultural debris, forest fires, and bioaerosols such as endotoxins, pollen, and fungal spores.[4,5,19,21,23,24] Currently, residential energy use is the primary contributor to global air-pollution-related mortality.[8,11] However, traffic pollution also has a substantial impact on ambient PM and public health.[5,11,16,17,19,21,24] Although legislative controls have reduced tailpipe emissions, other vehicle-related emissions from engine lubricating oil as well as road, tire, and brake wear also play a concerning role.[24] For example, in the United States, United Kingdom, and Germany, 20% of air-pollution-associated mortality (as compared to 5% globally) is attributable to land traffic emissions.[11] Due to an increasing occurrence of wildfires, some predict that these will become a more important contributor to global air pollution in the future, especially because wildfires can cause short-term elevations in ambient PM, exceeding levels produced by both traffic and industry.[21,25,26]

Depending on the source of the PM, there is variation in chemical composition, mass, size, number, reactivity, site and efficiency of pulmonary deposition, and toxicity.[4,10,19,20,27] Due to this inherent complexity, PM is typically classified and regulated by mass within three specific aerodynamic size ranges: coarse particles (PM_{10}), fine particles ($PM_{2.5}$), and ultrafine particles ($PM_{0.1}$) (table 9.15).[1,4,5,19,23,27]

Once deposited, these particles likely activate local sensory receptors and induce inflammatory and stress responses, which can extend beyond the lungs to the cardiovascular system. However, the smaller, more soluble particles may also cross the pulmonary epithelium into the circulatory system, inducing direct systemic effects.[1,4] Although evidence supporting the toxicity of the ultrafine particles is growing, $PM_{2.5}$ is primarily implicated in adverse health outcomes, with more than half of the health burden being cardiovascular in nature.[2,4-6,8,9,11,14,19,28] As such, both the American Heart Association and the European Society for Cardiology now formally acknowledge $PM_{2.5}$ as an independent risk factor for cardiovascular disease (CVD).[9]

Currently, attempts to determine exposure risks and hazard ratios associated with PM are crude due to the challenges of sampling accuracy and variability in regional PM composition. Nevertheless, a recent systematic review and meta-analysis indicated that for every 10 $\mu g \cdot m^{-3}$ increase in $PM_{2.5}$, global hospital admissions and mortality from cardiorespiratory diseases increase by 1.64% and 2.29%, respectively.[13] Moreover, the largest portion of global morbidity and mortality from $PM_{2.5}$ exposure is due to cardiovascular disorders.[4,5,8,9,11,13,19,28,29] To put the cardiovascular mortality risk into perspective, van der Zee and colleagues[29] estimate that each 10 $\mu g \cdot m^{-3}$ increment in $PM_{2.5}$ is equivalent in risk to the secondhand smoke of approximately 5.3 cigarettes. Although there is a disproportionate variation in pollution levels between the developed and developing world, with the highest concentrations reported in China and India, no safe threshold level for $PM_{2.5}$ is apparent: Exposure levels at or below the current recommended

Table 9.15 Particulate Matter Classification

Classification	Diameter (μm^{-3})	Composition	Site of pulmonary deposition
Coarse particles (PM_{10})	2.5-10	Natural and non-exhaust sources (e.g., soil and road dust, tire and brake wear, bioaerosols)	Upper airways
Fine particles ($PM_{2.5}$)	<2.5	Primarily combustion sources, including vehicle emissions (e.g., organic carbon; transition metals such as vanadium, nickel, zinc, iron, and copper; volatile organic compounds; ammonia; sulfate; and nitrite)	Small airways and alveoli
Ultrafine particles ($PM_{0.1}$)	<0.1	Combustion sources, primarily vehicular	Small airways and alveoli; may cross the pulmonary epithelium

limits (<10 $\mu g \cdot m^{-3}$) are still associated with significant threats to public health.[1,4,9,11,13,14,19,21,30-34]

Although the precise cause for the cardiovascular system's enhanced susceptibility to air pollution is unclear,[2] the adverse effects—both clinical and subclinical—can either occur following an acute exposure (of hours to days) or develop over time with chronic (months to years) exposure.[1,2,4,5,9] These pollutant-induced cardiovascular alterations appear to occur through various mechanisms and culminate in several similar outcomes, such as atherosclerosis, thrombosis, ischemia, and arrhythmogenesis, as well as potential alterations to cardiac or vascular structure and function.[1]

Effects of Short-Term Exposure

Although predominantly limited to individuals with underlying disease, many studies, systematic reviews, and meta-analyses report that short-term elevations in air pollution, particularly PM, NO_2, and volatile organic compounds (much of which are traffic derived), are associated with an increased risk of cardiac-related morbidity and mortality.[1,2,4,5,9,19,28] For example, pooled effects from multiple meta-analyses demonstrate transient elevations in $PM_{2.5}$ (per 10 $\mu g \cdot m^{-3}$ increases) over the previous few hours to days are associated with a 2.5% increased risk of an acute ST-segment elevated myocardial infarction (MI), as well as an increased risk of hospitalization or death from heart failure (2.1%), ischemic stroke (1.1%), and various arrhythmias and other electrocardiographic changes (1.0%) such as atrial and ventricular fibrillation, ventricular tachycardia, premature ventricular contractions, conduction disorders, ST-segment depression, altered heart-rate variability, and myocardial repolarization rates.[1,7,9,32] Short duration exposures to the major gaseous pollutants are associated with comparable levels of risk.[5,7,9,16,32,35,36]

The acute effects of air pollution can also be more subtle. A plethora of epidemiological studies note an association between acute exposure to air pollutants and subclinical markers of cardiovascular disease. Short-term exposure is sufficient to cause an acute elevation in markers of systemic inflammation, such as interleukin-6 and tumor necrosis factor alpha, which are likely a spillover from pulmonary inflammation and oxidative stress following pollutant deposition. The pro-inflammatory state within the vasculature may

subsequently cause other commonly reported alterations, including endothelial dysfunction, vascular injury, and hypercoagulability (from an increase in endothelial cell and platelet activation, and potentially increased hepatic fibrinogen production). Additionally, acute elevations in air pollution can cause rapid alterations in heart rate, decreased heart rate variability, increased systolic blood pressure, and narrowing of the retinal arterioles, an important predictor of future hypertension.[1,2,4,5,19,23] Air pollutants can trigger several lung receptors and nerve endings, resulting in sympathetic overactivation; this autonomic imbalance may explain the variations in heart rate and blood pressure. However, the inflammatory and autonomic pathways are not mutually exclusive: They share molecular cascades, and the physiological effects of air pollution are therefore more likely in response to a combination of the two pathways.[1,5,23]

Until recently, ozone (O_3) was typically viewed as a pollutant primarily involved in adverse respiratory effects,[21] particularly airway narrowing and reduced gas diffusion.[37] However, ozone is now understood to have independent cardiovascular effects, with short-term elevations being linked with increased markers of vascular inflammation as well as altered fibrinolysis, heart rate variability, and cardiac repolarization.[21] Although an acute fluctuation in ozone is also an important stimulus of stroke, heart failure decompensation, and overall cardiovascular mortality, the cumulative evidence for the association between ozone and acute MI risk is less consistent.[5,7,9,21]

Although effect estimates are not as strong as for the cardiovascular diseases, there is much evidence for an association between acute spikes in air pollution and the exacerbation of preexisting pulmonary diseases, including asthma, COPD, and cystic fibrosis.[24,31,38] The primary triggers are ozone and traffic pollutants,[31,38] and the respiratory system appears more reactive to short-term fluctuations in air pollutants than long-term exposure.[24]

Effects of Chronic Exposure

A number of large cohort studies now show that chronic exposure (of a few years to decades), especially to traffic pollution, is associated with the pathogenesis of cardiorespiratory diseases and elevated mortality from these diseases.[9,24,31] For instance, pooled estimates of chronic, persistent exposure to air pollution indicate that every 10 $\mu g \cdot m^{-3}$ increase in $PM_{2.5}$ is associated with an 11% increase in cardiovascular mortality, with the strongest association being for mortality from ischemic heart disease.[1,5,9] Mortality rates are also inversely proportional to residential distance from major roadways.[1,17,40-43] A large-scale and widely cited study of middle-aged and older American women followed over a 26-year period found that living within 50 m (~160 ft) of a major roadway increased the risk of sudden cardiac death by 38% when compared to those women living at least 500 m away. The hazard ratio for sudden cardiac death increased by 6% for every 100 m closer to a major roadway an individual lived, with these effects persisting following adjustment for potential confounders and cardiovascular risk factors.[42] Similar levels of relative risk were seen in a large cohort study of both men and women living within metropolitan Vancouver. In addition, the risk of cardiovascular mortality decreased by almost 12% in those who moved greater than 150 m away from traffic during the nine-year study period.[40]

In addition, there is strong evidence linking the persistent exposure to air pollutants and the development of chronic diseases, with heart failure and ischemic heart disease being the primary clinical outcomes.[1,2,9] Multiple recent reviews describe how chronic exposure alters several subclinical factors associated with both the onset and progression of disease, thus predisposing individuals to future or recurrent acute events. Importantly, susceptibility to the adverse effects of long-term exposure is noted in those with and without underlying cardiovascular disease. The most consistent findings include chronic low-level pulmonary and systemic inflammation and sympathetic activation, elevated blood pressure, microvascular (i.e., retinal arteriole) narrowing and risk of hypertension, reductions in ankle brachial index and increased likelihood of peripheral artery disease, increased right or left ventricular mass (thus predisposing individuals to the development of heart failure or exacerbating preexisting disease), and increased markers of atherosclerosis such as endothelial dysfunction, increased carotid intima-media thickness, and coronary artery calcification.[1,2,4,5,19,44] Arrhythmogenesis, however, appears to be more affected by

short-term fluctuations in pollution and is limited to those with cardiovascular disease.[1,5,9]

More recently, some have explored the plausibility for a link between chronic air pollution exposure and other adverse health outcomes related to cardiovascular disease such as type 2 diabetes mellitus (T2DM), epigenetic alterations, and potentially even obesity.[1,2,4,5,19,28,34,45,46] Although not all have seen an interaction effect, many epidemiological studies from North America, Europe, and Asia have noted a relationship between long-term air pollution inhalation (particularly traffic pollution) and insulin resistance.[5,28,34] For example, in a large cohort study of 62,012 nondiabetic adults living in Ontario, Canada, followed for a 14-year period, Chen and colleagues[47] demonstrated that the risk of incident diabetes increased by 11% for every 10 $\mu g \cdot m^{-3}$ increase in $PM_{2.5}$ concentration. Furthermore, animal models of chronic PM exposure exceeding recommended limits have noted insulin dysfunction in the vasculature, liver, and muscle.[48,49] Proposed pathogenic mechanisms include persistent sympathetic upregulation, inflammation, hepatic steatosis, and endoplasmic reticulum stress.[5,34] A limited number of studies suggest that chronic exposure to air pollution may also predispose individuals to obesity, a well-known risk factor for T2DM.[1,5] Although data for a confirmatory relationship are lacking, long-term exposure to air pollution is positively correlated with BMI in children and serum leptin concentrations in older adults.[50,51]

Air pollution can also cause alterations in gene expression, which can predict both the five-year incidence of and mortality from ischemic heart disease and stroke.[19] Animal studies reveal that these genetic alterations are stable, can accumulate over time, persist even in the absence of the initial trigger, and are transmissible for many generations.[19,45,46] If the same is true for humans, historical exposure to air pollution could have substantial ramifications on both current and future health.[19]

Susceptibility to Air Pollution

Because there is increasing evidence for an association between exposure to air pollution and cardiorespiratory diseases in those without a preexisting condition, and negative effects can occur at pollution levels below recommended limits, there are those who argue that no population is without risk. Nevertheless, there are several inherent characteristics with the potential to further increase susceptibility to air pollution.[31] Although sex, ethnicity, obesity (independent of T2DM), and certain genetic polymorphisms (associated with oxidative stress, inflammation, endothelial function, and the angiotensin pathways) are suggested to increase the risk of the adverse effects of air pollution, the results are inconsistent.[19,21] Evidence for an association with advancing age, lower socioeconomic status, and smoking habits, however, is better established.[2,4,9,13,21,31,52] Due to already chronically elevated levels of systemic inflammation, as well as vascular and autonomic dysfunction, individuals with preexisting cardiorespiratory diseases and T2DM are especially sensitive to the effects of air pollution.[21,52] Other environmental factors such as proximity to major roadways, excess noise, and extremes of temperature (at either end of the spectrum) can have additive effects with air pollutants, thereby further increasing vulnerability to air pollution.[2,21]

Metal Pollutants

Even though air pollution is deemed the leading environmental risk factor,[9-13] substantial epidemiological and experimental evidence supports the role of heavy metals in the onset of cardiovascular disease.[1,53-55] The metals arsenic and lead, which are the top two environmental chemicals of concern by the Agency for Toxic Substances and Disease Registry (ATSDR), have the most consistent associations with cardiovascular risk.[1,54-56] Cadmium is an additional metal of concern. However, because tobacco smoke is the principal source of cadmium, and current evidence has yet to determine adverse outcomes independent from the health effects associated with smoking,[1] cadmium will not be further discussed.

In contrast to cadmium, environmental sources of arsenic and lead are numerous, so the potential for human exposure is high. For example, arsenic can be found in soil, fertilizers, pesticides, crops, wood preservatives, and tobacco smoke, and it is emitted from smelting and coal-burning power plants. However, drinking water, particularly deep well groundwater, is considered the primary source of arsenic and constitutes a major environmental health problem in both the developed and developing world.[1,55] The primary sources of lead include airborne emissions from industry, combustion (including the combustion of gasoline still present in aviation fuel), tobacco smoke and dust, soil, food, drinking water, plumbing, paint, ceramic glazes, batteries, and alternative health or herbal remedies.[1,55,57]

Like airborne pollutants, metals such as arsenic and lead are believed to act via common physiological mechanisms, regardless of the specific source of exposure. The induction of oxidative stress and inflammation are the primary pathways proposed. However, there is also recent evidence for an association between these metals and altered gene expression.[1,54] Irrespective of the mechanistic pathway, exposure to these metals is positively correlated with hypertension, electrocardiographic abnormalities such as conduction delays (arsenic) and reduced heart rate variability (lead), endothelial dysfunction, atherogenesis, peripheral artery disease, dyslipidemia (lead), T2DM (arsenic), and an overall increased risk of mortality from CVD.[1,55] The use of chelation therapy as a strategy to protect against atherosclerosis from the influence of heavy metals has been experimented with for many years; emerging scientific evidence suggests that there are benefits for use in patients with CVD.[1,53,55]

Intervention Strategies

Risk reduction is challenging due to the pervasive nature of environmental exposure.[19] Pollution largely requires intervention at the legislative and community planning levels,[31,58,59] a discussion of which is beyond the scope of the current chapter. Although research on personal-level interventions is currently insufficient to support evidence-based guidelines, there are certain suggested strategies individuals, particularly susceptible individuals (e.g., those with cardiopulmonary diseases), could follow to help mitigate the risk specifically from air pollution (table 9.16).[9,31,59,60]

Although physical activity plays an important role in both the primary and secondary prevention of cardiorespiratory disease,[5,62-64] many of the most accessible and affordable forms of exercise, such as walking and cycling, occur outdoors.[5,61] Despite concerns about the potential effects of exercising in air pollution, for healthy individuals the long-term health benefits gained from exercise outweigh the adverse effects of air pollution, with

Table 9.16 Lifestyle Modifications Health and Allied Health Professionals Could Recommend to Their Patients to Reduce Exposure to Air Pollution

Suggested intervention	Specific recommendations or examples
Modify outdoor lifestyle	Limit the time spent outdoors when pollution levels are excessive (e.g., a designated Ozone Action Day) and avoid major roadways
Use face masks	N95 respirators are currently the most effective; however, surgical face masks may confer some benefit in heavily polluted regions
Reduce indoor and in-car air pollution	Use indoor and in-car air purifiers such as HEPA filter systems and particle traps, close windows, recirculate in-cabin air, use central air conditioning, and cook with cleaner-burning liquid fuel stoves with improved ventilation
Reduce overall burden of cardiorespiratory disease	Recommend already-established primary, secondary, and tertiary interventions such as medications to control hypertension and dyslipidemia; weight management; a healthy diet rich in vegetables, fish oils, and antioxidants; smoking cessation; and physical activity

the exception of the most polluted cities.[58,61,65,66] Whether the same is true for patients with preexisting chronic disease is currently not fully understood. Only a small number of lab-based and epidemiological experiments have suggested that exposure to CO or PM during exercise can cause premature ischemic responses (i.e., reduced time to the onset of angina and ST-segment depression) in CVD patients.[67] Therefore individuals with CVD who wish to exercise outdoors should be advised to follow local air quality forecasts, avoid peak exposure days and times such as rush hour, choose exercise locations away from traffic as much as possible, and opt for morning exercise in the summer months to avoid afternoon elevations in ozone levels.[5,61]

Summary

Patients enrolled in CR have various diseases, conditions, and exposures that put them at risk of a subsequent cardiac event. It is important to have an understanding of these and how to deal with them during CR participation so that patients can exercise safely and reduce their potential risk of having another cardiac event. Because CR participation offers consistent opportunities to interact with an individual patient for up to 12 weeks, it provides a unique and potentially efficacious setting in which to systematically educate, intervene, and change behavior where necessary to reduce the aforementioned risk.

Cardiac Disease Populations

Alison L. Bailey, MD, FACC; Alexis L. Beatty, MD, MAS; Brian Carlin, MD, FCCP, MAACVPR, FAARC; Dennis J. Kerrigan, PhD, FACSM; Steven J. Keteyian, PhD; Kirstine Laerum Sibilitz, MD, PhD; Karen Lui, RN, MS, MAACVPR; Ryan Mays, PhD, MPH; Jonathan Powell, MD; Ray W. Squires, PhD; Diane J. Treat-Jacobson, PhD, RN, FAAN

The specific components of a comprehensive CR program have been previously published[2] and reviewed in other chapters of this book. These programmatic core components should be applied and individualized to accommodate patients with various types of cardiac disease. In addition, program staff should have the aggregate knowledge and skills to safely and effectively implement programs in these patients.[3]

OBJECTIVES

This chapter provides an overview of the following:

- The various CVD populations commonly referred for CR
- Specific information about these groups with respect to developing and implementing exercise training:
  - Patients with CVD (MI, revascularization, and stable angina)
  - Patients with heart valve replacement or repair surgery
  - Patients with dysrhythmias
  - Patients with heart failure or left ventricular assist devices
  - Patients who have had a heart transplant
  - Patients with peripheral artery disease
  - Patients with chronic lung disease

CR for Patients With CVD (MI, Revascularization, and Stable Angina)

In the United States, approximately 580,000 new incidences of MI cases occur annually.[4] While care for the acute MI patient has improved, the morbidity and mortality remain high. Within five years after a first MI in people over 45 years of age, 36% of males and 47% of females will die. Annually, 210,000 recurrent MI still occur. Likewise, the number of patients undergoing procedures to improve coronary blood flow is considerable. The AHA recently reported the number of patients undergoing coronary artery bypass surgery (CABG) or PCI annually was 397,000 and 954,000, respectively. Males accounted for 70% of the procedures, and the majority of the procedures (60%) were performed on persons aged 65 years or older.

CR is a service covered by the Centers for Medicare and Medicaid Services for MI with or without stenting (within 12 months of the event), PCI, CABG, and stable angina or acute coronary syndrome (ACS).[5] Multiple analyses demonstrate reductions in morbidity and mortality in CR participants after an MI, PCI, or CABG when compared to nonparticipants.[6-8] The benefits appear to be dose-dependent; those participants who attend more sessions receive more benefits.[9,10] Additionally, reductions in hospital readmissions in the year after a cardiac event, improvements in quality of life, and ability to return to work are seen in CR participants.[11-14]

The use of CR and SP services is a Class I recommendation in the 2011 ACCF/AHA practice guideline for CABG; the 2011 ACCF/AHA/SCAI guideline for PCI; the 2013 ACCF/AHA guideline for the management of ST-elevation MI (STEMI); and the 2014 AHA/ACC guideline for the management of patients with non-ST-elevation ACS.[15-19] As such, referral to an outpatient CR program is an ACC/AHA performance measure for all patients with an ACS, MI, PCI, or CABG.[1] Unfortunately, only the minority of Medicare beneficiaries enroll in CR after an MI (13.9%) or CABG (31%), and of those enrolling only 18% attend all 36 sessions.[10-20] While referral rates to CR after PCI are better than those seen with MI and CABG, a recent study revealed that only 59.2% of the overall PCI population was referred to CR.[21] The use of an automatic referral strategy to outpatient CR at the time of discharge has been shown to improve referral rates significantly—especially if it is facilitated by adequate communication between the referring providers, CR program staff, and postdischarge contact with the patient.[22] A recent Million Hearts Collaborative estimated that increasing CR participation from 20% to 70% would save 25,000 lives and prevent 180,000 hospitalizations annually in the United States.[23]

Wait times for entry into CR are associated with likelihood of participation and program completion. In a large analysis of Medicare patients with MI or CABG in the United States, only 25% of patients enrolled in CR within 21 days of discharge, and over 25% initiated CR more than 2 months after hospital discharge.[20] Another analysis demonstrated that median wait time from referral to initiation of CR was 42 days. Efforts to minimize the time to CR enrollment are important; evidence suggests that for every day of delay after hospital discharge, a 1% reduction in participation rates occurs.[24] Longer wait time to start CR is also associated with less improvement in cardiopulmonary fitness, body fat percentage, resting heart rate, and poorer attendance to CR classes and completion rate.[25]

Revascularization

Several revascularization procedures are used to treat patients with significant symptomatic atherosclerotic lesions in the coronary arterial circulation. These procedures include traditional open-chest CABG, minimally invasive direct coronary artery bypass (MID-CAB), PCI, as well as hybrid approaches using both surgical and catheter-based revascularization techniques. The indications for revascularization are complex but in general can be considered in the context of either an ACS or for stable CVD.

ACS

- Approximately 60% of patients will receive PCI; the remainder will undergo CABG or receive medical therapy alone.[26]

- In patients with STEMI-ACS, primary PCI is the treatment of choice if it can be accomplished with a treatment time of 90 to 120 min (called *door-to-balloon* time).[26] The door-to-balloon time is the standard by which quality is judged in the catheterization laboratory, and the goal is <90 min from the time of first medical contact to the first balloon inflation in the culprit artery.[27]

Stable CVD

- PCI for single-vessel disease is indicated only when significant symptoms and ischemia are present despite maximally tolerated medical therapy.[16] Multivessel CVD can be managed by either PCI or CABG depending on individual patient characteristics.

- In general, patients who are candidates for revascularization with either PCI or CABG will have the following:
  - Fewer repeat procedures when they undergo CABG[26]
  - Higher stroke and atrial fibrillation rates and wound complications when they undergo CABG[26]
  - Faster recovery when they undergo PCI as compared to traditional CABG

- Patients with diabetes and multivessel disease have a lower long-term mortality rate with CABG than with PCI, assuming that they are suitable candidates for surgery and survive to at least 30 days.[28] Arterial revascularization with the left internal mammary artery to the left anterior descending artery (LIMA-LAD) protects the largest amount of myocardial tissue even in the setting of progressive CVD and is less likely to develop atherosclerosis compared to vein grafts, making it a more robust form of revascularization.
  - The mortality advantage for CABG over PCI takes approximately five years to manifest.
  - CABG is a more durable revascularization procedure in patients with multivessel CVD and increasing coronary lesion complexity.[28]

Exercise Prescription and Associated Outcomes

Expert opinion recommends that patients with CVD undergo symptom-limited exercise testing before initiating a CR program to establish a baseline fitness level, determine maximal attained HR, and confirm the safety of exercise by assessing symptoms and evaluating for severe ischemic ECG changes or cardiac arrhythmias.[29] However, it is not an absolute requirement, and most programs do not require testing in stable patients prior to initiation of the CR program. Exercise testing before CR is not designed for a diagnosis but rather typically performed for heart rate response and potential ischemic threshold identification. Therefore, patients should be tested while on their usual cardiac medications, including beta-blockers. If a patient is referred to CR without testing, the initial exercise session is used to determine the patient's baseline exercise capacity and any related symptoms.

Every patient entering CR should have an individualized exercise prescription containing both aerobic and resistance training. This prescription should be based on either a symptom-limited exercise test or estimated exercise capacity derived from the initial exercise session combined with comorbidities and patient goals.[2] A simple exercise prescription can be developed based on the FITT principle,[30] specifying frequency (F), intensity (I), Time (T), and type (T). Each session should include a warm-up and cool-down. More specific exercise prescription information can be found in *ACSM's Guidelines for Exercise Testing and Prescription*.[30] This prescription should be used as a dynamic blueprint with progression of exercise and modifications based on continuous monitoring of the patient's responses to the CR program.

Guideline 10.1 — Exercise Testing

Patients with CAD should undergo symptom-limited exercise testing before initiating a CR program to establish a baseline fitness level, determine maximal attained HR, and confirm the safety of exercise by assessing symptoms and evaluating for severe ischemic ECG changes or cardiac arrhythmias.[29]

Guideline 10.2 — Ischemic Threshold

In those patients with known ischemia from exercise testing, the heart rate should be monitored and kept at least 10 bpm below the ischemic threshold.

Timing of CR and Improvements in Exercise Capacity

In general, early enrollment in CR is safe and improves outcomes for both surgical and MI patients. In an analysis of patients who had cardiac surgery with a sternotomy and who were routinely enrolled in CR early postdischarge (<2 weeks; median of 10 days), there was no difference in major event rates between early and late enrollees.[31] Infection rates were similar between early and late groups, and CR-related adverse events were infrequent and rarely severe enough to require emergency management outside the CR program. Likewise, for post-MI patients with left ventricular dysfunction, earlier initiation of exercise training appears to be safe and associated with positive cardiac remodeling.[32] The largest improvements were seen when participants started the CR program around one week postdischarge for MI and lasted for six months. Each week that exercise was delayed required an additional month of training to achieve the same level of benefit on left ventricular (LV) remodeling. Importantly, no adverse events occurred during the six-month exercise training sessions initiated at the earliest juncture (around one week post-MI) in people with mild to moderate LV systolic dysfunction.

It is well established that exercise capacity is the strongest predictor of mortality in patients with prior MI or CABG.[33] It is becoming increasingly recognized that improvements in CRF seen during CR predict subsequent outcomes. In a recent analysis, patients referred to CR after ACS, PCI, or CABG showed improvements in cardiovascular outcomes only when improvements were seen in CRF.[34] About 23% of participants did not improve their fitness as measured by peak $\dot{V}O_2$ testing post-CR. Lack of improvement in peak $\dot{V}O_2$ was associated with significantly higher mortality than those who showed improvements in peak $\dot{V}O_2$. A 1 mL O_2/kg · m · min^{-1} improvement in $\dot{V}O_2$ was associated with a 10% reduction in all-cause mortality.

Alternatives to the traditional aerobic exercise prescription are associated with more favorable outcomes. High-intensity interval training (HIIT) has been compared to moderate-intensity continuous training (MICT) within CR programs in a recent meta-analysis.[35] All studies conducted exercise within the following intensity guidelines:

- HIIT: ≥85% $\dot{V}O_2$ peak or ≥85% heart rate reserve (HRR) or ≥90% heart rate maximum (HRM) interspersed with lower-level exercise
- MICT: 50%-75% $\dot{V}O_2$ peak or 50%–75% HRR or 50%–80% HRM. All participants were diagnosed with CVD, MI, PCI, and CABG making this a contemporary CR population.

HIIT was superior to MICT in improving peak $\dot{V}O_2$ in participants of CR and appeared to be as safe as MICT for CR participants in this analysis.

Complete Versus Incomplete Revascularization

In contemporary CR, some patients may not have undergone revascularization prior to entry into the program. It is important to know whether the patient has undergone a revascularization procedure that was complete or incomplete in order to ensure a full assessment of the patient's risk profile and associated symptoms. This information is generally available in a catheterization report, operative note, or discharge summary. Complete revascularization is defined as revascularization of all hemodynamically significant lesions and should alleviate all associated signs and symptoms of myocardial ischemia. Incomplete revascularization is more common in patients with complex coronary anatomy, diffuse CVD, and small vessel disease. There are many reasons why an incomplete revascularization may occur. For instance, in patients who present with an ACS and are found to have multiple vessels that are diseased, immediate revascularization of the culprit lesion (the vessel determined to be causing the immediate problem) alone improves outcomes in terms of patient morbidity and mortality when compared to patients receiving immediate complete revascularization of all lesions. Hence, patients may undergo culprit lesion intervention only and receive medical therapy to treat the rest of the CVD with the plan to intervene on the remaining lesions in a staged procedure process at a later date; the plan is in place if they continue to have chest pain or demonstrate signs of ischemia despite maximal medical therapy.[36] Incomplete revascularization may increase the likelihood of signs and symptoms of residual myocardial ischemia during exercise but is not a contraindication to exercise and, in fact, should be considered a viable therapy for angina. The COURAGE trial revealed that patients with stable CAD and evidence of inducible myocardial ischemia derive no additional benefit from invasive strategies when compared to optimal medical therapy and exercise for the endpoints of death or MI.[37] In addition, a small study in patients with a recent ACS and primary PCI and a second significant coronary artery lesion also revealed that CR was safe and well tolerated while waiting for a staged intervention.[38] No significant differences in workload capacities or need for urgent intervention between the two groups were observed.

Importance of SP

For patients who have experienced a prior CAD event, the likelihood of another event remains high despite contemporary therapy.[4] The goals for each patient in a CR program are to prevent another CAD event such as thrombosis and progressive atherosclerosis, optimize lifestyle factors and behaviors, include PA into their life for the long term, and reduce morbidity and mortality. A commonly encountered challenge for CR staff is to help participants understand that the procedure has not cured the disease and that SP is necessary for preventing subsequent clinical issues. All patients should be treated according to contemporary SP and risk reduction therapy for patients with coronary and other atherosclerotic vascular disease guidelines with an emphasis on tobacco cessation; weight control; control of BP, BG, and lipids to current guideline recommendations; the optimization of medical therapy with antiplatelets/anticoagulants, ACEi and ARBs, beta-blockers, and aldosterone antagonists as indicated; evaluation of depression; and education/administration of an influenza vaccine.[17] Of note, lipid values may be falsely low for several weeks following surgery or an ACS; thus, lipid lowering should be based on preoperative or postevent lipid profiles and current guidelines.

Practice Considerations for Patients Who Have Undergone PCI

Percutaneous revascularization of CVD has substantially changed since percutaneous transluminal coronary angioplasty with balloon inflation was introduced in 1977.[26] Bare-metal stents replaced balloon angioplasty as the treatment of choice but had a high rate of restenosis that required repeat intervention. First-generation drug-eluting stents (DESs) had a greater risk of stent thrombosis than bare-metal stents, especially when dual antiplatelet therapy was discontinued prematurely. Current generation DES have now overcome these problems and have lower rates of stent thrombosis than most bare-metal stents, decreased restenosis rates, and reduced the need for repeat revascularization procedures of the target vessel. Of the estimated 954,000 patients annually undergoing PCI procedures in 2010, 70% were males and 60% were 65 years of age or older.[4] When stents were implanted during PCI procedures, the majority were DES.

The route of intravascular access for a PCI procedure can be either transfemoral or transradial. Transradial access is growing in popularity; about 1/3 of contemporary procedures are performed via this route.[39] The radial approach has the benefits of less bleeding and usually a quicker recovery time. If the radial artery was used as the access site, the CR staff should ensure that the site is healing properly before the patient uses the arms for aerobic activity and progresses to heavier weights. If the groin was used for catheter access, care should be taken to ensure that the access site is healing appropriately before the patient begins lower extremity exercise. CR staff should confirm that the patient is receiving the prescribed antiplatelet therapy, which usually consists of aspirin as well as an additional antiplatelet agent. Special emphasis should be placed on the importance of adherence to these medications post-PCI to prevent thrombotic events and death. All post-PCI

Guideline 10.3   CR Participation Prior to Revascularization Procedures

For stable patients without progressive angina, CR combined with optimal medical therapy should be a first-line treatment prior to revascularization.

patients can begin exercise training as outpatients almost immediately after uncomplicated hospital discharge.

Practice Considerations for Patients Who Have Undergone CABG

Traditional CABG requires a median sternotomy and can be performed with or without the use of a cardiopulmonary bypass machine that delivers oxygenated blood through the circulatory system during surgery. CABG typically uses a section of an internal mammary artery (IMA) or saphenous vein (SVG) as a conduit to deliver blood distal to the lesion being bypassed. Radial or gastroepiploic arteries may also be used for this purpose. SVGs can develop intimal fibroplasia and vein graft atherosclerosis. Up to 25% of SVGs occlude within one year of CABG; an additional 1% to 2% occlude annually during years 1 to 5 after surgery and 4% to 5% occlude annually between years 6 and 10.[15] By 10 years after CABG, only 50% to 60% of SVGs are patent and the majority of these grafts have angiographic evidence of atherosclerosis.

In contrast, IMA grafts have a 10-year patency rate >90%. Studies suggest an improved survival rate in patients undergoing CABG when the left IMA (rather than a SVG) is used to graft the LAD artery and this is a Class I recommendation in current guidelines for CABG, meaning that this is the highest level of recommendation by a professional society because it is supported by high-quality research studies consistently showing a benefit. Additionally, left IMA to LAD grafting reduces the incidence of late MI, hospitalization for cardiac events, need for reoperation, and recurrence of angina.

MID-CAB involves access to the heart via small incisions between ribs on the left side of the chest and is performed without a cardiopulmonary bypass machine (off-pump) or median sternotomy. Compared to CABG, MID-CAB procedures have the clinical advantages of less blood loss, shorter hospital stays, and faster recovery. MID-CAB can also be performed using a robot while a surgeon controls the surgical instruments using robotic arms. In general, these patients should begin exercise directed at ADLs while inpatient (often guided by a physical therapist) and should be referred early to CR within two weeks of discharge.

A hybrid procedure for revascularization involves a direct surgical approach (usually for grafting the left IMA to the LAD artery through a MID-CAB approach) and PCI of the other diseased coronary arteries. The MID-CAB approach avoids a median sternotomy.

Timing of Exercise After Surgery

PA, including early ambulation and ROM, as well as walking and cycling, is indicated during hospitalization for CABG to help avoid the deleterious effects of bed rest, including decreased functional capacity and thromboembolic complications. Specific exercise prescription information for CABG inpatients can be found in the *ACSM's Guidelines for Exercise Testing and Prescription*.[30] The goals of early inpatient CR include assessing the patient's current clinical status, early mobilization, identification and education regarding CAD risk factors and self-care, and discharge planning with a home PA plan and referral to outpatient CR. Providing structured inpatient CR is a challenge because of the short hospital stay for uncomplicated patients, but multiple daily ambulation sessions for these patients are critical to recovery. Elderly patients and those with complicated postoperative courses are often transferred to postacute care programs, such as an inpatient rehabilitation facility or skilled nursing facility. In these programs, they receive continued medical care. They also receive occupational and physical therapy to improve endurance, strength, balance, and cognitive status for independence in self-care, household ambulation (including

---

Guideline 10.4 — Catheterization Access Location

If the radial artery was used as the access site, the CR staff should ensure that the site is healing properly before the patient uses the arms for aerobic activity and progresses to heavier weights. If the groin was used for catheter access, care should be taken to ensure that the access site is healing appropriately before the patient begins lower extremity exercise.

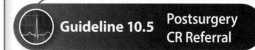

Guideline 10.5 — Postsurgery CR Referral

In general, postsurgery patients should be referred early to CR, within two weeks of discharge.

stairs), and home and food management activities. However, these programs do not provide the same education as the CR program, so these patients should be referred to and attend a CR program after they have completed the physical rehabilitation (occupational or physical therapy) in postacute care.

The rate of recovery for CABG patients depends on age, sex, and surgical techniques. Once enrolled into an outpatient CR program, exercise prescription methodology is generally the same as that for all other patients with CAD.[30] In general, while in CR, rhythmic upper limb activities such as arm ergometry should be encouraged. A general objective for patient care during CR for patients with a median sternotomy is to advance and progress through a pain-free ROM before focusing on regaining or improving muscle strength and endurance.

Role and Purpose of Sternal Precautions

As previously stated, the goal for patients with median sternotomy is to advance and progress while at the same time limiting sternal complications. Sternal wires are used to close the sternum after surgery and facilitate bone healing. Sternal complications following median sternotomy may include infection, nonunion, and instability.[40] Sternal instability is the abnormal motion of the sternum after either bone fracture or disruption of the wires reuniting the surgically divided sternum. Sternal instability is highly associated with the development of mediastinitis, a purulent deep sternal wound infection.[41] Most patients will heal without complications and achieve adequate sternal stability in approximately 6 to 10 weeks after CABG. The incidence of sternal complications remains relatively unchanged for the last two decades and is reported to be between 1% and 8% worldwide.[40] Several risk factors increase the risk of sternal instability and should be considered in the risk assessment of the CR patient.[41] An important role for the CR professional working with patients who have undergone median sternotomy is surveillance for any early signs or symptoms indicative of sternal instability.[30] This role requires routine assessment for pain and discomfort, excessive sternal movement or instability, and sternal clicking; if any findings are deemed to be clinically meaningful, informing the referring physician or surgeon is indicated.

Risk Factors Associated With Sternal Wound Complications

Primary Risk Factors

- Obesity
- COPD
- Bilateral IMA grafting
- Diabetes mellitus
- Repeat thoracotomy
- Increased blood loss/number of transfused units
- Higher disability classification
- Smoking
- Prolonged cardiopulmonary bypass/surgical time
- Prolonged mechanical ventilation
- Peripheral vascular disease
- Large breast size

Secondary Risk Factors

- Osteoporosis/decreased sternal thickness
- Longer intensive care unit length of stay
- Time of surgery
- Antibiotic administration >2 h presurgery
- Staple use for skin closure
- Impaired renal function
- Immunocompromised status
- Closure by non cardiovascular surgeon
- Cardiac reinfarction
- Inadvertent paramedian sternotomy
- Emergency surgery
- ACE use
- Use and duration of temporary pacing wires
- Septic shock
- Depressed left ventricular function

Cardiothoracic surgeons typically issue specific instructions for patients related to upper extremity exercise and resistance training, which; are known as sternal precautions. Restrictions in ROM and weight load are commonly advised for upper limb movement, are usually given prior to hospital discharge, and might vary based on the type of surgery and healing. These restrictions are usually set at a 5 to 10 lb (2.2-4.5 kg) limit for 8 to 12 weeks. Sternal precautions are almost universally given to patients following median sternotomy. However, the exact origin of these restrictions is difficult to find and no systemic reviews on this topic exist.[40,41] The goal of sternal precautions is to promote bone healing by minimizing the forces and the amount of micromotion between the sternal edges, which can promote progression to nonunion and/or infection.[40] To date, no direct evidence links postoperative activity level or arm movement to increased risk for sternal complications. Currently, many different protocols exist and frequently offer conflicting advice.[41] A recent survey looked at the top five sternal precautions reported by cardiothoracic surgeons and reported the following:

- Lifting no more than 10 lb (4.5 kg) of weight bilaterally
- Lifting no more than 10 lb (4.5 kg) of weight unilaterally
- Bilateral sports restrictions
- No driving
- Unilateral sports restrictions[42]

Likewise, in a survey of outpatient CR staff, 95% reported some form of restriction on upper extremity exercises following median sternotomy.[43] However, little agreement existed on the type and timing of these restrictions over the course of the outpatient CR programs, and most respondents drew on their clinical experience to inform the prescription and progression of exercises. Only about 40% of the respondents reported formally screening for sternal instability; and if it was diagnosed, there appeared to be little agreement on the modification of exercise program.

In an informative study, the push and pull force required to complete 32 ADLs was measured.[44] The majority of these activities (28/32) required forces greater than the 10 lb (4.5 kg) lifting restriction that is typically used to instruct patients after sternotomy. Interestingly, some of the greatest forces were necessary to open and close doors (~15-20 lb; 6.8-9 kg) and cough (~40 lb; 18 kg). A recent trial compared usual postoperative sternotomy restrictions to a less restrictive program based on pain and discomfort.[40] Starting on postoperative day 4, recommendations were given for traditional restrictions of upper limb use for four to six weeks after surgery and compared with instructions to encourage the use of upper limbs within the limits of pain or discomfort. Sternal complications did not differ significantly between these groups. Based on these trials, more specific instructions such as avoidance of exercises known to have increased risk for the poststernotomy patient (bench press, pectoral flys, and lat pulldowns) and avoidance of pain may be more helpful than an arbitrary weightlifting limit. Likewise, it may be appropriate to tailor the sternal precautions based on individual clinical characteristics and risk profile rather than restricting specific functional tasks and physical activity. The surgical team and the CR staff should discern an appropriate plan for each patient. It is important for CR staff to be knowledgeable about the poststernotomy instructions and to incorporate them into the exercise prescription for those patients.

The Post-CABG Patient

Common symptoms after cardiac surgery include incisional sternotomy pain and drainage; feelings of weakness; sleeping difficulties due to chest wall pain with side lying; problems with wound healing; dissatisfaction with postoperative supportive care; problems with eating; pain in the shoulders, back, and neck; and ineffective coping.[40] Persistent chest wall pain following median sternotomy is seen in nearly 50% of patients and has been termed *postcoronary artery bypass pain syndrome.* It is well documented that PA and upper limb exercises reduce sternal pain in the sternotomy patient and should be encouraged.[45] Initially, some patients may need lower-intensity or modified exercise prescriptions because of musculoskeletal discomfort or healing issues, but it should not be a routine policy. A recent trial determined that referral to CR early after open-heart surgery was safe and effective.[31] Patients who underwent open-heart surgery and started CR more than two weeks after discharge were prescribed lower extremity exercises such as walking or stationary cycling initially. After four to six sessions, patients usually started HIIT. Upper extremity exercises for those with sternotomy were restricted to general mobility, stretching, and upper extremity lifting of >10 pounds (4.5 kg) for six weeks after the operation. There was no difference in any adverse outcome, and infection rates were like those of patients who enrolled in CR later.

Staff should assess sternal and vein harvest site wound healing in all new patients referred after CABG. Signs of wound infection include redness, swelling, and drainage; patients with an infected wound require a sterile dressing to avoid cross-contamination of other patients in the program. Because of the possibility of early SVG closure, program staff should also be alert for new patient complaints of angina pectoris or angina-equivalent symptoms, signs and symptoms of exercise intolerance, and new ECG signs of myocardial ischemia. It is particularly important in patients with a remote SVG. Patients should be informed about and alert to these findings as well.

Dysrhythmias are not uncommon during the inpatient stay after CABG and can also occur during outpatient CR. One of the most common complications after CABG is atrial fibrillation (AF). Postoperative AF occurs in 20% to 40% of patients undergoing a cardiac surgery and generally occurs on postoperative day 2.[46] Up to 70% of cases of AF are seen in the first four days postoperatively, but it can first occur up to six weeks postoperatively. Antiarrhythmic drug therapy is commonly used to lower this risk in the immediate postoperative period. Complex dysrhythmias and new onset of atrial fibrillation should be reported promptly to the program medical director and referring physician.

Pleural and pericardial effusions may occur within the first several weeks after the operation. These conditions are generally related to postoperative inflammation and can be detected during early outpatient CR by evidence of decreasing exercise capacity, chest discomfort, and increasing dyspnea. These symptoms should be promptly reported to the program medical director, surgeon, and referring physician.

BOTTOM LINE

- CR is a service covered by the Centers for Medicare and Medicaid Services for MI, PCI, CABG, and stable angina as well as a Class I recommendation from the American College of Cardiology and the AHA for these diagnoses and an endorsed performance measure.

- Patients who attend CR have improvements in mortality as well as morbidity and QoL.

- Earlier entry into CR is safe for patients with an ACS, PCI, or CABG and is associated with improved outcomes.

Heart Valve Replacement and Repair Surgery

Heart valve disease is a global health problem. The incidence is growing, and in 2030 it is expected that valve related hospitalizations will increase dramatically compared with today.[1,2]

The overall incidence of heart valve disease is 63.9 per 100,000 person-years; the most common disease is aortic stenosis (AS) of almost 50%, followed by mitral regurgitation (MR) and aortic regurgitation (AR).[1] It is estimated that more than 280,000 prosthetic heart valves are implanted worldwide each year, and 90,000 are in the United States. Of these, 58% are performed on men and 64% on people aged 65 or older.[3] The annual number of hospital discharges in the United States for patients with a diagnosis

---

Guideline 10.6 Assessing Patients With Prior CABG

- All patients should be assessed for sternal and vein harvest site wound healing at entry into the program.

- All patients should be assessed for signs and symptoms of angina pectoris or angina-equivalent symptoms, signs and symptoms of exercise intolerance, and new ECG signs of myocardial ischemia.

of valvular heart disease (VHD) is nearly equal for aortic and mitral valve disease, an estimated 48,000 and 42,000, respectively.[3]

Etiology

VHD may involve either stenosis or regurgitation and can affect any of the four cardiac valves, although valve dysfunction on the higher-pressure left side of the heart (mitral, aortic) requires intervention much more frequently than the tricuspid or pulmonic valves in the lower-pressure right side.

Stenosis

Valvular stenosis is a narrowing or obstruction of the valve orifice, resulting in an inadequately opening valve. The causes of stenosis include degenerative calcification, rheumatic disease, congenital valve disease (e.g., bicuspid aortic valve), and radiation therapy.

Regurgitation

Regurgitation is a valve insufficiency resulting in retrograde flow. Valve regurgitation may be primary or secondary. It may be caused by rheumatic heart disease, infections, or congenital heart disease (e.g., Marfan syndrome). Aortic insufficiency can also be caused by an ascending aortic aneurysm and, in the case of the mitral valve, regurgitation can also be the result of mitral valve prolapse or myocardial infarction leading to ruptured chordae or papillary muscles.

Interventions

Valvular heart disease can be treated with either surgical- or catheter-based interventions. Surgical interventions are performed as open-heart surgery with sternotomy, whereas catheter-based interventions are percutaneous. Interventions for valvular dysfunction include annuloplasty or valve replacement using a prosthetic valve. Annuloplasty tightens the annulus to restore the competence of the valve. The criteria for either surgical or catheter-based interventions involve a multifactorial assessment of factors including comorbidities, age, valve dysfunction, frailty status, and functional capacity.

Prosthetic heart valves are divided into two main categories, bioprostheses and mechanical prostheses. Bioprosthetic valves are further classified as heterografts, homografts, and stentless heterografts. Types of mechanical prosthetic heart valves include the caged-ball, tilting-disk, and bileaflet valves.

Catheter-based procedures have emerged as alternatives to surgery for selected high-risk patients. Transcatheter aortic valve replacement (TAVR) compared to surgical replacement for high-risk patients was studied extensively in the PARTNER 1 study, and outcomes up to two years indicated that these two procedures resulted in similar mortality, reduction of symptoms, and valve hemodynamics[4,5] and confirmed in a recent meta-analysis.[6] Regarding intermediate-risk patients the FDA, since 2017, has approved replacement valves for use in intermediate-risk patients, whereas both European and American guidelines emphasize that the decision of TAVR versus surgery in intermediate-risk patients is based on each individual patient's frailty, preference, comorbidities, and surgical risk. In 2019, the FDA approved TAVR for low-risk individuals. Another type of catheter-based procedure involves repairing mitral regurgitation by percutaneously implanting a clip that realigns the mitral valve leaflets (MitraClip)[7] in selected high-risk patients.[8] Patients who undergo either of these procedures are not suitable for sternotomy.

Multiple Valve Disease and Cardiac Comorbidity

Heart valve disease can involve multiple valves requiring combined surgical or interventional management. Common combinations of valvular heart disease include mitral stenosis and tricuspid regurgitation, mitral stenosis and aortic stenosis, and aortic stenosis and mitral regurgitation. Valvular heart disease can also coexist with CVD, especially in older patients.

Follow-Up and CR After Heart Valve Surgery

Referral of patients to CR following valve replacement or repair is an AACVPR/AHA/ACC–endorsed performance measure[9,10] that is also recommended in a European position paper,[11] and it is a covered indication for Medicare patients.[12]

A follow-up program after valve surgery should include the components discussed next.

Echocardiography An essential part of follow-up includes echocardiography at latest six weeks after surgery.[13,14] The echocardiography should focus on prosthesis function, including any valve stenosis or regurgitation and paravalvular leakage.[15,16,17] Echocardiography should include assessment of pericardial and pleural effusion.[18] Left ventricular function, any changes in left ventricular remodeling, and ejection fraction should be reported. Echocardiography is recommended before commencing with CR exercise after valve surgery.

Clinical Assessment and Preventing Readmissions

Monitoring symptoms is essential after valve intervention in order to recognize possible HF, valve leakage, anemia, infection, and effusions. Further, tests for hemolytic anemia (Hb, LDL, haptoglobin, reticulocyte count, bilirubin), and HbA1c and cholesterol profile should be considered where relevant.[16]

The readmission risk should be considered.[19] Emerging evidence shows that the readmission rate of acute unplanned readmissions is high both after surgical and catheter-based interventions, with a 30-day all-cause readmission risk of about 25%, and in a recent review a combined overall 30-day risk of readmission of 16% for TAVR and 17% for surgerical aortic valve replacement (SAVR).[19-21]

The early CR phase should aim at avoiding preventable readmissions with increased symptom monitoring according to readmission risk.[21,22] Several trials are currently underway investigating intensified and individualized follow-up. In addition, future guidelines on valvular heart disease might aim at describing a more individualized triage of patients after valve surgery, with the aim of following patients at higher risk more closely and increasing patient empowerment.[23,24]

Assessment of Medication

Management of medication (including anticoagulation) is mandatory.[13,14] It requires individual indication assessment (e.g., for presence of atrial fibrillation[25]) and specific patient education depending on whether the patient is treated with warfarin/marcoumar, novel oral anticoagulants, or a platelet inhibitor.

Endocarditis Prophylaxis

Patients who have undergone valve replacement surgery or repair are not cured of valvular heart disease but have exchanged native valve disease for prosthetic valve disease.[16] Prevention of infections at prosthetic valve sites is crucial. Antibiotic prophylaxis and other preventive measures must be considered before every possible intervention, such as dental procedures and whenever a fever of unknown origin is present.[14]

Exercise Prescription

Several observational studies, a systematic review, three randomized trials, and one Cochrane Review (including a total of 148 patients in 2 randomized trials investigating the effect of exercise-based cardiac rehabilitation after valve surgery) show a beneficial effect on physical capacity measured by peak $\dot{V}O_2$ but cost-neutral effect for outpatient clinic visits.[26-31] However, the effect is based on short term data, and no effect of mortality and readmission has been reported. The exercise prescription and training of patients with valvular heart disease following valve replacement or repair are similar to those for CABG patients, however with restrictions and with the use of an individualized assessment before initiation.[32,33] Clinical issues, especially pericardial/pleural effusions, deleterious arrhythmias, and HF, should be handled before initiating exercise. For some patients, physical activity may have been restricted for an extended period due to symptoms before valve repair or replacement. The resulting low functional capacity requires these patients to progress slowly during early stages of an exercise training program. CR professionals should use standard exercise prescription methodology with these patients (e.g., exercise three times weekly at moderate to vigorous intensity, reaching 40%-80% HRR)[11,34] but should take care to avoid upper extremity exercise (including resistance training involving the upper extremities) for patients who have had open-heart surgery until the sternum is stable and no sternal wound healing issues remain (typically 6-10 weeks after surgery).[35,36] For more information, see Role and Purpose of Sternal Precautions earlier in this chapter. Until then, aerobic and resistance training can be performed with lower extremities. Patients who have had a catheterization procedure can begin upper and lower body resistance training almost immediately, although PA should be avoided the first four days after the procedure.

Risk Factor Management

Patients who have undergone combined valve replacement and CABG have the same SP issues regarding reducing CVD risk profiles (lipids, BP, diabetes, smoking, alcohol, diet, PA level) as presented earlier for patients undergoing isolated CABG.

The presence of anxiety and depression after valve surgery represent an important risk factor opposing compliance toward symptom monitoring, compliance to medication, and adherence to clinical follow-up, including physical training.[21,29,37,38] Studies show that up to 25% of patients have clinically relevant symptoms of anxiety and depression after surgery, and consideration should be given to monitoring or screening during follow-up,[29] such as using validated patient-reported outcome measures.

Follow-Up for Patients Without Valve Repair or Replacement

Patients with valvular heart disease, but without valve repair or replacement, may also be referred for CR for other coexisting conditions, such as MI, PCI, angina, or CABG. In general, worsening of any symptoms over time may indicate worsening valve disease and should be closely monitored. In cases, these contraindications exist:

• *Aortic stenosis.* The presence of critical aortic stenosis is a relative contraindication for both inpatient and outpatient CR. Patients with less severe aortic stenosis can exercise but may develop symptoms (e.g., dyspnea, angina, or syncope) during exercise. Exercise training intensity should be kept under the threshold that precipitates the onset of symptoms, because it indicates that cardiac output does not meet exercise demands. Severe, symptomatic aortic stenosis is an absolute contraindication to exercise.

• *Aortic or mitral valve regurgitation.* Severe regurgitation is a contraindication to physical exercise due to hemodynamic insufficiencies.

• *Mitral stenosis.* Dyspnea during exercise is the primary symptom of exercise intolerance with mitral stenosis, and exercise intensity should be below 75% of expected capacity.

• *Other syndromes.* Absolute contraindications for resistance training include Marfan syndrome, and patients with concomitant aortic disease (aneurysm, corrected or observed) should avoid resistance training and exercise at high intensity.

Dysrhythmias

Cardiac dysrhythmias are abnormalities in heart rhythm. They are also known as arrhythmias or irregular rhythms. Many CR participants have a history of cardiac dysrhythmias, and some experience dysrhythmias during CR participation.[1-3] Symptoms from dysrhythmias may or may not be present and vary from patient to patient. The effects of dysrhythmias can range from generally benign to potentially harmful. Most studies report a cardiac arrest rate of approximately 1/100,000 patient-hours of CR participation.[4-7] Although it is rare for dysrhythmias to have life-threatening consequences during exercise in CR programs, it remains important to recognize dysrhythmias and their features.

BOTTOM LINE

Cardiac dysrhythmias are common in CR participants. Life-threatening consequences of cardiac dysrhythmias are rare during exercise in CR programs.

The following are commonly encountered dysrhythmias and symptoms:

Cardiac Dysrhythmias in CR

Generally Benign

• Premature atrial complexes (PACs)
• Isolated premature ventricular complexes (PVCs)
• AF or atrial flutter with controlled ventricular rate (<110 bpm at rest)[8]
• Paroxysmal supraventricular tachycardia (SVT)
• Mild bradycardia (50-60 bpm)
• First-degree atrioventricular (AV) block and asymptomatic type I second-degree (also known as Wenckebach) AV block

Potentially or Likely Harmful

• AF or atrial flutter with a rapid rate (≥110 bpm at rest)
• Symptomatic or severe bradycardia (HR <50)
• Symptomatic or advanced AV block (type II second-degree AV block or complete heart block)
• Ventricular tachycardia
• Ventricular fibrillation

Symptoms Associated With Cardiac Dysrhythmias

Stable Symptoms

• Palpitations
• Dizziness or lightheadedness

- Shortness of breath
- Chest pain or discomfort

Nonspecific or Associated Symptoms

- Weakness or fatigue
- Sweating
- Blurred vision
- Nausea
- Anxiety
- Edema

Unstable Symptoms

- Hypotension
- Near-syncope or loss of consciousness
- HF
- Unstable angina or MI
- Cardiac arrest

Exercise induces many physiologic effects, which can have both direct and indirect effects on cardiac electrophysiology. Exercise intensity can be related to the occurrence of dysrhythmias. Some dysrhythmias diminish or disappear with increasing exercise intensity; others increase or appear with increasing exercise intensity; and still others have no observable relationship to exercise intensity. Factors that can contribute to dysrhythmias during exercise include autonomic nervous system activity, ischemia, genetic abnormalities, structural heart disease, medications with proarrhythmic side effects, electrolyte imbalance, dehydration, and certain environmental factors.

Atrial Fibrillation

Light-to-moderate activities, particularly leisure-time activity and walking, are associated with a significantly lower incidence of AF in older adults.[9] However, people who participate in extreme endurance training and sports activities may have an increased incidence of AF.[10,11] For those diagnosed with AF, regular moderate PA is known to increase exercise capacity and control ventricular rate.[12,13] In addition, exercise training increases exercise capacity and may reduce AF burden.[14,15] The following information provides specific information about CR participation in patients who have AF.

AF originates in the atrium and is the most common cardiac arrhythmia. It is characterized by irregular contractions of the muscle fibers of the atria resulting in a variable HR. Risk factors associated with developing AF include PA, obesity, advanced age, HTN, HF, diabetes mellitus, CVD and valvular heart disease, left ventricular and atrial enlargement, and hyperthyroidism.[43] Paradoxically, despite having few risk factors, athletes are also at increased risk for developing AF.

CR professionals will encounter these two types of patients with AF: patients who experience an initial (acute) onset (often noted during CR check-in or during exercise) and patients previously diagnosed and medically managed. Generally, AF is classified as (1) paroxysmal, (2) persistent, (3) long-standing persistent, or (4) permanent.[2]

AF should be considered when a patient presents with a rapid (often >110 bpm) "irregularly irregular" (no rhythmic pattern) resting HR. Patients experiencing an abrupt onset of AF may or may not report accompanying symptoms including palpitation, tachycardia, fatigue, shortness of breath, dizziness, and nausea. If AF is suspected, an ECG will confirm a diagnosis.

If new-onset AF is confirmed, the patient's physician should be consulted. Treating new-onset AF has three goals.[44,50] The first goal is to mitigate symptoms by initially focusing in on reducing HR. Typical therapeutic HR reduction options include beta-adrenergic and calcium channel blocking agents and antiarrhythmic

Guideline 10.7   Dysrhythmia Exercise Prescription

For patients with known dysrhythmias, the exercise prescription should be tailored to the individual, with predetermined goals and criteria for exercise termination. Exercise should be terminated when a patient experiences a potentially harmful dysrhythmia or dysrhythmia with unstable symptoms.

medication. The second goal is to reduce the risk for the development embolization of a blood clot (which the patient is at risk of developing due to atrial blood stagnation) through anticoagulation therapy. The third goal is to manage the patient's cardiovascular risk factors, which for overweight or obese patients is recommended to include weight loss and risk factor modification.[50]

Safety and rates of adverse event of exercise in patients have not been well studied. No large randomized control trials of exercise training and AF have assessed safety and efficacy. Guidelines for the treatment of patients with AF do not explicitly endorse specific exercise recommendations. Exercise, however, is not contraindicated in patients with AF. Moreover, exercise is effective treatment in multiple risk factors associated with AF, such as physical inactivity, HTN, diabetes mellitus, and obesity. Therefore, asymptomatic patients with AF who have received medical clearance should be encouraged to participate in an exercise program.

However, AF can profoundly impact the physiologic response to exercise training.[45] In particular, the rapid, irregular contraction of the atrium results in reduced ventricular output. To compensate for the reduced cardiac output there is a commensurate increase in the rate and irregularity of ventricular contraction. Despite the negative impact of AF, exercise training studies have demonstrated improvements in functional capacity, health status, and quality of life.[46]

The special consideration regarding exercise testing and prescription for patients with AF have been detailed elsewhere.[3] The following section is a brief review of special considerations regarding exercise testing and prescription for CR participants with AF.

Exercise Testing

As with all patients entering CR, undergoing a symptom-limited exercise tolerance test prior to initiating an exercise training program is optimal but not required. An exercise test is useful to assess for myocardial ischemia, evaluate chronotropic response, identify signs and symptoms, quantify functional capacity, and establish some general parameters for exercise training intensity.

Exercise Prescription for Patients With AF

Currently, no specific recommendations exist regarding exercise training for the treatment of AF. Studies of exercise training in patients with AF have employed a variety of protocols. Components of any exercise prescription include frequency, intensity, duration, modality, progression, and total volume. The exercise prescription for patients with AF should be individualized. A meta-analysis of exercise training studies involving people with AF recommends that a training regimen should include three or more sessions per week of a combination of moderate-intensity aerobic activity and resistance training. Session duration should be approximately 60 minutes, including adequate warm-up and cool-down.

By definition, the HR for a person with AF is irregular. Therefore, use of HR exclusively to assess exercise intensity is problematic. For aerobic training, in lieu of HR, use of RPE scale is an effective means to assess exercise intensity. A rating of 11 to 14 (on the Borg 6-20 scale) is typically associated with a moderate intensity that is approximately 70% to 85% of peak exercise capacity. Notably, very few studies have focused on the safety and efficacy of high-intensity aerobic training in patients with AF.

For overweight patients with AF, weight loss is recommended.[47,50] To facilitate weight loss, orienting the exercise prescription to maximize caloric expenditure is indicated. High caloric exercise training (e.g., treadmill walking at a moderate intensity for an extended duration) in CR is well tolerated and an effective strategy to promote weight loss and improve multiple cardiovascular risk factors.[48]

No specific guidelines exist for resistance training for patients with AF. Given the lack of recommendations, using professional discretion is necessary when providing guidance regarding resistance training. Following the resistance training recommendations for other, non-AF CR participants is advisable. General recommendations for resistance training are found in chapter 6.

Pacemakers

Modern cardiac pacemakers typically have pacing, sensing, and rate-responsive functions that are designed to maintain appropriate HR and improve functional capacity. Pacemakers can have leads in one or more chambers of the heart. AV (dual chamber) sequential pacing is common and allows the heart to maintain the normal sequence and timing of the contractions of the upper (atrial) and lower (ventricular) chambers of the heart. Recently, a leadless pacemaker has been developed that can be implanted into the right ventricle.

Rate-responsive pacing (also called rate-adaptive or rate-modulated pacing) has important applications related to exercise. Rate-responsive pacemaker programming increases the rate of pacing in response to patient activity. As a result, the physiologic response to exercise for patients with pacemakers can be like that of patients without pacemakers. Increasing HR during exercise is the single most important factor with respect to increasing cardiac output and oxygen uptake. For patients with chronotropic incompetence who cannot provide an appropriate intrinsic HR increase to exercise, a cardiac pacemaker can be programmed to increase HR and thus cardiac output can meet the physiologic demands of increased activity. Rate-responsive pacemakers can use several types of sensors to detect motion and physiologic and metabolic changes that occur with increased exercise, such as minute ventilation, body temperature, and intervals between heart beats from ECG waveforms. Many pacemakers combine or blend the input from multiple sensors to measure signs of increased workload and apply algorithms to produce a corresponding increase in HR to meet energy demands. If pacing rate does not increase appropriately with exercise, the patient's cardiologist should be alerted, and physical activity intensity may need to be gauged by a method other than pulse count, for example RPE or SBP response to a quantifiable or objectively measured workload. Pacemaker configuration and programming can influence exercise capacity[16-19]; in some patients, tailoring of pacemaker programming can be beneficial.[19]

Following a newly implanted cardiac device, vigorous upper body activity should be restricted for the first month after implantation to reduce the risk of lead dislodgment from the myocardium.[20] CR professionals must be aware of pacemaker configuration (chambers paced and sensed), rate responsiveness, and settings for upper and lower HR limits that, if exceeded, will trigger the pacemaker to respond with antitachycardic or antibradycardic pacing. Otherwise, typical precautions regarding exercise participation should be applied to this population.

Implantable Cardioverter-Defibrillators

Evidence suggests that exercise training in patients with an implantable cardioverter-defibrillator (ICD) is safe.[21-24] Studies of patients with ICDs have also reported that training improves exercise capacity.[21,23] Randomized clinical trials have demonstrated that patients with ICDs who participate in a CR program, compared to patients who do not participate, do not experience more ICD shocks.[22,23]

ICDs are programmed to detect ventricular tachycardia/ventricular fibrillation (VT/VF) and to deliver a shock when indicated. A key element of detecting VT/VF is HR. If HR exceeds programmed thresholds, the ICD interprets that VT/VF is present. Although ICDs are intended to deliver therapies in response to VT/VF, it is possible for ICDs to mistake high HR due to supraventricular tachycardia for VT/VF and deliver inappropriate VT/VF therapies. Some ICDs can include other VT/VF detection algorithms that consider other electrocardiographic features to discriminate VT/VF from rapid supraventricular tachycardia. VT/VF therapies can include both pacing and shocks. ICDs are often programmed to deliver antitachycardia pacing (ATP) to attempt to pace the patient out of VT/VF prior to delivering a shock. Programmed VT/VF HR thresholds and therapies can vary from patient to patient.

CR professionals must know the programmed settings for patients with ICDs. The CR referral and accompanying medical information should include the device manufacturer and programmed settings. CR professionals should confirm that the patient understands their device-related information. Baseline exercise testing is useful to ensure that the patient's peak HR is safely below the threshold at which the device will discharge. Results from a stress test are also useful for establishing a safe and appropriate exercise target HR zone and to determine whether exercise induces dysrhythmias. For some patients, adjusting medications may be necessary. The exercise prescription HR should be set at least 10 to 15 beats below the ICD VT/VF detection HR.[20] The widespread use of beta-blockers in patients with ICDs typically keeps HR, even at peak during an exercise test, below the VT threshold rate. In addition, low-intensity competitive sports that do not constitute a significant risk of trauma to the ICD device are permissible.[25]

Cardiac Resynchronization Therapy

Cardiac resynchronization therapy (CRT; also called biventricular pacing) is an adjunctive therapy for patients with advanced HF.[26] CRT includes an additional lead placed on the left side of the heart. Commonly, patients eligible for CRT have reduced ejection fraction and a left bundle branch block or an intraventricular conduction delay, resulting in left ventricular dyssynchrony. The benefit of CRT is based on reduced conduction delay between the right and left ventricles. CRT functions to maintain right and left ventricular synchrony by regulating the electrical impulses to each ventricle. CRT can improve ejection fraction, reduce mitral regurgitation, and promote left ventricular remodeling.[27-30] Total exercise time, 6-minute walk test distance, and peak $\dot{V}O_2$ are improved with CRT independent of exercise training.[27,29,31-33] Multiple studies have demonstrated that CRT improves symptoms and quality of life, and lowers rates of hospitalization and mortality.[27,34-36] Optimization, which involves adjusting the timing of CRT lead activation, may further improve outcomes.[37,38]

Exercise training may be used as an adjunct to CRT for improving cardiac and peripheral muscle function. Exercise training after CRT helps to improve exercise tolerance, hemodynamic measures, and quality of life.[39,40] Recommended typical precautions regarding exercise participation should be applied to this population.

BOTTOM LINE

- Exercise is generally beneficial and safe in patients with cardiac implantable devices.
- It is important to know the cardiac implantable device settings for CR program participants.
- Tailoring of device programming may have effects on exercise capacity for some patients.

Practice Considerations for Patients With Dysrhythmias and Devices

The goals of exercise for patients with cardiac dysrhythmias and devices vary widely. Therefore, baseline evaluation and treatment plans must be individualized. For lower-risk patients without a history of significant dysrhythmias, continuous ECG monitoring may not be required.[20,49] In some cases, patients with nonsustained ventricular dysrhythmias may require only a limited number of sessions of ECG-monitored exercise with subsequent serial assessments before transitioning to a nonmonitored or home exercise program. In other cases, higher-risk patients with severe myocardial dysfunction, ventricular arrhythmias, and ICDs may have limited functional capacity or be psychologically disabled by history of defibrillation. These patients may require more formal and prolonged ECG-supervised exercise programs.

Baseline evaluation at program entry should include a clear description of the dysrhythmias, the hemodynamic consequences of the dysrhythmias, possible inciting factors such as exercise or cardiac ischemia, and potential therapies should the dysrhythmia recur.[20,41,42] Before exercise is prescribed, the presence and severity of underlying heart disease should be evaluated, including the severity of CAD and LV function. Details about programmed pacemaker or ICD rates, detection parameters, and algorithms should also be obtained. The results of ECG monitoring or electrophysiologic stimulation studies, exercise testing results, and the most current medical regimen should be reviewed with the patient. For patients with a pacemaker, exercise testing can be used to guide the adjustment of the pacemaker settings, especially for active patients with rate-responsive pacemakers to ensure appropriate rate responses. Exercise testing is also helpful for ICD patients to evaluate any overlap of intrinsic HR and programmed VT/VF detection rate.

A common goal in the management of patients with dysrhythmias and devices is the early recognition of change of rhythm or signs and symptoms associated with dysrhythmias to prevent and treat these disorders. CR professionals are frequently the first to identify rest- or exercise-related dysrhythmias. Any new or change in the severity of a cardiac dysrhythmia should be brought to the attention of the program physician and/or referring physician for evaluation and management.

CR professionals can play an important role in the overall evaluation of the patient with an implanted device by providing feedback to the physician about HR, BP, and symptomatic responses to exercise. This information allows for programming the device in order to match the needs of the patient. In many cases, adjustments can improve exercise capacity and symptoms.

Cardiac rhythm disturbances are common in patients with heart disease, but it is rare for dysrhythmias to have life-threating consequences during exercise. The symptoms and presentation of dysrhythmias vary among patients, and the CR specialist is faced with the challenge of understanding the significance of the dysrhythmias, the corresponding hemodynamic consequences, and the resulting impact on exercise physiology. In addition, staff must have a clear knowledge of rhythm management devices, including pacemakers, ICDs, and CRT, in order to work with them and teach patients effectively. Standing orders should provide direction to individual staff members for responding to various rhythm disturbances and for providing limits to exercise levels. Table 10.1 lists common dysrhythmias and their corresponding implications for evaluation and exercise.

Heart Failure and Left Ventricular Assist Devices

This section provides an overview of patient evaluation considerations and strategies for successfully implementing secondary preventive services for patients with chronic HF, including those who have received a LVAD. Special emphasis is placed on practices that

- maximize patient safety,
- individualize rehabilitation services, and
- optimize patient outcomes.

Recent statistics on the prevalence of HF indicate that more than 6.4 million Americans are affected; the number is expected to increase by more than 40% over the next 12 years.[1] Additionally, the incidence of HF now stands at 1 million new cases annually, and it is often associated with repeated hospitalizations and numerous physician visits. In fact, more than 900,000 hospitalizations occur due to HF each year. HF remains a lethal condition, given that about 45% of people with the disorder die within five years after being diagnosed.[1] The estimated annual expenditure for the management of HF exceeds $30 billion. Therefore, therapies and methods aimed at decreasing the clinical manifestations and disability associated with HF remain areas of great interest.

HF is a condition characterized by a reduction in cardiac output (CO), such that it is insufficient to meet the metabolic demands of vital organs and physiological systems. The pathophysiology of HF involves an impairment in the ability of the ventricles to either appropriately contract (HF due to reduced ejection fraction [HFrEF]) or relax (HF with preserved ejection fraction [HFpEF]). The inadequate delivery of blood to match metabolic demands is associated with a variety of pathophysiological sequelae (table 10.2), many of which develop as compensatory mechanisms aimed at maintaining adequate CO. However, these mechanisms may improve or maintain heart function for only a temporary period, after which HF usually progresses. The pharmacologic management of patients with HFrEF currently targets these compensatory mechanisms through the routine use of a combination of beta-blocker, ACE inhibitor or angiotensin-receptor blocker (ARB), aldosterone antagonists, neprilysin inhibitor, and a diuretic as indicated.[2] Except for diuretic therapy, few treatments are effective for HFpEF. Because exercise-based CR is a covered benefit for Medicare beneficiaries with HFrEF, these patients are much more likely to participate in such a program compared to patients with HFpEF.

Clinical Manifestations of HF

The clinical manifestations of HF are as follows:

- Dyspnea and fatigue
- Tachypnea
- Paroxysmal nocturnal dyspnea
- Orthopnea
- Peripheral edema
- Cold, pale, and possibly cyanotic extremities
- Recent weight gain
- Hepatomegaly
- Jugular venous distension
- Lung crackles (rales)

Table 10.1 Dysrhythmias and Their Corresponding Recommendations for Evaluation and Exercise

Dysrhythmias	Clinical status	CR program recommendations
PACs	Asymptomatic	No restrictions
Sick sinus syndrome	Asymptomatic, pauses <3 s; HR ≥50 and increases with activity	No restrictions
	Symptomatic	Needs evaluation and physician recommendation.*
	Pacemaker	May participate with physician approval.^
SVAs (atrial flutter, atrial fibrillation, SVT)	Preexisting, asymptomatic, and HR <110 bpm at rest	May participate with physician approval.
	First detected, symptomatic, or HR ≥110 bpm at rest	Needs evaluation and physician recommendation.
	Postcardioversion or postablation	After 1 week, may participate with physician approval.
Frequent PVCs**	Asymptomatic and no worsening with exercise	May participate with physician approval.
	Symptomatic or worsens with exercise	Needs evaluation and physician recommendation.
Ventricular tachycardia	Stable, asymptomatic, <10 beats duration, monomorphic, HR <150 bpm	May participate with physician approval.
	First detected, symptomatic, or unstable	Needs evaluation and physician recommendation.
	Postcardioversion or postablation	After 3 months, may participate with physician approval.
	Post-ICD placement	Recovery time and restrictions vary; may participate with physician approval.
Ventricular fibrillation	Post-ICD placement	Recovery time and restrictions vary; may participate with physician approval.
First-degree AV block	Asymptomatic, normal QRS complex, PR interval <300 ms, no worsening with exercise	No restrictions
Type I second-degree AV block (Wenckebach)	Asymptomatic, normal QRS, no worsening with exercise	No restrictions
	Worsens with exercise, or symptomatic	Needs evaluation and physician recommendation.
	Pacemaker	May participate with physician approval.
Type II second-degree AV block or complete heart block	Preexisting or first detected	Needs evaluation and physician recommendation.
Complete right bundle branch block (RBBB)	Asymptomatic, no AV block with exercise, no ventricular arrhythmia	No restrictions
Complete left bundle branch block (LBBB)	Asymptomatic, no AV block with exercise, no ventricular arrhythmia	No restrictions

Abbreviations: PAC, premature atrial complex; SVA, supraventricular arrhythmia; SVT, supraventricular tachycardia; AV, atrioventricular; HR, heart rate; PVC, premature ventricular complex; ICD, implantable cardioverter-defibrillator; RBBB, right bundle branch block; LBBB, left bundle branch block).

*Needs evaluation and physician recommendation: Physician should evaluate the patient and provide recommendation. If dysrhythmia is observed with exercise, patient should terminate exercise.

^May participate with physician approval: Physician should review history to determine whether other evaluation or adjustments to exercise prescription are indicated.

**There is insufficient evidence to recommend a specific threshold of PVC frequency for stopping exercise. It is suggested that individual CR centers exercise their judgment for establishing protocols and addressing individual patients.

Based on Zipes et al. (2015).

Table 10.2 Physiological Consequences of Congestive HF

Organ/organ system	Effects
Cardiovascular	Decreased myocardial performance, with subsequent compensatory peripheral vascular constriction to maintain venous return (attempting to maintain stroke volume and cardiac output)
Pulmonary	Pulmonary edema because of elevated cardiac filling pressures, resulting from poor myocardial function and fluid overload
Renal	Fluid retention resulting from decreased cardiac output
Autonomic/neurohumoral	Increased sympathetic nervous system stimulation that eventually desensitizes the heart to beta$_1$ adrenergic receptor stimulation, thus decreasing the cardiac inotropic effect; attenuation of parasympathetic nervous system activity
Musculoskeletal	Skeletal muscle wasting and histochemical abnormalities, as well as osteoporosis resulting from inactivity or other accompanying diseases
Hematologic	Possible polycythemia, anemia, and hemostatic abnormalities resulting from a reduction in oxygen transport, accompanying liver disease, or stagnant blood flow in the heart chambers caused by poor cardiac contraction
Hepatic	Possible hypoperfusion resulting from an inadequate cardiac output or hepatic venous congestion
Pancreatic	Possible impaired insulin secretion and impaired glucose intolerance
Nutritional/ biochemical	End-stage heart failure can be associated with anorexia, subsequent malnutrition (protein, calorie, and vitamin deficiencies), and cachexia.

Adapted from *Essentials of Cardiopulmonary Physical Therapy*, L.P. Cahalin, "Cardiac Muscle Dysfunction," pg. 132, Copyright 1994, with permission from Elsevier.

- Tubular breath sounds and consolidation
- Presence of third (S3) or fourth (S4) heart sounds
- Sinus tachycardia

The two key clinical characteristics of HF are

- exercise intolerance as manifested by fatigue or dyspnea on exertion and
- fluid retention as evidenced by pulmonary or peripheral edema and/or recent weight gain factors.

Importantly, CR professionals need to evaluate changes in clinical status routinely to ensure that the patient can safely engage in exercise training.

Although clinicians often use New York Heart Association (NYHA) functional class to describe clinical status or severity of symptoms, use of that system alone has limitations in that it does not fully reflect the breadth of the disorder. Table 10.3 shows the stages in the development of HF as designated by the ACC and AHA.[3] This staging system covers all patients with left ventricular dysfunction, regardless of the presence or absence of symptoms. Note that patients experiencing symptoms (NYHA classes II-IV) fall only within stage C and stage D.

Determining the magnitude of the disability caused by HF involves assessing and tracking changes in signs and symptoms (e.g., dyspnea, fatigue, edema), functional status (e.g., walking, stair climbing, ADLs), and health-related quality of life (QoL). Evaluating exercise tolerance before, during, or in response to a CR program can be accomplished using distance walked during a 6-minute walk test, exercise duration from an exercise stress test, measuring peak oxygen uptake ($\dot{V}O_2$) during a cardiopulmonary exercise test, or calculating exercise training workloads (METs) during CR. Other exercise test–related variables to help determine a patient's response to CR can include change in HR or symptoms (e.g., dyspnea, angina) at a standardized or fixed submaximal.

Assessing QoL and health status before, during, and after CR can be accomplished using disease-specific questionnaires such as the Minnesota Living With Heart Failure Questionnaire (MLHFQ),[4] the Chronic Heart Failure Questionnaire, or the Kansas City Cardiomyopathy Questionnaire (KCCQ)[5]; as well as general health status questionnaires such as the Medical Outcomes Short Form (SF-36).[6]

The objective documentation of an individual patient's progress can (a) alert CR staff to main-

Table 10.3 Stages in the Development of Heart Failure (ACC/AHA Guidelines)

Stage	Description	Example	New York Heart Association functional class
A (patient at risk)	High risk for HF; no anatomic or functional abnormalities; no signs or symptoms	HTN, CAD, diabetes, alcohol abuse, family history	
B (patient at risk)	Structural abnormalities associated with HF but no symptoms	Left ventricular hypertrophy, prior MI, asymptomatic valvular disease, low ejection fraction	
C (HF present)	Current or prior signs or symptoms and structural abnormalities	Left ventricular systolic dysfunction with or without dyspnea on exertion or fatigue, reduced exercise tolerance	II or III
D (HF present)	Advanced structural HF with symptoms at rest and despite maximal medical therapy	Frequent hospitalizations, awaiting transplant, mechanical circulatory support, intravenous support	III or IV

Abbreviations; ACC, American College of Cardiology; AHA, American Heart Association; CAD, coronary artery disease; HF, heart failure; HTN, hypertension; MI, myocardial infarction.

Adapted from Jessup et al. (2009).

tain or modify the current regimen and (b) serve as a basis for database development either in an individual program or on a larger scale through local, regional, or national oversight.

CR for Patients With HF

The efficacy of CR in patients with NYHA class II to III HF has been previously described.[7,8] The major areas briefly addressed in this section are the physiological and clinical effects of cardiorespiratory exercise training and resistance training.

To date, little data exists regarding the formal exercise-related rehabilitation of patients while hospitalized for acute decompensated HF. Reeves and colleagues conducted a small, randomized pilot project in 27 older patients with acute decompensated HF and showed that a program of tailored physical rehabilitation started prior to hospital discharge and maintained afterward was feasible and was associated with favorable trends in rehospitalizations, physical function, and health status.[9] The remainder of this section summarizes studies involving patients engaged in home-based or supervised outpatient exercise programs.

BOTTOM LINE

The ideal scenario for both the patient and the CR professional might be to first provide exercise in a supervised setting, then begin to incorporate some home-based sessions, and finally progress to an all home-based program.[10] This approach may not be possible for all patients due to travel distance, so an entirely home-based program may be required.

Cardiorespiratory Training for Patients With HF

The 30% to 40% reduction in exercise capacity in patients with HFpEF and HFrEF[11,12] is caused by abnormalities in cardiac, pulmonary, peripheral vascular, and skeletal or respiratory muscle function[13-20] and can be quantified by measuring peak $\dot{V}O_2$. Of the numerous single-site randomized clinical exercise training trials that evaluated change in peak $\dot{V}O_2$ due to moderate-to-vigorous cardiorespiratory endurance–type training, most demonstrated improved peak $\dot{V}O_2$ of $1 \text{ mL} \cdot \text{kg}^{-1} \cdot \text{min}^{-1}$ or more, equating to an approximate 10% to 25% increase in exercise tolerance.[21,22] In the multicenter randomized HF-ACTION trial, the median increase in peak $\dot{V}O_2$ after three months of combined supervised and home-based exercise was $0.6 \text{ mL} \cdot \text{kg}^{-1} \cdot \text{min}^{-1}$ among patients in the exercise arm of the trial (vs. $0.2 \text{ mL} \cdot \text{kg}^{-1} \cdot \text{min}^{-1}$ change for patients in the usual-care group).[23] In addition to improvement in exercise tolerance, several important central and peripheral physiological adaptations occur as well, including an increase in peak HR, an increase in nutritive blood flow to the active skeletal muscle due to improved endothelial function, improved skeletal muscle function (e.g., oxidative capacity), and a downregulation of neurohormonal activity with exercise training.[20,21]

Over the past decade, several authors have used HIIT (as opposed to continuous moderate-intensity exercise) to improve exercise capacity. This method of training yields higher-intensity training levels (up to 95% of peak HR v. 75% of peak HR) and more total work during a single training session. Wisloff and coauthors[24] showed that aerobic interval training improved peak $\dot{V}O_2$ by 6 mL · kg^{-1} · min^{-1} (+46%). However, a subsequent larger randomized clinical trial showed no difference in change in exercise at 12 and 52 weeks when comparing HIIT to moderate continuous training.[25]

CR professionals should note that responses to exercise training do vary in patients with HFrEF. For example, Tabet and colleagues[26] demonstrated significant increases in both mean peak $\dot{V}O_2$ (14%) and mean percent predicted $\dot{V}O_2$ (13%) with exercise training; however, 50% of their subjects were classified as nonresponders, based on achieving a less than 6% increase in percent predicted peak $\dot{V}O_2$. As with other treatments, the response of each patient to exercise training varies, likely due to biologic factors, etiology of disease, and other clinical factors. CR clinicians should be prepared to identify and appropriately modify the exercise regimen of patients experiencing less than satisfactory improvement in fatigue and well-being.

With respect to regular exercise and clinical events, the 2014 Cochrane review reported a reduction in the risk of all-cause hospitalization (relative risk [RR] 0.75; 95% CI: 0.62 to 0.92) and HF-specific hospitalization (RR 0.61; 95% CI: 0.46 to 0.80).[8] HF-ACTION trial also showed beneficial effects, including an 11% reduction in the adjusted risk for all-cause mortality or hospitalization and a 15% reduction in adjusted risk for the combined endpoint of cardiovascular mortality or HF hospitalization.[23] More recently, the ExTra MATCH II meta-analysis showed that exercise-based CR did not have a statistically significant effect on all-cause mortality (HR 0.83; 95% CI: 0.67 to 1.04) or all-cause hospitalization (HR 0.90; 95% CI: 0.76-1.06).[27] In a subsequent analysis of the ExTraMATCH II data, the benefit of exercise training in patients with HF to improve both exercise capacity and quality of life was confirmed.[67] These results support the Class I and IIa recommendations that all patients with HF should participate in an exercise training and CR program, respectively.

Using data from HF-ACTION, Keteyian et al. also found exercise volume (defined as MET-h/week) to be a predictor for all-cause mortality or hospitalization.[28] Although not based on a formal analysis of treatment interaction, it endorses the concept that exercise dose is a potentially important consideration that is related to clinical benefit.

The 2014 Cochrane review reported a clinically important improvement in disease-specific health-related QoL on the MLHFQ (mean score −5.8 points, 95% CI: −9.2 to −2.4) compared to control at up to 12 months follow-up.[8] Using the KCCQ, the HF-ACTION trial examined the effects of exercise training on self-reported health status and showed a modest improvement in the total score at three months, which was maintained over two years.[29]

Cardiorespiratory Exercise Prescription for Patients With HF

With respect to prescribing aerobic-type exercise, the parameters pertaining to intensity, duration, and frequency of exercise must be considered (see table 10.4).[30] In all patients, the CR professional (e.g., clinical exercise physiologist) writing the exercise prescription and monitoring progress should adjust these parameters such that the total volume of exercise is gradually, safely, and consistently increased to 500 to 1,000 MET-min/week (e.g., 4 METs walking pace × 30 min per session × 5 sessions per week = 600 MET-min/week).[30] For most patients, increasing to this level of exercise should require no more than four weeks.

In general, the target levels for duration and frequency of exercise should be 20 to 60 min per bout and three (preferably most days of the week) sessions per week, respectively. For patients with an initially very poor exercise tolerance, it may be helpful to begin with intermittent instead of continuous exercise, such that one 30-minute bout of exercise is broken up into three or four separate bouts interspersed with brief rest periods. Over several weeks, the length of the rest periods is decreased while the exercise period is extended, until 30 continuous minutes can be completed. Regardless of which approach is chosen, both exercise duration and frequency should be increased to target levels before intensity of effort is increased.

With respect to guiding exercise training intensity, the most common approach involves progressively increasing effort to a training range between 40% and 80% of HRR.[31] Intensity is then modified as needed to achieve a rating of perceived exertion (RPE, scale range = 6 to 20) between 12 and 15. The measurement of peak HR is required for the HRR method and can be safely obtained

Table 10.4 Summary of Exercise Prescription for Patients With HFrEF or HFpEF

Type of training	Description	Intensity	Frequency	Duration
Cardiorespiratory endurance	Dynamic activities involving large muscle groups	40% to 80% of HRR RPE 11-14 (where HRR is not appropriate)	Minimum of 3 days/week, but preferably on most days of the week	20-60 min/session
Resistance training	8-10 muscle-specific exercises involving resistance bands, weight machines, handheld weights, or combination; begin with one set of 10-15 repetitions	50%-70% 1RM for lifts involving the hips and lower body; 40%-70% 1RM for lifts involving the upper body	2 or 3 days/week	20-30 min/session; contraction should be performed in a rhythmical manner at a moderate to slow controlled speed

Abbreviations: HRR, heart rate reserve, computed as (peak HR − seated resting HR) × training level in % + seated resting HR; RM, repetition maximum; RPE, rating of perceived exertion.

from a symptom-limited maximal exercise test.[32] As mentioned previously, higher-intensity aerobic interval training, with intensity during work bouts set to 85% to 95% HRR, may represent an effective alternate method for improving exercise tolerance in selected patients.[30] However, the results in the literature for improvement using interval training are mixed. For patients with a change in chronotropic therapy (e.g., beta-blockers), AF, or frequent ectopic beats that interfere with the accurate measurement of HR during exercise, training intensity can be guided by RPE alone or by using the talk test.[33] Regarding the talk test, it indicates that the intensity of exertional effort is excessive if an individual cannot comfortably carry on a verbal conversation during exercise.

Resistance Training for Patients With HF

Resistance can play a key role in recommended exercise guidelines for patients with HFrEF.[39] Regular resistance training improves both muscle strength and endurance without causing adverse effects on hemodynamics[34] or LV characteristics (LV ejection fraction [LVEF], LV end-diastolic volume [LVEDV]).[35-37] The increases in both muscle strength and endurance often exceed 30%[36-39]; however, whether resistance training improves aerobic exercise capacity in patients with HFrEF requires further investigation. Before the start of a resistance training program, patients should first demonstrate that they can tolerate the aerobic training component, which usually requires about three to six sessions to determine.

Similarly to the prescription for cardiorespiratory training, the prescription for resistance train-

ing needs to be increased in a progressive manner. For example, the intensity for upper body lifts should be progressively increased from 40% of 1RM to 70% of 1RM over several weeks.[30] Lower body lifts can begin at 50% of 1RM and progress similarly. Table 10.4 outlines the components of a resistance training regimen for patients with HF.[30,38-40]

Practice Considerations With HF

Following hospital discharge, all-cause 30-day and 90-day rehospitalization remains quite high (~20%-30%) in patients with HF; because of this and disease-related comorbidities, CR programs are well positioned and becoming increasingly involved in the comprehensive care of patients with HF. For Medicare beneficiaries with HF, impacting the 30-day rehospitalization rates through the use of CR is unlikely, given that these patients are currently required to wait six weeks before starting CR. That said, CR represents an ideal setting to address disease-specific education and medication reconciliation, as well as to provide clinical surveillance aimed at preventing rehospitalization by identifying signs and symptoms of cardiac decompensation and referring for treatment.[7] To ensure that the CR services are delivered appropriately, CR staff should review a recent history, results of medical and psychological tests, and results from disease-specific and general health status questionnaires.[41] Exercise test results can also provide important information about the severity of HF and the safety of exercise training and can help guide the development of an exercise prescription.

Table 10.5 summarizes several common safety, exercise, and educational strategies for patients with HF.[7] In addition to expanding their education and exercise strategies, CR professionals who work with the HF population need expanded assessment and communication skills. It is essential that CR professionals become proficient in assessing patients for early signs of HF exacerbation, including auscultation of heart and lung sounds, assessing for peripheral and central edema, and monitoring weight gain. They must establish strong communication links with attending physicians, home health nurses, specialty clinics, and other health care providers with a role in managing patient care.

Left Ventricular Assist Devices

Historically, heart transplantation was the only viable option for patients with end-stage HF on optimal drug therapy. However, due to both the limited availability of donor hearts and advances in technology, mechanical LVADs are now a standard therapeutic option as either a bridge to transplant or a destination therapy for patients with LV HF who do not qualify for transplant. More recently, for patients with both right- and left-sided HF, an option now exists for a total artificial heart (TAH). However, because of both a paucity of exercise studies and the small number of TAHs implanted (226 between 2013 and 2016), the remainder of this section focuses on the LVAD.

The REMATCH trial was the first to demonstrate improved survival for patients while on LVAD support; it showed a one-year survival rate of 52%, compared to 28% for patients receiving optimal medical care alone.[42] Current generation LVADs have advanced considerably as demonstrated by the most recent report from the

Guideline 10.8 CR and HF Disease Management

- Periodically report a patient's progress in CR to the referring physician, including program adherence and any changes in symptom status and functional capacity. Typically, the ITP is adequate to provide this information.

- Help monitor compliance to the overall medical plan, including compliance with diet, sodium and fluid intake, and medications.

- Routinely inquire about the patient's self-monitoring of daily weights, edema, and symptoms, and reinforce self-monitoring practices as needed.

Table 10.5 Safety, Exercise, and Educational Strategies for Patients With HF

Safety	Exercise	Education
• Uncompensated HF is a contraindication to starting an exercise program; decompensation is reason to discontinue the exercise program. • A focused patient assessment should be part of preexercise assessment of vital signs with each CR visit. • As part of the initial evaluation, patients should be asked about advanced directives; copies of such decisions should be placed in the patient's chart.	• Exercise stress tests should include, where possible, metabolic assessment using a progressive protocol (e.g., 1-2 MET/stage). • Patients are at higher risk for ventricular arrhythmias and decompensation. • Exercise protocol: Longer warm-up and cool-down; use interval exercise (1-6 min) as needed; encourage weight bearing for ADLs. • Use ECG and BP monitoring during exercise, as clinically needed; use subjective RPE and dyspnea scales. • After exercise, it is not uncommon for a patient to initially experience fatigue later in the day.	• Priority: Sign and symptom recognition and response, including fatigue, weakness, dyspnea, orthopnea, edema, weight gain (daily weighing). • Nutrition: Low-sodium diet (e.g., 1,500 mg/day), heart-healthy diet. • Drug regimen: Compliance monitoring, as well as medication education for common agents (e.g., diuretics, digitalis, ACE inhibitors, beta-blockers). • Psychosocial consult for depression symptomatology; HF support group and individual counseling. • Basic information regarding disease processes.

Abbreviations: ACE, angiotensin-converting enzyme; ADLs, activities of daily living; BP, blood pressure; HF, heart failure; ECG, electrocardiogram; MET, metabolic equivalent of task; RPE, rating of perceived exertion.

Interagency Registry for Mechanically Assisted Circulatory Support (INTERMACS), reporting a one-year survival for patients on LVAD support now at 80%.[43]

Current-generation LVADs have pumps that provide circulatory or hemodynamic support to underperfused organs and reverse the pathophysiological sequelae of HF.[43] In brief, the LVAD pump is implanted intra-abdominally or in a preperitoneal pocket external to the abdominal viscera. The LV is cannulated at the apex of the heart for inflow to the pump, which unloads the LV, sending blood into the ascending aorta distal to the aortic valve (figure 10.1). All continuous-flow (CF) LVADs operate at a set speed, as measured by revolutions per minute (RPM). However, carefully determining the operational speed is critical to prevent pulling of the septal wall (known as suction events) at higher RPM, which could lead to right-sided HF.

The technology of LVADs has evolved dramatically over the past 20 years. First-generation LVADs used in the early 1990s tethered patients to hospital floors for months while they awaited transplant.[44] These devices were replaced by battery-powered portable models, allowing patients the freedom to return to normal daily activities. However, these first-generation LVADs still had many limitations, including frequent mechanical breakdowns and a large internal pump, which made them incompatible for smaller patients, including most women and children. The second- and third-generation LVADs used today have smaller internal components, which have resulted in fewer mechanical device failures and a longer life span for the device.[45]

Exercise Considerations for Patients With LVADs

Participation in traditional aerobic-based exercise, including symptom-limited exercise testing, appears to be safe and well tolerated in patients with LVADs.[46-49] Despite operating at a fixed speed, CF LVADs have the capacity to increase CO during exercise up to approximately 10 L/min.[50] Factors contributing to the increase in cardiac output during exercise are a combination of increased preload, decreased afterload, and the native heart itself, as demonstrated by studies showing the aortic valve opening during exercise.[51] Limiting CO, and likely functional capacity during exercise, is the fixed speed of the LVAD. This relationship is illustrated in studies that show an increase in peak $\dot{V}O_2$ after the RPM settings are increased.[52,53] Parenthetically, it also may be a reason why peak $\dot{V}O_2$ tends to be lower in patients with LVADs compared to transplants.[54]

While peak exercise capacity may still be limited by the device itself, submaximal exercise and patient reported health improve significantly following LVAD implantation, showing increases in many patients that are comparable to changes observed following heart transplantation.[55,56] In a cohort of 281 patients with NYHA Class IV symptoms, 83% of patients receiving LVADs were reclassified as NYHA Class I or II at six months following implantation, with an increase of more than 70% in 6-minute walk distances.[55] In addition, improvements in functional status are associated with increased QoL and higher self-reported exercise ability.[56,57] In short, patients with an LVAD feel better and may be more willing to participate in a structured exercise program.

Participation in CR With LVAD

Although patients with an LVAD may have improved function, they are still likely to be

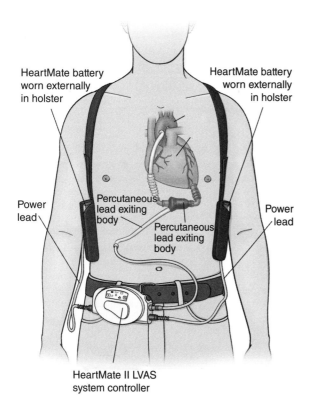

Figure 10.1 HeartMate II left ventricular assist system (LVAS).

Reprinted with permission from Thoratec Corporation.

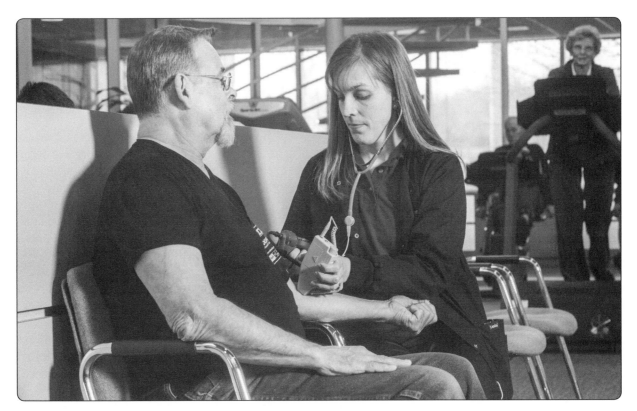

Participation in traditional aerobic-based exercise is beneficial for patients with LVADs and can lead to increased QoL.

extremely deconditioned and exhibit significant skeletal muscle atrophy secondary to extended periods of poor perfusion (prior to LVAD implant) and sedentary behaviors. Participation in CR improves functional capacity and exercise tolerance.[49,58,59] A meta-analysis of randomized control trials found that CR participation resulted in improvements of peak $\dot{V}O_2$ and 6-minute walk test by 23% and 28%, respectively, compared to usual care.[47] Additionally, CR studies report improvements in self-reported health status and muscular strength, which correlate with each other as well as with other important clinical outcomes such as disability.[60] Although more studies are needed, an observational study of 1,164 Medicare beneficiaries with LVAD support showed favorable clinical outcomes with CR participation, reporting reduced hospitalizations and one-year mortality.[61]

Another important role of CR is to provide surveillance and feedback to other clinicians regarding signs or symptoms. For example, as part of a multidisciplinary LVAD team, CR staff might report a paroxysmal dysrhythmia detected using ECG telemetry monitoring, one that

otherwise might go undetected. Other unique medical concerns requiring close surveillance by the CR staff are bleeding, infection (where the driveline inserts into the abdominal wall), device malfunction, and stroke.[62] However, despite the higher-risk nature of this patient population, the number of untoward events during CR appears to be very low, with few reported adverse events during exercise.[46,63] A study of 1,600 patient-hours during CR reported only a single training related event (nonsustained ventricular tachycardia).[63]

Exercise prescription. Similar to other CR patient populations, patients on LVAD support have a linear relationship between HR and $\dot{V}O_2$.[64] Thus, using 60% to 80% of HRR to guide exercise intensity is appropriate if a patient has undergone a recent exercise stress test and does not have a permanent implanted pacemaker. This range is appropriate because of the intact HR response of the native heart to exercise, even though the LVAD functions independent of exercise. However, in patients with an LVAD who are pacemaker dependent, a discordance exists in the HR to $\dot{V}O_2$ relationship due to chronotropic incompetence or another mechanism.[64] For these patients (or any patient without a graded exercise test), maintaining a moderate level of perceived exertion (RPE of 11-13) while gradually increasing exercise intensity represents a plausible and appropriate method for progressing the exercise prescription.

Initial exercise workloads for most patients with an LVAD will need to start at lower MET levels (≤2.5 METs), with modification guided by RPE and symptomatic response. Factors that can negatively influence the overall functional capacity of a patient and initial workloads chosen for CR include shorter time since LVAD implantation, low current PA habits, common comorbidities, and increasing age. Response of functional capacity to training can be safely and effectively evaluated using the 6-minute walk test.[62]

The safety and efficacy of resistance training in LVAD patients is another area in need of practical research. LVAD patients should wait 8 to 12 weeks after device implantation before beginning a light resistance training program primarily due to wound healing. Other considerations include avoiding activities that may dramatically increase intra-abdominal pressure (e.g., sit-ups) or that have the potential for physical trauma (e.g., contact sports); the latter could cause a fracture of the drive line or potentially create damage to the LVAD itself.

Special Considerations for Patients With LVADs

Extensive education is required for the LVAD patient. It includes knowledge of signs and symptoms of exercise intolerance and how to modify exercise, device console alarms (e.g., low battery, low flow), duration of the power supply, and who to contact during a medical emergency. CR staff should also be familiar with the LVAD and should work with the patient and LVAD coordinator at the institution where the device was implanted regarding emergency procedures and complications common with the device, such as the following:

Differential Diagnosis for a Low-Flow Alarm on the LVAD

- Obstruction
- Right ventricular failure
- Pulmonary embolism
- Hypovolemia
- Pump failure
- Bleeding cardiac tamponade
- Arrhythmias
- Systemic HTN

A brief review for clinical changes and assessment of vital signs should be performed before exercise, along with the patient's subjective response to exercise. However, due to the nonpulsatile flow of blood in the CF LVAD models, auscultatory BP assessment may be difficult and may not be reliable. Instead, the clinician should obtain the BP via Doppler ultrasound. This value is considered equivalent to the mean BP. Additionally, the system controller, which regulates the motor power and speed, has a monitor that displays any system alarms along with power output (W), flow (L/min), and pulsatility index (HeartMate II and III). These indicators have important clinical implications and should be recorded along with the vital signs during CR. For example, a significant rise in power above 10 W could be a sign of a pump occlusion (e.g., clot or twisted drive line) and would warrant immediate consultation with the LVAD coordinator or physician.[65]

Special considerations regarding exercise are like those for other CR participants, with particular attention to exercise tolerance.

Preexercise Doppler pressures >90 mm Hg are associated with increased clinical risks and complications, thus consultation with the LVAD team should be considered before starting an exercise bout.[65]

If a patient with an LVAD loses consciousness, emergency defibrillation for lethal arrhythmias may be performed. However, most LVAD patients typically have an implantable cardioverter-defibrillator (ICD). A current debate exists regarding chest compressions for unresponsive patients. While LVAD manufacturers do not recommend performing chest compressions due to the potential dislodgment of the LVAD, published cases describe chest compressions to be safe in these patients, leading some institutions to adopt the use of chest compressions.[65,66] Regardless of these cases, until further research, it is best to consult with your own LVAD and emergency response teams. CR programs that don't have an LVAD program but enroll patients with an LVAD should consider contacting an LVAD program coordina-

> **Guideline 10.9 Special Considerations for Patients With an LVAD**
>
> Exercise is contraindicated if preexercise mean arterial pressure is <66 mm Hg, if the low flow device alarm activates, or if the patient exhibits intolerance to the workload (regardless of BP findings).[60]

tor to arrange occasional continuing education for staff.

Heart Transplantation

Heart transplantation is the treatment of choice for eligible patients with advanced chronic HF with resulting markedly improved survival, functional status, and QoL compared to alternative treatments.[1] The Registry of the International Society for Heart and Lung Transplantation's 2017 report contained 135,387 heart transplantations (120,991 in adults) performed worldwide between 1982 and 2016 with median survival of 10.7 years for adults and 16.1 years for children.[2] One- and five-year survival is 82% and 69%, respectively.[1] It is not uncommon for some younger patients to survive more than 30 years after transplant. Forty-five percent of recipients were hospitalized at the time the donor heart became available; 40% received intravenous inotropes and 43% were on mechanical circulatory support (intra-aortic balloon pump, extracorporeal membrane oxygenation, LVAD, or total artificial heart).[2] Survival is similar for patients with and without circulatory support of an LVAD before transplantation. Causes of death for transplant patients include graft failure (primary graft dysfunction and acute rejection), infection, and multiple organ failure in the early years after surgery. Late mortality is due primarily to malignancy, cardiac allograft vasculopathy, and renal failure.[1]

For 2015, there were 4,390 adult and 684 pediatric (≤18 years) heart transplants reported to the Registry worldwide (approximately 2,500 in the United States).[2,3] The age of heart transplant recipients ranges from newborn to the eighth decade of life.[1] For adults, the average age at transplant is approximately 55 years, and 75% are men. Approximately 50% of children who receive a transplant are 5 years of age or younger. The average age of the donors is approximately 35 years. Combined organ transplant (heart and liver, kidney, or both; or heart and lung) accounts for 3% of transplants. Retransplantation also accounts for 3% of cases.[2]

The waiting time for an organ depends on blood type and the degree of medical urgency. Unfortunately, the number of potential candidates for heart transplantation greatly exceeds the available supply of donor organs. For example, for 2012 in the United States, 6,700 patients were eligible and listed for transplantation, but only 2,400 transplants were performed.[4]

Approximately 85% of adult patients who require transplantation suffer from cardiomyopathy (either nonischemic or ischemic).[2] Additional diagnoses leading to transplantation include HTN, valvular cardiomyopathy, myocarditis, acquired immunodeficiency syndrome (AIDS), complex congenital HD, and infiltrative diseases of the myocardium (amyloidosis, hemochromatosis).[1-4]

Orthotopic transplantation (figure 10.2) is the usual surgical technique with excision of the recipient's diseased heart and anastomosis of the donor heart to the great vessels and atria of the recipient.[5] The goals of cardiac transplantation are improved survival, reduced symptoms, improved QoL, and an increased exercise capacity. After recovery from surgery, most patients report a reasonable functional ability.[6] Many patients return to work, school, or their usual avocational activities, although aerobic exercise capacity generally remains below the age and sex specific average. Employment following transplantation for patients aged 25 to 60 years is approximately 50%.[7] However, due to immunosuppressant medications and other transplant-related factors, patients are prone to develop complications and comorbidities. HTN and dyslipidemia are extremely common.[7] Table 10.6 lists the prevalence of additional common medical problems observed in cardiac transplant recipients.

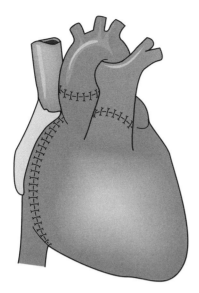

Figure 10.2 Orthotopic cardiac transplant technique.

Reprinted with permission from R.W. Squires, Exercise Training After Cardiac Transplantation," *Medicine and Science in Sports and Exercise* 23 (1991): 686-694.

Graft Dysfunction

The transplanted heart may fail soon after surgery due to primary graft dysfunction, pulmonary HTN, or hyperacute rejection. Primary graft dysfunction is caused by ischemia and reperfusion injury related to the transplant procedure and results in most early mortality.[8] Contributing factors include brain death of the donor, ischemic time, and hypothermia of the donor heart. The incidence is variable but occurs in at least 5% of patients. The pathophysiology includes both increased pulmonary vascular resistance and systemic inflammation.

Rejection

Rejection of the transplanted heart is a major cause of hospitalization and death in the first year after surgery.[9] There are four types of rejection: hyperacute, acute cellular, acute humoral (vascular), and chronic (cardiac allograft vasculopathy).

- Hyperacute rejection occurs shortly after surgery and is caused by preformed antibodies to the donor heart.[9] This type of rejection results in acute inflammatory infiltration with vessel necrosis of the transplanted organ and patient death. Fortunately, with immunologic matching of donor and recipient, hyperacute rejection is rare.

- Acute cellular rejection is most common during the first six months after transplantation and is due to T-lymphocyte and macrophage infiltration of the myocardium.[9] The diagnosis is made using routine, periodic transvenous endomyocardial biopsy of the right ventricle. If not treated promptly, myocardial injury and necrosis may occur, although mild acute cellular rejection may not require acute treatment.[1] Based on tissue sample analysis, acute cellular rejection is graded from mild to severe. The treatment of acute cellular rejection involves additional immunosuppressants and may require hospitalization. Severe acute rejection, resulting in substantial myocyte necrosis and fibrosis, may produce LV dysfunction and HF.[5]

- Acute humoral (vascular) rejection occurs within days to weeks of transplantation and is a relatively rare phenomenon.[9] Initiated by antibodies, the process may impair coronary

Table 10.6 Prevalence of Common Medical Conditions After Heart Transplantation

Condition	At 1 year	At 5 years
Renal dysfunction	26%	51%
Diabetes mellitus	22%	36%
HTN	50%	95%
Cardiac allograft vasculopathy	8%	29%
Malignancy	5%	16%
Osteoporosis	28%	n/a

Data from Institute of Medicine (2001); Sobal and Stunkard (1989).

Abbreviation: HTN, hypertension.

vasodilatory reserve resulting in ventricular dysfunction. Diagnosis is made by identifying immunoglobulins or complement in the vessels of the graft using biopsy material.

- Cardiac allograft vasculopathy (CAV), also called chronic rejection or accelerated graft coronary artery disease, occurs months to years after transplantation.[10] CAV is the major limiting factor in long-term survival after cardiac transplantation. CAV is present in 43% of heart transplant recipients at seven years.[11] The disease is an unusually accelerated form of coronary disease affecting epicardial and intramyocardial coronary arteries and veins.[10] The pathophysiology is incompletely understood but is thought to be associated with repetitive immunologic endothelial injury, ischemia-perfusion injury, viral infection, immunosuppressant medications, and traditional coronary risk factors, such as dyslipidemia, insulin resistance, and HTN. The lesions usually diffusely involve the entire vessel, although focal obstructive lesions sometimes occur. This disease process occurs in pediatric and adult recipients with equal regularity. Annual coronary angiography or imaging stress testing may be performed to detect the disease. Because of the diffuse nature of the typical lesions, retransplantation is the most common treatment. In patients with discrete focal lesions, revascularization (either catheter-based or coronary bypass graft surgery) may be effective.

Medications

Immunosuppressant medications are given to prevent acute rejection of the donor heart.[5] Maintenance drugs generally include combination therapy with a calcineurin inhibitor (sirolimus, tacrolimus, or cyclosporine), an antiproliferative agent (mycophenolate mofetil or azathioprine), and a corticosteroid (prednisone).[11,12] These powerful drugs enable the patient to tolerate the donor heart but are associated with several common side effects as listed in table 10.7. Prednisone, in the dose range used in transplantation, is particularly bothersome. It alters body fat distribution with resultant truncal obesity and a moon face (rounded appearance due to fat deposits in the sides of the face) for many patients. Prednisone may also cause mood swings as well as skeletal muscle atrophy and weakness, osteoporosis, and dyslipidemia. During the first one to two years after transplantation, an attempt is usually made to taper and stop prednisone.

Statin medications may slow progression of accelerated graft coronary disease and improve survival.[13-15] In addition, statins reduce the incidence of acute rejection and improve LV function.[14,15] These benefits appear to be independent of the drugs' effects in improving the blood lipid profile.

Common Nonrejection Medical Problems

Patients who have been transplanted are at risk for various other medical issues primarily related to the medications required to maintain immunosuppression.

Infection and Malignancy

Immunosuppressed transplant recipients are at a higher risk of opportunistic infections and malignancy than the general population of

Table 10.7 Common Immunosuppressant Drugs and Associated Side Effects

Drug name (brand name)	Potential side effects
Tacrolimus (Prograf)	Tremor, headache, diarrhea, HTN, nausea, renal dysfunction
Sirolimus (Rapamune)	Skin irritation, tremor, lightheadedness, weight gain, abdominal pain, diarrhea
Mycophenolate mofetil (Cellcept)	Diarrhea, leukopenia, sepsis, vomiting, infection, edema
Prednisone	Muscle atrophy/weakness, HTN, fluid retention, osteoporosis, asceptic necrosis of bone, moon face, truncal obesity, increased insulin resistance, cataracts, glaucoma, mood swings, personality change, insomnia, peptic ulcer disease
Cyclosporine (Gengraf, Neoral, Sandimmune)	Renal dysfunction, tremor, HTN, hirsutism, gum hyperplasia, muscle cramps, acne
Azathioprine (Imuran)	Nausea/vomiting, leukopenia, thrombocytopenia, anemia

Abbreviation: HTN, hypertension.

patients with CVD. During the first several weeks after surgery, pulmonary bacterial infections are common.[16] Late after transplantation, viral, bacterial, and fungal infections pose a threat. Special precautions should be taken to minimize the chances of exposure to patients with active infections. Patients are encouraged to wear a surgical mask and gloves as an infection barrier in public places, particularly during the first three months after surgery.

Malignancy risk is substantial for transplant patients. At seven years after surgery, the incidence of malignancy (primarily skin cancers) is 24%.[11] This risk is likely related to long-term immunosuppression.

Hypertension

HTN is common after transplantation and affects over 95% of patients at seven years.[11] The extremely high prevalence is thought to be due to the use of calcineurin inhibitors and their adverse effects on renal function.[11] Use of combination antihypertensive drug therapy is often required. BP after transplantation is usually sensitive to the dietary sodium load.

Obesity

Weight gain and obesity after cardiac transplantation are commonly observed. In a cohort of 95 patients, BMI averaged 28 ±1 kg/m² at the time of surgery.[17] The average increase in BMI and body weight by the first anniversary after transplantation was 2.1 ±3.6 kg/m² and 6.3 ±8.7 kg, respectively. Corticosteroid use plays a major role in posttransplant weight gain.

Dyslipidemia

Blood lipid abnormalities after cardiac transplantation are almost as universal as is HTN.[18] Immunosuppressants, diuretics prescribed for the treatment of HTN, and renal insufficiency all contribute to the problem. Statin medications are effective in treating dyslipidemia in these patients, although the risk of rhabdomyolysis is increased with concurrent statin and calcineurin inhibitor use.

Diabetes Mellitus

Diabetes is common after transplant and is present in 35% of patients at seven years.[11] Pretransplant diabetes, glucocorticoid and calcineurin inhibitor use, and obesity contribute to the high prevalence of the disease.[16] Diabetes is associated with a poorer long-term survival in cardiac transplant recipients.

Chronic Renal Insufficiency

Renal insufficiency, defined as creatinine levels >2 mg/dL, is a common side effect of calcineurin inhibitors.[16] Fortunately, <10% of transplant recipients develop end-stage renal disease.

Osteoporosis

Advanced HF is associated with osteopenia and osteoporosis before transplantation. Glucocorticoid use after transplantation results in additional loss of bone mineral. Osteoporosis resulting in vertebral fractures is common in heart transplant recipients, affecting up to 30% of patients.[16]

Depression

Depression has been reported in approximately 25% of heart transplant recipients at one to three years after surgery.[16] Therefore, many of these patients take antidepressant medications.

Psychological Factors

The psychological response to the transplant process is understandably intense for most patients.[19] While waiting for the operation, after acceptance as a transplant candidate emotions range from relief and happiness to anxiety (indefinite waiting time, lack of absolute assurance that the transplant will occur) and thoughts of death. Patients who require continuous hospitalization while waiting for an organ may find the environment supportive or merely tedious and boring. Immediately after transplantation, patients are usually relieved at the prospects for a longer, higher-quality life.

As the period of convalescence continues, patients must adjust to the tedium of medical appointments and procedures. As previously discussed, the immunosuppressant prednisone may cause mood swings and personality change. The first episode of acute rejection may result in heightened feelings of anxiety and transient depression. As the recovery from surgery progresses and the degree of medical surveillance decreases, patients generally shift their attention from transplant-related activities to becoming more independent, resuming family roles, and occupational and avocational pursuits. The readjustment to life after transplantation requires months, and the one-year anniversary is an important milestone in this process. Most patients can return to productive and meaningful lives.

Noncompliance as evidenced by inconsistent taking of medications, poor attendance at clinic appointments, smoking, lack of regular exercise or of attendance at CR classes, and dietary lapses are unfortunately common in transplant patients and result in poorer outcomes.[20] Predictors of noncompliance include young age at transplant, low level of formal education, depression, anxiety, hostility, substance abuse, and poor social support.

BOTTOM LINE

Transplant patients have complicated clinical courses before and after transplantation. Fortunately, contemporary surgical and medical care results in a favorable outcome for the majority of patients.

Responses to Exercise

The responses of heart transplant recipients to acute exercise are unique and related, in part, to the following factors[5,21,22]:

- With harvesting of the donor organ, the transplanted heart is surgically denervated and receives no direct efferent input from the autonomic nervous system, and it provides no direct afferent signals to the central nervous system. Months after transplantation, some patients demonstrate signs of partial cardiac reinnervation (discussed later in this chapter).

- During organ harvesting and with transplantation, the donor heart has experienced ischemic time and reperfusion.

- There is no intact pericardium.

- Diastolic dysfunction (elevated filling pressures at rest and with exercise) is common. Reasons for abnormal diastolic function include HTN, acute rejection episodes resulting in myocardial scarring and fibrosis, and cardiac allograft vasculopathy.

- Abnormal skeletal muscle histology and energy metabolism, developed during chronic heart failure, may continue after transplantation.

- Peripheral and coronary vasodilatory capacity may be impaired, in part, due to endothelial dysfunction.

Heart Rate and Exercise

Because of the loss of parasympathetic innervation of the donor heart with transplantation, HR at rest is elevated to approximately 95 to 115 bpm and represents the inherent rate of depolarization of the sinoatrial node.[19] With graded exercise, for most patients HR typically does not increase during the first several minutes (delayed increase), followed by a gradual rise with peak HR slightly lower than normal (~150 bpm) due to sympathetic nervous system denervation. Many patients achieve their highest exercise HR during the first few minutes of recovery from exercise, rather than at the point of maximal exercise intensity because of a lack of parasympathetic innervation to counteract circulating epinephrine. This also may result in HR remaining near peak values for several minutes during recovery before gradually returning to resting levels (delayed decrease). The chronotropic (HR) reserve (the difference between the maximal and resting HR) is less than normal. Figure 10.3 shows the HR response to graded exercise of the same patient one year before and three months after orthotopic transplantation. Note the delayed increase in HR during the first few minutes of exercise and the highest rate during recovery after transplantation.

With orthotopic cardiac transplantation, it is possible that the sinoatrial (SA) node of the recipient's heart may be left intact. The depolarization wave from the SA node generally does not cross the suture line in the right atrium, but the ECG may show two distinct P waves (one from the recipient and one from the donor SA nodes). Many patients have a RBBB conduction pattern.

Blood, Intracardiac, and Vascular Pressures

BP at rest is mildly elevated in heart transplant patients, even though most patients receive antihypertensive medications. During exercise, BP generally increases appropriately, although peak exercise BP is slightly lower than expected for otherwise healthy persons.[20] Vascular resistance is elevated, and intracardiac and pulmonary vascular pressures (particularly right-sided pressures) are elevated.[21]

LV Function

For most heart transplant patients, LVEF is normal at rest and during exercise.[21] However, as mentioned previously, LV diastolic function is often impaired, as evidenced by an elevated

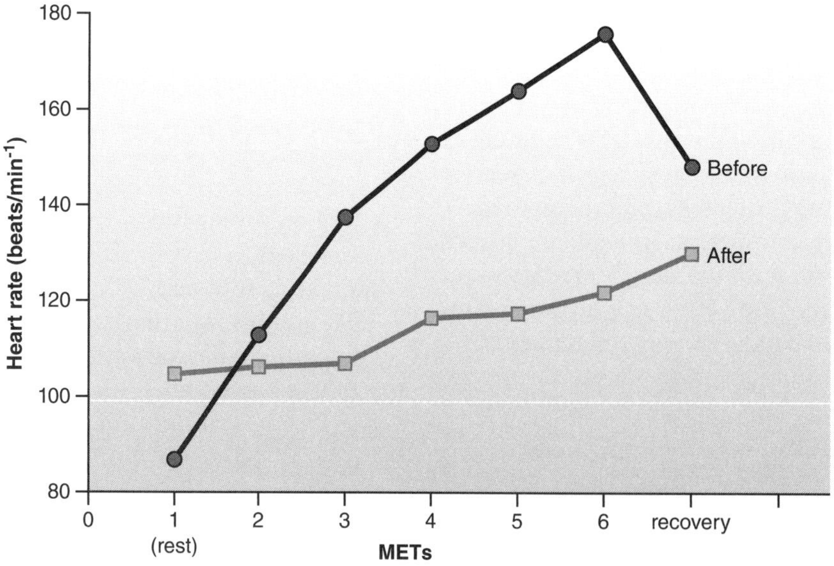

Figure 10.3 Heart rates measured during graded exercise in the same patient one year before and three months after orthotopic cardiac transplantation. Note the elevated resting HR and the delayed increase in HR during exercise after transplantation consistent with complete denervation.

Abbreviation: MET, metabolic equivalent.

Reprinted by permission from R.W. Squires, "Cardiac Rehabilitation Issues for Heart Transplantation Patients," *Journal of Cardiopulmonary Rehabilitation* 10 (1990): 159-168.

filling pressure for a given EDV. This impairment results in a below normal increase in stroke volume during exercise. The impaired rise in stroke volume, coupled with the below normal HRR, results in an impaired exercise CO.

Exercise CO

With the onset of exercise, CO in transplant recipients with complete cardiac denervation increases due to augmentation of stroke volume via the Frank-Starling mechanism. Later, increased HR also contributes to augmentation of cardiac output.[22] At rest and during exercise, the cardiac index is lower for transplant recipients than for nontransplant patients.

Skeletal Muscle Structure and Biochemistry

During the clinical course of chronic HF, several skeletal muscle structural and biochemical abnormalities develop; they include the following:

- Reduced aerobic metabolic enzyme activity
- Lower capillary density
- Endothelial dysfunction with impaired vasodilation during exercise

- Conversion of some slow-twitch motor units to fast-twitch motor units with greater reliance on anaerobic than aerobic energy production

These abnormalities generally persist after transplantation, with partial improvement after several months for some patients.[23,24]

Oxygen Uptake Kinetics, Peak Exercise $\dot{V}O_2$

With the onset of exercise, the rate of increase in oxygen uptake ($\dot{V}O_2$) kinetics is slower than normal as a result of both an impaired rise in cardiac output and a diminished oxidative capacity of the skeletal muscle (reduced arterial-mixed venous O_2 difference).[28] Figure 10.4 shows $\dot{V}O_2$ versus cycle ergometer power output during graded exercise for the same patient measured one year before and three months after cardiac transplantation. Although peak $\dot{V}O_2$ was 18% higher after transplantation, for any given submaximal power output, $\dot{V}O_2$ was consistently lower than before the transplant, consistent with slower $\dot{V}O_2$ kinetics.

Because of the dual abnormalities of an impaired exercise cardiac output and a reduced arterial-mixed venous oxygen difference just described, peak exercise $\dot{V}O_2$ is usually below normal for transplant patients. In a series of 95 patients with a mean age of 49 years who performed a cardiopulmonary exercise test approximately one year after transplantation, the mean peak $\dot{V}O_2$ was 20 mL·kg⁻¹·min⁻¹ (62% of age- and sex-predicted).[17] Marked variability in response was evident with a range for peak $\dot{V}O_2$ of 11 to 38 mL·kg⁻¹·min⁻¹ (39% to 110% of age- and gender-predicted). Some very highly trained transplant patients may achieve even higher values, such as the following:

- Mean peak $\dot{V}O_2$ of 40 mL·kg⁻¹·min⁻¹ in 14 men (mean age 43 years) with highest value of 54 mL·kg⁻¹·min⁻¹ [29]
- Mean peak $\dot{V}O_2$ of 45 mL·kg⁻¹·min⁻¹ in 12 men (mean age 47 years)[30]
- A 45-year-old male endurance athlete developed nonischemic cardiomyopathy with a pretransplant peak $\dot{V}O_2$ of 9 mL·kg⁻¹·min⁻¹. After transplantation he trained and completed three Ironman distance triathlons (peak $\dot{V}O_2$ 56 mL·kg⁻¹·min⁻¹, 149% of predicted).[31]

There are additional interesting abnormal exercise physiology findings in cardiac transplant recipients. These are the most common abnormalities:

- Increased resting HR
- Delayed HR increase at onset of exercise
- Blunted maximal HR
- Delayed return of HR to resting level after cessation of exercise
- Reduced HRR
- Increased exercise LVEDP (diastolic dysfunction)
- Increased exercise pulmonary artery pressure, pulmonary capillary wedge pressure, right atrial pressure
- Increased LV end-systolic and EDV indices
- Impaired increase in stroke volume during exercise
- Reduced exercise CO
- Decreased exercise arterial-mixed venous O_2 difference
- Slowed O_2 uptake kinetics during exercise
- Decreased $\dot{V}O_2$max
- Reduced maximal power output during exercise testing

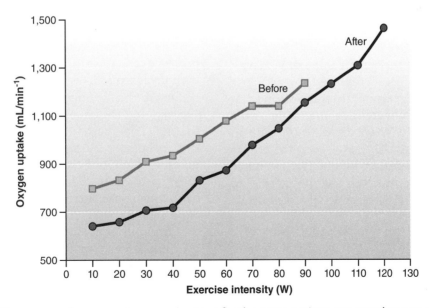

Figure 10.4 $\dot{V}O_2$ versus cycle ergometer power output for the same patient measured one year before and three months after orthotopic cardiac transplantation.

Reprinted by permission from R.W. Squires, "Cardiac Rehabilitation Issues for Heart Transplantation Patients," *Journal of Cardiopulmonary Rehabilitation* 10 (1990): 159-168.

- Decreased ventilatory anaerobic threshold
- Increased exercise ventilatory equivalents for O_2 and CO_2

Partial Cardiac Reinnervation

Occasionally, a heart transplant patient with cardiac allograft vasculopathy resulting in myocardial ischemia will report typical angina, suggesting at least partial afferent cardiac reinnervation.[32] It also appears that partial cardiac sympathetic efferent reinnervation occurs in many patients during the first several months to years after surgery. The evidence for this statement is based on neurochemical evaluation of autonomic nervous system activity in the heart and the observation of improved responsiveness of the HR during exercise.[32]

For instance, the HRR increases during the first six weeks after transplantation in many patients. In a subset of patients, the HRR increases further over the next 6 to 12 months.[33] A more rapid decline in HR from peak exercise to baseline is observed in some patients at one to two years after transplantation.[34]

HR responsiveness to maximal graded exercise was assessed in a group of 95 transplant recipients at one year after surgery.[17] About 1/3 of subjects exhibited at least partial HR response normalization. Figure 10.5 shows the HR responses to graded exercise for the same patient at 3 and 12 months after transplantation. Note the typical denervated response at 3 months and the partially normalized response at 12 months. The finding of a lack in improvement in peak $\dot{V}O_2$ with a larger HRR has been reported for pediatric heart transplant recipients.[35] In addition, in adult transplant patients, increasing the HRR with a novel high-intensity warm-up did not result in an increase in peak $\dot{V}O_2$.[36] However, the effects of partial normalization of the HR response during exercise on peak $\dot{V}O_2$ and the capacity to improve peak $\dot{V}O_2$ with training is not completely understood.[37]

BOTTOM LINE

Transplant patients demonstrate unique physiologic responses to acute exercise, especially HR. Over time, some patients demonstrate a more normal HR response during aerobic exercise.

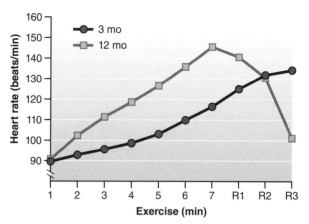

Figure 10.5 HR responses to graded exercise in the same patient at 3 months and 12 months after cardiac transplantation, demonstrating both denervation (at 3 months) and partial reinnervation (at 24 months).

Reprinted by permission from R.W. Squires et al., "Partial Normalization of the Heart Rate Response to Exercise After Cardiac Transplantation: Frequency and Relationship to Exercise Capacity," *Mayo Clinical Proceedings* 77 (2002): 1295-1300.

Graded Exercise Testing

Exercise testing is helpful in determining the exercise capacity, prescribing exercise training, and in counseling patients regarding the timing of return to work or school, or resumption of avocational pursuits. The ECG of transplant recipients commonly demonstrates RBBB and nonspecific repolarization abnormalities. The sensitivity of the exercise ECG in detecting the presence of CAD is poor (<25%) unless combined with myocardial imaging.[27]

Due to the healing and recovery process after surgery, and the usual deconditioned state prior to surgery, it is best to wait six to eight weeks after surgery before performing graded exercise testing to maximal effort. For patients with more complicated postoperative courses, an even longer period of recovery is recommended before performance of an exercise test.

Treadmill or cycle ergometer protocols, with continuous exercise (2 or 3 min stages) or ramp tests may be used. Arm cranking protocols may also be employed after adequate sternal healing, for a specific upper extremity fitness evaluation or an arm cranking exercise prescription.[38] The initial exercise intensity should be approximately 2 METs, with increments in intensity of 1 or 2

METs per stage.[38,39] Continuous multilead ECG monitoring with BP measurement and Borg perceived exertion ratings for each stage are recommended. For precise determination of aerobic capacity and the ventilatory anaerobic threshold, direct measurement of $\dot{V}O_2$ and associated variables is highly desirable. The endpoints of the graded exercise test should be maximal effort (symptom-limited maximum) or standard signs of exertional intolerance.[40]

Responses to Exercise Training

Cardiac transplant recipients are excellent candidates for progressive exercise training for several reasons, including the following:

- Pretransplant syndrome of chronic heart failure with poor exercise capacity due to central and peripheral circulatory abnormalities, as well as skeletal muscle pathology
- Deconditioning and the healing process with open-heart surgery similar to that observed with coronary or valvular surgery
- Posttransplant use of corticosteroid medications with resultant skeletal muscle atrophy and weakness

Aerobic Exercise Training

The first report of exercise training after heart transplant was published in 1983.[41] However, since that report, few reports have been published on the subject. Investigators have employed various approaches to exercise training with differences in intensity, session duration, frequency, and length of the training program. The time between transplant and starting exercise training has varied widely between studies. A systematic review and meta-analysis from 2013 reported only six randomized trials of exercise training after heart transplantation, which included a total of 175 subjects.[42] Training was safe and resulted in an average increase in peak $\dot{V}O_2$ of only 1 $mL \cdot kg^{-1} \cdot min^{-1}$. Another review of 12 observation studies reported a range of 1.3 to 5.6 $mL \cdot kg^{-1} \cdot min^{-1}$ improvements in peak $\dot{V}O_2$.[37] However, some individual trials demonstrated much better improvements in aerobic capacity.

Kavanagh et al. reported the results of a 16-month exercise training program in 36 transplant recipients (no control group).[43] Exercise training (walk/jog) began approximately seven months after surgery and was carefully supervised. Patients demonstrated many benefits after training, including an average 27% increase in peak $\dot{V}O_2$ (21.7-25.9 $mL \cdot kg^{-1} \cdot min^{-1}$). In a subset of subjects who performed a much greater amount of training, peak $\dot{V}O_2$ increased by 54% (21.3-32.2 $mL \cdot kg^{-1} \cdot min^{-1}$).

Kobashigawa et al. reported results of a six-month randomized controlled trial of exercise training in 27 transplant patients.[44] The exercise group underwent supervised training (aerobic and strengthening exercises), whereas the control group performed an unstructured home walking program. Peak $\dot{V}O_2$ improved to a greater extent in the supervised training group (+4.4 [49%] v. +1.9 [18%] $mL \cdot kg^{-1} \cdot min^{-1}$, P<0.01). However, baseline aerobic capacity was very limited (average peak $\dot{V}O_2$: 9.2 $mL \cdot kg^{-1} \cdot min^{-1}$). There were no differences between the two groups for number of episodes of acute rejection or infection.

On the other end of the spectrum of baseline fitness in transplant recipients, Rustad randomized 52 subjects into a one-year study of three times/week, high-intensity aerobic interval training (HIIT) versus no training in Norway.[45] Peak $\dot{V}O_2$ increased from 27.7 to 30.9 $mL \cdot kg^{-1} \cdot min^{-1}$ (10% increase) in the HIIT group and was unchanged in controls. Dall compared moderate continuous aerobic training (MCT) with HIIT in a randomized crossover trial and found that HIIT was superior to MCT for improvement in peak $\dot{V}O_2$ (+4.9 v. +2.6 $mL \cdot kg^{-1} \cdot min^{-1}$).[46]

Potential additional benefits of regular exercise for transplant recipients include the following[47]:

- Improved submaximal exercise endurance
- Increased peak treadmill exercise workload or peak cycle power output
- Increased maximal heart rate
- Decreased exercise HR at the same absolute submaximal workload
- Increased ventilatory (anaerobic) threshold
- Decreased submaximal exercise minute ventilation
- Reduced exercise ventilatory equivalent for CO_2
- Lessened symptoms of fatigue and/or dyspnea
- Reduced rest and submaximal exercise SBP and DBP
- Decreased peak exercise DBP

- Reduced submaximal exercise ratings of perceived exertion
- Improved psychosocial function
- Increased lean body mass
- Reduced body fat mass
- Increased bone mineral content

Resistance Exercise

Most cardiac transplant patients require prednisone, at least during the first several months after surgery, for immunosuppression. As previously mentioned, skeletal muscle atrophy and weakness are common side effects related to prednisone use. Resistance exercise training partially reverses corticosteroid-related myopathy and improves skeletal muscle strength. Horber and associates found definite evidence of skeletal muscle wasting and weakness in the lower extremities of renal transplant patients who received prednisone.[48] Fifty days of isokinetic strength training substantially increased muscle mass and strength in these patients. In addition, strength training has been shown to improve bone density and to reduce the potential development of osteoporosis (also caused by prednisone) in cardiac transplant recipients.[49]

BOTTOM LINE

Carefully designed and implemented resistance training is recommended to counteract the effects of pretransplant decline and post-transplant medications that can affect body composition, bone integrity, and muscle mass and strength.

Effect of Exercise Training on Immune Function, Longevity, CAV, and Hospital Readmissions

Traditional, moderate-intensity training does not increase or decrease the number or severity of episodes of acute rejection.[44] In addition, training does not require changes in immunosuppressant dosage or treatment. Exercise training does not change infection risk.

Rosenbaum et al. is the only study to date that addressed exercise training and longevity.[50] The number of CR exercise sessions attended during the first 90 days after transplantation predicted survival to 10 years (82% survival overall) with a hazard ratio of 0.31 (69% reduction) for mortality if patients participated in ≥8 sessions.

Nytroen et al. used intravascular ultrasound to assess CAV at baseline and after one year in patients randomized to HIIT versus standard care.[51] Although CAV progressed in both groups, HIIT resulted in a significantly reduced rate of progression of CAV.

Bachman and colleagues studied 595 Medicare patients who underwent transplantation in the United States and participated in CR. Participation in CR (55% participation rate) was associated with a 29% lower one-year risk of rehospitalization.[52]

BOTTOM LINE

Transplant recipients respond favorably to both aerobic and resistance exercise training. CR participation results in multiple impressive clinical benefits.

Exercise Programming Suggestions

As part of the evaluation process for transplantation, ambulatory patients usually undergo cardiopulmonary exercise testing. Peak $\dot{V}O_2$ is a powerful prognostic indicator. Patients with a peak aerobic capacity of <14 mL·kg^{-1}·min^{-1} (4 METs) experience a markedly reduced one-year survival, independent of LVEF.[53]

Based on the results of the exercise test, an exercise prescription may be developed for the patient with the goal of maintaining or even improving cardiorespiratory fitness while waiting for a donor organ (prehabilitation). See the section Cardiorespiratory Exercise Prescription for Patients With HF for exercise prescription specifics.

Early Mobilization and Inpatient Exercise Training

After surgery, patients are extubated expeditiously (usually within 24 hours). Passive ROM exercises for both the upper and lower extremities, sitting up in a chair, and slow ambulation may begin and progress gradually after extubation.[54] Walking or cycle ergometry should be increased in duration as tolerated. Exercise intensity is guided using the Borg RPE ratings of 11 to 13 (fairly light to somewhat hard), keeping the respiratory rate below 30 breaths per minute and arterial oxygen saturation above 90%. Exercise frequency is two or three sessions per day.[5] Patients whose postoperative courses are uncomplicated typically remain hospitalized for 7 to 10 days.

During inpatient rehabilitation and during the outpatient phases, episodes of acute rejection of a moderate or greater severity may require alteration of the exercise plan; it depends on the preferences of the transplant team. In general, if the rejection episode is graded as moderate, activity may be continued at the current level but should not progress until after the rejection has been adequately treated. Severe acute rejection necessitates suspension of all PA except for passive ROM exercises.

Outpatient Exercise Training

Cardiac transplant recipients may enter outpatient CR as soon as they are discharged from the hospital.[5] Generally the transplant team requires patients to remain near the transplant center for close follow-up for approximately three months. Ideally, they should exercise in both a supervised environment (three sessions per week) and independently (an additional three sessions per week).

Continuous monitoring of the ECG during the first few supervised exercise sessions is standard practice, although many weeks of ECG monitored exercise is not a requirement. It is not necessary to perform graded exercise testing before beginning the outpatient exercise program. Performing a 6-minute walk test is helpful in assessing functional capacity.

Exercise prescription for patients with cardiac transplant is similar to methods used with patients who have undergone other types of cardiothoracic surgery. The one exception is that a target HR is not used unless the patient exhibits a partially normalized HR response to exercise as discussed previously. The typical denervated heart increases in rate slowly during submaximal exercise, and the HR may either drift gradually higher during steady-state exercise or plateau after several minutes.[19] Borg 6-20 scale ratings of 12 to 14 (somewhat hard) may be used to prescribe exercise intensity.[5] Recently, HIIT has been used in exercise programs for transplant recipients and is well tolerated with favorable effects on fitness.[45,51] The exercise prescription should include standard warm-up and cool-down activities, a gradual increase in aerobic exercise duration to 30 to 60 minutes, with a frequency of four to six sessions per week. Typical modes of aerobic exercise used during the early outpatient recovery period include treadmill walking, cycle ergometry, stair climbing, and walking outdoors (or in shopping centers or at schools).

Because of the sternal incision, special emphasis on upper extremity active ROM exercises is recommended during early outpatient CR. Additionally, at approximately 6 to 10 weeks after surgery, when sternal healing is nearly completed, rowing, arm cranking, combination arm/leg ergometry, outdoor cycling, hiking, and jogging become additional options, depending on the patient's fitness level. Sports such as tennis and golf may be performed as early as six weeks after surgery if patient fitness is adequate (≥5 METs) and sternal healing is nearly complete. For more information, see the section titled Role and Purpose of Sternal Precautions earlier in this chapter.

Muscle strengthening exercises should be incorporated into the exercise program to counteract the skeletal muscle effects of deconditioning and corticosteroid use. For approximately the first 6 to 10 weeks after surgery (surgeon dependent), bilateral arm lifting is restricted to <10 lb (4.5 kg) to avoid sternal nonunion. During this early stage of CR, light hand weights are an excellent method of introducing resistance exercise. After at least six weeks of healing, patients may be started on standard weight machines, emphasizing moderate resistance, 10 to 20 slow repetitions per set, one to three sets of exercises for the major muscle groups, with a frequency of two or three

Guideline 10.10 ECG Monitoring

ECG monitoring is recommended for at least the initial several sessions of CR, but in most cases it does not need to be performed throughout the length of CR participation.

Guideline 10.11 Exercise Prescription Intensity

Because of denervation, HR should not be used to guide exercise intensity. Maintaining a perceived exertion between 11 and 14 on the Borg 6-20 scale is recommended.

sessions per week.[5,55] Resistance band exercises are another excellent mode of resistance training for these patients. Moderate intensities (Borg 6-20 RPE of 12 to 14) is recommended. Strength gains of 25% to 50% or greater commonly occur after eight weeks of strength training in these patients. Performance of the strengthening exercises immediately following the aerobic portion of the exercise prescription (after the cool-down) is recommended.

Encouragement to continue a lifelong exercise program should be a consistent message from the transplant team and the primary health care provider. Patients should continue in a supervised exercise program indefinitely or exercise independently, or use a combination of supervised and unsupervised exercise. Periodic adjustment of the exercise prescription should occur as needed.

Peripheral Artery Disease

Peripheral artery disease (PAD) occurs as a result of the development of atherosclerotic plaque in the arteries of the legs.[1] The partial or complete blockages due to plaque lead to a mismatch between oxygen supply and demand of the muscles of the lower limbs. Although patients may be asymptomatic or present with atypical symptoms as a result of comorbidities,[2] claudication is considered the hallmark symptom of the disease.[1] Claudication is often described by patients as pain, aching, discomfort, burning, or cramping in the muscles of the lower limbs during exercise that resolves with rest.[3] The most significant risk factors for developing PAD include cigarette smoking[4,5] and diabetes mellitus.[4,6,7] However, many other risk factors associated with the development of CVD are also strongly linked to the development of PAD.[6,7] Patients with claudication often lead sedentary lives, which subsequently results in poor walking ability, reduced functional performance, and a lower quality of life (QoL).[8,9] CR professionals have worked with patients with PAD because it is a common comorbidity along with CVD. The recent approval of reimbursement for supervised exercise training for those with PAD, and the allowance of CR programs to deliver supervised exercise therapy (SET) means that CR professionals will be working with more patients with PAD, including those without CVD. Because PAD patients are at a high risk for adverse cardiovascular and cerebrovascular events,[10] professionals must be aware of the challenges faced when using exercise to treat patients with PAD.

Diagnosis

A complete discussion of the diagnostic procedures in patients suspected of having PAD is beyond the scope of this chapter. Briefly, claudication may occur in the calves, thighs, and/or buttocks. The calf is the most common location of pain, but symptoms often present at the location of the proximal stenosis (partial blockage of the artery) or occlusion (completely blocked artery).[11] For example, aorta and iliac stenosis/occlusions typically result in thigh, hip, or buttock pain.[11] Claudication is typically consistent and reproducible, with the greater levels of pain as exercise intensity increases. Most patients have relief from pain within 10 minutes of resting.[1] For those who are asymptomatic, exercise intensity may not be great enough to elicit leg pain. For those with atypical pain presentations, the pain described may be exertional but does not resolve with rest. Other potential causes of non-PAD pain include (but are not limited to) orthopedic (e.g., arthritis) and neurogenic dysfunction (e.g., peripheral neuropathy), as well as venous insufficiency, which leads to pooling of blood and a feeling of pressure/fullness in the legs. If the patient description is consistent with signs and symptoms of PAD, the patient should be evaluated further via objective assessments. Diminished lower limb pulses can help confirm the diagnosis of PAD. Evaluation of the foot may provide further indication of the presence of disease. A lack of hair on the foot and dystrophic nails may be present in the patient with claudication. The most severe form of PAD is called critical limb ischemia (CLI); in these patients, perfusion of the limb is so limited they may experience ischemic pain in the distal lower extremity, usually the foot, while at rest.[12] Patients with CLI may also have rubor (redness of the skin) when the foot is in a dependent position (below the level of the heart) and pallor or paleness when the limb is elevated above the heart. Patients who have pain when the foot is elevated will often get relief when placing the leg in the dependent position. These patients may also have ulcerations and slow-healing or nonhealing wounds on the feet.

The ankle–brachial index (ABI) is the most useful, noninvasive, hemodynamic testing available to assess for PAD. The ABI compares the systolic blood pressure (SBP) of the legs and arms. Details of the procedure are described elsewhere.[3,13] Briefly, supine SBP is measured in the right and left brachial arteries of the arm and the dorsalis pedis and posterior tibial arteries of both feet. The ABI is a ratio of the highest pressure of each foot divided by the higher of the right or left brachial pressure. Table 10.8 provides the diagnostic criteria for the ABI. For patients with ABIs >1.40, additional tests such as the toe–brachial index (TBI) may be needed because of poor compression of the lower limb arteries due to calcification (e.g., as a result of diabetes or renal disease).[14-16] A TBI of ≤0.70 is abnormal and diagnostic for PAD.[12] For patients with equivocal (borderline) resting ABIs, postexercise ABIs can be useful for diagnosing PAD. Patients walk on a treadmill until they experience claudication symptoms. Walking is then stopped, and the ABI is repeated. Diagnosis of PAD is confirmed when a postexercise ABI is 0.99 or lower.[17] Other hemodynamic and physiological tests include segmental limb pressures, pulse volume recordings, transcutaneous oxygen pressure, and skin perfusion pressure.[18-21] Imaging is also a useful diagnostic procedure in PAD and includes computed tomography, magnetic resonance, duplex ultrasound, and invasive angiography.[22] If these tests are indicated, they are typically completed prior to referral to CR (as well as for follow-up with worsening symptoms), because they provide details on the anatomy of the stenosis/occlusion prior to determining the optimal treatment approach. It is recommended that CR specialists review the diagnostic testing algorithm within the AHA/ACC guidelines for PAD management.[22]

Preparticipation Evaluation and Baseline Outcome Assessments

Before beginning a program of exercise therapy, it is ideal for patients with claudication to complete baseline outcome assessments and determine whether it is safe for them to exercise. However, these assessments are not required by CMS for a patient with PAD to participate in supervised exercise programs. Claudication is not a contraindication to exercise; however, patients with PAD may have comorbidities that limit PA and could adversely impact the feasibility of program success.[67] Existence and severity of cerebrovascular disease or CVD, diabetes, arthritis, and other exercise-limiting diseases should be considered prior to development of the exercise prescription. The extent of PAD severity is also an important part of the initial evaluation and can be accomplished by assessing the walking ability and functional performance of the patient. Finally, baseline outcome assessments also allow for serial follow-up testing to evaluate whether progress is being achieved as a result of the exercise program. A brief review of the primary outcomes and testing procedures and protocols for patients with PAD who are entering a CR program are provided next.

Treadmill-Based Walking Ability

The objective evaluation of a patient's walking ability is an important first step when working with PAD patients. The evaluation could be a graded treadmill test, which is often accompanied by ECG and hemodynamic (e.g., BP, pulse oximetry) evaluation. Primary walking ability outcomes assessed using the treadmill are (1) claudication onset time or distance (point of initial presentation of leg pain) and (2) peak walking time or distance (time or distance at which leg pain severity is at maximal and forces the patient to stop walking). Several valid protocols are available, each starting at 2 mph and 0% grade.[23-25] In the event a patient cannot walk at 2 mph due to severe disease, a lower-intensity protocol such as a modified Naughton may be needed.[26] The stages for the various protocols are 2 or 3 minutes in duration and increase in speed and/or grade every stage thereafter. Patients should be asked

Table 10.8 Ankle–Brachial Index Diagnostic Criteria

Index value	Diagnosis
>1.40	Noncompressible vessels; TBI test recommended
1.00-1.40	Normal
0.91-0.99	Equivocal/indeterminate
≤0.90	Abnormal and diagnostic for PAD

Abbreviations: TBI, toe–brachial index; PAD, peripheral artery disease.

to report when the onset of claudication occurs and rate the severity of discomfort at each stage of the treadmill test using Likert scales with 5 or 6 category ratings (table 10.9).[23,27] Patients walk on the treadmill until they can no longer continue or until it is deemed unsafe. Patients with claudication are likely to reach severe levels of pain, which forces them to stop.

Community-Based Walking Ability

The most often used functional performance evaluation in PAD patients is the 6-minute walk test. The test was originally developed to test the function of patients with HF and respiratory disease,[28] and it has been validated in patients with PAD.[29] Patients are asked to walk for 6 min in a hospital corridor with known distances marked out (e.g., 100 ft).[29] The test can be conducted in other environments (e.g., community settings) as long as the distances walked by the patient can be quantified and the surface is level. Unlike the treadmill test, patients are allowed to stop and rest if needed. The timer continues uninterrupted for 6 min regardless of whether the patient is walking or not. Patients can elect to stand or sit during rest periods if needed. Key outcomes that the CR specialist should assess are (1) the distance walked prior to the onset of claudication and (2) the total distance walked.

Additional Functional Measures

Other objective measurements that may be used to assess changes in physical function, including balance, lower extremity strength, and fall risk are the Short Physical Performance Battery (SPPB) and the Timed Up-and-Go (TUG) test.

The SPPB consists of three measures: standing balance, 4 m (13.12 ft) walking velocity, and repeated chair rises.[30] The SPPB has been used extensively with older adults, including patients with PAD, to evaluate functional status and risk of falling.[31] The TUG test,[32] in which the patient is asked to rise from a chair, walk 10 ft (3 m), turn around, and return to their seat, is an assessment of both locomotion and balance.[33] Additionally, it may be useful to evaluate change in metabolic equivalents of task (METs) over the course of the exercise program as a measure of effectiveness. Change in MET level allows for the comparison of workloads from baseline to follow-up.

Patient-Reported Assessments

The subjective assessment of PAD patients' QoL and their perspective of their functional ability through the use of validated questionnaires can be a useful tool for CR specialists. They can perform this assessment with general and disease-specific questionnaires that have been studied extensively in patients with claudication.[34] The most often used questionnaire is the Medical Outcomes Study Short Form 36 (SF-36) questionnaire.[35,36] Because this questionnaire provides a snapshot of a patient's perceived health and functional status across a variety of domains (e.g., physical and mental health), it can be used to compare with other populations. The recently developed Patient Reported Outcomes Measurement Information System (PROMIS) measures multiple domains of functional status and health.[37] Disease-specific questionnaires for patients with PAD assess a number of domains including symptoms, functional limitations, mental health,

Table 10.9 Pain Rating Scales for Use During Exercise Training

Pain scale	Numerical ratings	Verbal descriptors
Claudication symptom rating scale[25]	0	No discomfort
	1	Onset of discomfort
	2	Mild discomfort
	3	Moderate discomfort
	4	Moderately severe discomfort
	5	Maximal claudication
ACSM Claudication pain scale[27]	0	No discomfort at all
	1	Minimal discomfort
	2	Moderate pain
	3	Intense pain
	4	Unbearable pain (person has to stop)

Reprinted by permission from D. Riebe, J.K. Ehrman, G. Liguori, and M. Maier, *ACSM's Guidelines for Exercise Testing and Prescription,* 10th ed. (Philadelphia, Lippincott Williams & Wilkinds, 2018).

and social and emotional well-being. Commonly used questionnaires in PAD include the Walking Impairment Questionnaire (WIQ),[38] the Peripheral Artery Disease Quality of Life (PADQOL) questionnaire,[39] the Vascular Quality of Life (VASCUQOL) questionnaire, and the Peripheral Artery Questionnaire (PAQ).[40] Questionnaires are either administered by the CR specialist or completed by the patient. Some questionnaire developers incur a cost for use of the tool and for interpretation of data, thus CR specialists should consider possible costs when selecting the metric for use in their respective clinics.

Structured Exercise Training for Claudication

The gold standard treatment option for patients with PAD is walking exercise training. These programs improve patients' walking ability, overall function, and self-reported QoL.[22,41,42] Walking programs are cost effective, and the AHA/ACC PAD management guidelines highly recommend them as key treatments for patients with claudication.[22] The following section includes detailed information on the location of training, exercise prescription, and modalities for consideration.

Supervised Exercise Therapy

Although hospital-based supervised exercise therapy for patients with PAD is effective, until recently these programs were largely unavailable. This scarcity was in large part due to a lack of insurance reimbursement, thus preventing widespread implementation. However, in 2017, the Centers for Medicare & Medicaid Services (CMS) approved reimbursement of supervised exercise therapy (SET) for patients with claudication. The decision memo and specific criteria for coverage and referral are described in the sidebar.[43] Importantly, CR was one of the settings allowed to provide SET.

Similar to CR patients, PAD patients should start with a standard low-intensity warm-up using any modality of their choosing (e.g., treadmill/track walking, leg ergometry). Light stretching of the major joints and muscle groups should follow standard guidelines.[44] Treadmill walking is the ideal modality. However, if the patient has any contraindications to walking exercise (e.g., balance problems, wounds on the feet), other modalities should be considered (see Alternative Modes of Exercise). Exercise bouts are intermittent and dependent on the claudication limitations of each individual patient. Patients are instructed to walk at a self-determined speed until experiencing moderate claudication (3 or 4 on a 5-point scale).[67] The time it takes for the patient to experience moderate claudication should be within 5 to 10 min. If the patient stops exercising before 5 min, the intensity is too great and the speed and/or grade of the treadmill should be reduced. Conversely, if a patient can walk beyond 10 min before experiencing moderate claudication, the intensity of the exercise bout should be increased.[67] For treadmill exercise, the ideal increase in percent grade should go up to 10% by increments of 1% or 2%, because most patients with PAD can more easily tolerate increases in grade than in speed. After a 10% grade is achieved, increases in speed should occur in 0.1 to 0.2 mph increments up to 3 mph before further increasing grade. However, when determining whether to increase grade or speed, the individual patient should be considered. When patients reach the target level of leg discomfort, they should rest (either standing or sitting) and resume walking when the leg pain completely subsides. These exercise and rest sessions are repeated for 30 to 45 min with a frequency of three times a week.[22] For those who cannot initially exercise for at least 30 min, duration of exercise should be increased until they reach 30 min before grade or speed is increased. Up to 36 sessions within a 12-week period are covered by CMS, and patients can opt in for another 36 sessions with a second referral from their physician. The lifetime limit is 72 sessions.

According to the CMS decision memo for coverage of SET for PAD, patients must experience claudication in order to receive the benefit. As previously mentioned, CR specialists may have patients referred to them who have previously received peripheral revascularization (endovascular and/or surgical bypass). Some of these patients still experience claudication; thus, they are eligible to participate in a SET program.

Community and Home-Based Exercise Programs

Although SET is the cornerstone therapy for claudication, the number of sessions available for patients is finite. Therefore, it is imperative that patients transition to community or home-based exercise programs so that the benefits derived from SET are maintained in the long term. Until

Regulatory Considerations for Delivery of SET for Symptomatic PAD

Evidence demonstrating the benefit of supervised exercise for PAD patients with symptomatic claudication has grown substantially over the past three decades. Clinical practice guidelines recommend exercise as a treatment for patients with symptomatic claudication.[1,2] In 2017, the CMS developed a coverage policy for qualifying Medicare beneficiaries. Some commercial payers have been covering SET for patients with PAD prior to the implementation of the Medicare coverage policy. (The following section reviews Medicare coverage considerations for SET services.) Private payers may vary in coverage policy decisions, so preauthorization is always prudent when providing services to non-Medicare patients.

The National Coverage Determination by CMS outlines Medicare requirements for physicians and institutions that provide SET to symptomatic PAD patients.[3] Accompanying CMS publications offer coding, billing, and operational instructions for a SET program.[4-8]

SET for patients with PAD is a separate and distinct service. While SET programs utilize shared space and equipment with other services, such as CR, Medicare regulations for SET are specific to SET services.

CMS requires an initial face-to-face office visit with a physician who is involved in managing the patient's PAD. The purpose of this visit is to confirm the presence of claudication symptoms. Prior to being referred to SET, a beneficiary must receive information regarding CVD and PAD risk factor reduction.

Patients may receive up to 36 exercise sessions of supervised exercise over a duration of 12 weeks in a hospital outpatient or physician office setting. SET is comprised of therapeutic exercise training sessions lasting 30 to 60 min. Progress is measured by reduced presentation of symptoms during exercise (progressively longer walk times before limiting pain). Patient progress should be tracked, updated, and documented.

Staffing for a SET program can be multidisciplinary, similar to that found in a CR program. CMS does not require a specific professional discipline to provide SET. The SET program must be under the direct supervision of a physician, physician assistant, or nurse practitioner trained in both basic and advanced life support techniques. Qualified personnel in a SET program should possess competence in the following:

- Assessing for cardiovascular risk factors

- Recognizing the presence of PAD

- Developing an individualized exercise prescription that is effective while accommodating existing comorbidities

- Understanding and practicing behavior change strategies that help patients achieve goals

PAD can severely limit lifestyle. However, appropriate exercise training in this patient population is potentially very effective in reducing claudication symptoms and can make a significant difference in a person's quality of life.

1. Gerhard-Herman MD, Gornik HL, Barrett C, et al. 2016 AHA/ACC guideline on the management of patients with lower extremity peripheral artery disease: A report of the American College of Cardiology/American Heart Association Task Force on Clinical Practice Guidelines. *J Am Coll Cardiol.* 2016;69(11):1465-1508.

2. Murphy TP, Cutlip DE, Regensteiner JG, et al. Supervised exercise, stent revascularization, or medical therapy for claudication due to aortoiliac peripheral artery disease: A randomized clinical trial. *J Am Coll Cardiol.* 2015;65(10): 999-1009.

3. Decision memo for supervised exercise therapy (SET) for symptomatic peripheral artery disease (PAD) (CAG-00449N). Centers for Medicare & Medicaid Services website. www.cms.gov/medicare-coverage-database/details/nca-decision-memo.aspx?NCAId=287. Published May 25, 2017. Accessed October 10, 2018.

4. Medicare National Coverage Determinations Manual, Chapter 1, part 1 (Sections 10-80.12) NCD 20.35. Centers for Medicare & Medicaid Services website. https://www.cms.gov/Regulations-and-Guidance/Guidance/Manuals/Downloads/ncd103c1_Part1.pdfPublished May 11, 2018. Revised Feburary 15, 2019. Accessed October 23, 2019.

5. Supervised Exercise Therapy (SET) for Symptomatic Peripheral Artery Disease (PAD), MLN Matters Number 10295. Centers for Medicare & Medicaid Services website. https://www.cms.gov/Outreach-and-Education/Medicare-Learning-Network-MLN/MLNMattersArticles/Downloads/MM10295.pdf Published 2017 Revised May 11, 2018. Accessed October 10, 2018.

6. Medicare Claims Processing Manual, Chapter 32-Billing Requirements for Special Services, Section 390. Centers for Medicare & Medicaid Services website. https://www.cms.gov/Regulations-and-Guidance/Guidance/Manuals/downloads/clm104c32.pdf. Revised February 8, 2019. Accessed October 23,2019.

7. Pub 100-03 Medicare National Coverage Determinations-Transmittal 207. Centers for Medicare & Medicaid Services website. https://www.cms.gov/Regulations-and-Guidance/Guidance/Manuals/Internet-Only-Manuals-IOMs-Items/CMS014961.html. Published May 11, 2018. Accessed October 23, 2019.

8. Pub 100-04 Medicare Claims Processing-Transmittal 4049. Centers for Medicare & Medicaid Services website. https://www.cms.gov/Regulations-and-Guidance/Guidance/Transmittals/2018Downloads/R4049CP.pdf. Published May 11, 2018. Accessed October 23, 2019.

recently, advice for patients to exercise was the standard of care for PAD. Patients were instructed to walk as much as possible, which was not effective.[45-48] However, recent trials have developed structured programs that occur at the home and in the community and consist of exercise components used in SET with occasional on-site visits (e.g., once per month).[49-51] Promotion of the optimal frequency, intensity, and duration of exercise is paramount to ensuring patients follow to the exercise prescription. Ideally, if resources permit, following up with patients (via phone calls or in-hospital visits) and objectively monitoring them remotely with activity monitors (e.g., pedometers, accelerometers) may aid in adherence to exercise. Discussions about the various barriers and facilitators to exercise should be discussed with patients to ensure that no regression in positive health changes is incurred following transition from SET to a community-based program.

Alternative Modes of Exercise

Treadmill walking is the cornerstone of rehabilitation exercise for people with claudication. However, in some cases walking exercise may not be feasible for the patient (e.g., safety concerns). Some patients may also prefer alternative modalities. Leg and arm ergometry are effective for improving claudication symptoms.[25,52,53] Total body recumbent stepping is another seated exercise that may be preferable to treadmill walking for some patients.[67] Resistance training may also be helpful for PAD patients,[54,55] but it is typically only considered as a complementary or optional component of the exercise program. PAD is an atherosclerotic disease, thus primarily aerobic-based exercise is recommended. The important point to consider is that both the patient and CR specialist will have the discretion to decide what is best for the patient given any special circumstances that exist. Of note, while it is required

that patients experience lower extremity ischemic symptoms in their daily lives, it is not required that claudication be induced during exercise training.

BOTTOM LINE

- SET is effective in improving functioning and QoL in patients with PAD and should be encouraged regardless of baseline functional ability.
- Intermittent treadmill or other walking is the most efficacious mode of exercise training and should be prioritized over other modalities.
- Alternative modes of exercise such as leg or arm cycling or total body recumbent stepping should be considered if treadmill exercise is not effective or contraindicated.
- SET is beneficial even for patients who have undergone revascularization procedures.
- Objective and patient-reported functional and QoL outcomes should be evaluated before and after completion of SET.
- Patients should be counseled on the best strategies to transition from SET to a home or community-based setting to promote lifelong participation in exercise.

Other Treatment Options for Claudication

A number of other therapies are available to treat PAD patients with ischemic lower limb pain. Treatment options can be partitioned into pharmacological therapy and peripheral revascularization.

Pharmacologic Therapy

Optimal medical therapy to reduce the risk of premature CVD is a mainstay in the treatment of patients with PAD. Patients may be taking antiplatelet agents (e.g., aspirin, clopidogrel), thus bleeding risk may be elevated in these patients. For patients with diabetes, glucose controlling agents (e.g., sulfonylureas, insulin) may be prescribed, thus the CR specialist should be aware of blood glucose levels before and after exercise for safety purposes. Other common medications prescribed to PAD patients as part of their medical management include (1) statins or other hypocholesteremia medications (e.g., niacin, fibrates), (2) ACE inhibitors for hypertension (others include diuretics and calcium channel blockers, and (3) bupropion and nicotine replacement therapies to support smoking cessation.

To date, the use of medications to improve claudication in patients with PAD is limited. Pentoxifylline was the first drug approved by the Food and Drug Administration (FDA) for claudication but has lacked significant benefit.[56,57] Side effects have also been noted (e.g., gastrointestinal distress) and are dependent on the dosage level. Cilostazol is the only other drug approved by the FDA[58] and has demonstrated consistent efficacy for treating claudication.[59,60] However, it is important to highlight that it has been given a black box warning (absolute contraindication) by the FDA and should not be used in patients with HF (as a result of higher mortality rates in other phosphodiesterase-III inhibitors).[61,62] Many investigational agents exist to treat claudication, but most have demonstrated mixed results or require more research to demonstrate safety and effectiveness before regulatory approval.[63]

Peripheral Revascularization

Peripheral revascularization performed by interventional cardiologists, radiologists, and vascular surgeons is an effective treatment option for patients with PAD. Technical success rates have improved considerably in the last decade. The goal of revascularization is intuitive in that a patent arterial vessel will likely result in improved blood flow to the lower extremities.[12] The seminal Claudication: Exercise Versus Endoluminal Revascularization (CLEVER) study evaluated the change in peak walking time for patients with PAD following a six-month study. Participants were randomized into one of three groups: (1) supervised SET plus optimal medical therapy; (2) peripheral revascularization (self-expanding or balloon-expandable stents and limited to only patients with aortoiliac disease) plus optimal medical therapy; and (3) optimal medical therapy alone.[64] The primary endpoint of peak walking time improved in both the SET group (+5.8 ±4.6 min) and peripheral revascularization group (+3.7 ±4.9 min) compared to optimal medical therapy alone (+1.2 ±2.6 min). Importantly, the exercise group showed the greater improvement in peak walking time compared to the peripheral revascularization group. However, the peripheral revascularization group showed a trend of greater improvement for claudication onset time compared to SET (+3.6 ±4.2 vs. +3.0 ±2.9 min, $p > 0.05$) and was significantly greater than the optimal medical therapy group (+0. ±1.1 min, $p < 0.05$). The two treatment groups were not statistically different for peak walking time at 18-month follow-up.[65,66] Finally, the group who received stenting was associated with significantly greater benefit across the majority of disease-specific QoL outcomes. This trial provides evidence to support the AHA/ACC PAD management guidelines giving a classification recommendation of I for SET prior to revascularization.[22] Regardless, many PAD patients referred to CR settings may have received or are planning to undergo this procedure.

Revascularization can be partitioned into endovascular therapy and surgical interventions; both have advantages and disadvantages. Patency rates for endovascular therapy and surgical bypass vary and are dependent on the arterial segment intervened upon, the length of the lesion, and the type of procedure.[22] While surgical procedures may provide more durable long-term patency outcomes, they are associated with higher rates of morbidity and mortality than endovascular procedures.[22] CR staff should be able to recognize when a patient may have had a restenosis of an artery following a lower extremity revascularization procedure (primarily by worsening symptoms), which warrants a referral back to the patient's health care provider.

BOTTOM LINE

- Physicians (and patients) should strongly recommend that their patients participate in an exercise program implementing SET prior to consideration of peripheral revascularization. Ideally it will take place in a CR setting.
- CR staff should evaluate the walking ability of all patients with symptomatic PAD referred to CR for SET. Those who can walk safely should begin exercise using a treadmill.
- For those patients with symptomatic PAD and comorbidities (e.g., obesity, orthopedic limitations) that prevent them from being able to derive benefit from treadmill walking, alternative modes of exercise should be considered (e.g., cycle exercise).

Chronic Lung Disease

A significant number of people who have cardiovascular disease (CVD) also have chronic obstructive pulmonary disease (COPD).[1] In many instances, the latter is the cause for a patient's exercise limitation. While the coexistence of both diseases has often been attributed to a common cause of cigarette smoking, it is now believed that systemic inflammation plays a central role in the pathogenesis of both COPD and CVD.[2] Recently researchers have learned that the more severe the COPD, the greater the severity of coronary lesions and presence of calcifications.[3] Often a significant lag time exists between the development of the underlying chronic lung disease (particularly COPD) and the occurrence of symptoms (which in some instances may be decades long), thus making an early diagnosis of the disease difficult.

Airway obstruction is often underdiagnosed, particularly in patients with CVD.[4,5] In fact, the prevalence of COPD not diagnosed in patients with CVD risk factors is extremely high.[6] It is important to consider the possibility of the presence of chronic lung disease for all patients who are entering a CR program, particularly in those with a greater than 10 pack per year smoking history or symptoms of dyspnea, cough, wheezing, or mucus production.

BOTTOM LINE

Consider assessing all patients entering CR for underlying chronic lung disease by examining symptoms and measuring oxygen saturation via pulse oximetry.

Diagnosis

Patients with comorbid pulmonary disease are likely to have shortness of breath (either at rest or with exercise) and may have cough and/or sputum production. Increases in respiratory rate, wheezing, chest hyperinflation, or generalized muscle wasting are often noted on examination. A variety of questionnaires exist that can help to determine whether a patient is at risk for the presence of COPD and dictate further diagnostic studies.[7,8] These questionnaires can be helpful in the initial assessment of patients referred for CR.

While the most commonly associated chronic lung disease in patients with CVD is COPD, a patient may have other types of chronic lung disease, such as obstructive (other than COPD), restrictive, or vascular. The diagnosis of COPD is confirmed based on spirometry testing. Current recommendations regarding the use spirometry for the role of case finding in COPD are available.[9] Complete pulmonary function testing (e.g., spirometry, lung volume measurements, diffusing capacity measurements) can be helpful to more fully determine the type of underlying lung process that is present, whether it be obstructive, restrictive, or vascular. This testing is also helpful to assess the disease progression as well as the response to therapy. Findings of spirometry for the various types of obstructive and restrictive lung diseases are noted in table 10.10.

Several other tests can be useful to help differentiate the type and severity of lung disease that is present. Arterial blood gases are helpful to determine whether gas exchange abnormalities (e.g., hypoxemia or hypercapnia) are present. Arterial oxygen saturation, as measured by pulse oximetry, is helpful to determine whether oxygen desaturation is present and is a less invasive test than arterial blood gas analysis. A chest x-ray may indicate the presence of lung hyperinflation or diaphragmatic flattening, as is seen in advanced COPD; or chest wall abnormalities, which can be seen in the case of kyphosis or scoliosis. A chest computed tomography (CT) scan can be used

Table 10.10 Spirometry Findings for Chronic Lung Disease Types

	COPD	Asthma	Restrictive lung disease
FEV1	Decreased	Decreased, normal	Decreased, normal
FVC	Decreased	Decreased, normal	Decreased
FEV1/FVC	Decreased	Decreased, normal	Normal, increased
TLC	Increased	Increased, normal	Decreased

Abbreviations: FEV1, forced expiratory volume in 1 s; FVC, forced vital capacity; FEV1/FVC, ratio of FEV1 to FVC; TLC, total lung capacity (cannot be determined from spirometry alone; will need lung volume measurements).

to determine whether interstitial lung disease is present. ECG is helpful to assess not only for LV or valvular heart disease but also for the presence of right ventricular dysfunction and is the noninvasive screening test of choice for the presence of pulmonary HTN.[10]

Cardiopulmonary exercise testing with the measurement of expired gases is helpful in the evaluation of a patient undergoing CR who is suspected to have underlying chronic lung disease. For a patient with chronic lung disease, decreased ventilatory reserve, increased dead space ventilation, hypoxemia, and increased respiratory rate at isotime (a standardized exercise period of time) may be noted. A pretest determination of the FEV1 can be useful to estimate the maximal ventilatory volume (MVV), which is used to determine the breathing reserve at peak exercise. In some circumstances, a pulmonary impairment may be the limiting factor to exercise. Although such exercise testing need not be performed in every patient who is entering a CR program, it can be very helpful for patients who have both cardiac and pulmonary disease to help determine the principal cause for the exercise limitation and to determine the exercise prescription. In addition, it is useful for developing a HR-based exercise prescription.[11] If a field test such as the 6-minute walk or shuttle walk test is used as part of the initial evaluation, continuous oxygen saturation monitoring during testing can uncover oxygen desaturation during activity. Guidelines have been developed for the use of these field walking tests.[12]

Types of Chronic Lung Diseases

COPD is characterized by the inability to exhale air fully on a forced maneuver. Early symptoms include the development of shortness of breath, cough, or wheezing. Exercise intolerance then develops secondary to the dynamic hyperinflation that is a result of the underlying airway and lung parenchyma abnormalities. The presence of hypoxemia or other comorbid conditions, such as skeletal muscle dysfunction or anemia, may also impact the patient's overall exercise tolerance.

Asthma, another type of obstructive lung disease, is characterized by variable airflow obstruction that is often reversible either spontaneously or with treatment. Asthma is characterized airway hyperresponsiveness, airflow limitation, and dyspnea. Patients often have a sensitivity to aeroallergens and worsening of symptoms with viral respiratory infections. These symptoms may be present seasonally and are often reversible. For some patients with asthma, long-term chronic airway disease may develop and overlap with COPD symptoms. This group of patients is now termed to have the asthma–COPD overlap syndrome (ACOS).[13]

Restrictive lung diseases are another type of chronic lung disease that can be seen in patients with CVD. These diseases impair the patient's ability to take a deep breath; they include interstitial pulmonary fibrosis, sarcoidosis, chest wall abnormalities, neuromuscular diseases (e.g., myasthenia gravis, amyotrophic lateral sclerosis), or kyphoscoliosis. Pulmonary vascular disease (e.g., primary pulmonary HTN, chronic thromboembolic pulmonary HTN, veno-occlusive disease) is another type of chronic lung disease that may be present. The underlying pathophysiology of the disease may impact the patient's exercise tolerance. As with COPD, hypoxemia associated with the disease may adversely affect that person's exercise tolerance.

Medical Management

Optimal management for a patient with chronic lung disease includes both pharmacologic and nonpharmacologic therapy. For patients who continue to smoke, smoking cessation should be undertaken as a first step in the management process. For a patient with COPD, optimal pharmacologic management is the cornerstone of treatment. Appropriate use of inhaled bronchodilator therapy to include one or more long-acting agents (e.g., a long-acting beta-agonist or long-acting anticholinergic agent) should be afforded. Short-acting bronchodilators are usually used for rescue or during exacerbations. Inhaled corticosteroid therapy should be reserved for severe COPD with frequent exacerbations or for patients with persistent asthma. These medications are administered either in an inhaled form (metered-dose inhaler, dry powder inhaler, slow mist inhaler) or an aerosolized form. In some instances, these medications, particularly the beta-agonist or anticholinergic agents, used in the treatment of COPD, may be associated with cardiovascular side effects particularly in those patients with HTN, CVD, or cardiac dysrhythmias.

Pharmacologic therapies are also available for patients with interstitial pulmonary fibrosis and pulmonary HTN. Medications used for interstitial pulmonary fibrosis include tyrosine kinase inhibitors or growth factor production downregulators. A variety of medications are available for pulmonary HTN and include prostaglandins, endothelin receptor antagonists, phosphodiesterase type 5 inhibitors, and soluble guanylate cyclase activators. Most of these therapies can be administered orally, but some are administered intravenously or by aerosolization. Hypoxemia can be present in any patient with chronic lung disease. Supplemental oxygen therapy should be considered for those patients who have resting or exercise-induced hypoxemia.[14]

Nonpharmacologic therapy for every patient with chronic lung disease should be considered and individualized. The cornerstone of non-pharmacologic treatment is pulmonary rehabilitation.[15] Breathing retraining techniques (e.g., pursed-lip breathing; for some, diaphragmatic breathing), energy conservation measures such as pacing, and self-management techniques such as prevention and early management of exacerbations, should be discussed with each patient. Bronchial hygiene techniques (e.g., postural drainage, chest physical therapy, secretion clearance devices) should be included for patients who have chronic sputum production and retained secretions.[16,17] Influenza and pneumococcal vaccination should be a standard part of the treatment regimen.

Exercise Training

Standard exercise prescription regimens can be used for most patients with CVD and chronic lung disease. For patients who have exercise limitation primarily related to underlying chronic lung disease, an exercise prescription based on symptom-limited endpoints can be used. For patients who have undergone cardiopulmonary exercise testing, an exercise prescription can be developed based on the findings from that testing. Both lower extremity and upper extremity training should be included as part of the treatment regimen. Weakness of the upper extremities is frequently noted in patients with chronic lung disease. Specific upper body exercises, including resistance training, should be part of the training; this therapy has been shown to improve functional ability during ADLs in these patients. Specific training regimens and ancillary interventions for specific patient populations (e.g., COPD, interstitial lung disease, and pulmonary HTN) have been developed.[18,19,20,21]

Guideline 10.12 Exercise Prescription Development

Use of standard exercise prescription methods is recommended unless the patient has underlying signs or symptoms (e.g., oxygen desaturation, severe dyspnea, chest pain, dizziness/lightheadedness) that warrant a reduction in exercise training intensity. Training intensity can be guided by oxygen saturation (maintain at or above 90% SaO_2), HR, or subjective RPE.

Summary

The range of CVD types and severity eligible for and ultimately participating in CR is vast. For the CR professional to adequately and safely care for these patients during exercise and to provide adequate lifestyle and behavior change education for preventing a future cardiac event, they should understand basic exercise physiology responses and have the ability to develop a personalized exercise prescription. The goal is to help patients adequately recover, progress, and to recognize issues related to nonresponse to CR programming. Therefore, strategies to understand the individual patient in order to apply specific and effective CR programming methods are necessary.

Special Demographic Populations

Justin M. Bachmann, MD, MPH, FACC; Daniel Forman, MD;
Naomi Gauthier, MD; Alexander Opotowsky, MD, MPH, MMsc;
Marta Supervia, MD, MSc, CCRP; Carmen Terzic, MD, PhD

Although an emphasis has been in place to recruit all eligible patients to participate in CR programs, traditionally it is heavily attended by the white male population; it has lower enrollment of eligible women, racial minorities, and younger and older individuals. Thus, much of what is known about CR adherence, progression, and outcomes has been gathered from a limited demographic population. As the emphasis on overcoming barriers to participation in all demographics continues, it is important to consider the particular subsets of patients who may enroll in CR. This chapter aims to provide an overview of specific considerations in these patient subsets.

OBJECTIVES

This chapter discusses the following:

- Definitions of the following subgroups of CR participants: younger and older ages, sex and gender categories, racial and cultural categories, and socioeconomic status

- Specific CR participation data, where available

- Information for the subgroups with respect to specific group characteristics that can affect participation in CR

- Recommendations for CR program assessment and delivery of programming

Younger Adults

It is critically important to consider the impact of patient age on program development, delivery, and effectiveness of CR services. Characterizing patients based solely on age is an oversimplification and is unproductive when considering a specific patient. Nonetheless, some general considerations are reasonable in the probability of potential special needs of patients in general, particularly on both ends of the age continuum.

CR in Younger Patients

Younger patients (<40 years old) constitute a small proportion of the CR population, because CVD is uncommon in this age group. However, the emergence and growth of particular groups who may benefit from CR, such as adults with congenital heart disease, may increase the demand among younger patients as evidence for its benefit accrues.[2] Younger patients have issues that can be characterized in general by a higher priority on and demand by vocation and family, but these issues also differ substantially between patients. Given the extended time horizon, the importance of risk reduction and long-term exercise adherence in these patients needs to be emphasized. Obesity is common,[3,4] but muscle mass, strength, and physical functioning are more often normal compared to older people. Time constraints and anxiety are typical in the context of unexpected illness and related lifestyle adjustments, with additional stresses in younger patients related to employment requirements and dependent family. The time required for traditional CR program participation may be prohibitive. Some have reported a trend toward decreasing rates of CR participation among younger and male patients over the past several decades (although younger people and men are still more likely to participate in CR compared with older and female patients).[5] Younger patients with CVD often present with complex risk factor profiles and an urgency with regard to decreasing risk-associated behavior. Those with congenital heart disease often carry a lifetime history of multiple surgeries and interventions, along with an increased burden of various comorbidities. Some young people may feel uncomfortable in groups of mainly much older patients; this should be considered when designing programs and scheduling patients. For example, creative solutions to CR scheduling can be important for younger patients given that employment and family issues often preclude twice- or three-times-weekly sessions at the CR center. Less-frequent visits with prescription of home-based CR exercise combined with alternative arrangements for preventive teaching are preferable to no CR services delivered at all. Alternative modes of exercise training principles, such as HIIT, may appeal to younger patients without an apparent sacrifice in efficacy or safety.[6,7] Integration of newer technology into CR programs (e.g., text messages, social media, activity monitors, video-based education) could also appeal to a younger generation who use these tools in their daily lives already.[8,9] More research on the additive benefit of newer technology is needed.

Younger Women

Women with an indication for CR are less likely to be referred to or attend a program.[10] Women overall compose roughly 25% of CR participants in contemporary programs, and participation of women <40 years old is rare (~1%-2% of all participants).[1] Indications other than obstructive CHD are more frequent among younger women referred to CR. These include congenital heart disease, chronic heart failure, pulmonary arterial hypertension, and microvascular coronary disease, or coronary artery spasm in the absence of obstructive atherosclerotic coronary disease. Younger women with obstructive CHD are characterized by high rates of obesity, T2DM, and cigarette smoking.[5] Depression and anxiety are common, and patterns of psychosocial risk and reasons for nonadherence may be different in younger, compared with older, women.[11]

Younger Men

Younger men constitute about 4% to 5% of all patients attending CR.[1] Compared with older men, younger men with CVD have higher rates of obesity, associated insulin resistance (or T2DM), dyslipidemia, and HTN.[1] Weight loss is a priority since it is associated with greater improvements in insulin resistance, hyperlipidemia, and HTN.[12] Younger men also tend to have more anxiety, anger, and hostility.[13] For younger men whose employment involves physical work, such as construction, reproducing work requirements in the CR setting with close cardiovascular monitoring often addresses patient anxiety regarding return to the workforce.

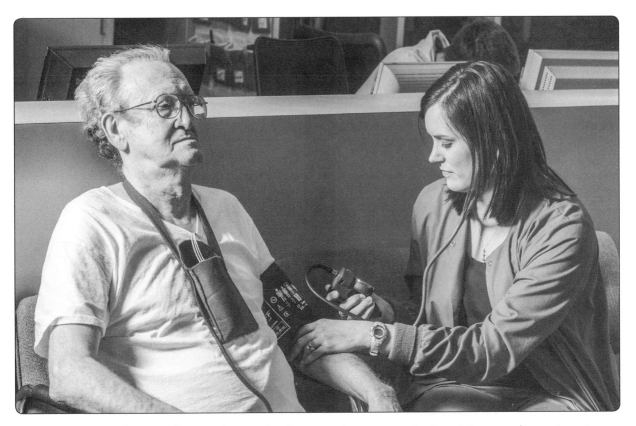

In the CR setting, close cardiovascular monitoring may decrease patient anxiety regarding return to normal activities and the workforce.

Older Adults

Amidst widespread improvements in health care, nutrition, antibiotics, and sanitation, average life span has lengthened. More adults are surviving into old age, when their predisposition to CVD increases.[1] Adults who were once likely to die after a CVD event early in their lives are now more likely to survive into their senior years, when recurrent events and chronic CVD morbidity become likely. Furthermore, otherwise healthy older adults become increasingly prone to CVD, because aging is conducive to biological changes that essentially catalyze CVD pathophysiology. Prevalence of coronary artery disease, HF, valvular heart disease, PAD, and arrhythmias all increase in older adults.[2,3] To an extent, CR enrollment already reflects these demographic shifts. Studies from diverse CR programs indicate the average age of patients in the United States is progressively increasing, including more who are aged in their 70s and older.[4,5]

Nonetheless, only a small portion of older adults who are eligible for CR tend to enroll. Suaya et al. studied Medicare patients to show that only about 14% of eligible older adults with acute MI participated,[6] with percentages dropping much further among women and minorities. Remarkably, in the years since Suaya published this analysis, underenrollment of older adults has persisted even as CR eligibility expanded to include HF and valvular HD.[7]

Underenrollment cannot be attributed to a lack of efficacy. Multiple studies demonstrate that older adults benefit from CR with advantages that include increased aerobic function, reduced risk factors, better adherence, improved insights regarding disease, and enhanced mood.[8,9] Beyond these data-driven accounts, CR provides the capacity of vital surveillance, both to patients themselves as well as their providers; this surveillance is a critical enhancement to care as patients adapt to new medications, devices, and elements of recovery after an acute hospitalization.

Still, the majority of older candidates eligible for CR are not referred, and even among those who are, few participate.[10] Multiple studies have attributed underenrollment to system factors, including poor physician referral, geographic maldistribution of programs, and lack of automatic referral,[11,12] but fundamental dynamics of aging are also relevant. Aging itself is associated with distinctive circumstances and experiences of patients that also significantly impact upon their interest and capacities for CR.[13]

Geriatric Domains Pertinent to CR

Some factors that are relevant to CR participation are specific to the older patient. Not all patients have the same issues; they may be related to conditions, diseases, limitations, and the age of an individual. This section addresses these factors.

Multimorbidity

While younger patients typically experience CVD as a dominant medical condition, older adults are more likely to experience their cardiovascular problems as part of a constellation of chronic conditions (e.g., diabetes, COPD, arthritis).[14] Conventional precepts regarding optimal CVD care are often altered by the context of comorbidities. For example, symptoms typically attributed to CVD (e.g., fatigue, pain, dyspnea) may derive from multiple etiologies, with persistence after CVD therapy that can seem discouraging and even depressing.

While many older patients with multimorbidity often opt not to attend due to the complexity of their circumstances, CR may serve as a way to better cope with their circumstances. CR provides opportunities to better understand symptoms, organize medications, and generally integrate dynamics that can otherwise become debilitating.

Polypharmacy

The prescribing of many medications is widespread among older CR patients. It is often because older adults are prescribed comprehensive evidence-based regimens for multiple diseases, which are usually related to multiple CVDs (e.g., AF, HF, coronary artery disease) as well as non-CVDs (e.g., arthritis and chronic obstructive lung disease).[15] Not only are the cumulative number of medications difficult for many older adults to arrange and to take as prescribed, but even if medications are taken perfectly, polypharmacy still often predisposes to iatrogenesis through drug-drug (clopidogrel and epixaban exacerbating GI bleeding) and/or drug-disease (beta-blockers exacerbating depression) interactions.[16] Issues attributed to poor adherence can often be resolved by helping patients to streamline medications and determine which are the most helpful and necessary.

CR offers opportunities to evaluate medication effects and to provide important information back to primary providers. For patients who may be experiencing untoward symptoms or signs (e.g., confusion, excessive fatigue, hypoglycemia, and hypotension), CR enables potential medication adjustments.[17] CR providers can coordinate with referring clinicians, providing them with accounts of medication effects (accounts that are often more sensitive over multiple CR sessions than those that can be achieved during intermittent doctor visits). CR also enables ongoing surveillance if regimens are modified.

Frailty

Frailty implies a state of vulnerability to stressors, with limited reserves to stabilize declines across multiple physiologic systems.[18] Adults who are frail are prone to developing CVD, and they also have worse disease outcomes and greater risks for harmful sequelae from standard therapies. Prevalence of frailty ranges from 10% to 60%, depending on the particular population being assessed as well as the assessment tool used to define it. Increased inflammation and muscle atrophy are key instigating factors. Small studies have suggested that exercise and diet may help modify and even reverse frailty.[19] Strength and balance training provide particular benefit to counter muscle atrophy and weakening[20] and, for most frail adults, these trainings are new types of activity that require guidance and coaching. Molino-Lova et al. specifically investigated older adults exhibiting frailty after participating in acute rehabilitation following cardiac surgery.[21] They found significant improvements using a physical activity intervention focused on strength, flexibility, balance, and coordination.

Loss of lean body mass contributes to frailty and weakening. Nutrition supplementation with a high-protein diet or supplement also helps frail CR patients,[22] especially in combination with exercise. Notably, the loss of muscle (sarcopenia) in older adults is often not apparent; many older adults have a high percentage of body fat that obscures muscle atrophy.[23] Both ideal-weight and overweight patients can have severe lean muscle depletion.

Key differentiations in frailty assessment metrics are important to highlight. Fried et al. advanced the premise of a frailty phenotype by identifying these five specific physical characteristics by which it could be standardized: weakness, low energy, slowed walking speed, decreased PA, and weight loss.[24] In contrast, Rockwood et al. advanced the premise of frailty as an index of deficits (morbidities, disabilities, and other clinical variables that accumulate and progressively burden a person).[25] The magnitude and speed that deficits accumulate are used to gauge vulnerability and risk.

The value of contrasting Fried's and Rockwood's general approaches to frailty (a phenotype versus deficit accumulation) is not to critique their respective merits but to recognize the inherent uncertainty regarding an element of assessment that is extremely important for older CVD patients. Patients assessed as frail by Fried's criteria may not seem frail when assessed using a Rockwood-based metric. Yet despite these methodologic inconsistencies, the underlying premise of inherent susceptibility is similar in each. Frail adults merit greater attention to amassed health circumstances, and they may particularly benefit from CR.

In addition to emphasis on exercise and nutrition, frail patients warrant added attention to medications (e.g., greater consideration of deprescribing for patients who are more likely to be weakened or confused by medications), added psychosocial support (e.g., helping to minimize tendencies for isolation and depression), and other parameters that, while not directly linked to CVD, still contribute significantly to improved CVD outcomes, particularly in those who are frail.

Screening for frailty is an important consideration for CR.[26] While frailty can be assessed in many ways, measuring gait speed is popular; it is convenient, reliable, and well validated,[18] and it usually fits well as part of a busy CR program. Although persuasive arguments can be made for different frailty tools, and many

assert the value of one versus the other, certain broad-spectrum principles are uncontroversial. Multifaceted assessments (such as the Short Physical Performance Battery [SPPB], which combines gait speed with specific measurements of sit-to-stand and balance) provide relatively greater sensitivity and specificity compared to single-assessment indices (such as gait speed or hand grip strength),[18] but the implementation of multifaceted approaches typically entails more time, space, and patient burden. Whatever tool is used, consistency of technique is paramount in order to apply them as reliable standards (which can be difficult to achieve amidst multiple providers and variable assessment spaces), as well as its consistent application into ITPs used in CR.

Cognitive Decline

Screening for cognitive decline is another important consideration for older adults who enroll in CR. Executive cognitive losses are highly prevalent among older adults with CVD, and often they are particularly subtle. Even cognitively challenged patients benefit from CR with respect to their own physical function capacities, mood, and symptoms, as well as to reduced readmissions for patients who usually tend to become more adherent and safety oriented.

While formal neurocognitive testing to assess for cognition is long and unrealistic for typical CR programs, many simpler screening tools are practical and effective. The Mini-Cog is easily administered and can be integrated as a standard assessment for older CVD patients.[27] Once cognitive limitations are recognized, many elemental aspects of CR must be modified to accommodate these patients' needs. For example, affected patients may benefit from educational reinforcements (e.g., more visual prompts and reminders), a support system, and simplified approaches to care.

Functional Decline and Posthospitalization Syndrome

Even in adults who are not frail, functional decline is often disproportionate in older adults with CVD, and it can have a detrimental impact on long-term recovery outcomes.[28] Intrinsic chronotropic and inotropic declines, as well as increases in afterload impedance, are predictable physiological changes with aging. They lead to characteristic declines in cardiorespiratory fitness independent of disease, and to disproportionate functional decrements if CVD also develops. Ischemia, diminished cardiac output, and vascular perfusion impairments are among the many facets of CVD that tend to exacerbate the already embedded functional declines of so-called typical aging. Furthermore, changes in body composition (e.g., loss of muscle mass and function, increase in adiposity) and high prevalence of comorbid disease (e.g., anemia, pain, renal insufficiency, arthritis, and depression) are among the many non-CVD factors that compound functional losses.

Hospitalizations usually exacerbate age-related functional declines, often due to the combined effects of bed rest leading to deconditioning, sleeplessness, anxiety, malnourishment, and oversedation. A general period of increased risk after hospitalization has become known as posthospitalization syndrome,[29] highlighting the particular importance of interventions to improve functional capacity after hospitalization.

A key value of CR is the opportunity it provides to evaluate for the distinctive functional limitations in older populations. Training regimens may need to start with extended periods of very low-intensity activity, including high proportions of strength and balance training in those who are severely functionally incapacitated at the onset. Moreover, regimens that emphasize seated activities (e.g., cycle ergometer, seated stepping ergometer) may be much more effective and safer than those that rely on standing or ambulating. It merits highlighting that even the most functionally limited older patients are likely to benefit from CR; in fact, they often make very high relative gains.[30] CR staff need to have goals that are proportional to the limited capacities of many older patients, as well as the patience to guide recoveries that can be slow in spite of the patient's motivation and hopes.

Other Relevant Geriatric Issues

Many other physical limits are widespread in older adults. Approximately 33% have mobility limitations, 20% have vision problems, and 33% have hearing impairments.[31] Incontinence, depression, and poor sleep are also often commonly present. While none of these factors directly confound precepts of CR, each makes them harder to initiate and sustain. If CR is to be effective, programs must make careful provisions for the needs of these patients. Moreover, for patients to feel comfortable, safe, and not ostracized, these responses must be a seamless part of standard care.

Underenrollment into CR is also affected by factors that are not directly related to age but often become particularly impactful in the context of old age.

- *Sex.* Women are underreferred to CR at any age, but CVD tends to be disproportionate in older women than men, increasing the implications of underreferral.[32] Furthermore, older women usually have relatively less muscle mass than men, and they are more susceptible to frailty.[33] The goal to better extend CR to the rising population of older women is a particularly important one.

- *Socioeconomics.* Older adults usually must contend with shrinking financial resources. Even modest copayments are often a disproportionate deterrent. Similarly, requisite paperwork and logistics for CR are often contingent on a patient's sophistication and family and community resources. Typically, older patients who are socioeconomically challenged are less likely to participate in CR, especially those who are also struggling with cognitive changes, bereavements, social isolation, and other burdens of old age.[34] In order to be effective, programs must usually make special efforts to reach out to anticipate the needs and limitations of older candidates.

Tailoring CR to Meet the Needs of Older Adults

Whereas CR was conceived and organized relative to younger adults (often as a means to expedite their return to work), the needs and goals of older adults considering CR are usually quite different. While most younger adults see CR primarily as a means to recover from a CVD event, older adults are usually struggling with other health challenges, such that the suggestion of recovery is more subtle. For older adults, CVD recovery overlaps with complexities such that the fundamental concept of therapeutic goal is more vague.

An important first step for achieving adherence and satisfaction in CR for older patients is to approach it as a shared decision,[35] and to clarify personal goals of care. For many older candidates,

CR is less compelling as a means to overcome CVD than it is as a program that can enhance quality of life, physical function, independence, and other lifestyle priorities. If these goals can be clarified and framed as the objectives of CR, it is more likely the program will be personally meaningful, engaging, and sustained.

Consistently, the standard evaluation of CR for older adults with CVD should go beyond the standard clinical review, stress test, and risk factor review performed in younger adults. Elements of evaluation must focus on a broader range of functional attributes (e.g., strength, balance, aerobic fitness) as well as other domains that affect function (e.g., frailty, multimorbidity, both the primary and secondary CVDs, as well as non-CVDs), cognition, depression and anxiety, sensory (e.g., vision, hearing) impairments, medications, nutrition, sleep, psychosocial dynamics, and lifelong habits.[36] Considerations regarding where and with whom the patient lives and how they will travel to the CR program are usually integral to the potential success of the program, and often they determine critical aspects of safety, adherence, mood, and logistics.

Evaluating Functional Capacity

Not all patients enrolling in CR require an exercise test. However, the utility of exercise testing for CR is well established, both as the basis of exercise prescription, but also to monitor for ischemia, hemodynamics, arrhythmia, symptoms, HR dynamics and, when cardiopulmonary exercise testing is available, ventilator measurements. Testing provides a collection of insights that are relevant for CR exercise prescription and safety. The growing tendency of cardiology providers to order pharmacological stress tests to assess for ischemia in their older patients should not be substituted for exercise tolerance testing; they serve very different purposes.[37]

Nonetheless, severely deconditioned adults are often unable to perform a standard exercise tolerance test, and the consideration of submaximal evaluations (such as a 6-minute walk test [6MWT]) are often pursued instead. For many older adults, a 6MWT has been shown to be a physiological maximum workload, but it is still relatively more achievable than treadmill or bicycle protocols. In general, walking is usually regarded as relatively familiar and comfortable to anticipate. In order for the 6MWT to best assess patients for CR, it is helpful to standardize technique (particularly in regard to consistent cuing and layout), and include telemetry (to rule out arrhythmia), hemodynamics, and symptom assessment as parts of the walking protocol.

Exercise Training Considerations

Exercise goals need to be tailored to a patient's unique capabilities. For frail adults, exercise training often centers on strength and balance training before progressing to aerobic modalities. When frailty or a chronic condition prohibits specific activities, exercise should be tailored to capacities that are preserved, and aim to slowly foster capacities that are absent.

Warm-Up and Cool-Down Activities

Warm-up and cool-down activities are particularly important for older patients. Warm-ups prompt gradual increases in heart and breathing rates and limb blood flow before higher-intensity exercises are undertaken.[38] Warm-up for strength training entails similar movements with less weight. For older adults, warm-ups have added benefits to optimize HR responses, to increase perfusion to muscles and joints, and to optimize joint flexibility. Cool-downs are also particularly important for older adults, given that they attenuate vascular pooling in a population prone to hypotension, and to lessen arrhythmias and ischemia.

Strength Training

Strength training is particularly important in older patients, because they are inherently vulnerable to deconditioning and weakening after a cardiovascular event. Frail older adults may require extended strength training before aerobic training is even feasible. Resistance training increases muscle strength and mass through muscle hypertrophy and neuromuscular adaptation, facilitating improvements in gait, balance, functional capacity, and resistance to falls.[39] Strength training also increases bone mineral density and content,[40] increases metabolic rate, assists with maintenance of body weight by decreasing fat mass and increasing lean mass, and improves insulin sensitivity.[38]

Muscle-strengthening exercises should be generally oriented to the legs, hips, chest, back, abdomen, shoulders, and arms, because these muscle groups are all highly engaged during ADLs. In addition, these exercises enable aerobic training goals in patients who are often particularly debilitated when CR begins.

In general, resistance training should be adapted to progressive weights, targeting adaptations in muscle size and force. Power (a dimension of velocity integrated with force) training can help reduce risks of falls.[41] Muscle endurance is the ability of muscle to maintain force and power over an extended period of time. It often plays a distinctive role in maintaining independence and QoL in older adults.[41]

For most older adults, resistance training machine-type equipment may be safer to use than free weights, because it better ensures proper body position and safety. In select patients, free weights may provide more flexibility and individualization, particularly at lower weight levels.

Flexibility Training

Flexibility plays an important role for older adults, especially to compensate for natural bone, joint, and muscle changes that occur with aging. Generally, the exercises consist of static stretches lasting 10 to 30 s per stretch, with three or four repetitions each. ROM exercises usually focus on all the major muscle and tendon groups (all the major joints of the body including hip, back, shoulder, knee, trunk, and neck region). Performing them in conjunction with aerobic or resistance training is usually well tolerated. Static stretching and dynamic movements are recommended.

Balance Training

Balance training complements strength and flexibility training with potential to mitigate or reverse frailty and risks of falling.[42] It is particularly useful for older adults with CVD whose age-related falling risks (e.g., sarcopenia, frailty, vision impairments) are commonly exacerbated by circumstances related to their CVD (e.g., hypotensive medications, deconditioning). Balance assessments are particularly useful in older patients as part of CR programming. As previously noted, the SPPB is a composite assessment tool that is commonly used to gauge frailty,[18] but it includes a subset of balance assessments that also identify falling risks.[43]

A lack of balance can be improved with both balance and strength training,[44] which are particularly valuable for older patients contending with deconditioning, new medications, and perhaps even fluid restrictions in the weeks after CVD hospitalizations. Balance training options include static and dynamic modalities. Static options are often relatively easier to initiate in the older adult, and they can then be advanced to dynamic modes in those who are able (e.g., walking activities [backward, sideways, heel to toe], standing activities [one-legged stand, heel stand, toe stand], and dynamic movements [circle turns]).

Aerobic Training

Aerobic training entails repeated movements of large muscle groups. In CR it usually entails walking (treadmill or indoor track), bicycle ergometry, arm ergometry, rowing, or recumbent stepping. Seated aerobic activities are also especially useful for patients who are unable to perform ambulatory activities. While aerobic training is the customary mainstay of CR, its utility is only achievable in older patients who have sufficient strength, flexibility, and balance to enable such movement and capacity. Thus, aerobic training goals of older adults often start with nonaerobic training requirements.

Enhanced aerobic capacity, cardiac output, peripheral oxygen utilization, vascular responsiveness and perfusion, neuromuscular responses, muscle strength, proprioception and balance, glucose metabolism, and reduced inflammation have all been described with regular aerobic exercise.[45] Although the absolute magnitude of exercise training benefit is usually greater among older adults who are robust, even frail and infirm older adults can derive physiological gains that translate into meaningful benefits, including enhanced independence, confidence, and QoL.[45]

Older patients with a low exercise capacity often best tolerate exercise dosed in short durations. Given the high prevalence of chronotropic incompetence in older populations, often then compounded by use of beta-blockers, it is often useful to guide exercise intensity by the ratings of perception that feel moderate to somewhat hard. Intermittent walking bouts on the treadmill with rest periods and weight-supported exercises, such as those on a seated stepper cycle or rowing ergometer, are usually sufficient to gradually advance the duration and intensity of exercise based on RPEs.

HIIT or moderately high-intensity interval training (short bouts of vigorous exercise separated by periods of rest or active recovery) is a form of exercise that incorporates physiologic principles well-suited to many older adults. The conceptual advantage is that the higher intensity maximizes physiologic benefit and, when coupled with a rest interval, maximizes recovery and stabilization.[46] In some instances, it is well-suited to the structure and supervision of a CR program.[47] Nevertheless, such training programs require that patients be highly motivated, and that they also have capacities for proper exercise form, precise exercise timing, and reliable self-organization. Patients who are cognitively impaired or who lack sufficient capability are less likely to be successful. Likewise, CR programs also need to provide requisite capacities for interval training to be successful, including comprehensive instruction and vigilant monitoring. These services may not be practical or feasible for many CR programs.

Ensuring Program Success

Certain parameters ensure program success for older adults, including assistive devices, appropriate and varied staffing models, safety measures, and optimized social and education opportunities for patients.

Integration of Assist Devices

Older patients often benefit from assessment for assistive devices (e.g., walkers, canes) at program entry with their continued integration in the activity thereafter. These devices can help many patients to better ambulate and advance in exercise and lifestyle goals. Therefore, integrating physical therapy with CR often generates synergies that better ensure an older patient's success.

Developing Staffing Models Accommodating the Variability of Patients

Severely deconditioned older patients, especially those with baseline frailty or who are experiencing posthospitalization syndrome, need to be closely monitored and guided. Staffing models must be sufficiently flexible to accommodate the needs of such debilitated patients. Limiting the number of adults who are relatively more frail or debilitated at any one session is often practical in terms of staffing capacities and safety.

The presence of a cognitive impairment and fall risk usually requires greater supervision. The role of spouses or other family members in assisting the patient can be a help or a hindrance, but it can be considered.

Optimizing Safety

CR provides critical opportunities for older adults to overcome many hurdles attributable to disease and aging. Seizing these opportunities may mean addressing the personal needs of individual patients, but in other respects it implies broader programmatic priorities.

Older patients may have concerns that respond to reassurance, meticulous monitoring, redundancy, written prompts (cue cards), as well as clear, loud, and direct articulation. It is mandatory that staff anticipate the limitations and anxieties, and guide care with added patience and scrutiny.

Beyond addressing the personal needs of each older patient, the physical infrastructure of CR is also important. Lighting should ideally be bright and without glare. Flooring should be designed to minimize slipping and falls. Exercise areas must be cleared of clutter, such as seated walkers or canes. Exercise equipment, such as rowing and cycle ergometers, should be stabilized to avoid tipping, loss of balance, and injuries. Safety accessories for mounting and dismounting (step stool for bike, grab bar for rower) are useful, along with ample space allowed for these maneuvers. Extra time should also be structured into the progression of each patient's activities to allow for recovery and to minimize overuse.

Emphasis on Long-Term Social Benefits and Activity Goals

Social benefits of outpatient CR, as well as longer-term maintenance, are often especially important to older adults, particularly among those contending with social isolation or depression. Improvements in depression can result from social engagements as well as from the gains in physical functioning derived from CR.[48]

Over time, goals to maintain PA are usually more successful than goals to merely continue exercise training. CR also provides opportunity to direct older patients to sustainable activities, particularly because many may lack insights or resources to achieve these goals. Long-term participation in a CR maintenance program is an attractive option when available; but for many who are eligible, the logistics and costs for a maintenance program are disproportionate, and community programs (e.g., Silver Sneakers, GeroFit) may be relatively more accessible. Related principles of long-term safety (e.g., footwear, hydration, nutrition) are important to highlight.

Adapting Education to the Capacities of Patients

Effective educational strategies for older adults usually entail the identification of barriers and initiating steps to overcome them. Impairments in cognition, vision, and hearing are among the many important considerations. It helps to routinely integrate related assists such as printed instructions for hearing impaired people and large-type print for visually impaired people. Furthermore, content is usually best delivered in small amounts, repeated often, and individualized to maximize learning. In many instances, involving family and personal caregivers in the personal education programs helps to enhance their efficacy.

Many times these deficits may not have been previously recognized or addressed, and patients often benefit from feedback to their primary care providers that facilitates referral to the appropriate clinical services (e.g., audiology consult).

Controlling Risk Factors

In general, trial data have suggested that older adults with CVD benefit from risk reduction similarly to young adults, but the age-specific domains of multimorbidity, polypharmacy, frailty, and limited life expectancy are rarely incorporated into these investigations. Therefore, while some patients with advanced stages of frailty and comorbidity may benefit from risk factor reduction using an intense pharmacological regimen, others may not. Approaches should be tailored to each individual's aggregate circumstances. The following sections discuss risk factors specific to older patients. General information about risk factor reduction is found in chapter 9.

Dyslipidemia

According to trial data, beneficial results of lipid lowering in older patients with CVD are similar to those in younger patients, but given the underlying risks associated with coronary artery disease in old age, the absolute risk reduction from statins for both all-cause and CHD risk is approximately twice as high for older patients.[49] Nonetheless, the benefits of aggressive pharmacological management are offset by concerns regarding polypharmacy and other risks associated with statins (e.g., myalgia and associated exercise intolerance).

Whereas diet is usually considered the safest and most important initial step in lipid management, steps to modify nutrition are rarely simple in older adults amidst concurrent challenges of lipid management, losses of lean body mass (raising consideration of increasing protein and calories), increases in insulin resistance (raising considerations of reducing unrefined sugars), increases in obesity (raising consideration of weight loss), and HTN (raising consideration of reducing salt). Most older patients benefit from nutrition education that emphasizes these broader principles and strategies of self-care. Furthermore, many older patients, especially those with T2DM and clinical indications for weight reduction, likely benefit from individualized nutritional consults. Notably, the vulnerability of older patients to malnutrition as well as sarcopenia commonly leads to prioritization of hypercaloric intake before long-term cholesterol-reducing dietary goals can be addressed.

Multiple cohort studies have shown that both total cholesterol and LDL-C correlated significantly with fatal CVD in both sexes across a broad age range.[50,51] Therefore, rationale for pharmacological therapy to lower cholesterol is strong. A meta-analysis of 26 randomized controlled trials (RCTs), including data from 170,000 patients, indicates safety of statins in older patients.[52] The most common side effect observed with statins was myalgia, which occurred in about 5% of patients.[53] Myopathy occurred in only 0.01% to 0.05%, and rhabdomyolysis in only 3.4/100,000 person-years. Age was not an independent risk factor for these complications.

Furthermore, even in a population with fundamental risks of polypharmacy and complexity, rationale for high-intensity statin therapy is an important consideration. In the Pravastatin or Atorvastatin Evaluation and Infection Therapy trial, atorvastatin 80 mg reduced major CVD events by 16% compared to pravastatin 40 mg in patients hospitalized with acute coronary syndrome; similar risk reduction occurred with higher-intensity treatment in an older subgroup.[54]

Similarly, in a study of over 500,000 veterans (mean age 68.5 years; 98% men) with CVD, a graded association was observed between intensity of statin therapy and all-cause mortality.[55] In older patients intolerant of statins or who cannot achieve their LDL-C goal on maximal statin doses, ezetimibe may be a useful adjunct.[56]

Hypertension

HTN is the most common CVD risk factor among older men and women, with prevalence rates of about 70% in those aged 75 years and older.[50,57] HTN has the greatest population-attributable risk for CVD, cerebrovascular disease, and PAD among older adults.[58]

Multiple clinical trials in older cohorts have shown benefits of HTN treatment.[59] Whereas the target of BP reduction in older adults has been controversial, several recent trials have raised compelling rationale for aggressive BP targets, with new guidelines now calling for broad primary and secondary BP goals <130/80 mm Hg[60] in older adults. Systolic Blood Pressure Intervention Trial showed a 34% reduction in CVD events and 33% reduction in mortality in 2,636 patients aged ≥75 years with SBP >130 mm Hg treated with a variety of BP lowering medications, but particularly chlorthalidone and amlodipine to reach a target of 120 mm Hg versus 140 mm Hg.[61] An associated study demonstrated the value and safety of such stringent BP reduction even in subsets of frail older adults.[58] Yet the relatively higher targets in the guidelines implicitly acknowledge residual concerns about such aggressive BP reduction in a population also prone to falls, syncope, exercise intolerance, dehydration, and other sequelae that could be aggravated by intense BP reduction.

The role of CR in BP control includes the opportunity (as needed) to monitor BP in a wide variety of clinical contexts, and to communicate with the primary physician if safety or efficacy are concerns. CR also enables interventions including weight loss when appropriate, aerobic exercise, and diet, usually the DASH diet, which effectively overlaps with heart-healthy nutrition.[62]

Diabetes, Insulin Resistance, and Obesity

Advancing age is accompanied by reduced insulin sensitivity and secretion, contributing to greater glucose intolerance and higher rates of T2DM in older adults. Furthermore, T2DM, insulin resistance, and abdominal obesity often occur in combination[63] as part of a continuum of metabolic disease, which also tends to include dyslipidemia, HTN, inflammation, and clotting abnormalities. The metabolic syndrome is common in patients with CVD and is strongly and inversely related to age. Approximately 22% to 33% of adults older than 65 years have diagnosed T2DM, and it is undiagnosed in approximately 33%.[64] Older adults with T2DM and CVD are at high risk for adverse macrovascular and microvascular outcomes as well as functional disability and geriatric syndromes (e.g., frailty and falls).

The primary treatment goal of older adults with T2DM is lifestyle modification. CR provides an optimal opportunity for lifestyle modification, because patients have essentially agreed to participate in the requisite exercise and lifestyle program. Weight loss can reduce insulin resistance and improve glycemic control. Dietary interventions that optimize macronutrient content as well as calorie count also help improve glycemic control that is independent of weight change. Regular aerobic and resistance exercises lower HbA1c by 0.5% to 1.0% in older adults, even without changes in body weight or fat mass. Similar to younger adults, an optimal goal is low-intensity, longer-duration, high-frequency (almost daily) PA (such as walking), which is usually coordinated with healthful diet.[65]

CR provides important opportunities for education and guidance, encouragement, as well as surveillance. A key concern is that exercise and weight loss can predispose a patient to hypoglycemia. CR provides important opportunities to monitor these levels, and to coordinate with a patient's physician if therapies merit adjustment. While rationale exists for medications to lower glucose, among older patients with diabetes, several large clinical trials have found either no effect or even increased mortality in patients receiving intensive glycemic therapy.[66] Therefore, a less-intensive target HbA1c of 7% to 7.9% is recommended for most older adults. Even less stringent targets may be considered for older patients who are frail.

Metformin is favored as a first-line therapy due to its low risk for hypoglycemia and other adverse effects. Additional options include the short-acting sulfonylurea, glipizide, and the short-acting insulin secretagogue, repaglinide.[50] Two newer agents are the sodium–glucose cotransporter 2 inhibitor empagliflozin and the glucagon-like peptide-1 analogue liraglutide, both of which reduced CV events in large RCTs. The reduced CV risk with empagliflozin was especially prominent in patients ≥65 years old.[67] If insulin therapy is needed, ultra-long-acting basal and very short-acting prandial insulins are strongly preferred over intermediate-acting insulin formulations. Although tighter glycemic control in T2DM may help to avoid microvascular complications, greater CVD risk reduction may be achieved from control of concurrent risk factors such as HTN and dyslipidemia.[50]

Physical Inactivity

Physical inactivity is a risk factor for the development as well as the progression of CVD. Older patients with CVD who begin PA have an improved overall health status and prognosis.[50] Notably, most older patients entering CR, particularly women, have remarkably low fitness. The effects of sedentary lifestyles is often inadvertently compounded by medications, sleep disruption, deconditioning, and other hazards that mount in the course of standard care.[68] Recommendations for increasing exercise participation should not be limited to structured CR sessions but should employ a broader interpretation of PA programming and include leisure activities, as well as integrating daily activities such as taking stairs, yard and housework, grocery shopping, and other activities of normal living. The harmful effects of prolonged sitting (e.g., thromboembolism risk, joint stiffness, orthostatic hypotension) should be emphasized, and patients should be encouraged to interrupt periods of sitting at 20 to 30 min intervals with brief (even 2-3 min) episodes of activity.

Psychosocial Dysfunction

Rates of depression, social isolation, and anxiety are high in older patients with CHD.[69] These factors not only affect QoL but are significant predictors of long-term medical outcomes and may be influenced by psychosocial interventions and exercise.[70,71] CR programs need to screen for these factors at baseline using instruments such as the Geriatric Depression Scale[72] or the Patient Health Questionnaire-9 (PHQ-9).[73] Patients who are depressed need to be monitored closely as they proceed through CR, with appropriate referral of high-risk and nonresponding individuals for counseling or medical therapy. CR providers should also address end-of-life issues, including resuscitation (code/no-code) status and advance directives (end of life).[74]

Tobacco Use

Smoking cessation reduces cardiac morbidity and mortality even when accomplished in very old age.[75] Thus, while some older adults assume that they are naturally protected, in fact the health value of tobacco cessation persists in old age, and it can enable health benefits with respect to reduced symptoms and events as well as extended longevity. Interventions that have proven effective in younger patients, such as nicotine replacement therapy and group and individualized counseling, have also been shown to be safe in patients with CVD, including those who are older.[76]

Skilled Nursing Facilities

Many older adults who dwell in retirement communities and become debilitated as a result of CVD hospitalizations are referred to skilled nursing facilities (SNFs). While SNFs provide structured training to reinforce transfers, they are not designed to promote the multifaceted goals of CR. While many patients would presumably benefit from a continuum of care after SNF discharge that extends into CR, it often does not occur.[77] This dimension of care remains an important one to target and facilitate.

Facility-Based Versus Home-Based CR

A recent trend in CR is the growing interest in home-based models of care. A Cochrane review comparing facility- and home-based CR analyzed 17 trials, including 2,172 patients with AMI, revascularization, or HF, and concluded that no difference in outcomes existed between the two modes of delivery based on functional metrics.[78] Importantly, this review did not address the impact of older age on these findings, nor did it comment on any differences in safety between home- and facility-based programs. Given the distinctive complexities of older adults, much research is essential to best understand the implications of home-based care across the spectrum of older adults. Most of the patients studied had low cardiac risks, and little attention was paid to issues relevant in older populations.

A related dimension to home-based options is escalating interest in telehealth, wearables, and smartphone-based delivery of CR. A recent study suggests that a smartphone app was effective in increasing CR utilization and improving health outcomes.[79] However, it was a small study with a mean age of 55, and it remains unclear if and how technological options will respond to the complex needs across the wide spectrum of older adults.

Women and Men

CVD is the leading cause of death in women and men in United States.[1] However, the total number of deaths from CVD is higher for women than for men, in spite of the fact that the mean age at manifestation of CVD is about 10 years older. Besides mortality rates and age of onset, differences by sex are observed when considering other related clinical aspects (e.g., symptom presentation, management, and outcome, as well as traditional and sex-specific risk factors). Also, clinical aspects in the prevention, diagnosis, and treatment of CVD and differential social determinants of health burdens play a role in an increasingly diverse CVD population.[2]

Men have a higher risk of obstructive disease, while women more often develop nonanatomically obstructive CVD (microvascular disease), such as sex-specific CVD (e.g., spontaneous coronary artery dissection or Takotsubo cardiomyopathy). Also, women present with an increased prevalence of angina, along with a higher rate of MI compared to men. Women have a higher rate of mortality (being 1.5 times more likely to die within the first year after MI) and rehospitalization because of CVD.[3-5]

The reasons for these facts remain unclear. It is particularly puzzling because there has been a stagnation of improvements in incidence and mortality of CVD among women younger than 55 years),[2] during a time of considerable declines in cardiac disease mortality for both sexes, especially in the >65 year age group.[6,7] Thus, it is very important to understand the biological and behavioral variables that contribute to worsening risk factor profiles, especially in younger women, to attempt to reduce future CVD morbidity and mortality rates (table 11.1).

Despite the demonstrated benefits of pharmacological interventions and CR, these therapies are often underutilized in populations with existing CVD, particularly in women.[8-11] Among men it may be due to a preconditioned inattention to self-care based on age, occupation, and relationship status.[12]

Although some risk factors for CVD, such as elevated BP, overweight and obesity, and elevated cholesterol, are well known to have a similar impact among women and men, some differences are observed when prevalence and subsequent hazardous effects are analyzed by sex.[13]

Risk factors for CVD that are common for both men and women present differently when the level of burden by sex is considered. For example, T2DM has a higher incidence among women younger than 50 years compared to men, with a 44% greater risk for CVD in women. The rate of T2DM is double in Hispanic women compared to Hispanic men.[14] According to the Framingham Heart Study, obesity increases the relative risk of CVD by 46% in men, as opposed to 64% in women.[15] The 2011 National Health Interview Survey (NHIS) showed that sedentary behavior was higher among women than men, and this difference increases with age; over 50% of female adults over the age of 75 are inactive.[16] No apparent differences exist between men and women for hypertension prevalence.[17] However, hypertension is poorly controlled in older women compared to men.[18]

After menopause, dyslipidemia is the most prevalent CVD risk factor among women.[19] According to data from the CDC, only 45% of all adults eligible for cholesterol treatment take medication consistently, and women are less likely to be treated with statin therapies.[20] In addition to the typical risk factors, many nontraditional risk factors disproportionately affect women, including preterm delivery, hypertensive pregnancy disorders, gestational diabetes, a higher prevalence of autoimmune diseases such as rheumatoid arthritis and lupus erythematous, chemotherapy and radiation for breast cancer, and depression.[2]

Recent research has led to a new understanding of the pathophysiology of CVD in women,[2,21] which might help to identify CVD symptoms that are different from the classic pattern described based on males (e.g., absence of chest pain in young women who have a more aggressive CVD prognosis). Despite unique symptomology and more physical limitations, women often present with less obstructive CVD than men. This difference is most evident along the spectrum of

Table 11.1 Physiological Presentations of Women With CVD Compared to Men

	Premenopausal women	Postmenopausal women
PHYSIOLOGICAL		
Less obstructive CVD	✓	✓
Less Q-wave MI	✓	✓
Prevalent congestive HF		✓✓
RISK FACTORS		
Diabetes mellitus	✓✓	✓
Obesity	✓✓	✓
HTN	✓	✓✓
Tobacco consumption	✓✓	✓
Musculoskeletal limitations	✓	✓✓
Inactivity	✓✓	✓
Dyslipidemia	✓	✓✓
Depression	✓✓	✓
Family history	✓✓	✓
Elevated C-reactive protein	✓✓	✓
ISCHEMIC SYMPTOMS		
Unusual fatigue	✓✓	✓✓
Dyspnea	✓✓	✓
Nausea or vomiting	✓✓	✓
Chest pressure	✓✓	✓
Sleep disturbance	✓✓	✓✓
Anxiety	✓✓	✓
Weak or heavy arms	✓✓	✓
Hand or arm tingling	✓✓	✓
Dizziness or fainting	✓✓	✓

Note: Check marks indicate that the presentation or symptom is more common in women than men; two check marks indicate a greater incidence.

Abbreviations: CVD, cardiovascular disease; MI, myocardial infarction; HF, heart failure; HTN, hypertension.

Data from Garcia et al. (2016); Canto et al. (2012).

acute coronary syndromes and when referred for revascularization.[2,21] In part due to these differences, coronary angiography has been used less in women. Coronary plaque erosion occurs more frequently among younger women with sudden cardiac death; whereas plaque rupture is more common in men and in older women.[22]

Psychosocial, Sociocultural, and Environmental Considerations

It is well known that sex differences in the cardiovascular system are due to differences in gene expression; by contrast, gender differences arise from sociocultural practices that may require a different approach.

Socioeconomically disadvantaged patients (e.g., women who belong to certain minority groups or live in economically depressed communities) are particularly confronted with psychosocial stressors that interfere with the self-management of CVD.[23] It is clear that stressors differ by gender (family responsibilities, job stress[24]) and can manifest in people as fear, anger, social isolation, and a perceived burden to family and friends. These stressors often lead to the presentation of depressive symptoms, particularly in younger women.[25] In turn, these symptoms lead to distinctive gender-based needs and gender-specific assessment (see table 11.2), such as measurement of patients' perceptions of their health (poorer among women with CVD), which may lead to worse outcomes when not identified, addressed, and intervened upon.[26]

Depression confers an increased risk of CVD mortality[27] and the development of more adverse cardiovascular outcomes in women compared to men.[28] Women tend to have a lower adherence to depression treatment, resulting in poorer outcomes.[29,30]

In order to address the depression component, the use of the Patient Health Questionnaire (PHQ-2) is recommended as a routine screening of all patients with CHD upon CR entry.[31] When a positive result for depression occurs using the PHQ-2, the nine-item PHQ-9[32] can be used to determine whether a behavioral health referral is needed. Patients should also be assessed for psychological or psychosocial considerations such as anxiety, anger or hostility, social isolation, marital or family distress, sexual dysfunction, and substance abuse. If psychosocial issues are identified, referrals for psychiatric or psychological care should be provided.[33]

Public awareness campaigns such as Go Red for Women from the AHA, in addition to other efforts for public education by the AHA, ACC, and the National Heart, Lung and Blood Institute (NHLBI) are focused on increasing the awareness of CVD as the leading cause of death among women, with a special focus on minorities, seeking improvement on its management and outcomes.[34,35]

Gender-Specific Barriers to CR Participation

CR is a Class IA recommendation for patients with CVD.[36,37] Despite international endorsement[38-40] and strong evidence of improved morbidity and mortality with participation,[36,37] CR utilization remains low,[41,42] especially among women.[43-45]

Patient, provider, and social/environmental factors for referral, enrollment, and CR completion exist for both sexes.[46,47] Recent interest has emerged in female-specific referral factors, including those that are considered modifiable and nonmodifiable (table 11.3).[48,49]

Lack of information and familiarity about CR and unfounded fear of physical pain associated with exercise likely are participation barriers among both men and women. Additionally, a lack of physician endorsement of CR, which is more prevalent among women, is a strong

Table 11.2 Psychosocial Considerations for Women With CVD Compared to Men

Psychosocial considerations	Premenopausal women	Postmenopausal women
Depressive symptoms	✓✓	✓
Anxiety disorder	✓✓	✓
Anger or hostility	✓	✓
Marital or family dysfunction	✓✓	✓
Social isolation	✓	✓✓
Substance abuse	✓✓	✓
Suboptimal QoL	✓✓	✓
Sexual dysfunction	✓	✓
Low self-efficacy	✓	✓
Sleep disruption	✓	✓
Fear	✓	✓

Note: Check marks indicate that the presentation or symptom is more common in women than men; two check marks indicate a greater incidence.

Abbreviation: QoL, quality of life.

Data from Mead et al. (2010); Beckie et al. (2008); Berger et al. (2009); Whooley et al. (2008); Kramer et al. (2010); Szerencsi et al. (2012); Hamm et al. (2011); Mosca et al. (2006); Heran et al. (2011); Wenger (2008); Balady et al. (2007); Balady et al. (2011); Piepoli et al. (2016); Aragam et al. (2011).

predictor of poor attendance.[49,50] Other factors, including family obligations, financial concerns, transportation problems, and lack of adequate insurance coverage, are also associated with a lower participation rate among women (table 11.3). On the other hand, men frequently report work responsibilities as a barrier.[46]

Table 11.3 Factors Associated With Lower CR Participation for Women

Levels of barriers	Factors associated with less likelihood of participation
REFERRAL	
Patient	CABG, PCI, and valve surgery as reason for CR referral Older age
Health care provider	Lack of physician referral to CR
Social/environment	Individuals from underrepresented minority groups, particularly those with financial barriers Lack of CR insurance
ENROLLMENT	
Patient	Perception of exercise as being tiring or painful Lack of CR awareness Multiple comorbidities Percutaneous intervention as reason for CR admission Higher exercise barriers as measured by the EBBS score History of MI 70 years or < 55 years old
Health care provider	Lack of strong endorsement to attend to CR Lack of health care provider support
Social/environment	Education level over 12 years Transportation issues Numerous family responsibilities or home- related stress Lack of support system (friends, family) Individuals from underrepresented minority groups, particularly those with financial barriers Unemployed
COMPLETION	
Patient	Multiple comorbidities <55 years old Obesity Depression as measured by the BDI-II score Diabetes Previous MI High level of anxiety as measured by STAI score Current smoker Physically inactive previous CR Lack of history of CVD
Social/environment	Divorced/separated Transportation problems Long distance between CR program and place of residence Numerous family responsibilities Lack of CR insurance

Abbreviations: CABG, coronary artery bypass graft; PCI, percutaneous coronary intervention; EBBS, exercise benefits and barriers scale; MI, myocardial infarction; BDI-II, Beck Depression Inventory-II; STAI, state-trait anxiety inventory.

Data from Supervía et al. (2017).

Solutions to CR Referral, Enrollment, and Completion

The need exists to address the low CR referral, enrollment, and completion for both sexes. Although the existence of evidence-based barriers by sex is well known, there is not enough evidence to report specific solutions by sex.[49] Systematic approaches to improve CR delivery may help to reduce most types of barriers for males and females (table 11.4). Contact between automated CR referral systems, clinician (nurse or clinical exercise physiologist CR liaison), and patient, as well as early CR enrollment, may help to increase referral and participation rates. Additionally, increasing the awareness of CR among health care providers and patients may also increase referral and participation rates.

Incentive programs, flexible hours, and alternative delivery models of CR might contribute to increased enrollment rates and at the same time avoid dropout prior to CR completion. New CR delivery models that offer more flexible and personalized options (e.g., home based programs) might present a good opportunity to guarantee an optimal treatment at the same time as a tailored gender-based pathophysiological and psychosocial management.[49] To date there is a paucity of research on new CR delivery models.

Table 11.4 Recommendations for Improving CR Referral, Enrollment, and Completion for Men and Women

Intervention	Description	Guideline determined strength of recommendation
CR REFERRAL EVIDENCE-BASED SOLUTIONS		
Early access	Integration of early access clinic increased referral	IIA
Automatic referral and/or liaison referral	Systematic referral methods (e.g., preapproved strategy) and/or liaison intervention (e.g., nurse)	I
Peer navigation	Bedside visit, education material, encouragement to get CR referral before discharge	IIB
Increase awareness	Increase awareness about CR among health care professionals	I
CR ENROLLMENT/PARTICIPATION EVIDENCE-BASED SOLUTIONS		
Increase awareness	Increased awareness among patients and health care providers	I
Patient navigation	Education about CR and support by phone and mail	IIA
Referred to site closer to home	Referring patients to the closest CR program	IIB
Physician recommendation	Strong endorsement by a nurse or physician	IIA
Early access	Early appointment in CR	I
Automatic referral and/or liaison referral	Systematic referral methods (e.g., preapproved strategy) and/or liaison intervention (e.g., nurse)	IIA
Letter	Theory-based invitation letter	IIa
Alternative program models	Home-based programs/community programs	I/IIc
Nursing phone call and/or home visit	Nursing assessment and encouragement	IIa/IIb
Motivational interviewing	Personalized motivational interviewing	IIa
CR COMPLETION/ADHERENCE EVIDENCE-BASED SOLUTIONS		
Early access	Integration of early access to clinic and increased referral rate	IIA
Automatic referral	Systematic referral methods (e.g., preapproved strategy)	I
Incentive programs	Motivational programs	IIa
Alternative programs	Home based/telemedicine supported/smartphone/web-based model	IIa/IIb/I

Data from Supervía et al. (2017).

Race and Culture

CVD is the principal cause of death worldwide. In 2015, it accounted for more than 17.9 million deaths/year.[1] By 2035, more than 45.1% of adults in the United States population are expected to have CVD.[2] A challenging issue for the health care system is the fact that in the next 35 years, non-Hispanic whites (NHW) will no longer comprise the majority of the U.S. population due to the increased numbers of Hispanic and Asian Americans.[2] More than 53 million Hispanics (approximately 18% of the total U.S. population) live in the United States, making them the largest racial/ethnic minority in the country.[3-5] However, by 2050 Hispanics are expected to represent approximately 30% of the total U.S. population.[3-6] The numbers of African Americans and Asians are also expected to increase and constitute 22% and 10% of the total U.S. residents, respectively.[3-6] Because current racial and ethnic minority groups will constitute an increasingly larger proportion of the U.S. population in the coming years, improving the cardiovascular health of these groups is important and supports the AHA's 2020 Impact Goals "to improve the cardiovascular health of all Americans by 20% while reducing deaths from CVD and stroke by 20%."[6(p.1)] In addition to racial and ethnic minority populations, other portions of the population experience health disparities. These groups include people with physical, emotional, and behavioral disabilities and lesbian, gay, bisexual, and transgender (LGBT) populations. However, whether these disparities extend to CR is not known at this time. Figure 11.1 summarizes racial and ethnic population distribution in the United States.

CVD and Risk Factors Among Different Racial and Ethnic Groups

The IOM defines health disparities as "differences in the quality of health care that are not due to access-related factors or clinical needs, preferences, and appropriateness of interventions."[7(p.32)] Health disparities in the United States exist by ethnicity, race, geography, and socioeconomic status. Although progress in disparities has occurred (e.g., the black–white disparity gap in CVD mortality rate has declined from 27.6% in 1999 to 22.2% in 2015), differences in cardiovascular health and CVD rates continue to exist.[8]

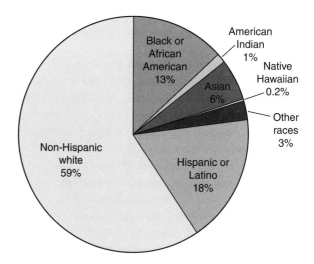

Figure 11.1 U.S. population by race and ethnicity.

Data from Tabulation of US Census Bureau Statistics; 2017 Population Estimates.

Some of these disparities arise from differences in major CVD risk factors among several racial groups. In this regard, black Americans continue to have the highest burden of CHD mortality among all ethnic groups in the United States despite an overall decline in CHD related mortality among the general population. These people as a group have a higher prevalence of untreated or unrecognized CVD risk factors such as high cholesterol, obesity, diabetes, and HTN, putting them at high risk for developing HF and cerebrovascular diseases.[2,9]

Hispanics are a racially diverse group.[5] The Hispanic subpopulations are linked by the Spanish language and geographic origin with ancestry related to nations from Europe, the Caribbean, and Central/South America. Despite having a higher prevalence of CVD risk factors, Hispanics demonstrate lower rates of CVD mortality when compared with non-Hispanic whites, a phenomenon referred to as the Hispanic paradox.[10-11] Hispanic culture includes strong social and familial support and a sense of optimism that can be stress-buffering, potentially explaining the paradox.[10-11] This phenomenon is controversial and not fully understood, and it may not apply equally to all Hispanic groups or across all types of CVDs. In addition, as Hispanic immigrants assimilate to the host culture and are exposed to living in U.S. communities, they may adopt high-risk behaviors such as smoking, consuming a poor diet, consuming alcohol, and abusing illicit substances.[12] Hispanics with African backgrounds may have more similarities to black Americans regarding CVD risk factors.[12] Hispanics, together with black Americans and Asians, have higher rates of diabetes. Mexican Americans and Puerto Ricans have twice the prevalence of diabetes than non-Hispanic whites.[8] Mexican Americans have a higher incidence of high BP than non-Hispanic whites. Puerto Rican Americans had the highest number of HTN-related death rates compared to the other Hispanic subgroups.[12]

Another racially and ethnically heterogeneous group is Asian Americans. Six Asian American subgroups (Asian Indian, Chinese, Filipino, Korean, Japanese, and Vietnamese) make up approximately 90% of all Asian Americans. Little data exists to evaluate CVD among Asian Americans. The most representative data comes from the National Health Interview Survey (NHIS).[13] The NHIS shows that the prevalence of traditional CVD risk factors appears to vary greatly across all Asian subgroups, which could affect CVD risk assessment and prevalence rates among them.[13,14] Filipinos and Asian Indians have high prevalence rates of traditional risk factors for CVD.[13] Korean Americans, Vietnamese Americans, and Filipino American males have some of the highest smoking rates, indicating the importance of having targeted interventions to address this CVD risk factor for these subpopulations.

Approximately 4.5 million American Indians and Alaskan Natives live in the United States. In this combined racial group, CVD is the leading cause of death and at younger ages than other racial and ethnic groups, with approximately 36% of those dying before age 65. Diabetes is an extremely prevalent risk factor for CVD among American Indians.[15] Table 11.5 summarizes risk factors for CVD by race and ethnicity in the United States.

Racial, Ethnic, and Geographical Disparities in CR Care

Disparities are defined as preventable differences in the incidence, prevalence, prevention, treatment, morbidity, and mortality rates of CVD and related risk factors. Also included in the definition of disparities are differences in access to health care and the quality of care delivered among different social and ethnic groups and races.[16]

Despite the overwhelming evidence that supports referral to CR programs, overall participation remains low and substantial gaps in sex and race exist, especially for female, black, Hispanic, and Asian patients, who were respectively 12%, 20%, 36%, and 50% less likely than white male patients to receive CR referral.[17-19] Variables associated with reduced referrals for nonwhites included language barriers; transportation problems; lack of culturally appropriate information on nutrition, lifestyle modification, and other educational topics; learning styles and values and beliefs relating to adherence; need to return to work; and funding for people in financial need.[17-19]

Although CVD inequalities by race and ethnicity have been recognized for decades, sociodemographic factors and geographic disparities have only recently begun to receive more attention. Recent data show that referral and participation (adherence) rates are significantly low among people from lower socioeconomic status (SES), lower employment rates, lower educational level, and lower income.[20] In addition, people from the geographic areas extending from southeastern Oklahoma along the Mississippi River Valley to eastern Kentucky and Appalachia have high CVD mortality and lower CR referral and participation rates when compared to the general population.[20-22] These geography-based differences could be explained by access to health-promoting resources and quality health care, behavioral patterns (poor diet, decreased PA, and tobacco use), psychosocial issues (stress, depression, opioid use, and lack of social support), and cultural factors (acculturation and dietary patterns).[22]

Inequities in Access to Health Care and Quality of Care

Black American and Hispanic American patients continue to experience inequities in the receipt of effective interventional therapies for acute coronary syndromes, including cardiac catheterization, PCI, and surgical revascularization. These inequities exist because they are more likely to be treated at institutions with limited revascularization capabilities, and health centers with poor MI outcomes and high surgical mortality.[26] The differences in cardiac outcomes between black, Hispanic, and white Americans[26,27] might be explained, in part, by the quality of the care provided in hospitals. For instance, when cardiac surgery is performed in a high-volume, high-quality medical center, no difference in operative mortality exists between those groups.[26]

Table 11.5 Cardiovascular Risk Burden (Prevalence of Disease or Risk Factor Expressed in Percentages)

	U.S. population	Asian and Pacific Islander	American Indian and American Native	Hispanic	Non-Hispanic white	African American
CAD						
Overall	2.7%		9.3%			
Males	2.4%	5%		5.9%	7.7%	7.1%
Females	2.9%	2.6%		6.1%	5.3%	5.7%
HTN						
Overall	34.0%		26.5%			
Males	34.5%	28.8%		28.9%	34.5%	45%
Females	33.4%	25.7%		30.7%	32.3%	46.3%
DIABETES MELLITUS						
Overall	9.1%		7%			
Males	9.4%	11.8%		12.6%	8%	14.1%
Females	8.9%	9.1%		12.7%	7.4%	13.6%
OBESITY						
Overall	36.3%		28%			
Males	34.3%	11.2%		39%	33.6%	37.5%
Females	38.3%	11.9%		45.7%	35.5%	56.9%
SMOKING						
Overall	15.1%	7%	21.9%	10.1%	16.6%	16.7%
Males	16.70%					
Females	13.60%					
STROKE						
Overall	6.3%	2.5%	3%			
Males	7.4%			2%	2.2%	3.9%
Females	5.3%			2.6%	2.8%	4%
HF						
Overall						
Males	2.4%	1.3%		2%	2.4%	2.6%
Females	2.6%	0.3%		1.3%	2.5%	3.9%
PA (ACTIVE TRANSPORTATION)						
Overall	10.3%			11%	9.2%	13.4%
Males						
Females						
METABOLIC SYNDROME						
Overall		33%				
Males	29%			34%	22.9%	27%
Females	34.4%			36%		40%
CHOLESTEROL >200 MG/DL						
Overall	39.7%		30%			
Males		39.9%		43.1%	37%	32.6%
Females		40.5%		41.2%	43.4%	36.1%

Abbreviations: CAD, coronary artery disease; HTN, hypertension; HF, heart failure; PA, physical activity.

Additional inconsistencies exist regarding prescription and adherence to medications between races. Hispanic and black Americans are 20% and 15%, respectively, less likely than white Americans to receive statin treatment for high serum cholesterol and 30% less likely than white Americans to have their dyslipidemia under optimal control.[23-24] In addition, black Americans exhibit less compliance with prescribed cardiac medications than white Americans.[25] These results could not be explained by biological differences alone, because there was attenuation of the disparity when these metrics were corrected for SES and access to health care.[23-25]

Besides inequities in access to health care and quality of care, disparities in awareness and access to information about a healthy cardiovascular lifestyle play also a key role in cardiac outcomes. An AHA survey revealed that black and Hispanic American women have the lowest awareness of CVD risk factors of any racial or ethnic group.[25]

Barriers to Attending CR Programs in Nonwhite Patients

Systems
- Physician referral
- Availability of CR programs

Socioeconomic
- Insurance status
- Access to transportation
- Working hours and access to CR programs (flexible CR hours)
- Cost of missing work days to participate in CR

Linguistic
- Ability to speak English
- Difficulty understanding written information in the English language

Cultural
- Causal beliefs about CVD
- Understanding lifestyle changes and their impact in CVD
- Preference to be treated by physicians
- Family support

Cultural and Diversity Competence

The definition and conceptualization of culture vary across disciplines. However, culture in the context of health science has been defined as "unique shared values, beliefs, and practices that are directly associated with a health-related behavior, indirectly associated with a behavior, or influence acceptance and adoption of the health education message."[28] Cultural competence is defined as "a set of congruent behaviors, attitudes, and policies that come together in a system, agency, or professional and enable that system, agency, or professional to work effectively in cross-cultural situations in order to understand, communicate with, and effectively interact with people across cultures."[29] Cultural competence can be conceptualized and operationalized in a variety of ways, and this variance leads to disagreement about the training needed for health care providers to attain adequate cultural competence. The populations to which the term *cultural competence* applies are also not well defined. Often, *cultural competence* is used only in reference to racial and ethnic minority populations, omitting other groups, such as LGBTQ and people with physical and mental disabilities who have different health care needs and are at risk for discrimination. Therefore, cultural competence must continue to evolve, and interventions to train and educate a culturally competent health care workforce are essential to ensuring the delivery of a comprehensive CR program to an increasingly multicultural and diverse society. Health care professionals need to consider the impact of culture and ethnicity on healthy cardiac behaviors and, ultimately, on cardiac outcomes.[30]

However, although changes in CR provider knowledge, attitudes, and skills are necessary to translate into culturally competent behaviors, the structures and culture of CR care systems and organizations must also evolve. In addition, cultural competence interventions targeting patient–provider relationships are also of critical importance. Interventions focused on improving language, communication skills, or shared decision making may change the relationship between the patient and the CR provider. It is also important to tailor and develop culturally relevant strategies in order to engage minorities in their health promotion, and cultivate a larger workforce of medical providers and researchers with the goal of reducing CVD prevalence and burden among diverse populations.[31-33]

Although culture is a valid clarifying variable for ethnic and racial differences in cardiac health outcomes, medical providers and researchers need to recognize that knowing the ethnic identity or national origin of a patient does not reliably predict that patient's beliefs and attitudes. Therefore, CR service providers need to continue to engage in self-awareness, self-reflection, and self-critique when caring for patients who are not culturally compatible with the provider in race and ethnicity. This process is termed *cultural humility,* and it is essential to creating an honest and trustworthy environment.[34]

BOTTOM LINE

Recommendations to address race and cultural issues and improve participation and adherence to CR programs include the following:

- The initial CR assessment should address race and cultural issues and preferences, level of family and community support, education level, and socioeconomic and insurance status.

- CR staff should be free to ask questions, such as "What is _____ like in your culture? How do you interpret this recommendation on the discharge papers?" Open conversations about matters of race and ethnicity stimulate an atmosphere of trust.

- Ethnocultural background match between health care providers and patients is an important component of culturally responsive care and a key factor in improving participation and adherence to medical recommendations. In this regard, it will be essential to have a diverse CR professional workforce with a background that represents the population served in the program.

- CR centers should have access to language interpreters either face to face or with the use of phone line or other electronic devices (video interpreters).

- CR programs must be prepared to provide ethnoculturally sensitive services personalized to the patient and cultural needs (e.g., exercise areas or CR classes for women only).

- Involve social workers and patients' community, when appropriate, to support patients' needs and adherence to CR programs.

- CR standards and competencies for health care providers must include training in cultural competence. It is expected that the CR team be proficient in recognizing cultural preferences and potential barriers that may impair successful participation in a CR program.

Socioeconomic Considerations

Socioeconomic status (SES) is a combined measure of a group or person's economic and social position relative to others, generally based on income, wealth, educational attainment, and occupation.[1-3] SES is a complex construct that is assessed by a range of factors and at a variety of levels, ranging from individuals to households, neighborhoods, and larger groups (table 11.6). At the individual level, SES is most often measured by income, net worth, years of formal education, terminal degree, and occupation.[4-6] At the group level, SES is often evaluated in terms of population-level or other geographic characteristics.[4-6] For example, neighborhood deprivation indices describe neighborhood poverty, access to transportation, and home ownership.[7] Whether at the individual or group level, most indicators of SES are strongly associated with race and ethnicity, and SES is a significant determinant of health disparities.[8] However, SES is also an independent predictor of health outcomes within racial and ethnic groups.[9,10] Accordingly, SES is an important consideration for CR practitioners for the following reasons: (1) Lower levels of SES are linked with an increased burden of CVD risk factors; (2) a direct association exists between SES and cardiovascular outcomes; (3) low SES is linked to lower CR enrollment and attendance; and (4) evaluation of SES in CR programs allows for patient-centered interventions to increase CR participation and effectiveness.

National CLAS Standards

The National Standards for Culturally and Linguistically Appropriate Services (CLAS) are intended to advance health equity, improve quality, and help eliminate health care disparities by establishing a blueprint for health and health care organizations.

Principal Standard

1. Provide effective, equitable, understandable, and respectful quality care and services that are responsive to diverse cultural health beliefs and practices, preferred languages, health literacy, and other communication needs.

Governance, Leadership, and Workforce

2. Advance and sustain organizational governance and leadership that promotes CLAS and health equity through policy, practices, and allocated resources.

3. Recruit, promote, and support a culturally and linguistically diverse governance, leadership, and workforce that are responsive to the population in the service area.

4. Educate and train governance, leadership, and workforce in culturally and linguistically appropriate policies and practices on an ongoing basis.

Communication and Language Assistance

5. Offer language assistance to individuals who have limited English proficiency and/or other communication needs, at no cost to them, to facilitate timely access to all health care and services.

6. Inform all individuals of the availability of language assistance services clearly and in their preferred language, verbally and in writing.

7. Ensure the competence of individuals providing language assistance, recognizing that the use of untrained individuals and/or minors as interpreters should be avoided.

8. Provide easy-to-understand print and multimedia materials and signage in the languages commonly used by the populations in the service area.

Engagement, Continuous Improvement, and Accountability

9. Establish culturally and linguistically appropriate goals, policies, and management accountability, and infuse them throughout the organization's planning and operations.

10. Conduct ongoing assessments of the organization's CLAS-related activities and integrate CLAS-related measures into measurement and continuous quality improvement activities.

11. Collect and maintain accurate and reliable demographic data to monitor and evaluate the impact of CLAS on health equity and outcomes and to inform service delivery.

12. Conduct regular assessments of community health assets and needs and use the results to plan and implement services that respond to the cultural and linguistic diversity of populations in the service area.

13. Partner with the community to design, implement, and evaluate policies, practices, and services to ensure cultural and linguistic appropriateness.

14. Create conflict and grievance resolution processes that are culturally and linguistically appropriate to identify, prevent, and resolve conflicts or complaints.

15. Communicate the organization's progress in implementing and sustaining CLAS to all stakeholders, constituents, and the general public.

Reprinted from The Office of Minority Health (OMH) at the U.S. Department of Health and Human Services (HHS) https://www.thinkculturalhealth.hhs.gov/clas/standards

Table 11.6 Measures of SES

INDIVIDUAL			
Financial resources	**Education**	**Occupation**	**Group**
Income	Years of education	Occupation type (e.g., white collar, blue collar, service)	Area poverty (e.g., city, zip code, neighborhood)
Net worth	Terminal degree	Occupational status	Regional access to personal and public transportation
Medicaid eligibility			Neighborhood deprivation index[7]
Home ownership			
Access to transportation			

SES and CVD Risk Factors

Significant evidence details the link between low SES and a higher burden of CVD risk factors. Smoking is associated with SES,[11] and the majority of current smokers in the United States are of low SES.[12] Indeed, tobacco marketing has often focused on low SES segments of the population.[13] Hypertension is also associated with low SES, particularly low educational levels.[14] Socioeconomic inequalities exist in dietary quality; low SES populations are less likely to eat fruits and vegetables and more likely to eat less nutritious, calorie-dense foods.[15] These dietary habits translate to higher obesity rates in low SES populations within developed countries.[16] The dietary gradient within SES also results in poorer lipid profiles (higher total cholesterol levels) in low SES populations.[17] Diabetes mellitus is highly associated with SES.[18] Patients with low SES have a higher prevalence of depression,[19] which is closely linked with poor cardiovascular outcomes[20] due to deleterious effects on health behaviors.[21] Lower SES patients are generally two to four times less likely to make positive behavior changes, including smoking cessation and medication adherence, after a MI.[22]

SES and Cardiovascular Outcomes

Socioeconomic status is a particularly powerful predictor of CVD outcomes. In the Women's Health Study, there was an 11% decrease in risk of incident CVD per category increase in level of education.[23] Low SES is associated with a more than 50% increase in ischemic heart disease mortality across 10 western European populations.[24]

The association of SES with CVD mortality is much stronger than for other disease conditions such as cancer.[25] Lower levels of SES are also associated with CVD morbidity, particularly hospital readmissions. After adjusting for demographic variables, one study identified a 30% increase in HF readmissions in the lowest quintile of SES as compared to the highest quintile.[26]

Myriad factors underlie the strong link between SES and CVD outcomes. A higher burden of CVD risk factors in low SES populations as described previously translates into a greater severity of CVD. Patients of low SES also face structural disadvantages to health care access. Patients who experience acute MI and are in the lowest quintile of income have a 45% longer waiting time for coronary angiography as compared to those in the highest quintile.[27] Patients in the lower strata of SES also receive lower rates of evidence-based medical therapy. For example, a significantly lower proportion of low-income Medicare patients hospitalized for acute MI receive aspirin, beta-blockers, and smoking cessation counseling.[28] These findings reinforce the importance of considering SES in the context of cardiovascular therapies such as CR.

SES and Participation in CR

SES is clearly associated with CR enrollment and attendance. Patients who enroll in CR are more likely to be employed and have higher educational attainment than those who do not.[29-31] Patients who do not attend CR are also more likely to have lower income levels.[32] For example, median county income has been directly associated with Medicare beneficiaries' odds of attending

CR programs.[33,34] Eligibility for Medicaid is strongly associated with decreased CR enrollment and attendance in numerous analyses.[35-37] A recent study of over 1,600 patients referred to CR in Vermont demonstrated that Medicaid eligibility was one of the strongest predictors of the number of CR sessions completed, nearly as powerful as age.[38] In addition to individual SES, neighborhood socioeconomic context also affects the probability of CR participation. Patients from deprived neighborhoods are much less likely to attend CR, even after adjusting for individual SES.[39] Neighborhood deprivation is generally assessed through a composite measure focusing on area poverty levels and access to transportation.[7] The latter is critically important for CR attendance, because the resources necessary to travel to and from up to 36 CR sessions are significant. Many qualitative studies have identified lack of transportation as a significant barrier to CR attendance.[40]

Costs of CR Although prior work has evaluated CR participation in the context of many different definitions of SES, it is not surprising that a lack of financial resources is an impediment to attending a CR program. Beyond the transportation costs described, the cost of CR services is often prohibitive for patients of lower SES. The proposed Medicare reimbursement rate for CR services in 2019 is an average of $118.79 per session.[41] Thus, Medicare patients without supplemental coverage will have a copayment of $23.76 per session, or $855.36 total cost for the generally recommended course of 36 sessions. Copayments for CR patients enrolled in Medicare Advantage programs are highly variable; some programs pay the full cost of CR, and others require a copay higher than the 20% copayment for fee-for-service Medicare beneficiaries.

Using Socioeconomic Considerations to Increase CR Participation The development of interventions to increase CR enrollment and adherence is notoriously difficult due to the myriad barriers to CR participation.[42] However, a study in Vermont encouragingly demonstrated that patients receiving financial incentives tied to CR participation ($20 for the first session, and $4 per subsequent session with a $2 increase for each consecutive session, up to a maximum of $70/session) had a 77% attendance rate compared to a 25% attendance rate in the control group.[43] As cost is one of the major considerations for patients of low SES referred to CR, programs can quickly identify patients at risk for nonattendance simply by payer status. Medicaid is a clear surrogate for low SES, and CR centers are familiar with CR coverage levels for various Medicare Advantage programs in their areas. Potential incentives can be deployed on this basis. Further cost–benefit analyses are needed in order to evaluate the potential of financial incentives as an effective strategy to increase CR participation in patients of lower SES.

Educational attainment can also be used as a potential target for interventions to increase CR enrollment and attendance. Patients of low SES are more likely to have low levels of health literacy[44,45] and may not be aware of the potential of CR to improve health outcomes. Clinicians should be cognizant of the importance of explaining the benefits of participating in CR when referring patients of low SES to CR programs.

SES and Effectiveness of CR

Given the relationship between SES and CVD risk factors, outcomes, and CR participation, most CR programs will find an assessment of patients' SES upon enrollment to be useful. There are several options for evaluating SES in this setting.

Measuring SES at CR Enrollment Many programs participate in the AACVPR Outpatient Cardiac Rehabilitation Registry. This registry has data fields for the type of health insurance plan as well as the patient's education level.[46] CR programs that wish to obtain more specific data regarding SES for the purpose of research and patient-centered interventions can use validated questionnaires for this purpose. Two well-known instruments for assessing barriers to CR participation also collect data on SES in addition to other psychosocial characteristics. The Beliefs About Cardiac Rehabilitation Scale[47] inquires as to whether the cost and availability of transportation would prevent a patient from attending CR, as well as whether it would be financially difficult for a patient to take time off from work to attend CR. The Cardiac Rehabilitation Barriers Scale[48] also evaluates whether patients would find it difficult to attend CR due to cost, transportation, or work responsibilities. Each of these instruments can be included with other questionnaires regarding diet and physical activity that are incorporated into the CR intake process.

Using Socioeconomic Considerations to Increase Effectiveness of CR Once assessed, SES can be used to optimize CR effectiveness through two chief considerations, health literacy and self-efficacy. Health literacy is strongly associated with knowledge gains from CR programs.[49] Apprised of the fact that patients with lower educational attainment are likely to have lower health literacy,[44,45] CR practitioners can modify their instruction techniques accordingly. Recommended strategies for communicating clearly with patients who may have low health literacy include avoiding the use of jargon, emphasizing key points, encouraging patients to ask questions, using teach-back methods to confirm understanding, and writing down important instructions.[50]

Self-efficacy is a patient's belief in their ability to perform specific tasks, such as medication adherence or exercise.[51] Patients of low SES frequently have low self-efficacy levels for a variety of health behaviors, particularly exercise.[52,53] Self-efficacy is particularly important in CR, because it affects patients' ability to internalize and sustain positive health behaviors after the completion of CR.[54] A full discussion of this psychological construct and the use of theory-based interventions to support self-efficacy is outside the scope of this chapter. However, motivational interviewing is a counseling technique that is par-

ticularly effective at improving self-efficacy.[55-57] Motivational interviewing encourages patients to discover their desire to make positive change and develop motivation to take action toward this change.[55-57] Accordingly, motivational interviewing is taught to many CR practitioners and is particularly useful for supporting self-efficacy for exercise.[58]

Summary

Within the universe of patients with CVD are subgroups that are at risk of not participating in CR or not completing CR. Each of these groups presented in this chapter (younger and older patients, those of differing sex or gender, the various races and cultures, and those of lower socioeconomic status) have their own unique challenges that affect their overall health care and specifically their ability to participate in CR. The CR staff member who attempts to understand, assess, and adapt practices to adjust to the individual patient will likely be best at delivering effective CR programming and SP. In addition, the expanded application of CR is a critical opportunity to improve value and quality of health care, and to address patient-centered priorities for the prominent and distinctive clinical challenge of a diverse population. It is also important to understand that these differences in CR patients are likely to continue to evolve over time based on ongoing changes in U.S. society.

Program Administration

Karen Lui, RN, MS, MAACVPR

Providing excellent service to patients requires effective leadership. CR programming should foster an environment that helps patients develop the long-term solutions to reinforce positive health behaviors. Programs should strive for ongoing quality improvement (QI) to optimize patient outcomes and program efficiencies. The application of standards and guidelines to improve clinical efficacy and cost-effectiveness requires a sophisticated approach to management and administration. (For more information, search for AACVPR Resources for Professionals at aacvpr.org.)

OBJECTIVES

This chapter reviews the following administrative considerations for program operation:

- Program priorities
- Facilities and equipment
- Organizational policies and procedures
- Insurance and reimbursement
- Documentation
- Personnel
- Continuum of care and services

Effective administration requires knowledge of the following:

- Performance and quality measures
- Core program components and professional competencies
- Data collection and analysis of patient-centered outcomes
- Clinical practice guidelines and position statements
- Budget
- Policy and procedure formation and implementation
- Productivity and utilization
- Regulatory opportunities for patient-centered delivery
- Insurance and managed-care contracting
- Quality and performance improvement issues

Program Priorities

The AACVPR has identified important programming related priorities. To highlight these priorities, performance measures have been established regarding referral to and enrollment in CR and for specific clinical outcomes. The *Core Components of Cardiac Rehabilitation/Secondary Prevention Programs*[1] detail the key elements of a comprehensive program. The *Core Competencies for Program Professionals*[2] integrate specific knowledge and skills into the implementation of the Performance Measures as well as the Core Components. Through establishing exams for Program Certification and Certified Cardiac Rehabilitation Professional, AACVPR endorses these priorities to which programs and CR professionals should aspire. This chapter addresses administrative issues that all CR programs need to consider.

Applying CR Performance and Quality Measures

The emergence of performance measures in all areas of health care has been embraced by governmental entities and providers seeking to promote and deliver both efficacious and cost-effective services. Significant underutilization of CR[3,4] has led to the development of performance and qual-

ity measures that promote physician referral and enrollment in early outpatient CR.[3] The inclusion of the measures discussed in chapter 2 are examples of clinical and programmatic actions taken as a result of scientific evidence. The integration of the CR performance and quality measures into program operation should be prioritized.

Maximizing Program Utilization

One strategy for enhancing program enrollment is the application of referral performance measures in CR programs. Automation of the referral process results in significant improvement in referral patterns.[6] Other effective strategies to address underutilization of the service include taking an active role in facilitating referrals and initiating patient participation in a CR program within one to three weeks after hospital discharge.[7,8] Barriers to utilization due to capacity restraints may be addressed through various methods, including expanding days of operation, adding sessions at more convenient times, expanding or relocating to a larger space, adding a satellite site, and changing the program model to an open gym design rather than limited class slots. The program director and staff must consider many factors and continually assess for optimal utilization and program growth opportunities.

Outcomes-Based Programming

Currently in health care, providers, payers, and consumers have an ever-increasing focus on clinical outcomes of procedures and treatments. While the reasons for this focus are multifactorial, the result has been a heightened emphasis on scientific research and evidence-based guidelines to justify medical interventions. One illustration of this transition in CR is the Medicare-added designation of Intensive Cardiac Rehabilitation (ICR), which is reimbursed for significantly more CR sessions. The Centers for Medicare and Medicaid Services (CMS) made this designation based on identified clinical outcomes demonstrated by these ICR programs.[9-12] Measurement and attainment of significant clinical patient outcomes upon completion of CR should be a top priority for all programs. The most relevant and clinically meaningful evidence-based patient and program outcomes are addressed in chapter 13.

Ensuring Program Comprehensiveness

CR services are typically provided by a multidisciplinary team of health professionals. This model has served the profession well by providing a broad spectrum of expertise through the combined use of various professional disciplines. The AACVPR Core Competencies assist a program director in building a comprehensive team (see table 12.1).[1] Mastery of core competencies by individual CR staff members enables the team to be successful in meeting the scientifically based AACVPR Core Components of a comprehensive CR program.[2]

BOTTOM LINE

Integrating the CR Performance and Quality Measures into program operation should be a priority.

- Programming should include all of the AACVPR Core Components of CR and SP.
- To effectively deliver the core components, staff members must exhibit the skills outlined in the AACVPR Core Competencies for CR/SP.
- The AACVPR Cardiac Rehabilitation Program Certification process is designed to promote adherence to standards and guidelines.
- The Certified Cardiac Rehabilitation Professional is a certification aligned with the published CR core competencies.

Contemporary Models of CR Delivery

A changing clinical profile of patients entering CR over recent years has significant implications for contemporary CR programs. CR patients are older, more overweight, more likely to have diabetes mellitus and HTN, and relatively less fit than their predecessors.[13] Moreover, patients with chronic systolic HF are now eligible to participate in CR.[14]

Consequently, CR programming should target specific patient needs including low levels of CRF and obesity-related metabolic disorders.[15] Attention should be paid to applying current principles of exercise physiology in the early outpatient and maintenance CR settings. Strategies have moved beyond the early outpatient CR model established in the 1970s to be more effective given additional research and the demographic trends of patients enrolling in CR.

Current knowledge of adult learning and behavior change theory (discussed in chapter 8) suggests that an individualized approach to education is more effective than the historical approach in CR using preselected topics that are delivered in a set number of educational classes for all CR participants. A CR program can provide critical tools and support in fostering self-efficacy and behavior change if these concepts are understood and supported, and if the entire CR staff puts them into practice.

The longstanding paradigm for early outpatient CR patients has been 1 h sessions of primarily aerobic exercise, two or three times per week. If this routine is not provided in combination with an emphasis on a concurrent progressive home exercise prescription, it fails to successfully integrate science into practice. The evidence that a dose >250 min/week of physical activity is most effective in eliciting clinically significant weight loss should be considered in the development and progression of the exercise prescription.[16] Most participants in early outpatient and maintenance CR programs fail to perform significant amounts of activity on non-CR exercise days.[17,18,19] These findings reinforce the importance of the CR team in providing exercise, PA, and educational components that will assist in achieving the best possible outcomes for each patient. In addition, the importance of resistance training, as well as its safety and efficacy for patients with CVD, is well substantiated,[20] and it is one of the fundamental interventions for CR programs.[12] A delivery model for exercise prescription that provides for individualized exercise components—that is, exercise frequency, intensity, duration, modality, volume, and progression—promotes increased PA that is consistent with evidence-based recommendations.[21] Specific recommendations regarding PA are discussed in chapter 6. On an ongoing basis, program directors should evaluate program delivery models in order to provide those clinical outcomes that are the foundation of CR and are based on the science of exercise physiology and behavior change.[22]

Table 12.1 Core Competencies for CR and SP Professionals

Competency	Knowledge	Skills
Patient assessment	Demonstrate an understanding of the following: • Cardiovascular anatomy, physiology, and pathophysiology • Process of arteriolosclerosis and pathogenesis of cardiovascular risk factors • Cardiac arrhythmias (e.g., complex PVCs, AF, SVT) and their influence on physical activity and symptoms • Cardiac device therapies (e.g., pacemakers, defibrillators, and LVADs) • Cardiovascular assessments, diagnostic tests, and procedures • Signs and symptoms of CVD • Appropriate emergency responses to changing signs and symptoms • Effective lifestyle management of CVD and associated risk factors • Pharmacologic approaches for CVD and risk factor management • Comorbidities limiting or otherwise influencing function or treatment strategies • Side effects from pharmacologic therapies • Psychosocial factors related to CVD • Adult learning principles, theoretical models for behavior change, adherence, coping, and disease management strategies • Compliance and adherence to therapeutic regimens • Effective communication to referral sources and the interdisciplinary team to promote care coordination • Principles and methods for outcome assessment and reporting	Ability to perform the following: • Obtain a comprehensive medical, social, and family history through interview, review of medical records, and questionnaires. • Conduct physical examination of cardiovascular system (e.g., measure HR, BP; auscultate heart and lung sounds; palpate and inspect extremities for edema, pulses, signs of DVT and PAD; inspect surgical wound). • Develop risk factor profile and CVD risk reduction strategies. • Basic tests and assessments: 12-lead ECG, oximetry, BG, and blood lipids. • Obtain information on patient preferences and goals. • Interactive communication and counseling with patient and family on treatment plan through shared decision making. • Develop an ITP. • Document and communicate ITP and progress reports to physicians and interdisciplinary team. • Quantify patient outcome assessment through pre- and postprogram assessment.
Nutritional counseling	Demonstrate an understanding of the following: • Role and impact of diet on CVD progression and risk factor management • Analysis of diet composition with specific emphasis on total caloric intake and dietary content that influences risk factors (e.g., total fats, cholesterol, refined and processed CHOs, sodium) • Potential risks and benefits of nonprescription nutritional supplements and alcohol intake • Target goals for dietary modification and nutrition interventions for identified risk factors and comorbidities (e.g., dyslipidemia, HTN, diabetes, obesity, HF, kidney disease) • Effective behavior change strategies based on common theoretical models and adult learning strategies	Ability to perform the following: • Assess dietary intake to estimate total calories; amounts of saturated fat, trans fat, cholesterol, sodium, fruits and vegetables, whole grains, fiber, and fish; number of meals and snacks; portion sizes; frequency of eating out; alcohol consumption. • Provide education and counseling on specific dietary modifications needed to achieve target goals. • Conduct behavioral interventions to promote adherence and self-management skills in dietary habits. • Measure and report outcomes of nutritional management goals at the conclusion of the program.

Competency	Knowledge	Skills
Weight management	Demonstrate an understanding of the following: • Physiological and pathological effects of overweight and obesity and those of low body weight • Principles of weight management through the balance of caloric intake and caloric expenditure • Awareness of fad diets and possible risks to CVD patients • Current guidelines and recommendations for healthy body weight and secondary prevention • Weight loss interventions that promote gradual, sustainable weight loss (5%-10%) over 3 to 6 months • Medications and surgeries for weight loss • Nutritional and medical risks associated with rapid weight loss and cyclical weight gain and weight loss • Recognition that weight loss and weight maintenance is often complex and difficult and requires ongoing dietary management, PA, and behavioral management • Importance and efficacy of regular PA, modification of dietary patterns, changes in caloric balance, and drug therapy in weight management • Effective behavior change strategies based on common theoretical models and adult learning strategies	Ability to perform the following: • Measure body weight, height, and waist circumference. • Calculate BMI and determine proper category: normal, overweight, or obese. • Develop short- and long-term weight loss goals for those in overweight or obese categories. • Assess nutritional and dietary habits as well as daily energy intake and expenditure to help guide individualized education and counseling for weight management. • Conduct behavioral interventions to promote adherence and self-management skills in weight management. • Measure and report outcomes of weight management at the conclusion of the program.
BP management	Demonstrate an understanding of the following: • HTN as a risk factor for AVD and potential end-organ damage • Signs and symptoms of hypotension and HTN • Normal range of BP at rest and during exercise • Current BP targets for SP • Role of home BP monitoring in BP management • Actions of classes of antihypertensive medications and common side effects • Postural and postexercise hypotension • Elements of the DASH diet for treating HTN • Principles of measurement and operation for different devices used to measure BP • Recognition that BP control is often complex and difficult and may require ongoing medication adjustments, dietary management, PA, and behavioral management • Importance and efficacy of sodium restriction, weight management, PA and exercise, smoking cessation, alcohol moderation, and drug therapy in the control of BP	Ability to perform the following: • Calculate accurate BP determinations at rest (seated, supine, and standing) and during exercise. • Recognize significant BP deviations from the expected range or targeted outcome. • Assess compliance with BP medications and management plan. • Measure and report outcomes for BP management at the conclusion of the rehabilitation program.

(continued)

Table 12.1 *(continued)*

Competency	Knowledge	Skills
Lipid management	Demonstrate an understanding of the following: • Definitions of LDL-C, HDL-C, VLDL-C, TG, non-HDL-C • Physiological role of lipids in the atherosclerotic disease process • Elements of the Therapeutic Lifestyle Changes diet and the MEDIT diet • Actions of classes of antihyperlipidemic medications, including nonprescription, and side effects • Types of dietary fats and simple CHOs and their effect on serum lipid levels • Current serum lipid target values for SP • Importance and efficacy of weight management, PA and exercise, smoking cessation, alcohol moderation, and drug therapy in the control of serum lipids	Ability to perform the following: • Interpret LDL-C, HDL-C, non-HDL-C, VLDL-C, and TG values in light of secondary prevention target values. • Assess compliance with antihyperlipidemic medications and management plan. • Assess compliance with lifestyle interventions for the management of serum lipid values. • Provide patient education information concerning serum lipids. • Develop a risk reduction plan for abnormal serum lipids and communicate the plan to the patient and family. • Measure and report outcomes for serum lipids at the conclusion of rehabilitation.
Diabetes management	Demonstrate an understanding of the following: • Type 1 and type 2 diabetes • Fasting and casual BG values that define hypoglycemia and hyperglycemia • Importance of and recommended target value for HbA1c • Complications related to diabetes: micro- and macrovascular; autonomic and peripheral neuropathy; nephropathy; and retinopathy • Signs and symptoms related to hypoglycemia and hyperglycemia • Use of CHOs for hypoglycemia • Actions of glucose-lowering medications and insulin • Importance of monitoring BG values, especially before and after exercise • Contraindications to exercise based on BG values • Importance of compliance with diabetic medications and dietary, body weight, and exercise recommendations • Importance of recognizing and managing the metabolic syndrome and the associated CVD risk factors • Importance and efficacy of weight management, PA and exercise, alcohol moderation, and drug therapy in the control of BG	Ability to perform the following: • Record history of complications related to diabetes, including frequency and triggers of hyperglycemia and hypoglycemia. • Calibrate and properly use glucometers. • Assess signs and symptoms of hyperglycemia and hypoglycemia and take appropriate actions. • Provide patient education concerning the effects of lifestyle and medications on glycemic control. • Refer the patient to a diabetic educator or clinical dietitian, as needed. • Measure and report outcomes for glucose control at the conclusion of rehabilitation, including episodes of hyperglycemia and hypoglycemia during and after exercise.

Competency	Knowledge	Skills
Tobacco cessation	Demonstrate an understanding of the following: • Current guidelines for treating tobacco use and SP goals • Biochemical and physiological consequences of smoking on CVD • Exposure to secondhand smoke as a risk factor for cardiovascular events • Effective behavior change strategies based on common theoretical models • Available services to support smoking cessation (e.g., community smoking cessation programs, counselors, psychologists) • Physiological and psychological aspects of tobacco addiction • Efficacy of pharmacologic interventions, including risks and benefits	Ability to perform the following: • Assess use and categories of tobacco use: never, former, recent, or current. • Conduct behavioral interventions to promote tobacco cessation and long-term tobacco-free adherence. • Measure and report outcomes of tobacco cessation at the conclusion of the program.
Psychosocial management	Demonstrate an understanding of the following: • Influence of psychosocial factors on the pathophysiology of CVD and adherence to treatment • Depression and its major association with recurrent CAD events, poorer outcomes, and adherence to treatment • Other psychological indicators that may affect treatment response, such as anxiety, anger or hostility, and social isolation • Actions of pharmacologic and lifestyle interventions for psychological distress • Socioeconomic factors that may serve as barriers to treatment adherence, such as educational or income level, lack of resources, or lack of support • Available support services to augment psychological interventions (e.g., psychologists, counselors, social workers, clergy) • Effective behavior change strategies based on common theoretical models and adult learning strategies[17]	Ability to perform the following: • Screen and assess for psychological distress, especially depression, anxiety, anger, or hostility; social isolation; marital or family distress; sexual dysfunction; and substance abuse. • Provide appropriate referrals for psychiatric or psychological care when needs are recognized as beyond the scope of usual care. • Provide individual and group education and counseling interventions that address stress management and coping strategies. • Measure and report outcomes of psychosocial management at the conclusion of the program.[7,18]

(continued)

Table 12.1 *(continued)*

Competency	Knowledge	Skills
PA counseling	Demonstrate an understanding of the following: • Lack of regular PA and sedentary behavior as a risk factor for CAD • Negative health consequences of time spent being sedentary • Current recommendations for intensity, frequency, and duration for regular PA in persons with CVD • Preexisting musculoskeletal and neuromuscular conditions that may affect PA • Identifying activities that may increase the risk for an untoward cardiovascular event and environmental conditions that may also increase the risk • Barriers to increasing PA • Metabolic requirements for recreational, occupational, and sexual activities • Recommendations to avoid musculoskeletal injury related to PA • Effective behavior change strategies based on common theoretical models and adult learning strategies	Ability to perform the following: • Assess current PA level using both questionnaires and available activity-monitoring devices. • Assist patients in setting realistic incremental goals for future PA. • Provide recommendations for increasing the level of safe and appropriate daily PA and structured exercise. • Assess physical and metabolic requirements for ADLs and occupational and recreational activities. • Use communication and behavioral strategies that will improve compliance with regular PA recommendations. • Measure and report outcomes for PA at the conclusion of rehabilitation.
Exercise training evaluation	Demonstrate an understanding of the following: • Normal and abnormal responses to exercise including signs and symptoms of exercise intolerance, MI, ACS, and VAs • Physiological responses to acute exercise and adaptations to chronic exercise • Risk stratification according to patient assessment and exercise test results • Exercise prescription methodology for cardiovascular endurance exercise and resistance training in a broad range of patients with heart disease • Absolute and relative contraindications for exercise • Absolute and relative indications to terminate an exercise session	Ability to perform the following: • Recognize life-threatening cardiac arrhythmias, myocardial ischemia or MI, hypoxemia, hypotension, hypoglycemia, and other signs and symptoms of exercise intolerance. • Risk stratify each patient according to AHA and AACVPR criteria. • Develop an individualized, safe, and effective cardiovascular endurance exercise prescription, including modes, intensity, duration, frequency, and progression. • Develop an individualized, safe, and effective exercise prescription for resistance training, including load, number of repetitions, frequency, and progression for appropriate muscle groups. • Include warm-up, cool-down, and exercises for flexibility and balance in the exercise prescription. • As needed, accommodate existing comorbidities within the exercise prescription. • Skin preparation and electrode placement for exercise ECG telemetry monitoring. • Measure and report outcomes for exercise training at the conclusion of rehabilitation.

Abbreviations: AACVPR, American Association of Cardiovascular and Pulmonary Rehabilitation; AF, atrial fibrillation; ACS, acute coronary syndrome; AHA, American Heart Association; BG, blood glucose; BP, blood pressure; CAD, coronary artery disease; CVD, cardiovascular disease; DASH, Dietary Approaches to Stop Hypertension; DVT, deep vein thrombosis; ECG, electrocardiogram; HbA1c, glycosylated hemoglobin; HDL-C, high-density lipoprotein cholesterol; HF, heart failure; HR, heart rate; HTN, hypertension; ITP, individual treatment plan; LDL-C, low-density lipoprotein cholesterol; LVAD, left ventricular assist device; MI, myocardial infarction; PA, physical activity; PAD, peripheral artery disease; PVCs, premature ventricular contractions; SVT, supraventricular tachycardia; TG, triglycerides; VA, ventricular arrhythmia; VLDL-C, very low-density lipoprotein cholesterol.

Reprinted by permission from L.F. Hamm et al., "Core Competencies for Cardiac Rehabilitation/Secondary Prevention Professionals: Update. Position Statement of the American Association of Cardiovascular and Pulmonary Rehabilitation" *Journal of Cardiopulmonary Rehabilitation and Prevention* 31 (2010): 2–10.

Quality improvement (QI) are critical. However, QI projects are advantageous only if used as more than a perfunctory process to satisfy regulatory, accreditation, and internal institutional requirements. The AACVPR program certification process is useful for promoting program quality. It is the obligation of the program director to maintain an atmosphere of continuous QI (guideline 12.1) through continuous oversight of operations relative to objectives in striving to consistently elevate program quality and ultimately add value to the patient experience.

Fiscal Accountability

Operating a fiscally sound CR program requires analysis of barriers to participation and opportunities to increase utilization, innovative programming, strategic hiring, prudent control of costs, and maximizing use of space. In the past, Medicare regulations restricted varied program paradigms. In contrast, now outpatient CR programs are able to offer flexible participation at a time when the importance of identifying individual patient needs has been emphasized by both regulating bodies and payers.[23,24] Continuous analysis of referral and enrollment rates to track program utilization and removing barriers to program participation result in increased utilization.[25] It is essential to maintain good communication with the business office and administration to ensure accurate assessment of program performance by all decision makers and to ensure full awareness of administrative expectations. Hospital and facility administrators should be regularly provided with evidence-based summaries of the value of CR with respect to program outcomes including mortality, morbidity, and cost-effectiveness analyses.[26-29]

BOTTOM LINE

Program administration of a CR program requires knowledge and the application of the following:

- *Current* regulations
- *Current* science
- Best practice strategies to address program deficiencies
- Programmatic strategies to ensure fiscal sustainability
- A well-qualified, multi-disciplined CR staff
- Strong communication skills with payers, patients, staff, hospital administration, and all departments that intersect with CR
- Willingness to change and leadership skills to lead change

Facilities and Equipment

Policies and procedures regarding the management of the facility are aimed at providing a safe, functional, and effective environment. Many of the requirements for services provided within institutions are regulated by federal, state, and local agencies. The components of these policies should include

- planning of space utilization,
- maintenance of equipment,
- reduction and control of environmental hazards and risks,
- maintenance of safe conditions, and
- climate control.

Guideline 12.1 Continuous Quality Improvement

Program staff should develop a process for all of the following:

- Annual review of department policy and procedure manuals to ensure that they are current, comprehensive, and accurate
- Utilization of published CR performance and quality measures, including but not limited to program referral, enrollment, and participation rates

- Evaluation of client satisfaction
- Continued scrutiny of related research to compare program outcomes with national, regional, and local programs

Specific AACVPR delineations are provided here to better ensure safe and effective CR programming, facilities, and equipment. These guidelines are organized into these four areas:

- General—Apply to all CR service facilities and equipment.
- Inpatient—Specifically address the needs of inpatient services.
- Outpatient—Specifically address the needs of outpatient CR, both early and long-term services.
- Stress testing—Specific to programs that provide stress testing services.

Inpatient Exercise Facilities

In the current era of short hospital stays and very limited time for the patient to receive even a basic evaluation of CVD risk and initiation of preventive therapies, specific inpatient exercise facilities and equipment are not necessary components to inpatient CR program services. Nonetheless, the environment for such services should allow safe and easy patient movement. Exercise services may be conducted in patient rooms, hospital hallways, and stairwells. All areas should be free of obstruction, with access to handrails; and distances should be measured. Equipment needs depend on the services provided, but they might include 1 to 3 lb (0.45-1.3 kg) dumbbell weights or low-level resistance bands, cycle ergometers, and treadmills with low-speed capabilities. A primary focus of IPCR is referral to early outpatient CR. This focus offers perhaps the best opportunity to improve referral and enrollment rates. Effective strategies to increase the referral of patients to CR include the following:

- Electronic medical record discharge order set with referral for qualifying diagnoses, preferably using an option-out automatic order
- Referral accompanied by a liaison referral in the hospital with follow-up shortly after discharge; often most effectively provided by CR staff
- An enrollment date for outpatient CR established before discharge when possible; ideally within 21 days of hospital discharge[3]
- Reinforcement of the benefits and importance of participation from the patient's referring physicians and advanced practitioners

Outpatient Facilities and Equipment

Facilities should provide separate space for patient reception and waiting, patient consultation and education, exercise, confidential chart storage, safekeeping of valuables, and easily available rest rooms, which may include showering facilities. Outdoor exercise areas may also be included. Participants with disabilities should have full access to all CR facilities in adherence with requirements of the Americans with Disabilities Act (ADA). Outpatient facilities should provide for the following[30]:

- Program and safety information that is accessible and prominently posted
- Open-access circulation, avoiding blind corners, unnecessary doors, pointless partitions, and other hazards that present a safety risk to users
- Space for program operation, storage, and maintenance that is separate from that used for PA (Floor surfaces in PA areas should provide the proper level of absorption and slip resistance to minimize the risk of impact- or fall-related injuries.)
- Exercise floor space of 40 to 60 ft² (12-18 m²) per piece of equipment, as well as adequate floor space for stretching activities
- PA spaces with sufficient air circulation and outside air to maintain air quality, room temperatures, and humidity at safe and comfortable levels during times of PA
- A patient consultation area with adequate space, privacy, and amenities for interviewing, counseling, teaching, and physical examination
- Rest rooms and showering facilities that are equipped with nonslip surfaces that are cleaned and disinfected regularly
- A regularly tested emergency call system in rest rooms and shower facilities

Specific equipment selection depends on individual program preference, available space, and budget. Exercise equipment should provide multiple modalities for safe and effective aerobic and resistance training (see chapter 6). Examples of such equipment are motorized treadmills with speed and grade control; calibrated upright or recumbent cycle ergometers; and calibrated upper body ergometers, rowers, or elliptical trainers that display accurate ergonomic units. Possible resistance training equipment includes weight training machines representative of what patients will encounter in fitness facilities (stack, plate-loaded, cable or pulley), adjustable benches, dumbbells of a variety of weight, and elastic bands.

Patient characteristics, safety, and financial considerations should influence decisions concern-

---

Guideline 12.2   General Facility Considerations[30]

- Space must meet the requirements for the activities and services provided and the unique needs of patients. There must be emergency access to all patient areas, and floor space must allow easy access of personnel and equipment. Floor space should be approximately 40 to 45 ft² (12.2-13.7 m²) per patient.

- All areas should provide temperature and humidity control that allow for a comfortable environment. Humidity should be at or below 60%; temperature should be 68 to 72 °F (20-22 °C).

- Sound levels should be kept at a comfortable level that is conducive for conversations between patients and health care professionals.

- Ceiling height in exercise areas must allow for full, unrestricted activity with a minimum height of 10 ft (3 m).

- A water source should be immediately available to all exercise areas. Food and drink should not be allowed on or near exercise or monitoring equipment.

- All facilities must provide for confidentiality of patient records and privacy.

- A regularly tested telephone and emergency call system should be available in all exercise areas and an emergency phone list available at all phones. (Emergency delivery system guidelines are discussed in chapter 14.)

- Basic first aid should be available to all exercise areas.

Guideline 12.3   General Equipment Considerations

- Equipment requirements may vary depending on the patient population and the staff training.

- All equipment should be commercial grade with stringent maintenance guidelines to ensure patient safety.

- Scheduled maintenance and cleaning programs for all exercise equipment must be documented.

- Equipment that is not functioning properly or that is damaged and may cause a hazard should be designated as out of service until repairs are complete.

- Equipment such as treadmills or cycle ergometers should be regularly calibrated and maintained as recommended by the manufacturer.

- Staff should be thoroughly trained in the proper use of all equipment and manufacturer information for correct use and calibration, and troubleshooting should be readily available.

- The CR facility should provide equipment that can be accessed by people with physical limitations, including the use of a wheelchair, with at least one modality for CRF and resistance training exercise.

- Equipment should be of sufficient quantity and quality to adequately meet the purpose and intended function for the participating patient population.

- A chair and an exam table or a cart suitable for supine and recumbent positions should be available in the area.

- Equipment for patient assessment, including a quality stethoscope, portable sphygmomanometer, ECG monitors, pulse oximeter, portable oxygen, and a posted and clearly visible RPE scale, should be available to all exercise areas.

ing facilities and equipment for programming. Providing equipment that patients are likely to encounter in a community fitness setting helps adherence to a new setting. For example, gradually moving patients from arm ergometers and recumbent cross-trainers (where appropriate) to elliptical and stair machines can facilitate a successful transition to a new exercise facility in the future.

Additional facility and equipment (materials) recommendations for program operations include the following:

- Emergency equipment (see chapter 14)
- Clearly visible scales for RPE, angina and other pain, and dyspnea
- HR monitoring technology that patients can use on home exercise days
- BG meter and glucose supplements (e.g., fruit juice and crackers)
- Education area with comfortable chairs; and access to computers with Internet, a resource library, and anatomical models or diagrams

Stress Testing Facility and Equipment

Areas used for exercise testing should comply with guidelines 12.2 and 12.3. A treadmill and leg-alone or arm–leg cycle ergometer with measurable, calibrated workload are the equipment most often used in a testing facility. Rowing ergometers with wattage display are also effective as exercise testing options for some patients with physical limitations.

Some CR programs perform a 6-minute walk test as a pre- and post-assessment of functional improvement in exercise capacity. For this test a premeasured distance is utilized for purposes of reproducibility. An area that minimizes turns is advantageous. It is important to follow proper test protocol to ensure validity and reliability of outcomes.

Organizational Policies and Procedures

All health care providers come under the purview of regulatory bodies, including federal and state regulatory boards. In Medicare terminology, *providers* include patient care institutions such as hospitals, critical access hospitals, hospices, nursing homes, and home health agencies. The Social Security Act (SSA) mandates the establishment of minimum health and safety standards

that must be met by providers participating in the Medicare and Medicaid programs. These standards are published in Title 42 Code of Federal Regulations (CFR) Part 482.[31] The U.S. Department of Health and Human Services (HHS) has designated the Centers for Medicare and Medicaid Services (CMS) to administer the standards compliance process. State survey agencies carry out the Medicare certification process on a contractual basis. Title XVIII of the SSA, Section 1861, contains Conditions of Participation (CoP) and Conditions for Coverage (CfC) that health care organizations must meet in order to participate in the Medicare and Medicaid programs. CMS ensures that the standards of accrediting organizations recognized by CMS meet or exceed the Medicare standards in the CoP and CfC. All accrediting entities must have first completed a CMS application process to obtain "deemed status." For example, a hospital accredited by the Joint Commission (TJC) or Det Norske Veritas Healthcare (DNVHC) is deemed to meet all Medicare requirements for hospitals (excluding special conditions for psychiatric hospitals and other specified services). Most accrediting entities are independent and hold nonprofit status. Other examples are the Commission on Accreditation of Rehabilitation Facilities (CARF) and the National Committee for Quality Assurance (NCQA). Hospital-affiliated programs must meet Occupational Safety and Health Administration (OSHA) regulations for safety of personnel. National Patient Safety Goals (NPSG) is an important component of TJC accreditation that is periodically reviewed and revised. The web resource contains a list of websites containing information on regulatory and accrediting organizations.

Policies and Procedures

Institutional policies and procedures must conform to regulatory standards regarding infection control and hazardous waste, human resource management, nursing practice, performance improvement, emergency and disaster response, administrative policy and procedures, and safety.

Departmental policies and procedures are subordinate to institutional policies and function to define numerous aspects of the CR program philosophy, processes, and plans of action. These policies and procedures should be reviewed annually and revised as frequently as necessary for maintaining relevance. Citing the evidence that is the foundation for a specific department policy or procedure helps provide the rationale for the policy. Policies and procedures are helpful resources for new staff members and are useful in fostering consistency of care provided in the CR program. Policies, procedures, current research, and professional guidelines should be easily accessible with the expectation that all CR staff be familiar with them.

Information Management

Information management involves oversight of the storage, transmission, use, and tracking of patient information. The passage of the Health Insurance Portability and Accountability Act of 1996 (HIPAA) led to the development of the Privacy Rule in 2000. National standards were set for the protection, use, and disclosure of certain health information by organizations subject to the Privacy Rule and standards for the privacy rights of individuals. Policies and procedures related to information management should include storage and access to

- patient records, patient privacy and confidentiality, and outcome data;
- financial records and analysis, budget allocation, capital and operational expenses;
- insurance billing, precertification, and reimbursement;
- provision of charity and scaled remunerative services; and
- patient registration and procedure scheduling.

The policies for management of information are usually developed and implemented by the institutional management team in a centralized area or department.

Insurance and Reimbursement

Continuous change in health care management and reimbursement patterns for CR is evident in nearly all markets across the United States. Advances in technology will continue to affect all areas of medicine through

- proliferation of electronic medical records (EMR) and consequent enhanced health information communication between health care providers;

- use of telemedicine in the treatment of chronic disease and targeted patient populations; and
- growth of evidence-based treatment decisions through greater integration of endorsed performance measures, appropriateness criteria, and guidelines.

The escalating cost of health care in the United States is one of the major driving forces behind the direction of these advances. Demonstration projects funded and implemented by government and private insurance companies seek treatments that result in effective patient outcomes at lower cost to deliver while maintaining quality. Payers and providers will continue to seek technological changes in medicine that demonstrate improved patient care.

Health Insurance Companies

Health insurance companies can be divided into two distinct sectors, private and public. The private sector contracts with individuals or groups to offer a variety of plans. These plans provide a range from no coverage or minimum coverage with copays and deductibles to 100% coverage with no copays or deductibles. The enrollee may make these contracts directly with an independent insurance company or through the employer. Managed-care plans may be promulgated by integrated delivery systems, hospital systems, insurance companies, and private for-profit companies.

Public sector insurance is administered under a government-sponsored program. Examples of public sector entities are Medicare and Medicaid, Federally Qualified Health Centers, TRICARE for military and public health service workers, and the Bureau of Vocational Rehabilitation.

Medicare

The CMS is the governing body within the Department of HHS, which is responsible for the enactment of congressional laws that oversee the government public medical insurance plan. CMS administers coverage and payment guidelines for the following categories of Americans who qualify for Medicare:

- People age 65 or older
- People under age 65 with certain disabilities
- People of all ages with end-stage renal disease (permanent kidney failure requiring dialysis or a kidney transplant)

Medicare is relatively comprehensive in its coverage for hospital inpatient, outpatient, and physician services. Outpatient benefits for CR are summarized here:

- *Part A, Hospital Insurance.* Most people do not pay a premium for Part A if they or a spouse already paid for it through their payroll taxes while working. Medicare Part A (Hospital Insurance) helps cover inpatient care in hospitals, including critical access hospitals, inpatient rehabilitation facilities, and skilled nursing facilities (not custodial or long-term care). Beneficiaries must meet certain conditions to qualify for these benefits.

- *Part B, Medical Insurance.* Most people pay a monthly premium for Part B. Medicare Part B (Medical Insurance) assists with physician services and hospital outpatient care when medically necessary. The original Fee-for-Service (FFS) Medicare insurance is often accompanied by the purchase of supplemental health coverage policies by Medicare beneficiaries as secondary insurance, also known as Medigap policies.

- *Part B, Medicare Replacement Plans.* Medicare Advantage (MA) Plans (sometimes called Part C) are offered by private companies approved by and regulated by CMS as an alternative to traditional FFS Medicare insurance. MA Plan coverage replaces the need for a supplemental insurance plan and includes Medicare prescription drug coverage (Part D).

CMS has established geographical jurisdictions and currently awards Medicare contracts to insurance companies through competitive procedures. Medicare Administrative Contractors (MACs) for Parts A and B Medicare jurisdictions administer Medicare services and process Medicare claims for the jurisdictions. Although MACs may not deny coverage of services covered by CMS, latitude is allowed in the interpretation of these rules. As a result, local coverage rules for CR may vary among local Medicare contractors. MAC instructions to providers are typically issued via bulletins and articles and for some services through local coverage determinations (LCD), although LCDs are not required. It is, therefore, imperative that each program be familiar with federal, state, and regional (MAC) policies that govern CR.

Medicare Provision for CR and Intensive CR Services

In 2008, the U.S. Congress passed Public Law 110-275, which included the addition of coverage for CR and intensive CR (ICR) services in the Social Security Administration (SSA) Title XVIII, Section 1861. From that mandate, CMS promulgated the Medicare provision for early outpatient CR services, titled "Cardiac Rehabilitation Program and Intensive Cardiac Rehabilitation Program: Conditions of Coverage."[32]

The CMS definition of early outpatient CR is "a physician-supervised program that furnishes physician-prescribed exercise, cardiac risk factor modification, psychosocial assessment, and outcomes assessment."[32] Medicare provisions are subject to modification and shifting interpretation

---

Guideline 12.4 Cardiac Rehabilitation Staffing and Monitoring Requirements

- There is no specific professional discipline required or recommended in order to be part of the CR staff (except where mandated by state law). There is no requirement that a CR staff include a specific professional discipline such as a registered nurse, clinical exercise physiologist, or physical therapist.

- There is no required or recommended staff-to-patient ratio (except where mandated by state law).

- CR is not prohibited from combining with other services to share space, staff, equipment, and hours of operation.

- Use of ECG monitoring in CR is not a Medicare requirement; AACVPR recommendation is to use ECG monitoring as needed on an individual patient basis. However, private insurance coverage may mandate ECG monitoring.

- CMS does not regulate self-pay services, including maintenance CR (i.e., phase III or IV).

- There is no minimum or maximum number of days per week a patient can receive CR.

- Medicare regulations and AACVPR recommendations are subject to change.

Medicare Requirements for Early Outpatient Cardiac Rehabilitation

The Medicare provisions for CR require the following components:

- Physician referral with Medicare-eligible diagnosis identified
  - Medical documentation to support the diagnosis—should be available to the CR program upon request

- Medicare accepts the following diagnoses (Medicare regulations may change, so periodic review of the regulations is essential):
  - Acute MI within the preceding 12 months*
  - Coronary artery bypass surgery
  - Current stable angina pectoris
  - Heart valve repair or replacement
  - Percutaneous transluminal coronary angioplasty (PTCA) or coronary stenting
  - Heart or heart–lung transplant
  - Chronic HF (LVEF of ≤35% and NYHA Class II to IV) symptoms despite being on optimal HF therapy for at least six weeks. (Stable patients are defined as patients who have not had recent or planned [≤6 months] major cardiovascular hospitalizations or procedures.)
  - Other cardiac conditions that would require specification through a national coverage determination

- Individualized treatment plan:
  - Details on how components of CR are provided for each patient
  - Description of the diagnosis
  - Type, amount, frequency, and duration of services furnished under the plan
  - Physician-prescribed (aerobic, strength, stretching) exercise as appropriate, provided each day the patient receives CR services
  - Agreed-upon goals and outcomes
  - Must be established, reviewed, and signed by a physician at program entry, every 30 days, and upon program completion

- Outcomes assessment that evaluates progress from entry to completion of the CR course:
  - Includes objective clinical measures of exercise performance
  - Includes self-reported measures of exertion and behavior

- Cardiac risk factor modification, tailored to individual needs, that includes education, counseling, and behavioral interventions
- Psychosocial assessment that includes a description of the tool, interpretation of the score, and a plan of action with an identified time line, based on the assessment outcome
- One or more medical directors who are responsible for the program and are involved (in consultation with staff) in directing the progress of individual patients in the program
- Physician supervision that is immediately available and accessible for medical consultations and medical emergencies at all times during which CR is being furnished
  - See Medicare policies for interpretation and requirements for compliance with this standard.

*12-month window applies only to postacute MI in the federal regulation. Other diagnoses have no time window *unless additional requirements are stipulated in local Medicare policies.*

by CMS. Therefore, it is important to remain current on regulatory aspects of program delivery. CR program professionals can stay current through active participation in local, state, and national professional organizations. Networking at this level ensures that accurate and timely information is received. Erroneous or outdated information can lead to detrimental consequences.

CMS has designated two areas as appropriate for delivery of CR and ICR services, namely, physician office and hospital outpatient setting.

As the applicability of telemedicine expands, CR could be an appropriate outpatient service to use this emerging technology. Some private payers recognize the patient benefits of telemedicine to improve CR utilization and reimburse for hybrid or home CR. At this time, CMS does not reimburse for CR services that use this alternative model.

The Medicare provision lists required components of a CR program. Eligible diagnoses are subject to change; therefore, they should be obtained from current CMS regulations. Medical emergencies and equipment necessary for appropriate preparedness are discussed in chapter 14.

Documentation

The ITP should be a clear, concise, logical, and organized evaluation and intervention plan, which is essential for capturing the comprehensive components that are provided. Relevant documentation includes subjective and objective information and measurable indices for describing outcomes (see chapter 13). For Medicare beneficiaries, outcomes assessment evaluates progress related to the CR treatment and includes the following:

- Assessments based on patient-centered outcomes measured from entry to completion of CR
- Objective clinical measures of exercise performance and self-reported measures of exertion and behavior

The following considerations should influence the documentation format and the use of terminology:

- Clarity of information—Information should be accessible and understandable.
- Consistency of information—The type and extent of information should be consistent from patient to patient and staff member to staff member.
- Simplicity of language—Use of medical jargon, abbreviations, and acronyms should be minimized.
- Efficiency of information—Essential information should be recorded accurately and succinctly, without duplication of documentation, using acceptable abbreviations and terminology.
- Reliability and consistency of records—Electronic medical records and computerized documentation methods are preferred.

An ITP tailored to each patient is developed prior to or at the initial CR session. Guideline 12.5 lists information that should be included in the ITP. The ITP is CMS-required documentation that must be completed or revised at program

---

 Guideline 12.5 Individualized Treatment Plan (ITP)

The initial, periodic, and discharge ITP should be individualized to each patient and include the following:

- A description of the patient's diagnosis
- Type, amount, frequency, and duration of the items and services furnished under the plan
- Physician-prescribed exercise (aerobic, strengthening, and stretching) appropriate for the individual patient

- Goals set for the patient under the plan
- Development and timely progression of the ITP by the CR staff with direction, review, and signature of the medical director

entry, every 30 days, and upon program completion. A physician develops, reviews, and updates the initial exercise prescription every 30 days. All members of the CR team should be familiar with and provide input on the ITP as the patient progresses through CR. The ITP tells the patient's story and documents progress during CR. Programs should determine which outcomes need to be measured at program entry and completion versus those collected more frequently, such as weekly or monthly. Patients may have different needs in regard to frequency of measurement for specific outcomes. MAC-specific regulations may dictate the timing for the administration of some outcomes measurements.

All communications with physicians, other health care professionals, and families that may affect patient outcomes must be documented in compliance with general guidelines. Communication includes telephone conversations with physicians or physician extenders regarding adverse reactions to exercise therapy, progress on risk factor modification, and formal physician communications. Any occurrences related to clinical status, including those away from the program, should be documented; examples include changes in medical therapy, new signs or symptoms, physician visits, or other information that could be relevant to patient progress or outcome.

The program director should be knowledgeable of the rules and regulations regarding reimbursement. Before enrollment, it is important to verify the insurance coverage for CR services, including billing codes, reimbursement amounts, copayments and coinsurance, and specific plan limitations and requirements. Variations in commercial insurance plans are numerous, and eligible diagnoses may vary. In situations where coverage rules are a barrier to participation or are clinically inappropriate, intervention and education by the CR staff and medical director would be important to communicate to the payer. It could be beneficial for CR program staff to identify the common private insurance plans in the geographical location and provide them information on program operations and goals, including meaningful patient outcomes. Ultimately, insurance verification, proper coding and billing practices, and successful and accurate payment require close oversight by the program director in collaboration with the institution's business office personnel. Thorough training of CR staff is essential.

Personnel

Qualified health care personnel, including the program medical director, are integral to a successful program. The collective knowledge, skills, and clinical experience of the professional staff reflect the multidisciplinary competencies necessary to affect the desired treatment outcomes (see guideline 12.6). The clinical skills and medico-legal authority required for patient safety can be ensured by following appropriate requirements and recommendations for individual staff positions.

The knowledge and technical skills required for optimal care are derived from several disciplines and health care professions. No federal requirements or organization guidelines exist in regard to staff–patient ratios or specific disciplines in the composition of the staff. However, individual state laws might dictate staffing requirements. Given the multidisciplinary nature of the

---

Guideline 12.6   Medical Director Qualifications

- Every outpatient CR program shall have a medical director or team of medical directors who share the responsibility.
- Standards for the physician(s) responsible for a CR program are as follows:
  - Expertise in the management of patients with cardiac pathophysiology,
  - cardiopulmonary training in basic life support or advanced cardiac life support, and
  - license to practice medicine in the state in which the CR program is offered.

program, this flexibility allows even small clinical facilities to meet program competency guidelines. Each program and facility should select personnel with professional specialties that fit the model and policies of the institution and the human resource department. Additionally, title and level of positions are a function of the institution and program. Nevertheless, the collective knowledge base of the staff should include a comprehensive understanding of CVD, cardiovascular emergency procedures, nutrition, exercise physiology, pharmacology, behavior change strategies, health psychology, and medical and educational strategies for CVD risk factor management. Licensed and nonlicensed health care professionals may be included on the CR team. Any existing individual state laws would take precedence over these guidelines.

The professions most frequently represented in the essential staff positions include specially trained registered nurses, clinical exercise physiologists, dietitians, health educators, health psychologists, vocational rehabilitation counselors, physical therapists, occupational therapists, pharmacists, and physicians. Staff should participate in multidisciplinary patient care continuing educational activities. Ongoing education and certification of staff also ensures the maintenance of competence. The competency guidelines for program personnel specified here agree with standards published in the AACVPR Core Competencies document[11] (see table 12.1).

Core Functions

Core functions for CR programs include the provision and coordination of a broad range of services and adequate emergency response capability. In addition, each program professional should possess a common core of professional and clinical competencies regardless of academic discipline. The following are recommended minimum qualifications for all CR staff:

- Bachelor's degree in a health field such as exercise science or licensure in the jurisdiction, such as for a registered nurse or physical therapist; or designation as registered respiratory therapist, per state practice laws that regulate respiratory therapists

- Experience or specialty training in CR as outlined in the AACVPR Core Competencies document

- Successful completion of basic life support (BLS) course with training in advanced cardiac life support (ACLS) preferred

Staff recommendations and core competencies specific to emergency services in CR are discussed in chapter 14.

Program Staff

This section outlines specific personnel and associated core competencies typically found in program settings. AACVPR offers a voluntary certification (Certified Cardiac Rehabilitation Professional [CCRP]) for CR professionals, based on the AACVPR Core Competencies.[11] Successful obtainment of this certification reflects an advanced knowledge of exercise physiology, nutrition, risk factor modification strategies, counseling techniques, and uses of behavioral change programs and technologies as applied to CR and SP services. The CCRP, exclusively for CR professionals, is the only certification aligned with the CR core competencies. This voluntary certification is appropriate for staff with various degrees working in CR who meet the qualifications to take the examination. It is the preferred certification for CR staff members.

Medical Director

Guideline 12.6 presents qualifications mandated by CMS for medical directors. The primary responsibilities are as follows[33]:

- Ensuring that the CR program is safe, comprehensive, cost effective, and medically appropriate for individual patients

- Ensuring that policies and procedures are consistent with evidence-based guidelines

- Ensuring that the program complies with regulatory standards

The interactive role of multiple physicians and team members involved in patient care is strengthened by active leadership of the medical director.

Program Director: Preferred Qualifications

- Master's degree in an allied health field, such as exercise physiology, or licensure as a health care practitioner in a related health care discipline such as a registered nurse or physical therapist (or both master's degree and licensure)

- Mastery of the AACVPR Core Competencies, as indicated by current certification as a CCRP
- Experience in staff coordination and delivery of CR services to patients
- Successful completion of AHA BLS and, where applicable, ACLS courses

Registered Nurse: Preferred Qualifications

- License to practice as a registered nurse in the jurisdiction
- Where applicable, successful completion of an ACLS course
- Mastery of the AACVPR Core Competencies, as indicated by current certification as a CCRP

Exercise Specialist: Preferred Qualifications

- Bachelor's in exercise science or related field
- Where applicable, successful completion of an ACLS course
- Mastery of the AACVPR Core Competencies, as indicated by current certification as a CCRP

Clinical Exercise Physiologist: Preferred Qualifications

- Master's degree in exercise science or related field
- Where applicable, successful completion of an ACLS course
- Mastery of the AACVPR Core Competencies, as indicated by current certification as a CCRP

Physical Therapist: Preferred Qualifications

- License to practice physical therapy in the jurisdiction
- Where applicable, successful completion of an ACLS course
- Experience in the identification and physical remediation of various musculoskeletal limitations that may be present in CR patients
- Mastery of the AACVPR Core Competencies, as indicated by current certification as a CCRP

Respiratory Therapist: Preferred Qualifications

- Licensure or registration (per state law) for practice in the jurisdiction as a respiratory therapist

- Successful completion of an ACLS course
- Mastery of the AACVPR Core Competencies, as indicated by current certification as a CCRP

Registered Dietitian: Preferred Qualifications

- Master's degree in nutrition
- Registered dietitian status with the American Dietetic Association
- Experience in practicing therapeutic dietetics in a clinical or community setting, particularly in areas of lipid disorders, obesity, diabetes, and hypertension

Mental Health Professional: Preferred Qualifications

- License for practice in the jurisdiction as a clinical social worker, counselor, psychologist, or psychiatrist
- Experience in psychological assessment, administration of behavioral health interventions, and counseling with CR or chronic disease

Health Educator: Preferred Qualifications

- Certification as a health education specialist
- Master's degree in health education
- Experience in providing individual and group educational programs for patients and family members to reduce CVD risk factors and promote health self-maintenance
- Experience in the wide range of available technologies to provide individual health self-monitoring and promote positive health behaviors

Occupational Therapist: Preferred Qualifications

- Master's degree in occupational therapy
- License to practice as an occupational therapist in the jurisdiction, if applicable
- Registration with the American Occupational Therapy Association
- Experience in providing occupational therapy to CVD patients or related field

Vocational Rehabilitation Counselor: Preferred Qualifications

- Master's degree in vocational rehabilitation counseling

- Experience in vocational counseling with CR patients

Staff Education and Performance Review

All professional staff should strive for full and independent functioning in the content areas described in the AACVPR Core Competencies document. It is recognized that mastery of all knowledge and skills criteria is an ongoing process. Policies should be in place regarding the number of continuing education hours, in-services, and educational experiences required of staff. TJC and most other surveying organizations require documentation of monthly emergency education and skill in-services, department meetings, agendas, education programs, and completed certifications and certificates. The policies and procedures manual should describe the department's continuing education process.

Continuum of Care and Services

Policies delineating the integration of all activities directly or indirectly related to the continuum of care from entry through exit should be in place. The needs of patients should be matched with the appropriate appraisals, programs, and services. Policies in this section should establish the process by which the patient is able to move through the SP program, affording a minimum of difficulty and excess time involvement, with a clear understanding of the process and expectations. These policies should address

- appointment scheduling,
- parking,
- registration,
- insurance preauthorization and enrollment,
- participation barriers addressed through program options to meet patient's treatment needs,
- informed consent,
- intermittent progress evaluations, and
- communication between the program and primary caregiver(s) throughout CR, including discharge planning and follow-up.

Establishing a program does not require a large facility with state-of-the-art equipment, a large staff, and the most expensive monitoring equipment. A menu of program options should be available to best meet each patient's CR needs. Innovative programs could include such designs as these:

- Telephonic health coaching and similar supplemental phone software applications
- Less-frequent center-based CR sessions with a well-structured home exercise regimen for patients who travel from a farther distance or have other barriers to more frequent weekly participation
- A higher-frequency program, for example five days/week, for patients who are able and eager to progress more rapidly or have a short-term window for program participation
- Flexible attendance options for patients with other obligations that prohibit a rigid schedule of attendance

There are opportunities for facilitating a successful transition through partnering early outpatient CR programs with maintenance programs in existing facilities such as high school and elementary school gymnasiums, YMCAs, Jewish Community Centers, and other fitness facilities.

Summary

A knowledgeable and well-trained multidisciplinary team that can provide guidance and support is critically important to the successful, long-term management of patients with CVD. The synergism of effective exercise training principles coupled with the application of behavior change strategies are vital components of this well-established disease management program known as CR. The science supporting CR interventions has advanced dramatically and should continue to be the foundation of departmental policies and procedures. Continual assessment of program paradigm and patient outcomes is fundamental to the primary goal of delivering a valued, cost-effective, patient-centered service to diverse populations.[34,35] The medical community and health insurance industry recognize CR as a treatment that has demonstrated significant, positive patient outcomes with respect to mortality, morbidity, risk factor reduction and management, and QoL.

Outcomes Assessment and Utilization

Sherry L. Grace, PhD, FCCS, FAACVPR, CRFC

Major CR societies, including AACVPR, recommend outcome assessment as a standard of care, including degree of program utilization (i.e., enrollment, adherence, and completion).[3-6] Outcomes reflect program performance and quality. Therefore, the process of measuring, collecting, and analyzing patient outcomes is a critical component of the successful provision of health care services. Ideally, outcomes applied should reflect therapeutic goals and drive tailored approaches to disease management.[7]

OBJECTIVES

This chapter aims to do the following:

- Define outcome domains based on the Cardiac Rehabilitation Outcomes Matrix[1,2] (table 13.1), including utilization indicators, and provide examples of tools that can be used to measure these outcomes in CR.

- Forward recommendations for creating a comprehensive, systematic approach for collecting, tracking, analyzing, and reporting outcomes data within routine clinical practice such as through AACVPR's registry.

- Introduce how outcomes are used to plan and implement quality improvement (QI) projects in CR.

An outcomes-focused approach to patient care occurs at two levels: (1) measuring clinical variables for individual patients at program entry and at subsequent intervals to assess individual patient outcomes, and (2) evaluating aggregate patient outcomes at periodic intervals to assess program effectiveness. Health status is assessed at CR program entry to determine priorities and objectives in order to develop an ITP. Utilization indicators such as referral, enrollment, adherence, and completion enable ascertainment that indicated patients are accessing and taking full advantage of CR, to achieve the associated benefits.[8,9] Formal assessments should be repeated during the program as appropriate and at program exit. Outcomes measured during the program are used to evaluate patient progress and guide discharge and long-term goal planning (guideline 13.1).

Purposes for Measuring Outcomes

Measuring, reporting, and comparing outcomes are important steps toward improving patient health outcomes.[10] Simply providing service to patients at a reasonable cost without assessing the benefit does not establish program efficacy. In addition, measuring various parameters without careful consideration of the outcomes assessment process can result in misleading conclusions.

While measuring outcomes is a requirement for AACVPR program certification and recertification, it should not be the sole purpose for tracking outcomes. Programs are encouraged to benchmark (evaluate or compare to a recognized standard) outcome findings externally with comparable programs. The AACVPR offers the CR Registry for this purpose,[11] providing a mecha-nism for evaluating program effectiveness. Once programs have been benchmarked externally or internally, staff is encouraged to use the findings to assess further opportunities for quality assurance.

Emphasizing the importance of program outcome measurement to administrators, medical directors, and clinicians creates buy-in at all levels. Securing administrative support for measuring program outcomes increases the likelihood of a successful outcomes tracking program. Value is measured by results; thus, outcomes measurement becomes significant to consumers and third-party payers (entities that reimburse and manage health care expenses).

BOTTOM LINE

Measuring patient and program outcomes is necessary because

- it is a requirement of CMS.
- it provides objective data regarding program effectiveness.
- it results in data used to inform and educate patients, referring physicians and other clinicians, hospital administrators, and third-party payers.
- it allows for benchmarking results against recognized standards.
- it is required for AACVPR program certification.

Outcomes Matrix

The CR Outcomes Matrix (table 13.1)[2] is the model that the AACVPR suggests for classifying and organizing measurable patient outcomes in CR (see guideline 13.2). The AACVPR Registry also offers data elements and recommended validated scales to assess patient outcomes in these domains.[11]

Guideline 13.1 Outcomes Assessment

Program professionals should uniformly measure outcomes across all domains of the core CR components and use these analyses to develop, monitor, and drive QI projects in order to promote effective treatments and optimal outcomes. The resulting data provide valuable information for quality improvement, accreditation, certification, and reimbursement.

Guideline 13.2 CR Outcomes Matrix

AACVPR recommends using the CR Outcomes Matrix as a guide for a systematic approach to assess patient outcomes.

Table 13.1 AACVPR CR Outcomes Matrix

Core components of care	Clinical	Behavioral	Health	Service
Overall management	Risk factor profile Evaluation of symptoms Hemodynamic responses ADLs assessment	Self-efficacy 1. Improved knowledge and application of self-care actions 2. Return to desired PA level 3. Desire to return to work Cardiac disease knowledge score Appropriate response to symptoms and complications Medication adherence, compliance Accessibility to needed resources Session attendance rate	Morbidity and mortality Health care utilization: 1. Hospitalizations, readmissions 2. Emergency room visits 3. Physician sick visits Untoward events during supervised sessions Health-related QoL Return to work, loss of work days	Patient satisfaction 1. Satisfaction with the care received 2. Progress toward goals Performance measures 1. Cost per patient 2. Program cost 3. Enrollment rate 4. Dropout rate 5. Completion rate 6. Admission rate
Exercise testing and training[2]	Exercise testing 1. Maximal exercise test 2. Submaximal exercise test or functional assessment (e.g., 6-minute walk test) Resting, exercise, and recovery responses 1. Heart rate and rhythm 2. Blood pressure 3. Rating of perceived effort 4. Peak METs 5. Rating of perceived dyspnea 6. Oxygen saturation level	Exercise compliance 1. Supervised sessions 2. Home or outside sessions 3. Adherence to exercise prescription Energy expenditure 1. Min of PA/week 2. Calorie expenditure daily, weekly PA stage of change		
Strength and flexibility training[2]	Strength measures (e.g., 1RM, 5RM, grip strength) Flexibility measures (e.g., sit-and-reach test, goniometer)			
Lipid management[3]	Lipid levels Initiation of or adjustment in medication dosage	Adherence to diet, exercise, and medications Diet and exercise stage of change		
Hypertension management[3]	Resting BP Exercise and recovery BPs Initiation of or adjustment in antihypertension medication dosage	Adherence to diet, exercise, and medications Diet and exercise stage of change Self-monitoring behaviors		
Diabetes management[3]	BG levels HbA1c Initiation of or adjustment in hypoglycemic medication dosage	Adherence to diet, exercise, and medications Diet and exercise stage of change Self-monitoring behaviors		

(continued)

Table 13.1 *(continued)*

Core components of care	Clinical	Behavioral	Health	Service
Nutrition and weight management[3]	Anthropometric measures 1. Height, weight, BMI 2. Body fat, lean body weight measures 3. Abdominal circumference 4. Sum of skinfolds, girths Nutritional biochemical markers, bone mineral density test	Adherence to diet and exercise Diet and exercise stage of change Diet recording logs PA recording logs Diet habit scores		
Psychosocial management[3]	Measurements of mood Depression, anxiety, hostility, emotional distress Measurements of cognitive function Memory, orientation, judgment	Coping mechanisms Stress management and relaxation skills Social support network Sexual dysfunction		
Smoking cessation[3]	Serum cotinine levels Exhaled carbon monoxide Number of cigarettes or cigars smoked per day Duration of smoking habit (pack-years)	Smoking stage of change		

Abbreviations: ADLs, activities of daily living; BG, blood glucose; BP, blood pressure; BMI, body mass index; HbA1c, glycosylated hemoglobin; MET, metabolic equivalent; PA, physical activity; RM, repetition maximum; QoL, quality of life.

Adapted from Sanderson, Southard and Oldridge (2004).

The CR Outcomes Matrix[2] was developed by the AACVPR Outcomes Committee and is designed to link outcomes assessment to the evidence-based core components of CR and SP.[12] *Core components* are elements of patient care that have strong scientific evidence of their ability to optimize CVD risk reduction, reduce disability, and promote healthy behaviors. The matrix provides a standardized method for categorizing outcome measures for each component across these four domains: clinical, behavioral, health, and service. The clinical, behavioral, and health domains are based on Green's PRECEDE Model.[13] The service domain was created by the AACVPR as a category to measure patient satisfaction and service utilization. Examples of outcome measures in each domain are shown in sidebars Examples of Clinical Domain Measures and Relevant Instruments, Behavioral Domain Measures and Relevant Instruments, Health Domain Measures and Relevant Instruments, and in the service area as well.

The rationale for the measurement of multiple outcomes across each domain is the inherent value in assessment of effectiveness of patient care and individual progress toward achieving goals.[14] Given the number of risk factors that must be controlled in order to achieve optimal secondary prevention,[15] multiple outcomes used collectively best define success for patients and programs.[7] For example, if assessment of a clinical outcome related to exercise capacity (e.g., change in MET level during or following CR) indicates that a patient or program has not achieved the goal, then staff can evaluate the processes of providing PA or specific exercise programming to more effectively influence the clinical outcome.

Outcomes should be clinically relevant, measurable, patient-centered, and consistent with patient care goals as set forth in the ITP. Depending on available program resources, program directors should select from the measures best suited for their population. All outcome measures selected for assessment should be within the means of the CR program, not only to adequately and reliably assess, but also to influence and manage. Burden to staff and patients to collect the outcome measures should also be considered.

Outcomes should be assessed systematically, at a minimum, at program entry and at discharge. It is very important to collect discharge data in as many patients as possible so that outcome assessment is not biased. The AACVPR Registry website puts forth strategies to assist programs to optimize follow-up data collection.[11] Programs should consider inviting patients who do not complete the program to return so that outcomes can be assessed. Alternatively, patients could be contacted by phone or by mail (electronically or otherwise) to assess patient-reported outcomes. Ideally, outcomes should also be assessed during the program (as applicable) and at later follow-up, such as six months and one year after the program.

BOTTOM LINE

- Outcomes data should be gathered and recorded in a systematic and predetermined fashion.
- Outcome measures should be obtained from the following four domains: clinical, behavioral, health, and service.
- Outcomes should be clinically relevant, measurable, patient centered, and consistent with patient care goals.
- It is important that a proper balance be established between the resources required of the staff to measure and record outcomes and the burden (time and otherwise) placed on patients.

Clinical Outcomes Domain

This domain includes physical and psychosocial outcome variables that relate to the evaluation of disease status and the effects of therapy. Clinical outcomes include the results of tests used for the assessment of risk factors (e.g., physiological measurements and laboratory values), and the prognostic evaluation of the disease. Physical or biometric variables such as measured or estimated exercise capacity,[16] BP, blood lipids, HbA1c, and anthropometric measurements are common clinical measures.[2] Tobacco use can be assessed via self-report, but the potential exists for socially desirable responding (see Behavioral Domain, later in this chapter).

The results of surveys, questionnaires, or other instruments used to assess psychosocial function are also included in this domain. Psychological measures include assessments of depression, anxiety, and anger or hostility.[17] The reliability of these findings increases when scientifically valid and reliable questionnaires and instruments are used and, in the case of depression and anxiety, when a structured clinical interview is performed by a regulated mental health care professional. The AACVPR Registry has several accepted measures for depression.[11] Examples of clinical outcomes are shown in the sidebar Examples of Clinical Domain Measures and Relevant Instruments.

Behavioral Domain

Outcomes within this domain are individualized and reflect knowledge, adherence to medical and behavioral therapies, and return to previous roles and activities (e.g., work, domestic, relationship).[2] This domain includes core components such as individual behavioral management of exercise, nutrition, smoking, and medication adherence. These measures reveal the patient's ability to make and maintain recommended lifestyle changes that lead to goal achievement in the clinical and health domains. Behavioral interventions offered to the patient are determined as a result of abnormal or unsatisfactory clinical findings. For example, if a patient has hyperlipidemia and a BMI of 31 kg/m², behavioral interventions such as a dietary consult and weight loss program will be recommended. Provision of these services or components should also be documented.

Behavioral measures are typically obtained through the use of standardized questionnaires or logs or diaries to characterize adherence to a prescribed regimen of PA, diet, or medications. It is important to review the ITP with each patient to determine adherence to the plan. The ITP follow-up is an opportunity for reassessing individual behavioral goals and determining patient progress. Adherence to healthy lifestyle behaviors and to medication therapies is integral to the attainment of sustained benefits. Examples of additional behavioral outcomes are provided in the sidebar Behavioral Domain Measures and Relevant Instruments.

Health Domain

The health domain represents general or primary indicators of health outcomes that include morbidity, mortality, and QoL. Outcomes related to the overall health of the patient include the occurrence, recurrence, or exacerbations of the primary disease or comorbid conditions, either fatal or nonfatal; the impact of the disease on QoL; and use of health care resources in response to these events. Unfortunately, changes in morbidity and mortality associated with CR participation are generally not readily available to most CR programs, particularly once the patient has been discharged from the program.

Examples of Clinical Domain Measures and Relevant Instruments

- Cardiorespiratory fitness:
    - Functional MET level (and change)
    - Graded exercise test MET level[16]
    - 1RM (strength) or equivalent (e.g., 5RM)
    - Joint-specific ROM
    - 6-minute walk test distance[18]
    - Balance and mobility tests[19]
    - Duke Activity Status Index[20]
- Smoking:
    - Blood cotinine level
    - Carbon monoxide level
- BP
- Lipids (TC, LDL-C, HDL-C, TG)

- Anthropometric data:
    - Waist circumference
    - BMI
    - Percent body fat
- Diabetes:
    - BG level
    - Fasting glucose
    - HbA1c
- Psychosocial assessments:
    - Beck Depression Inventory-II (available on the Pearson Assessments website)[a,21]
    - Center for Epidemiologic Studies-Depression[22]
    - Hospital Anxiety and Depression Scale[23]
    - Patient Health Questionnaire-9[24]
    - Psychosocial Risk Factor Survey[a,25]

[a]Requires licensing or usage fee.

Behavioral Domain Measures and Relevant Instruments

- Step counts per day (log)
- Home exercise diary
- International Physical Activity Questionnaire[26]
- Tobacco use (e.g., number of cigarettes smoked per day, packs per day, or other forms of tobacco)
- Frequency of exposure to secondhand smoke
- Medication adherence (pill counts, filled prescriptions)
- Morisky Medication Adherence Scale[a,27]

    - Diet Habit Survey[a,28]
    - MEDFICTS[29,30]
    - Block Food Frequency Questionnaire[a]

- Coronary Artery Disease Questionnaire (CADE-Q)[31]

[a]May require a licensing or usage fee.

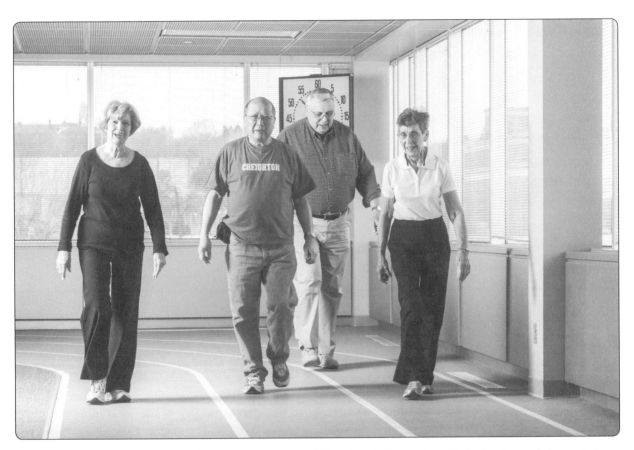

Patients should be encouraged to assume responsibility for their own health behaviors while participating in CR.

Health status and health-related quality of life (HRQoL) are important to the patient and, unlike morbidity and mortality, can more easily be measured; thus, the AACVPR recommends that HRQoL be measured by CR programs.[32] HRQoL tools that measure various aspects of health affected by disease and treatment provide a global health profile.[33] The three main dimensions of HRQoL are (1) physical function, (2) psychological well-being, and (3) social functioning. Tools used to measure HRQoL may be disease specific or generic. The disease-specific instrument provides an indication of the patient's perception of health with regard to specific disease components such as symptoms. Generic tools can be used when one is comparing patient health status to that of an apparently healthy or other diseased population. If resources allow, both types of tools should be used. Examples of other common health outcomes are provided in the sidebar Health Domain Measures and Rel-

evant Instruments, and the AACVPR Registry has several accepted tools.[11]

Service Domain

QIs relate to program-level outcomes, structure, and processes.[37] This domain captures measures related to patient satisfaction, service utilization, cost of providing services, and program performance in meeting evidence-based goals (outcomes as previously mentioned, but at the program level). When the aggregate of individual service domain outcomes is analyzed, the quality of the services provided can be evaluated and future program needs can be better identified and prioritized.

A patient's satisfaction with personal progress toward goals and with the CR program is an outcome that merits greater attention. Programs should assess patient satisfaction with care or services received while attending and at the end of the program. Patient satisfaction is inherently

---

Health Domain Measures and Relevant Instruments

- Mortality following CR discharge (all-cause and cardiovascular)
- Morbidity—emergency department visits and hospital admissions related to primary diagnosis, all-cause, or both[a]
- Progression of HF
- Stroke or transient ischemic attack
- Health-related quality of life instruments:
  - Dartmouth Primary Care Cooperative (CO-OP) charts[34]
  - EuroQol EQ-5D[b]
  - Ferrans and Powers Quality of Life Index-Cardiac Version
  - MacNew Health-Related Quality of Life Instrument[b]
  - Medical Outcomes Study SF-36/12 Health Status Questionnaire[35,b]
  - Nottingham Health Profile[36]

---

[a]As program resources allow.

[b]Requires licensing or usage fee.

---

subjective and based on personal experience. However, validated scales assessing CR satisfaction, as well as generic satisfaction with chronic illness recovery are available and should be used.[38] Examples of recommended measures are provided in the sidebar Service Domain Instruments for Patient Satisfaction.

To evaluate program performance, individual observations are compiled and aggregated, then evaluated for internal or external benchmarking purposes, such as through the AACVPR Registry.[11] Performance measures (PMs) and QIs to measure overall program performance have been developed by AACVPR;[41,42] the ACC and AHA;[43] as well as the Australian,[6] Canadian,[44] British,[45] and European[46] CR associations. Those measures have been reviewed elsewhere.[47] Utilization indicators such as CR referral rate, enrollment, wait times, adherence, and completion rates are also important outcomes (see sidebar titled CR Utilization Indicators). Indeed, some of these utilization PMs were endorsed by the National Quality Forum in 2010.

Service Domain Instruments for Patient Satisfaction

- CR Preference Form-Revised[39]
- Patient Assessment of Chronic Illness Care[40]

Numerator and denominator specifications are provided for the measures. Exclusion criteria for patients who should not be counted are specified. Other measures such as the fiscal value of services provided for CR patients may also be assessed when one is evaluating program outcomes.[32]

Measuring, Documenting, Analyzing, and Reporting Program Outcomes

An effective program of measuring CR outcomes requires a systematic, coordinated team approach. Ensuring that team members are informed about that process is critical to achieving a quality outcomes program. Protocols and policies defining the outcome assessment process will increase the likelihood of accurate outcomes reporting. Program staff should recognize that factors outside of CR, including the recovery process itself and medical oversight, can affect the results.[48]

The process begins with data collection and measurement. Outcome assessments can be documented using customized program spreadsheets, CR electronic patient records, or the AACVPR Registry.[11] Following documentation, data analysis provides for interpretation of the results. The final step in the process is the reporting phase, which may include several audiences. Generally, outcomes are reported at staff meetings, on QI

CR Utilization Indicators

CR patient referral from the inpatient setting:

- All appropriate patients hospitalized with a primary diagnosis of an acute MI or chronic stable angina or who during hospitalization have undergone coronary artery bypass graft surgery, a percutaneous coronary intervention, cardiac valve surgery, or cardiac transplantation are to be referred to an outpatient CR program.

---

teams, in administrative and clinical committees, and at professional conferences.

Data Collection and Measurement

Outcomes measurement is a core component of CR. Hence, data collection should not be viewed as an extra or laborious task. In fact, many of the data points are included in the standard measurements obtained during the patient intake and discharge assessments. Taking advantage of this connection can significantly reduce the time required to track outcomes and minimize data entry errors.

CR referral is a key metric. Capturing it accurately requires linking with cardiology practices and inpatient units in the surrounding area. While it can be labor intensive and requires partnership, it is very worthwhile for CR programs to understand the proportion of indicated patients that are being referred,[49] and whether inequities exist in the characteristics of patients being referred.[50] Indeed, it has been demonstrated that CR referral can be reliably measured.[51]

Several sources for obtaining CR outcome data exist. They include referral forms, medical records (from CR but also from health care encounters for the referral event), patient interviews, observation, surveys, registries, and administrative databases. Medical records are one of the preferred sources for collating lab results, BP, and other clinical outcomes. CR charts should be scrutinized to ascertain structure and process measures such as patient receipt of each core component, including patient education and stress management (e.g., smokers received a cessation intervention, depressed patients received mental health care). Although not routinely possible, linkage to hospital records or administrative databases can enable assessment in the health domain.

The surveys selected for data collection should (1) be appropriate for the cardiac population, (2) be reliable and valid, (3) be appropriate to the context of CR services, (4) be sensitive to change during the course of CR, (5) place minimal burden on the patient, and (6) be easily scored and interpreted. As much as possible, instruments should provide objective endpoints of the outcome(s) they purport to assess. Questionnaires assessing psychosocial aspects of the clinical domain, such as hostility, anxiety, or depression, are typically self-reported. When the patient's primary language is other than English, a validated translation should be sought or the tool should not be administered.

Sustainability of patient outcomes demonstrates program benefit; therefore, collecting outcome data up to 12 months postdischarge is strongly encouraged. Not only is follow-up desirable; it is also important because adherence to lifestyle behaviors diminishes within the first three to six months after the end of treatment. Follow-up outcome data can be acquired by clinic visit, phone, mail, or electronically. Clinic visit or electronic chart audit at associated clinics with patient consent is required in order to collect biochemical outcomes. Patient-reported outcomes such as health behaviors and HRQoL can be collected by phone, by mail, or electronically. Again, linkage to hospital or administrative databases enables objective assessment of long-term morbidity and mortality.

Documentation

Documentation of the initial assessment and reassessments of patient outcomes throughout the program and at discharge is a requirement set forth by the CMS. Ultimately, it is the responsibility of the program director or manager to ensure that team members are properly familiarized with documentation forms, as well as with the process for accurately documenting outcome measures.[52] Direct oversight or audits are recommended in order to ensure correct outcome documentation and accurate reporting, along with associated policies for data rectification and training to prevent recurrent errors.

To promote accuracy, the implementation of written standards and data definitions for describing the process of data acquisition cannot be overemphasized. Forms for documenting outcomes are available through position statements such as the papers on performance measures.[41] These forms are intended to simplify outcomes documentation. Assessment forms that make liberal use of check boxes and option lists ease the process of recording outcome information. The ITP can serve as a ready guide for outcome documentation and simplifies the process for data entry before analysis of the data. Forms may serve dual roles as data management systems and as reporting tools to health care providers. More powerful tools, such as database applications, electronic medical records, and registries, can use error detection, validation, and reminder algorithms to ensure complete and accurate data entry.

Consideration should be given to who is most responsible and accountable for documenting each of the outcomes. Attention should be made to clinical knowledge requirements and also cost efficiency. Where data points are not already captured, another consideration is whether an administrative assistant or clinician should be extracting or entering it. Accountability for the various outcomes should be delegated clearly and kept consistent as much as possible, while maintaining cost and time efficiencies. If clinicians are entering the information, patient rapport should not be impacted, which may require documentation or entry after, rather than during, a clinical encounter.

Data Analysis

Outcomes data analysis should take place when sufficient quantities of data have been collected. Preferably, a review of aggregate program outcome data should take place quarterly. Program staff should review data for completeness and for change in values from entry to discharge to follow-up, as well as for trends in measures over time. To calculate percentage change for an individual patient, the difference between the entry and discharge values is divided by the entry value. Simple outcome calculations provide valuable feedback with regard to patient progress toward individual and program goals. This analytic process high-

lights patient outcomes at a single point in time; however, the true value of outcomes assessment is in using the data to track changes over time.

It is preferable to report outcomes for all patients enrolled in CR; separate analysis should also be done on those patients who do not complete the program and the reasons for noncompletion. At a minimum, report values should include sample size (number of patients included in the analysis) and means or percentages, depending on the specific measure. More advanced programs may wish to report standard deviations, median values, or other statistical comparisons as needed to inferentially convey the significance of the outcomes.

After individual change scores are assessed, group data can be analyzed to assess outcomes of the CR group as a whole. The mean values for the entire group can be compared internally to determine program effectiveness. Aggregated outcome results can also be compared externally, such as when programs participate in the AACVPR registry.[11] Programs may wish to enlist or collaborate with a scientist to undertake more advanced analyses, including inferential tests and adjustments for patient characteristics.

Reporting and Interpreting Outcomes

Results from outcome assessments and patient questionnaires or surveys should be shared with the patient and health care provider(s), including CR providers as well as referring and primary care physicians. In addition, opportunities should be sought to communicate outcome findings to program administrators and health care payers to demonstrate program effectiveness or, conversely, treatment gaps that can be improved.

For patients, a review of outcomes allows them to see the improvements they have made, and the degree to which they have achieved their short- and long-term goals. This information must be presented in such a way that takes into account their health information literacy.[53] Outcomes review can support discussion with patients regarding risk factors that may not yet be at guideline target, and hence to revisit goals and associated behaviors. Patients can also celebrate their successes, which will promote long-term maintenance and hence optimal health outcomes.

Guideline 13.3 Benchmarking Program Outcomes

Outcomes should be benchmarked to historical data, published studies of comparable programs, published policy statements,[49] or through the AACVPR registry[11] to understand program quality.

Clinicians, managers, and administrators understand that it is not sufficient merely to collect outcomes. In order to make positive improvements to systems and processes, it is necessary to analyze outcome findings at the programmatic level; compare findings to those outcomes with selected benchmarks; and, when the findings are suboptimal, to initiate QI projects.[10] The outcomes observed are the result of the way in which programs are designed.[54] Therefore, suboptimal programs lead to suboptimal outcomes; highly effective programs produce optimal outcomes. Measuring and analyzing outcome findings can assist staff in ascertaining the quality of a program.

A program must first establish a benchmark by which to compare the effectiveness of care delivery (see guideline 13.3). Benchmark data can come from a number of sources. Programs can establish a historical baseline by using samples of their data aggregated over a specified period of time. These values then serve as internal benchmark measures from which the effects of any procedural changes can be compared. Outcomes from published studies may also be used as a benchmark. However, it is important to first evaluate whether results of a study can be generalized to a specific program population.

Finally, CR registries provide real-world benchmarks.[55] Registries attempt to capture demographic, clinical, and treatment data on individual patients in a standardized fashion over time. Data elements and time frames for measurement are strictly defined and consistently adhered to. Data from the registries are combined across numerous participating sites in order to develop aggregated mean values for each demographic, clinical, behavioral, and health outcome measured. Subsets of data can be created within the registry for further analysis of various demographic and clinical characteristics within specific populations. These data can be helpful when evaluating the outcomes of treatments and disparities observed based on differences in sex, age, race, and socioeconomic status, among other patient-level characteristics. The advantage of participating in a registry is that questions about program processes and structure can be tested using the registries' aggregated data as a benchmark for comparative purposes.

QI Using Program Outcomes

QI has previously been successfully applied in CR programs,[56] and many programs do engage in QI activities.[57] Following the analysis and reporting of outcome findings, team members should identify opportunities for program improvement based on the lowest-performing outcome scores.

Measurement of outcomes is a learning process that helps a program understand what can be improved and clarifies the reasons for improvement. The aim of QI should be learning about a process and should not be about passing judgment.[54]

Many projects suffer from inertia and delay and ultimately failure because of a perceived need to create an ideal project at the outset. Tackling too many outcomes at one time is not advisable. When a program consistently meets the threshold of quality care (which can be viewed in the AACVPR Registry[11] reports), then it is time to move to another outcome or add an outcome to the assessment of program effectiveness.

Once a system or process of care has been targeted for change, programs may select one of many QI models or approaches.[58] They should use evidence-based approaches where possible, such as are synthesized by the Cochrane Collaboration. Interventions to increase CR program utilization in particular would be useful to programs.[59,60] The following discussion highlights the use of Deming's Plan-Do-Study-Act (PDSA) model for planning and implementing a QI project.[61]

Once program outcomes have been analyzed, the planning for the QI project begins. The *planning* phase involves targeting an outcome for improvement and studying aspects of the system or process leading to that outcome. The specific goal of the QI project, its duration, the data required to assess change, how the data will be measured, and those responsible for collecting the data are considered during this stage.

It is in the *do* phase that the so-called experiment is performed and the applicable outcomes continue to be gathered. Some key approaches to improve quality should include patient and provider education, reminder systems, and organizational change.[47] When the planned duration of the study has been reached, the outcome data are analyzed (*study* phase) and results are summarized to determine whether the QI approach was successful.

Lastly, the result of the QI project is used to refine the CR system or procedure (the *act* phase). Lessons can be learned from adopting promising changes and rejecting others. The process of QI is not a singular occurrence but is instead a continuous cycle of study, change, and refinement until the most effective process is formed, resulting in the best outcome for the patient or program.

When the QI study is evaluated, questions like the following are addressed:

- To what extent were strategies employed and adhered to in the project?
- To what extent did program processes change as a result of the QI project?
- What processes were kept or discarded as a result?
- What is the next structure or process that can be evaluated or improved?

Resources

The AACVPR has developed a national CR registry that is available to programs to assist in outcome evaluation and accreditation.[11] Detailed information about the CR registry, including data elements, frequently asked questions, and directions for participation, can be found on the AACVPR website. CR registries in other countries have also been used successfully to assess program outcomes.[45,62,63]

While the actual surveys and questionnaires for the domains are not provided within the CR Outcomes Matrix, recommendations for valid and reliable surveys or questionnaires are identified and listed according to the individual outcome domains that were discussed earlier in this chapter. Additional tools include publications regarding outcome calculations, and considering factors such as reaching guideline targets versus degree of change from pre- to postprogram.[44]

Summary

While the processes and structure for outcome data collection, measurement, and reporting will continue to evolve, outcomes measurement and assessment form an important component of CR performance assessment. Programs should have written policies in place for systematic outcomes assessment and management and should regularly use data for quality assurance and improvement projects. As a result of outcome tracking and reporting, the value of CR programs becomes transparent to patients, providers, and health care payers.

Management of Medical Problems and Emergencies

Jason L. Rengo, MS, FAACVPR

A critical responsibility of a CR program is to provide patients a safe environment while anticipating and preparing for situations involving medical problems and emergencies. This responsibility is important whether the site of service is a hospital, freestanding center, community-based location, or home. It is imperative that the plan for responding to medical problems and emergencies be individualized to the level of professional training of the health care provider and be particular to the site where care is delivered.

OBJECTIVES

The purpose of this chapter is to do the following:

- Describe the response to urgent and emergent medical situations in CR.
- Identify procedures for assessment and screening for potential problems.
- Identify procedures for medical intervention for emergencies, including the use of emergency equipment and standing orders.
- Delineate staff training requirements.
- Describe documentation procedures.

Potential Risks in Outpatient CR

The safety of CR exercise programs is well established, with very low mortality and MI rates during exercise training. An analysis of four reports of exercise-related cardiovascular complications reveals 1 cardiac arrest per 116,906 patient-hours, 1 MI per 219,970 patient-hours, 1 fatality per 752,365 patient-hours, and 1 major complication per 81,670 patient-hours. The low fatality rate is attributed to medically supervised programs that are equipped and prepared to manage adverse events and emergencies, the practice of preprogram medical evaluations, and highly trained staff that are able to identify and treat potential problems.[1] However, even when patients are thoroughly screened at program entry, the potential for adverse medical events before, during, or after exercise is ever present, particularly as more high-risk patients are entering CR programs. Demographic trends indicate that participants in CR are very unfit and increasingly older with a higher prevalence of CVD risk factors and comorbid conditions.[2]

Services offered in health care facilities that have been accredited by the TJC must meet the specific quality and safety standards.[3-6] Guidelines described in this chapter for the management of medical problems and emergencies do not supersede TJC standards but rather complement and further detail the preparation for and delivery of care in CR.

Advance Directives

Advance directives are documents that patients prepare in order to direct their future health care should they become unable to make such decisions. The most common types of advance directives are living wills and durable power of attorney or health care proxy. When a patient enrolls in CR, the staff should ascertain if an advance directive exists; if so, their wishes related to cardiovascular care should be documented and communicated to all staff members. In accordance with the Patient Self-Determination Act, all institutions serving Medicare and Medicaid patients are required to provide information to patients and train health care providers about advance directives and to facilitate completion if a patient so desires. The outpatient CR setting pro-

vides an opportunity for offering this education. Discussions with health care providers regarding patient wishes and desires may lead to a higher prevalence of completion of advance directives.[7,8]

Patient Assessment and Screening

Although patients need to be evaluated and receive medical clearance before entering the CR program, the clinical status of a patient may change. In addition, risk stratification models and routine diagnostic procedures, such as exercise stress testing, may not identify all patients at risk for exercise training–related adverse events. Consequently, it is important to observe and assess patients carefully prior to, during, and after an exercise session.

Staff must anticipate and recognize impending medical problems by evaluating a change in patient condition and providing appropriate intervention. In many cases of impending emergency, patients exhibit warning signs and symptoms. A change in the usual clinical status of a patient should alert staff to the possibility of a developing medical problem (guideline 14.1). The best approach to managing clinical emergencies is through the early recognition of these signs and symptoms that prompt intervention and treatment. Additionally, it is imperative that CR staff regularly train to respond to emergency situations. Creating and responding to real-life scenarios is critical to maintain staff readiness to address medical emergencies when they occur. It is important that the CR team's response to mock or actual emergencies be thoroughly evaluated. Deficiencies need to be identified and provisions put in place to allow for an optimal response in future emergencies.

Guideline 14.2 lists clinical problems CR professionals should recognize and for which they should be prepared to provide immediate intervention. CR program policies and procedures and standing orders should describe specific treatment guidelines (see appendixes A and B for examples). When indicated, new or changing signs and symptoms should be reported to the supervising physician, referring physician, or both.

Angina and Ischemia

Both quality and quantity of chest discomfort or angina equivalent (e.g., atypical chest discomfort,

Guideline 14.1 Routine Patient Assessment and Documentation

All patients should be screened before each exercise session for changes in clinical status including, but not limited to, the following:

- Recent medical history and symptoms (including hospitalizations) since the last patient visit
- Heart rate and rhythm
- ECG (when indicated)

- BP
- Body weight
- Medication compliance and changes in medication regimen

All screening must be documented regardless of the findings.

Guideline 14.2 Clinical Problems Requiring Intervention

Guidelines for managing the following conditions, including standing orders for urgent situations and emergency interventions where appropriate, should be included in program policies and procedures:

- New or changing pattern of angina
- New or changing patterns of dysrhythmia
- Decompensated HF
- Hypoglycemia or hyperglycemia

- Syncopal or near-syncopal episodes
- Hypotension or hypertension
- Dyspnea
- Decreased exercise tolerance
- Depression
- Cardiac or respiratory arrest
- Cerebrovascular accident

shortness of breath), as well as frequency, duration, and triggers for angina (e.g., physical exertion, exposure to cold, the postprandial period, emotional stressors), should be noted. If angina or ischemic changes with ECG monitoring occur during an exercise session the workload, HR, and BP should be recorded as well as associated signs or symptoms (e.g., lightheadedness, diaphoresis, decreased BP, increased dysrhythmias). For patients with stable chronic angina, the medical director should provide clearance according to established program guidelines. Generally, prescribed exercise intensity should be no more than slightly above the ischemic threshold.[9]

Dysrhythmias

Frequency, duration, and type of dysrhythmia(s), including accompanying signs and symptoms, should be noted (e.g., ECG findings of ischemia, lightheadedness, dyspnea, poor perfusion). Dysrhythmias to be documented include, but are not limited to, the following: new onset or symptomatic resting and exercise-induced atrial or ventricular ectopy, tachyarrhythmia, atrioventricular block, symptomatic bradycardia, and intraventricular conduction delays (see Dysrhythmias section in chapter 10).

Heart Failure

Despite having higher overall morbidity and mortality rates, the event rates in exercise training studies in patients with chronic HF have been low. The most common adverse events are postexercise hypotension, atrial and ventricular dysrhythmias, and worsening of HF symptoms.[10,11] Signs and symptoms, such as shortness of breath at rest or with usual activity, weight gain, edema, or decreased exercise tolerance, may indicate worsening HF and should be noted. Patients with decompensated HF should not exercise and need to be referred to their physician or health care provider for evaluation and treatment.

Hypoglycemia or Hyperglycemia

Note pre- or postexercise hypoglycemia or hyperglycemia (in patients with type 1 or 2 diabetes mellitus) and whether the patient is symptomatic. Glucose monitoring equipment should be available along with glucose tablets or gel or other sources of carbohydrate. Patients using either oral agents or insulin should target a BG of ≥100 mg/dL during the pre- and postexercise period until a BG pattern and response have been established. Thereafter, evaluation and treatment of BG response should be individualized for each patient. Patients with hypoglycemia unawareness or frequent hypoglycemia episodes may require a higher BG target or more frequent testing. Factors to consider during exercise or prior to discharge include, but are not limited to, timing of most recent insulin dose relative to food consumption, and previous BG responses to exercise and carbohydrate intake. Avoid exercise in patients with type 1 diabetes with a BG >300 mg/dL, and use clinical discretion in T2DM.[12]

Episodes of Syncope or Near-Syncope

Documentation should include the onset, duration, and severity of the episode, along with BP and cardiac rhythm.

Hypotension or Hypertension

Note pre- or postexercise hypotension that is associated with signs and symptoms or persistent resting or exercise hypertension.

Dyspnea

Feelings of dyspnea can be an angina equivalent or a symptom of respiratory distress. Note the level of activity when symptoms occur as well as lung sounds and oxygen saturation.

Exercise Intolerance

Abnormal hemodynamic response, increasing fatigue, abnormally elevated RPE, or an inability to tolerate usual levels of activity should be noted.

Depression

Depression screening at entry to the CR program is recommended because depression is associated with adverse events, increased mortality, and a worse prognosis in cardiac patients.[13] Depression may also increase the risk of nonfatal cardiac events and double the risk of cardiovascular mortality after MI. Approximately 20% of hospitalized cardiac patients meet criteria for major depression, and more show subclinical levels of depressive symptoms.[14] Patients who have abnormal screenings, persistent depression, or changes in affect should be assessed further to determine necessity for treatment and to rule out risk of self-harm. Referral to the primary care physician or a professional qualified in the diagnosis and treatment of depression may be indicated. Screening for depression is an AACVPR performance measure, and programs should perform repeat assessments as indicated.

Cardiac or Respiratory Arrest

Medical evaluation and risk stratification before starting the CR program and a thorough assessment and screening prior to each exercise session can assist with identifying unstable patients. Prompt recognition of adverse signs and symptoms during the exercise session is essential, and the exercise session should be terminated when indicated. Quarterly emergency drills are required to ensure that the staff will be able to respond efficiently and effectively when a cardiac or respiratory arrest occurs.

Cerebrovascular Accident

Patients demonstrating signs and symptoms of a cerebrovascular accident (CVA) should be immediately evaluated with a rapid out-of-hospital stroke assessment such as the Cincinnati Prehospital Stroke Scale. If a CVA is suspected, EMS should be contacted immediately for rapid transport to a stroke center. Note the time when a patient was last at neurological baseline, and check BG. Maintain airway, breathing, and circulation; and provide supplemental oxygen if the patient has hypoxemia (<94%) or if oxygen saturation is unknown.

Intervention Summary

When an untoward event occurs, follow-up should include documentation of interventions or changes in medical therapy. Patients involved in an adverse event should be educated and provided with counseling about the signs and symptoms of the clinical findings. During assessment of a clinical problem or emergency and for the general purposes of patient evaluation, CR staff should document the clinical status of the patient. Appropriate interventions may then be applied. Assessment of clinical status should include the following:

- Self-reported history describing symptoms— the degree and type, precipitating and relieving factors, and any change in pattern
- HR
- BP
- ECG monitoring
- 12-lead ECG if diagnostic-quality monitoring is not available
- Results of the most recent exercise or pharmacological stress test
- Auscultation of the heart and lungs
- Assessment of peripheral pulses and perfusion
- Pulse oximetry
- Assessment of level of consciousness
- BG level

Based on these assessments, interventions may include the following, as appropriate:

- Not initiating, or terminating the exercise session
- Assisting the patient to a comfortable sitting or lying position
- Comforting the patient
- Monitoring BP and HR-ECG
- Administering supplemental oxygen
- Administering sublingual nitroglycerin
- Administering glucose
- Establishing intravenous IV access and administering IV fluids
- Administering BLS[15]
- Administering ACLS[16]
- Transporting to a hospital or providing emergency services for immediate care
- Notifying the supervising physician, program medical director, and the referring physician
- Notifying family

Documentation of Emergencies

Emergencies must be documented according to the standards set forth by the organization's risk management or legal department. All incidents must be documented in the patient's medical record. Other documentation may include an incident or adverse event form (see appendix C).

With increased utilization of electronic medical records, documentation included in appendix C may contain electronic orders or signatures and is not required to be in hardcopy format. The AHA recommends that community- and hospital-based programs systematically monitor cardiac arrests to improve performance and outcomes using a cycle of evaluation, benchmarking, and developing strategies to address deficiencies. Benchmarking can be facilitated by existing cardiac arrest registries, such as the AHA Get With the Guidelines (GWTG-R) or the Cardiac Arrest Registry to Enhance Survival (CARES), and further information can be obtained from their respective websites. The Utstein guidelines are a useful template for measuring key aspects of the resuscitation process and outcomes that can be used for quality improvement processes.[17,18]

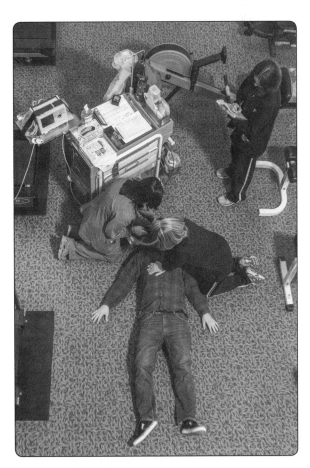

The emergency cart, resuscitation equipment, and medications must be checked regularly.

BOTTOM LINE

- While occurring infrequently, medical emergencies will happen in CR.
- CR professionals need to be prepared to respond to a wide variety of medical emergencies.
- To minimize the chances of medical emergencies, participants in CR should be assessed prior to, during, and after completing an exercise session.

- Every CR program needs to develop clinic-specific policies and procedures for medical emergencies.
- The response to medical emergencies should be thoroughly reviewed, and deficiencies must be identified and rectified.

Guideline 14.3   Emergency Equipment and Maintenance

Emergency equipment should be immediately available and include the following:

- Telephone, medical alert signal, or other emergency signal system to call for emergency medical services (EMS) or code team as applicable
- Portable, battery-operated defibrillator with ECG printout and monitor that may have external pacemaker capability (essential for programs with moderate- to high-risk patients)
- Direct current (DC) capability in case of battery failure (for the defibrillator, monitor, and ECG printout)
- An automatic external defibrillator (AED), which is especially useful for programs serving low-risk participants and is strongly recommended in areas of the hospital or in facilities where early defibrillation could be delayed (<3 min from collapse)
  - Depending on the individual facility's policies, an AED may be used in place of a manual defibrillator.
  - Continued use of an AED (or the automatic mode) when a manual defibrillator is available and provider skills are adequate for rhythm interpretation is not recommended, because rhythm analysis and shock administration may result in prolonged interruptions in chest compressions.[16]
- Portable oxygen and tubing with nasal cannula and face masks
- Adult oral and nasopharyngeal airways in various sizes as well as bag valve mask and pocket face masks, which should be standard equipment on all emergency carts
- Intubation equipment, including air adjuncts such as Combitube or laryngeal mask airway (If intubation equipment is available for use, personnel who are certified and licensed to perform intubation and continuous quantitative waveform capnography should be accessible.)
- Additional equipment for medical emergencies and maintenance policies, including the following:
  - Portable suction equipment
  - Intravenous access and administration equipment and fluids
  - Sharps container
  - ACLS medications as noted in the AHA standards and based on community standards and medical advisory committee recommendations
  - BP measurement equipment (sphygmomanometer and stethoscope)
  - Cardiac board
  - Personal protective equipment—gloves, masks, gowns, face shields
  - General medical supplies
  - Emergency documentation forms
- Cart or mobile storage unit for emergency equipment and medications, which should be appropriately stored, locked, and secured out of reach of the general public when not in use
- Biomedical engineering check of equipment for maintenance and performance should be performed every six months or as TJC standards or state regulations require. Documentation of such maintenance is required.
- Defibrillators should be checked daily for discharge capability.
- Medications should be checked per organization policy by designated professional staff for outdates.

Emergency Equipment

Emergency equipment availability is site dependent and is presented in guideline 14.3. The emergency cart, resuscitation equipment, and medications must be checked regularly. Examples of forms in appendixes D, E, and F may be used to document equipment checks and maintenance.

Staff Training and Site Preparation

The AHA provides the recommended training courses for emergency cardiac care (ECC) for CR personnel. ECC includes treatments for sudden and life-threatening events affecting the cardiovascular and pulmonary systems. The 2015 AHA Guidelines for CPR and ECC provide the treatment recommendations based on current and comprehensive resuscitation literature. The AHA curriculum for BLS or ACLS for Healthcare Providers are typically recommended depending on personnel training requirements (guideline 14.4).[15,16]

The concepts of high-quality CPR and early defibrillation are of utmost importance to improving resuscitation outcomes in CR programs. Staff members successfully completing BLS and AED training may provide for chest compressions, ventilation, and immediate defibrillation, if indicated.[19-21] CR personnel should be authorized, trained, equipped, and directed to operate an AED if their professional responsibilities require them to respond to patients in cardiac arrest, regardless of whether ACLS providers are immediately available. For example, ACLS-trained providers may not be available in early-morning or evening CR maintenance programs. Because CR services, whether hospital or freestanding, are medical facilities and under the auspices of a physician medical director, they are not subject to public access defibrillation regulations but rather to the policies and procedures of the supervising physician and parent medical facility.

Qualified professional staff may administer medications to cardiovert patients as allowed by state licensure laws. Only trained health care providers may perform tracheal intubation. Therefore, most health care providers should use alternative, noninvasive techniques for airway management, such as a bag valve mask device, laryngeal mask airway, esophageal–tracheal Combitube, or pharyngeal-tracheal lumen airway. If tracheal intubation is used, continuous quantitative waveform capnography is recommended during the resuscitation period, because it is useful for confirming tracheal tube placement, monitoring CPR quality, and detecting return of spontaneous circulation. ACLS training emphasizes assessments and interventions that improve outcomes. However, while vascular access, drug delivery, and advanced airway placement are

Guideline 14.4 Personnel and Emergency Care in Outpatient Cardiac Rehabilitation: Hospital-Based or Freestanding Center

- All professional staff will successfully complete the AHA curriculum for BLS or ACLS for Healthcare Providers.

- Physicians and appropriately trained professional staff who have successfully completed the AHA curriculum for BLS or ACLS for Healthcare Providers and have met state or facility medicolegal requirements for defibrillation and other related practices will provide medical supervision for moderate- to high-risk patients.

- All professional staff will be aware of the specific emergency procedures required by the organization for inpatients, outpatients, and specific patient care units.

- Standing orders or policies and procedures for all emergency situations will be in effect and reviewed regularly by the staff and the program medical director.

- Regularly scheduled emergency procedure in-services including mock codes (at least four per year) for all staff involved in patient care will be performed and documented.

- Regularly scheduled reviews (monthly is recommended) of emergency cart equipment, emergency medications, and supplies will be performed and documented.

recommended, they should not cause significant interruptions in the delivery of high-quality chest compressions or delay defibrillation of ventricular fibrillation or pulseless ventricular tachycardia, two critical links in the chain of survival.[21]

Within each facility, the emergency plan must address transportation of patients to a hospital emergency room or other destination (e.g., catheterization lab, coronary care unit). Such a plan must include telephone access to call a code, 9-1-1, or local EMS. For programs not operating within a hospital, staff should be familiar with the emergency transport teams in their geographic area so that access and location of the center are clearly identified. The emergency response team should be met at the entrance of the facility so that they can be most expeditiously guided to the site of the emergency situation while the patient remains under the direct observation of an appropriate staff member at all times. A number of publications provide the basis for guidelines regarding professional staff and emergency care.[17,20]

Inpatient (also known as "Phase 1") programs have a wide range of standing protocols for the treatment of medical emergencies. All staff should be properly trained in BLS or ACLS and be prepared to respond in case of an emergency.

Phase 3 CR Programs

Phase 3 CR maintenance programs began in the late 1970s as gymnasium-based programs with or without ECG monitoring.[30] Due to lesser need for either ECG monitoring or direct physician supervision, programs tended to be less formal and less expensive to set up, with safety assumed based on studies in Phase 2 (also known as "early outpatient") CR populations.[31,32] Studies have highlighted the low-risk nature of Phase 3 CR programs with participants displaying decreases in the occurrence of clinical events, rates of nonfatal MI and cardiovascular mortality, and lower Framingham Risk Scores.[33-35] While limited research has been conducted on the medical benefits of Phase 3 CR programs, the value is self-evident because it fosters long-term adherence in a group environment that is almost certainly safer than isolated exercise.

While Phase 3 CR participants are classified as lower risk, programs should employ proper assessment and screening prior to entry as well as periodic reevaluations. Initial assessments may include consultations with a medical provider and

exercise testing in patients with CVD, HF, or multiple cardiovascular risk factors, as determined by the medical director and program policy. Exercise tolerance testing is the gold standard for medical evaluation and provides the program with information on ischemic changes, anginal thresholds, BP response, aerobic capacity, and target heart rates, all important considerations for exercise prescriptions (see chapter 4). Medical evaluations may not be required if patients are moving directly from Phase 2 CR or from pulmonary rehabilitation programs. All participants should be oriented to the exercise facility by staff and provided with safety guidelines. If exercise testing is not performed, it is recommended that staff assess functional capacity (e.g., 6-minute walk test) prior to providing recommendations regarding PA. Reevaluations should occur on at least a yearly basis and include review of medical records, symptoms, medications, and exercise history. Consultations with a medical provider and/or exercise testing may be required as directed by the medical director and program policy. More frequent participant assessment and screening (monthly, quarterly) with staff may increase participant satisfaction and provides an opportunity to update exercise prescriptions.

Phase 3 CR personnel requirements depend on program location. Emergency policies and procedures are similar to those employed in Phase 2 CR or community-based programs, and staff should be prepared to treat potential medical issues highlighted in guideline 14.3. Without the need for physician supervision, programs that operate in the early-morning or late-evening hours should have policies that address single rescuer situations.

BOTTOM LINE

- Phase 3 CR participants are generally considered to be lower-risk patients than Phase 2 patients.
- Proper assessment, screening, and periodic reevaluations should occur regularly.
- Exercise prescription is similar to Phase 2 CR.
- Emergency policies and procedures should address the potential for single rescuer situations.

Alternative Models of SP

To be able to offer CR and SP services to more patients, alternative models of care are offered through Internet-based risk factor reduction and community- or home-based settings. Some existing programs have also incorporated home-based CR as a service option.[22-24] The exercise portion of these programs may be managed by remote ECG monitoring, conducted in a supervised setting, or self-managed by patients following recommended exercise prescriptions.[25] These options are addressed in the following subsections.

Remote ECG Monitoring

Remote ECG monitoring is used primarily in patients who require monitored exercise programs but are unable to participate at an outpatient exercise facility.[26-28] The prime example of such monitoring is at-home programming, but it may be used in exercise facilities such as community centers, health clubs, or gymnasiums. The professional staff member monitoring the ECG is responsible for identifying problems, evaluating changes in medical condition and symptoms through patient interview, and providing counseling to the patient. Patients should be trained in proper use of the equipment used to transmit the ECG and signal accuracy confirmed prior to at-home programming. Additionally, exercise prescriptions should be similar to those provided in the outpatient setting. Ideally, the exercise prescription is based on exercise tolerance testing. When patients are exercising in a facility where health personnel are providing direct supervision, such staff members should meet personnel requirements as described for outpatient program staff for emergency care. However, in situations where patients are exercising without health care staff supervision, the plan for the course of action is much different (guideline 14.5).

Home Setting

Rehabilitative and SP services performed in the home may be subject to different personnel requirements inherent in the unique delivery of care. Whereas home health nurses and physical therapists are not typically ACLS prepared and do not carry an ECG monitor or a defibrillator to the patient home, those providing CR should be similarly qualified to those providing care in a hospital or outpatient setting. Personnel requirements for staff are listed in guideline 14.6. Other recommendations relative to guideline 14.6 include the following:

- Family members should be familiar with the signs and symptoms of a cardiac event, how to notify EMS, and how to administer BLS.
- The home should be evaluated for ease of emergency access.
- A plan should be established and reviewed, including labeling of telephones with the local EMS number and home address.

Evidence is insufficient to recommend for, or against, the deployment of an AED in homes at this time.[29]

Community-Site Programming

Patients are encouraged to make their exercise program a lifelong commitment, so many of them eventually use a community-based facility. The AHA/ACSM scientific statements Recommendations for Cardiovascular Screening, Staffing, and Emergency Policies at Health/Fitness Facilities, and Automated External Defibrillators in Health/Fitness Facilities; and the book *ACSM's Health/Fitness Facility Standards and Guidelines, Fourth Edition,* offer guidelines for emergencies within these facilities.[9,19,20] Guideline 14.7 is based on these documents.

Guideline 14.5 Remote Supervision of Exercise in the Absence of On-Site Health Care Providers (in the Home or Nonsupervised Center)

- An open phone line to provide access to the patient will be available not only for routine communication but also in times of an emergency situation.

- A plan should be developed to address access of emergency cardiac care in the home or nonsupervised facility.

Guideline 14.6 Home Health Personnel Requirements Related to Emergency Care

- According to department policy, all staff responsible for direct patient care, either while exercising or during education sessions, should complete BLS or ACLS training.
- Health care professionals providing CR services should be familiar with how to provide care to people with CVD.

- Health care professionals providing direct patient care will be familiar with how to contact local EMS and, at a minimum, have immediate access to a sphygmomanometer, a stethoscope, an emergency plan, and possibly an AED.

Guideline 14.7 Community-Site Requirements Related to Emergency Care

- All staff will have completed BLS and AED training.
- The facility will have a designated coordinator to oversee emergency planning. In medically supervised exercise programs and facilities that serve clinical populations, emergency planning should be developed by a licensed physician.
- The facility will have written emergency policies and procedures (e.g., staff training, emergency instructions).
- Staff will document the review and performance of emergency plan practice drills at least twice yearly or more often as indicated.
- Standards for such programming should comply with those for hospital-based centers and are also subject to the particular oversight of the community program director.
- Emergency equipment for such programming should comply with guidelines for freestanding centers and include an AED and medical supplies, as determined by the program director, that may be required to treat reasonably foreseeable complications including, but not limited to, cardiac arrest, MI, hypoglycemia, stroke, heat illness, or common orthopedic injuries.
- Phones will be available and labeled with the local EMS number, building address, and locations of entrances and exits.

Summary

It remains the ultimate responsibility of the medical director and professional CR staff to provide emergency care to the patient, regardless of the site of service. Regular review of emergency plans and appropriate modifications to enhance patient outcomes are required. The foundation of emergency care in CR is continued assessment and recognition of changes in patient condition to avert an emergency. The role of early defibrillation with BLS and ACLS is paramount. It is important that all CR programs have emergency plans and properly trained professionals in place for the early recognition of adverse events and prompt, effective delivery of emergency care.

Appendix A

Example of Standing Orders to Initiate Outpatient CR

1. Initiate monitored exercise program per outpatient CR policies and procedures.

2. Determine target heart rate (THR) via sign- or symptom-limited graded exercise testing (GXT) or sign- or symptom-limited responses to submaximal exercise.

3. Begin with a training duration of up to 30 min to tolerance, one to five times a week.

4. Gradually increase duration of training exercise if patient cardiovascular and physiological responses are within normal limits.

5. Observe participant for signs of exercise intolerance and adapt or terminate exercise as indicated in policies and procedures.

6. Assess lipid profile approximately six weeks postevent.

7. Administer nitroglycerin 0.3 or 0.4 mg sublingually every 5 minutes × 3 as needed for angina discomfort or ischemic symptoms.

8. Provide regular, periodic progress reports to the referring physician. Provide copies of reports to other physicians as needed.

9. Initiate patient education and counseling sessions as patient needs indicate.

10. Consult patient's personal physician or CR supervising physician for any necessary orders.

11. Consult with the CR dietitian to provide individualized nutrition education for each participant.

12. Enter the patient into a non–ECG-monitored maintenance program upon completion of early outpatient CR program.

Physician's signature

Date

From American Association of Cardiovascular and Pulmonary Rehabilitation, *Guidelines for Cardiac Rehabilitation Programs,* 6th ed. (Champaign, IL: Human Kinetics, 2021).

Appendix B

Example of Outpatient CR Emergency Standing Orders*

Table of Contents

Protocols for Urgent Situations and Emergency Interventions in the Cardiac Rehabilitation Area

   I. Cardiopulmonary arrest

  II. Angina pectoris

 III. Hypoglycemia

 IV. Hyperglycemia

   V. Hypotension

 VI. Hypertension

VII. Dysrhythmias

VIII. Dyspnea

 IX. Cerebrovascular accident

  X. Placement of intravenous line

 XI. Patient transportation

I. Cardiopulmonary Arrest

A. Identify responsiveness and determine if breathing is absent or abnormal (gasping).

B. Call out for help/activate emergency medical system (EMS).

   1. Call out for help from coworker. If no one responds and if no other staff member is available to assist, go to the nearest phone and activate EMS. (Emergency numbers with specific scripted instructions are posted at each phone.) Get defibrillator/automated external defibrillator (AED). If no pulse, attach defibrillator/AED and shock if indicated. Begin cardiopulmonary resuscitation (CPR) with compressions.

   2. If a second responder is available to assist, that person should activate EMS and then get the defibrillator/AED while the first responder stays with the patient to begin compressions.

   3. Staff will meet the EMS team at the appropriate entrance and direct them to the patient.

First Responder

1. Determine responsiveness and absent or abnormal breathing.

2. Send someone to activate EMS and get defibrillator/AED.

3. If pulseless, begin chest compressions at a depth of at least 2 in. and a rate of at least 100 compressions/min until defibrillator/AED arrives. Allow for complete chest recoil, minimize interruptions to <10 s, use a compression to ventilation ratio of 30:2 and avoid excessive ventilation.

Second Responder

1. After activating EMS, take cart with defibrillator/AED to the patient. Place defibrillator pads or AED on patient and assess cardiac rhythm.

2. Shock if indicated, resume compressions. Follow appropriate algorithm according to ACLS guidelines.

Third Responder (if Available)

1. Direct remaining patients to another area.

2. Direct and control incoming emergency response team and patients.

3. Obtain extra supplies and equipment as needed.

4. Act as the recorder of events until EMS arrives.

5. Prepare records to be sent with patient to the emergency department if needed.

6. Notify patient physician/cardiologist and family.

---

*Appendix B should be used only as an example of standing orders that might be considered and adopted for use in freestanding outpatient or community-based programs.

From American Association of Cardiovascular and Pulmonary Rehabilitation, *Guidelines for Cardiac Rehabilitation Programs,* 6th ed. (Champaign, IL: Human Kinetics, 2021).

Emergency in Other Locations

7. Protocols should be developed for emergencies occurring in locations other than the cardiac rehabilitation gym including but not limited to:

- Locker room/restrooms
- Lobby/waiting area
- Patient education area
- Parking lots

II. Angina Pectoris

A. If a patient develops unstable angina while in the exercise area, the patient should immediately discontinue exercise and sit or lie down. Note the exercise workload, HR, and BP at which the symptoms occurred.

B. The following protocol should be followed by the CR staff:

1. Check pulse, BP, cardiac rhythm (attach telemetry monitor if not already monitored), and oxygen saturation.

2. Rate angina on a scale of 1 to 10.

3. If no relief with 1 to 3 min of rest, give 1 nitroglycerine (NTG) 0.4 mg SL or spray.

4. Obtain 12-lead ECG and call supervising physician.

C. If pain is relieved:

1. If this angina is of new onset, the patient should be evaluated by the supervising physician. The primary care physician should be notified of the results of the evaluation and recommended treatment, if any.

2. If the patient experiences chronic stable angina, exercise intensity should be decreased or halted until the angina is relieved. Patient may resume exercise at a lower workload dependent on the clinical judgment of the medical director and professional staff.

OR

The patient can be discharged but should be instructed to report any increase in frequency or severity of angina to their physician.

D. If pain is not relieved:

1. Monitor pulse, BP, cardiac rhythm, and oxygen saturation closely.

2. Place on oxygen at 2 to 4 L per nasal prongs if oxygen saturation is <94%.

3. Patient to chew aspirin 160 to 325 mg.

4. Repeat NTG 0.4 mg SL or spray every 5 min for unrelieved angina symptoms.

5. The supervising physician will evaluate and determine the course of action.

III. Hypoglycemia

A. If patient displays any symptoms of hypoglycemia:

1. Obtain finger-stick blood glucose level.

2. If BG results are <70 mg/dL or the patient is symptomatic, give 15 g CHO, juice, or three glucose tablets.

3. Retest BG in 15 min. If BG is not >90 mg/dL, repeat 15 g CHO and recheck BG in 15 min.

4. If patient is uncooperative or unconscious, contact supervising physician, give glucose gel or establish IV access and give 50 cc (1 amp) 50% dextrose solution. Arrange for transport to ED.

IV. Hyperglycemia

A. A participant with a BG >300 mg/dL should not exercise unless the patient's referring physician and the program medical director give their consent.

B. Frequency of BG checks should be determined according to the patient profile and ITP.

C. BG evaluations may be performed by rehabilitation staff or the patient according to the ITP.

---

*Appendix B should be used only as an example of standing orders that might be considered and adopted for use in freestanding outpatient or community-based programs.

From American Association of Cardiovascular and Pulmonary Rehabilitation, *Guidelines for Cardiac Rehabilitation Programs,* 6th ed. (Champaign, IL: Human Kinetics, 2021).

D. The CR staff may request a blood glucose evaluation on any patient based on suspected signs and symptoms of hyperglycemia (nausea, flushing, polyuria, polydipsia, fruity breath, tachypnea).

V. Hypotension

A. Remove the patient from the exercise area if possible.

B. Place patient in a supine position. Consider elevating legs or placing in Trendelenburg position.

C. Attach a telemetry monitor if not already monitored.

D. Check BP, pulse, cardiac rhythm, and oxygen saturation.

E. If no response to the position change, call the supervising physician. If the patient condition continues to deteriorate or becomes progressively symptomatic, or if BP continues to drop, start an IV of normal saline at 100 mL/h and arrange for transport to the ED. After evaluation and treatment of the patient, the supervising physician should notify the patient's primary care physician of the hypotensive episode and discuss any further treatment if necessary.

F. If patient responds to the supine position, keep supine until SBP is >100, then gradually assist to sitting position. Continue to monitor BP, pulse, and rhythm. Encourage fluids. Notify the patient's primary physician of the episode.

VI. Hypertension

A. Check every patient's BP before exercise and compare with previous recordings.

B. If the SBP reading is >170 mm Hg or the diastolic reading is >100 mm Hg, have the patient sit and recheck the BP in 5 min.

C. If the BP remains elevated, do not have patient exercise. Notify the primary care physician or supervising physician to evaluate and determine course of action.

D. Patients may exercise with elevated BP if directed by the primary care physician and medical director.

E. Investigate whether patient is complying with medications and sodium restrictions.

VII. Dysrhythmias

Premature Ventricular Contractions (PVCs)

A. Observe for the following:
  1. Frequency
  2. Whether multifocal or unifocal
  3. Pairs or runs, sustained or paroxysmal
  4. Associated signs or symptoms
  5. Palpate pulse to evaluate for peripheral perfusion

B. Document any new arrhythmias or increase in severity with a rhythm strip and make notation on chart. Notify supervising physician and referring physician, where appropriate, to discuss treatment.

C. Discontinue exercise if PVCs become symptomatic and check pulse, BP, and oxygen saturation. Provide oxygen at 2 to 4 L if hypoxemic, and obtain IV access if directed by a physician.

D. Notify the supervising physician for evaluation and treatment.

Bradycardia

A. If patient develops symptomatic bradycardia, stop exercise.

B. Monitor HR and rhythm, BP, and oximetry. Provide oxygen at 2 to 4 L if hypoxemic. Obtain 12-lead ECG if available.

C. Assess for symptoms of instability or altered mental status, ischemic chest discomfort, HF, or hypotension and notify supervising physician for evaluation and treatment. Notify the supervising physician and if available, obtain IV access, and prepare to administer atropine or external pacing per ACLS guidelines.

D. Prepare for transfer to ED.

---

*Appendix B should be used only as an example of standing orders that might be considered and adopted for use in freestanding outpatient or community-based programs.

From American Association of Cardiovascular and Pulmonary Rehabilitation, *Guidelines for Cardiac Rehabilitation Programs*, 6th ed. (Champaign, IL: Human Kinetics, 2021).

Tachycardia

A. If patient develops a new wide or narrow complex tachycardia, stop exercise.

B. Monitor HR and rhythm, BP, and oximetry. Provide oxygen at 2 to 4 L if hypoxemic. Obtain 12-lead ECG if available.

C. Assess for symptoms of instability or altered mental status, ischemic chest discomfort, HF, or hypotension, and notify supervising physician for evaluation and treatment. If directed by a physician, obtain IV access and prepare for synchronized cardioversion. If stable, may utilize vagal maneuvers or antiarrhythmic agents per ACLS guidelines.

D. Prepare for transfer to ED.

VIII. Dyspnea

A. If patient develops acute dyspnea, stop exercise and have patient sit down.

B. Monitor heart rate and rhythm, BP, respiratory rate, lung sounds, and oximetry. Provide oxygen at 2 to 4 L for oxygen saturation <94%.

C. If patient has a metered-dose inhaler, it may be administered as prescribed.

D. If condition deteriorates, notify supervising physician to evaluate for treatment options and possible transfer to ED.

E. If condition improves, notify primary care physician for further recommendations.

IX. Cerebrovascular Accident

A. If patient develops signs and symptoms of a stroke such as sudden arm or leg weakness, confusion, trouble speaking, dizziness, loss of balance or coordination, severe headache, or facial droop, immediately evaluate with rapid out-of-hospital stroke assessment.

B. If stroke is suspected, initiate EMS for immediate transport to a stroke facility.

C. Establish time of last known neurological baseline.

D. Maintain airway, breathing, and circulation.

E. Provide supplemental oxygen if hypoxemic or if oxygen saturation is unknown.

F. Check blood glucose.

G. Alert receiving hospital when patient is in transport.

X. Placement of IV Line

Purpose: To provide immediate access to administer emergency medication and IV fluids.

A. An attempt will be made to notify the supervising physician.

B. Place a saline lock in participant when one or more of the following apply:

   1. Angina pectoris protocol has been followed and chest pain persists.

   2. ECG, vital signs or participant appears to be clinically unstable or symptomatic.

   3. Physician directs the placement of IV line.

XI. Patient Transportation

Staff will meet and direct ambulance personnel to the patient treatment area.

Staff will prepare medical records to be sent with the patient as needed.

Staff will alert the emergency department of the patient transfer.

Cardiac Rehabilitation Department Emergency Procedures and Standing Orders Were Reviewed and Approved

_____

Physician's name

_____

Signature

_____

Date of most recent review

*Appendix B should be used only as an example of standing orders that might be considered and adopted for use in freestanding outpatient or community-based programs.

From American Association of Cardiovascular and Pulmonary Rehabilitation, *Guidelines for Cardiac Rehabilitation Programs,* 6th ed. (Champaign, IL: Human Kinetics, 2021).

Appendix C

Cardiac Rehabilitation Untoward Event—
Physician Notification

Patient name:_____ DOB:_____ Date:_____

To: Physician _____ Date physician notified: _____

Time physician notified: _____

Phone: _____

Fax: _____

Physician orders:

____May resume CR at next scheduled visit

____May not resume CR until _____

____Limit exercise as directed below

____Will be evaluated on _____

____No follow-up needed

Additional physician orders or comments: _____

_____

_____

_____

Signature: _____ **Date:** _____

Please return this page, completed and signed, to Cardiac Rehabilitation.

_____

Patient name: _____ DOB: _____ Diagnosis: _____

Date of event: _____ Time: _____ Rehab week/visit #:_____

Reason for report:

____New sign or symptom

____Change from previous condition

____Findings exceed acceptable parameters

____Other:_____

Type of event:

____Angina symptoms

____Dysrhythmia or ECG changes

____BP abnormality

____Dyspnea or abnormal O_2 saturation

From American Association of Cardiovascular and Pulmonary Rehabilitation, *Guidelines for Cardiac Rehabilitation Programs,* 6th ed. (Champaign, IL: Human Kinetics, 2021).

____ HF symptoms

____ BG abnormality

____ Other:_____

Description of occurrence: _____

_____

_____

_____

Description of action:

____ Managed by rehab staff

____ Seen in rehab by supervising physician

____ Transferred to emergency room

____ Sent to clinic or physician office

____ Appt made with _____ on _____

Treatment:

____ NTG _____ mg × _____

____ Oxygen @ _____ L/m

____ 12-lead ECG

____ Aspirin _____ mg

Recommendations: _____

_____

_____

_____

Disposition:

____ ER

____ Physician's office or clinic

____ Home

Accompanied by:

____ Self

____ Spouse/family

____ Rehab staff

____ Other

Status upon departure:

____ Stable

____ Unstable

____ Other

Report completed by:_____

Attach appropriate physiological data such as 12-lead ECG, BP measurement, code form, and so on.

Appendix D
Daily Emergency Cart Checklist

Month _____ Year _____

1. Defibrillator discharges appropriate test Joules (unplugged)

1	2	3	4	5	6	7	8	9	10	11	12	13	14	15	16	17	18	19	20	21	22	23	24	25	26	27	28	29	30	31

2. Defibrillator plugged in

1	2	3	4	5	6	7	8	9	10	11	12	13	14	15	16	17	18	19	20	21	22	23	24	25	26	27	28	29	30	31

3. Defibrillator battery registers full capacity

1	2	3	4	5	6	7	8	9	10	11	12	13	14	15	16	17	18	19	20	21	22	23	24	25	26	27	28	29	30	31

4. Monitor display records ECG accurately (extra roll of paper available)

1	2	3	4	5	6	7	8	9	10	11	12	13	14	15	16	17	18	19	20	21	22	23	24	25	26	27	28	29	30	31

5. Electrode patches and fast patches available

1	2	3	4	5	6	7	8	9	10	11	12	13	14	15	16	17	18	19	20	21	22	23	24	25	26	27	28	29	30	31

6. O₂ tank registers full capacity

1	2	3	4	5	6	7	8	9	10	11	12	13	14	15	16	17	18	19	20	21	22	23	24	25	26	27	28	29	30	31

7. Ambu bag, oral airway, O₂ mask/cannula available

1	2	3	4	5	6	7	8	9	10	11	12	13	14	15	16	17	18	19	20	21	22	23	24	25	26	27	28	29	30	31

8. Suction machine functions with appropriate suction capacity

1	2	3	4	5	6	7	8	9	10	11	12	13	14	15	16	17	18	19	20	21	22	23	24	25	26	27	28	29	30	31

From American Association of Cardiovascular and Pulmonary Rehabilitation, *Guidelines for Cardiac Rehabilitation Programs*, 6th ed. (Champaign, IL: Human Kinetics, 2021).

9. Suction canister, tubing, Yankauer suction tip available

1	2	3	4	5	6	7	8	9	10	11	12	13	14	15	16	17	18	19	20	21	22	23	24	25	26	27	28	29	30	31

10. Emergency code documentation sheets available

1	2	3	4	5	6	7	8	9	10	11	12	13	14	15	16	17	18	19	20	21	22	23	24	25	26	27	28	29	30	31

11. Sharps container present

1	2	3	4	5	6	7	8	9	10	11	12	13	14	15	16	17	18	19	20	21	22	23	24	25	26	27	28	29	30	31

12. Personal protective equipment available (gloves, eye/face shield)

1	2	3	4	5	6	7	8	9	10	11	12	13	14	15	16	17	18	19	20	21	22	23	24	25	26	27	28	29	30	31

13. Signature of reviewer (Name):

1	2	3	4	5	6	7	8	9	10	11	12	13	14	15	16	17	18	19	20	21	22	23	24	25	26	27	28	29	30	31

Appendix E
Monthly Emergency Cart Checklist

1. The entire emergency cart is to be checked monthly and following any time the contents are accessed.

2. The defibrillator, monitoring equipment, and oxygen equipment are to be checked by staff before the first exercise session of the day. (See daily emergency cart checklist.)

3. If there is any problem with the equipment, the staff checking it is responsible for calling the appropriate office and seeing that the equipment is restored to full function as soon as possible.

4. The following monthly checklist is an example of emergency supplies. Availability should match the policies of the particular site where care is delivered as determined by the medical director (e.g., inpatient versus outpatient).

	Quantity	Jan	Feb	Mar	Apr	May	Jun	Jul	Aug	Sep	Oct	Nov	Dec
Date checklist completed													
TOP OF CART													
Defibrillator	1												
Extra rolls ECG paper	2												
ECG cable and fast patch cable	1												
Electrode sets and fast patches	2												
Adult oral airways (small/medium/large)	3												
ACLS algorithms	1												
Clipboard, pen, resuscitation documentation form	1												
Ambu (bag valve mask)	1												
Pocket face mask	1												
O_2 nasal prongs	2												
O_2 mask/tubing	1												
O_2 extension tubing	1												
Box of gloves	1												
Face shields/masks	2												
Sharps/contaminated box	1												
DRAWER #1: PHARMACY DRUGS													
Adenosine 6 mg/2 mL	2												
Amiodarone 150 mg/3 mL	2												
Atropine sulfate 1 mg/10 mL	3												
Aspirin chewable	2												
Dextrose 50%, 25 g/50 mL	1												
Glucose gel	1												
Epinephrine HCl (1:10,000) 1 mg/10 mL	4												
Lidocaine HCl 100 mg/5 mL	3												
Magnesium sulfate 5 g	1												
Metoprolol 5 mg/5 mL	3												
Nitroglycerin 0.4 mg SL tablets or spray	1												
Sodium bicarbonate 50 mEq/50 mL	4												
Vasopressin 20 u/1 mL	2												

From American Association of Cardiovascular and Pulmonary Rehabilitation, *Guidelines for Cardiac Rehabilitation Programs,* 6th ed. (Champaign, IL: Human Kinetics, 2021).

	Quantity	Jan	Feb	Mar	Apr	May	Jun	Jul	Aug	Sep	Oct	Nov	Dec
DRAWER #2: GENERAL SUPPLIES													
Latex-free tourniquets	2												
IV start kits	4												
#18 g. IV catheter	4												
#20 g. IV catheter	4												
#22 g. IV catheter	4												
10 cc syringes	5												
5 cc syringes	5												
3 cc syringes	5												
50 cc syringes	2												
50 cc Toomey syringe	1												
#18 needles	5												
#19 needles	5												
#22 needles	5												
Plastic anti-stick needle/connectors	10												
Normal saline 20 mL vials or prefilled saline syringes	4												
Silk suture 3-0	2												
Scissors (pair)	1												
Alcohol wipes	30												
1 in. tape (roll)	1												
2 in. tape (roll)	1												
2 × 2s (packages)	2												
4 × 4s (packages)	2												
Sterile gloves: sizes 6, 6 1/2, 7, 7 1/2, 8 (2 of each size)	10												
Suture set	1												
Disposable razor	1												
Saline lock	4												
DRAWER #3: IV SUPPLIES													
Macrodrip IV tubing	3												
Minidrip IV tubing	3												
Infusion pump tubing	2												
Normal saline 1,000 cc	2												
D5W 1,000 cc	1												
Lactated ringers 1,000 cc	1												
D5W 100 cc	2												
D5W 250 cc/400 mg dopamine	1												
IV extension tubing	2												
Three-way stop cocks	2												
Cut-down tray	1												
Arrow introducers	2												
Triple lumen catheters	2												

(continued)

From American Association of Cardiovascular and Pulmonary Rehabilitation, *Guidelines for Cardiac Rehabilitation Programs*, 6th ed. (Champaign, IL: Human Kinetics, 2021).

(continued)

	Quantity	Jan	Feb	Mar	Apr	May	Jun	Jul	Aug	Sep	Oct	Nov	Dec
RESPIRATORY DRAWER													
Goggles/shield	1												
ABG kits	2												
1 in. tape	1												
Laryngoscope handle	1												
#2 Miller laryngoscope blade	1												
#3 Miller laryngoscope blade	1												
#2 McIntosh blade	1												
#4 McIntosh blade	1												
Oral airways, 80, 90, and 100 mm (1 each size)	3												
7.0 cm nasal airway	1												
#14F suction catheter	2												
Extra bulbs	2												
Stylette	1												
Flow meter	1												
Endotracheal tubes 6.5, 7.0, 7.5, 8.0, 8.5 cm (1 each size)	5												
12 mL syringe	1												
Water-soluble lubricant	1												
Americaine spray	1												
Extra batteries	2												
Magill forceps	1												
CO_2 detector	1												
BOTTOM DRAWER													
Sterile water or normal saline 1,000 cc	1												
Blood pressure cuff	1												
Stethoscope	1												
Flashlight	1												
Blanket	1												
SIDE OF CART													
Oxygen tank	1												
Portable suction machine	1												
Disposable suction canister	1												
Suction tubing	1												
Yankauer suction tip	1												
Back board	1												
Electrical extension cord	1												
Signature of reviewer:													

From American Association of Cardiovascular and Pulmonary Rehabilitation, *Guidelines for Cardiac Rehabilitation Programs,* 6th ed. (Champaign, IL: Human Kinetics, 2021).

Appendix F

Emergency Equipment Maintenance Log

Date of most recent maintenance check:_____

Date due for next maintenance check: _____

1. Defibrillator

    • Batteries replaced: _____   _____

1. Electrocardiographic monitor: _____

2. Oxygen tank: _____

3. Suction apparatus: _____

Maintenance problems noted: Date corrected: _____

    1. _____
    2. _____
    3. _____

Other: _____

Program director notified   (yes/no)   Date corrected: _____

    1. _____
    2. _____
    3. _____

Other:_____

From American Association of Cardiovascular and Pulmonary Rehabilitation, *Guidelines for Cardiac Rehabilitation Programs,* 6th ed. (Champaign, IL: Human Kinetics, 2021).

References

Chapter 1

1. Balady G, Ades PA, Bitner V, et al. Referral, enrollment and delivery of cardiac rehabilitation/secondary prevention programs at clinical centers and beyond. *Circulation.* 2011;124:1-10.

2. King M. Affordability, accountability, and accessibility in health care reform: Implications for cardiovascular and pulmonary rehabilitation. *J Cardiopulm Rehabil Prev.* 2013;33(3):144-52. doi:10.1097/HCR.0b013e31828f5602.2013

3. Heidenreich P, Trogdon JG, Khavjou OA, Butler J, Dracup K, Ezekowitz ME. Forecasting the future of cardiovascular disease in the United States: A policy statement from the American Heart Association. *Circulation.* 2011;123(8):933-944.

4. Ades PA, Keteyian SJ, Wright JS, et al. Increasing cardiac rehabilitation participation from 20% to 70%: A road map from the Million Hearts Cardiac Rehabilitation Collaborative. *Mayo Clin Proc.* 2017;92(2):234-242. doi:10.1016/j.mayocp.2016.10.014.

5. About the Affordable Care Act: Key features of the Affordable Care Act by year. U.S. Department of Health and Human Services website. www.hhs.gov/healthcare/ facts-and-features/key-features-of-acaby-year/index.html. Published December 7, 2017. Accessed August 1, 2018.

6. Arena R, Williams M, Forman DE, et al. American Heart Association Exercise, Cardiac Rehabilitation and Prevention Committee of the Council on Clinical Cardiology, Council on Epidemiology and Prevention, and Council on Nutrition, Physical Activity and Metabolism. Increasing referral and participation rates to outpatient cardiac rehabilitation: The valuable role of healthcare professionals in the inpatient and home health settings: A science advisory from the American Heart Association. *Circulation* 2012;125(10):1321-1329. doi:10.1161/CIR.0b013e318246b1e5

7. Berwick, D, Noan, T, Whittington, J. The triple aim: Care, health, and cost. *Health Aff.* 2008;27(3):759-769.

8. Benjamin EJ, Virani SS, Callaway CW, et al. Heart Disease and Stroke Statistics-2018 Update: A Report From the American Heart Association. *Circulation.* 2018 Mar 20;137(12):e67-e492. doi: 10.1161/CIR.0000000000000558.

9. Kiindig DA. Understanding population health terminology. *Milbank Q.* 2007;85(1):139-161.

10. Spring B, Ockene JK, Gidding SS, et al. Better population health through behavior change in adults: A call to action. *Circulation.* 2013;128(19):2169-2176.

11. Institute of Medicine (IOM). *Crossing the Quality Chasm: A New Health System for the 21st Century.* Washington, D.C: National Academy Press; 2001.

12. Institute of Medicine (IOM). *Performance Measurement: Accelerating Improvement.* Washington, D.C: National Academy Press; 2005.

13. Thomas RJ, King M, Lui K, Oldridge N, Piña IL, Spertus J. AACVPR/ACC/AHA 2007 performance measures on cardiac rehabilitation for referral to and delivery of cardiac rehabilitation/secondary prevention services. *Circulation.* 2007;116(14):1611-1642.

14. Thomas RJ, King M, Lui K, et al. AACVPR/ACCF/AHA 2010 update: Performance measures on cardiac rehabilitation for referral to cardiac rehabilitation/secondary prevention services. *Circulation.* 2010;122(13):1342-1350.

15. Thomas RJ, Balady G, Banka G, et al. 2018 ACC/AHA clinical performance and quality measures for cardiac rehabilitation: A report of the American College of Cardiology/American Heart Association Task Force on Performance Measures. *Circ Cardiovasc Qual Outcomes.* 2018;11(4):e000037. doi:10.1161/HCQ.0000000000000037

16. Porter ME. What is value in health care? *N Engl J Med.* 2010;363(26):2477-2481.

17. Stiefel M, Nolan K. Measuring the Triple Aim: A call for action . *Population Health Management.* 2013;16(4):219-220.

18. Sumner J, Harrison A, Doherty P. The effectiveness of modern cardiac rehabilitation: A systematic review of recent observational studies in non-attenders versus attenders. *PLoS One* 2017;12:e0177658. doi:10.1371/journal.pone.01776583

19. Dunlay SM, Pack QR, Thomas RJ, Killian JM, Roger VL. Participation in cardiac rehabilitation, readmissions, and death after acute myocardial infarction. *Am J Med.* 2014;127:538-46.

20. Leggett LE, Hauer T, Martin BJ, et al. Optimizing value from cardiac rehabilitation: A cost-utility analysis comparing age, sex, and clinical subgroups. *Mayo Clin Proc.* 2015;90(8):1011-1020.

21. About the National Quality Strategy. Agency for Healthcare Research and Quality website. www.ahrq.gov/workingforquality/about/index.html. Published March, 2017. Accessed August 1, 2018.

22. Lamb G, Newhouse R. Care Coordination: A Blueprint for RNs. First Edition. American Nurse Associations, Inc.; 2018

23. National Voluntary Consensus Standards for Coordination of Care across Episodes of Care and Care Transitions. National Quality Forum website. https://www.qualityforum.org/Projects/c-d/Care_Coordination_Endorsement_Maintenance/Care_Coordination_Endorsement_Maintenance.aspx (published date unknown). Accessed October 12, 2019

24. Lamb, G. (Ed.). *Care Coordination: The Game Changer: How Nursing Is Revolutionizing Quality Care.* Silver Spring, MD: American Nurse Association; 2013.

25. Morley M, Bogasky S, Gage B, Flood S, Ingber MJ. Medicare post-acute care episodes and payment bundling. *Medicare Medicaid Res Rev.* 2014;4(1):1-13.

26. Farmer SA, Darling ML, George M, Casale PN, Hagan E, McClellan MB. Existing and emerging payment and delivery reforms in cardiology. *JAMA Cardiol.* 2017;2(2):210-217. doi:10.1001/jamacardio.2016.3965

27. BPCI Advanced. Centers for Medicare & Medicaid Services (CMS) website. https://innovation.cms.gov/initiatives/bpci-advanced. October 2, 2019. Accessed October 4, 2019.

28. Mechanic R, Tompkins C. Lessons learned preparing for Medicare bundled payments. *N Engl J Med.* 2012;367(20):1873-75. doi:10.1056/NEJMp1210823

29. Anderson L, Sharp GA, Norton RJ, et al. Home-based versus centre-based cardiac rehabilitation. *Cochrane Database Syst Rev.* 2017;30:6. doi:10.1002/14651858.CD007130.pub4

30. Thomas RJ, Beatty AL, Beckie TM, et al. Home-based cardiac rehabilitation: A scientific statement from the American Association of Cardiovascular and Pulmonary Rehabilitation, the American Heart Association, and the American College of Cardiology. *J Cardiopulm Rehabil Prev.* 2019;39(4):208-225. doi:10.1097/HCR.0000000000000447

Chapter 2

1. Berwick DM, Nolan TW, Whittington J. The Triple Aim: Care, health, and cost. *Health Affairs.* 2008;27(3):759-769.

2. Bodenheimer T, Sinsky C. From Triple to Quadruple Aim: Care of the patient requires care of the provider. *Ann Fam Med.* 2014;12(6):573-576. doi:10.1370/afm.1713

3. The Medicare Access and CHIP Reauthorization Act of 2015. https://fas.org/sgp/crs/misc/R43962.pdf. Published (November 10, 2015). Accessed October 9, 2019.

4. Brant-Zawadzki M, Perazzo C, Afable RF. Community hospital to community health system: a blueprint for continuum of care. *Physician Exec.* 2011;37:16-21.

5. Evashwick CJ. Creating a continuum. The goal is to provide an integrated system of care. *Health Prog.* 1989;70:36-39, 56.

6. Oelke ND, Cunning L, Andrews K, et al. Organizing care across the continuum: primary care, specialty services, acute and long-term care. *Healthc Q.* 2009;13:75-79.

7. Chrysant SG. Stopping the cardiovascular disease continuum: Focus on prevention. *World J Cardiol.* 2010 Mar 26;2(3):43-9. doi: 10.4330/wjc.v2.i3.43

8. Kay D, Blue A, Pye P, Lacy A, Gray C, Moore S. Heart failure: Improving the continuum of care. *Care Manag J.* 2006;7:58-63.

9. Miranda MB, Gorski LA, LeFevre JG, Levac KA, Niederstadt JA, Toy AL. An evidence-based approach to improving care of patients with heart failure across the continuum. *J Nurs Care Qual.* 2002;17:1-14.

10. Rockson SG, deGoma EM, Fonarow CG. Reinforcing a continuum of care: In-hospital initiation of long-term secondary prevention following acute coronary syndromes. *Cardiovasc Drugs Ther.* 2007;21:375-388.

11. Bundled Payments for Care Improvement Advanced (BPCI Advanced or the Model). https://innovation.cms.gov/initiatives/bpci-advanced. (October 9, 2019). Accessed (October 9, 2019).

12. Blackburn H. Population strategies of cardiovascular disease prevention: Scientific base, rationale and public health implications. *Ann Med.* 1989;21:157-162.

13. Capewell S, Lloyd-Jones DM. Optimal cardiovascular prevention strategies for the 21st century. *JAMA.* 2010;304:2057-2058.

14. Thomas RJ, Balady G, Banka G, et al. 2018 ACC/AHA clinical performance and quality measures for cardiac rehabilitation: A report of the American College of Cardiology/American Heart Association Task Force on Performance Measures. *J Am Coll Cardiol.* 2018;71(16):1814-1837. doi:10.1016/j.jacc.2018.01.004

15. McNamara RL, Wang Y, Herrin J, et al. Effect of door-to-balloon time on mortality in patients with ST-segment elevation myocardial infarction. *J Am Coll Cardiol.* 2006;47:2180-2186.

16. Fonarow GC, Gawlinski A, Moughrabi S, Tillisch JH. Improved treatment of coronary heart disease by implementation of a Cardiac Hospitalization Atherosclerosis Management Program (CHAMP). *Am J Cardiol.* 2001;87:819-822.

17. Peters AE, Keeley EC. Trends and predictors of participation in cardiac rehabilitation following acute myocardial infarction: Data from the Behavioral Risk Factor Surveillance System. *J Am Heart Assoc.* 2017;7(1). pii:e007664. doi:10.1161/JAHA.117.007664

18. Dunlay SM, Witt BJ, Allison TG, et al. Barriers to participation in cardiac rehabilitation. *Am Heart J.* 2009;158:852-859.

19. Grace SL, Gravely-Witte S, Brual J, et al. Contribution of patient and physician factors to cardiac rehabilitation enrollment: A prospective multilevel study. *Euro J Cardiovasc Prev Rehabil.* 2008;15:548-556.

20. Grace SL, Gravely-Witte S, Brual J, et al. Contribution of patient and physician factors to cardiac rehabilitation referral: A prospective multilevel study. *Nat Clin Pract Cardiovasc Med.* 2008;5:653-662.

21. Grace SL, Russell KL, Reid RD, et al. Effect of cardiac rehabilitation referral strategies on utilization rates: A prospective, controlled study. *Arch Intern Med.* 2011;171:235-241.

22. Witt BJ, Thomas RJ, Roger VL. Cardiac rehabilitation after myocardial infarction: A review to understand barriers to participation and potential solutions. *Eura Medicophys.* 2005;41:27-34.

23. Choudhry NK, Winkelmayer WC. Medication adherence after myocardial infarction: A long way left to go. *J Gen Intern Med.* 2008;23:216-218.

24. Shah ND, Dunlay SM, Ting HH, et al. Long-term medication adherence after myocardial infarction: Experience of a community. *Am J Med.* 2009;122:961.e7-13.

25. Thomas RJ. Cardiac rehabilitation/secondary prevention programs—A raft for the rapids: Why have we missed the boat? *Circulation.* 2007;116:1644-1646.

26. Grace SL, Krepostman S, Brooks D, et al. Referral to and discharge from cardiac rehabilitation: Key informant views on continuity of care. *J Eval Clin Pract.* 2006;12:155-163.

27. Riley DL, Stewart DE, Grace SL. Continuity of cardiac care: Cardiac rehabilitation participation and other correlates. *Int J Cardiol.* 2007;119:326-333.

28. Giannuzzi P, Temporelli PL, Marchioli R, et al. Global secondary prevention strategies to limit event recurrence after myocardial infarction: Results of the GOSPEL study, a multicenter, randomized controlled trial from the Italian Cardiac Rehabilitation Network. *Arch Intern Med.* 2008;168:2194-2204.

29. Hammill BG, Curtis LH, Schulman KA, Whellan DJ. Relationship between cardiac rehabilitation and long-term risks of death and myocardial infarction among elderly Medicare beneficiaries. *Circulation.* 2010;121:63-70.

30. Oldridge NB, Guyatt GH, Fischer ME, Rimm AA. Cardiac rehabilitation after myocardial infarction. Combined experience of randomized clinical trials. *JAMA.* 1988;260:945-950.

31. Squires RW, Montero-Gomez A, Allison TG, Thomas RJ. Long-term disease management of patients with coronary disease by cardiac rehabilitation program staff. *J Cardiopulm Rehabil Prev.* 2008;28:180-186.

32. Suaya JA, Stason WB, Ades PA, Normand SL, Shepard DS. Cardiac rehabilitation and survival in older coronary patients. *J Am Coll Cardiol.* 2009;54:25-33.

33. Taylor RS, Unal B, Critchley JA, Capewell S. Mortality reductions in patients receiving exercise-based cardiac rehabilitation: How much can be attributed to cardiovascular risk factor improvements? *Euro J Cardiovasc Prev Rehabil.* 2006;13:369-374.

34. Williams MA, Ades PA, Hamm LF, et al. Clinical evidence for a health benefit from cardiac rehabilitation: An update. *Am Heart J.* 2006;152:835-841.

35. Witt BJ, Jacobsen SJ, Weston SA, et al. Cardiac rehabilitation after myocardial infarction in the community. *J Am Coll Cardiol*. 2004;44:988-996.

36. Gupta R, Sanderson BK, Bittner V. Outcomes at one-year follow-up of women and men with coronary artery disease discharged from cardiac rehabilitation: What benefits are maintained? *J Cardiopulm Rehabil Prev*. 2007;27:11-18.

37. The Six Domains of Health Care Quality. Agency for Healthcare Research and Quality website. www.ahrq.gov/professionals/quality-patient-safety/talkingquality/create/sixdomains.html. Published (November 2018). Accessed March, 2019.

38. Riggio JM, Sorokin R, Moxey ED, Mather P, Gould S, Kane GC. Effectiveness of a clinical-decision-support system in improving compliance with cardiac-care quality measures and supporting resident training. *Acad Med*. 2009;84:1719-1726.

39. Gravely-Witte S, Leung YW, Nariani R, et al. Effects of cardiac rehabilitation referral strategies on referral and enrollment rates. *Nat Rev Cardiol*. 2010;7:87-96.

40. Mueller E, Savage PD, Schneider DJ, Howland LL, Ades PA. Effect of a computerized referral at hospital discharge on cardiac rehabilitation participation rates. *J Cardiopulm Rehabil Prev*. 2009;29:365-369.

41. Suaya JA, Shepard DS, Normand SL, Ades PA, Prottas J, Stason WB. Use of cardiac rehabilitation by Medicare beneficiaries after myocardial infarction or coronary bypass surgery. *Circulation*. 2007;116:1653-1662.

42. Thomas RJ, Miller NH, Lamendola C, et al. National survey on gender differences in cardiac rehabilitation programs. Patient characteristics and enrollment patterns. *J Cardiopulm Rehabil*. 1996;16:402-412.

43. Tricoci P, Peterson ED, Roe MT. Patterns of guideline adherence and care delivery for patients with unstable angina and non-ST-segment elevation myocardial infarction (from the CRUSADE Quality Improvement Initiative). *Am J Cardiol*. 2006;98:30Q-35Q.

44. Jacobson PD. Legal and policy considerations in using clinical practice guidelines. *Am J Cardiol*. 1997;80:74H-79H.

45. Spertus JA, Eagle KA, Krumholz HM, Mitchell KR, Normand SL. American College of Cardiology and American Heart Association methodology for the selection and creation of performance measures for quantifying the quality of cardiovascular care. *J Am Coll Cardiol*. 2005;45:1147-1156.

46. Fonarow GC, Abraham WT, Albert NM, et al. Association between performance measures and clinical outcomes for patients hospitalized with heart failure. *JAMA*. 2007;297:61-70.

47. Fonarow GC, Peterson ED. Heart failure performance measures and outcomes: Real or illusory gains. *JAMA*. 2009;302:792-794.

48. Artham SM, Lavie CJ, Milani RV. Cardiac rehabilitation programs markedly improve high-risk profiles in coronary patients with high psychological distress. *South Med J*. 2008;101:262-267.

49. Milani RV, Lavie CJ. Impact of cardiac rehabilitation on depression and its associated mortality. *Am J Med*. 2007;120:799-806.

50. Oldridge N, Guyatt G, Jones N, et al. Effects on quality of life with comprehensive rehabilitation after acute myocardial infarction. *Am J Cardiol*. 1991;67:1084-1089.

51. Piotrowicz E, Piotrowicz R. Cardiac telerehabilitation: Current situation and future challenges. *Eur J Prev Cardiol*. 2013;20(2 Suppl):12-6. doi:10.1177/2047487313487483c

52. Sandesara PB, Lambert CT, Gordon NF, et al. Cardiac rehabilitation and risk reduction: Time to "rebrand and reinvigorate". *J Am Coll Cardiol*. 2015;65(4):389-395. doi:10.1016/j.jacc.2014.10.059.

53. Gordon NF. New methods of delivering secondary preventive services: The promise of the Internet. *J Cardiopulm Rehabil*. 2003;23:349-351.

54. Vandelanotte C, Dwyer T, Van Itallie A, Hanley C, Mummery WK. The development of an internet-based outpatient cardiac rehabilitation intervention: A Delphi study. *BMC Cardiovasc Disord*. 2010;10:27.

55. Varnfield M, Karunanithi MK, Särelä A, et al. Uptake of a technology-assisted home-care cardiac rehabilitation program. *Med J Aust*. 2011;194:S15-19.

56. Bradley EH, Holmboe ES, Mattera JA, Roumanis SA, Radford MJ, Krumholz HM. A qualitative study of increasing beta-blocker use after myocardial infarction: Why do some hospitals succeed? *JAMA*. 2001;285:2604-2611.

57. Curry LA, Spatz E, Cherlin E, et al. What distinguishes top-performing hospitals in acute myocardial infarction mortality rates? A qualitative study. *Ann Intern Med*. 2011;154:384-390.

Chapter 3

1. Mechanic R, Tompkins C. Lessons learned preparing for Medicare bundled payments. *N Engl J Med.* 2012;367:1873-1875.

2. National and regional estimates on hospital use for all patients form the HCUP National Inpatient Sample (NIS). HCUP website. www.hcup-us.ahrq.gov/nisoverview.jsp. Published September 18, 2019. Accessed October 21, 2019.

3. Sud M, Qui F, Austin PC, et al. Short length of stay after elective transfemoral transcatheter aortic valve replacement is not associated with increased early or late readmission risk. *J Am Heart Assoc.* 2017;6(4):1-10. doi:10.1161/JAHA.116.005460

4. Wertheimer B, Jacobs RE, Iturrate E, et al. Discharge before noon: Effect on throughput and sustainability. *J Hosp Med.* 2015;10:664-669.

5. Johnson AM, Henning AN, Morris PE, et al. Timing and amount of physical therapy treatment are associated with length of stay in the cardiothoracic ICU. *Sci Rep.* 2017; 7(1):1-9. doi:10.1038/s41598-017-17624-3

6. Gruther W, Pieber K, Steiner I, et al. Can early rehabilitation on the general ward after an intensive care unit stay reduce hospital length of stay in survivors of critical illness?: A randomized controlled trial. *Am J Phys Med Rehabil.* 2017;96(9):607-615. doi:10.1097/PHM.0000000000000718

7. Schweickert WD, Pohlman MC, Pohlman AS, et al. Early physical and occupational therapy in mechanically ventilated, critically ill patients: Randomized controlled trail. *Lancet.* 2009;373:1874-1882. doi:10.1016/S0140-6736(09)60658-9.

8. Nakamura K., Nakamura E, Niina K, et al. Outcome after valve surgery in octogenarians and efficacy of early mobilization with early cardiac rehabilitation. *Gen Thorac Cardiovasc Surg.* 2010;58:606-611. doi:10.1007/s11748-010-0665-0.

9. Ahluwalia SC, Enguidanos S. Advance care planning among patients with heart failure: A review of challenges and approaches to better communication. *Journal of Clinical Outcomes Management.* 2015;22(2):73-82.

10. Vollman KM. Introduction to progressive mobility. *Crit Care Nurse* 2010;30(2):53-55.

11. Bassett RD, Vollman KM, Brandwene L, et al. Integrating a multidisciplinary programme into intensive care practice (IMMPTP): A multi-center collaborative. *Intensive Crit Care Nurs.* 2012;28:88-97.

12. Hodgson C, Stiller K, Needham D, et al. Expert consensus and recommendations on safety criteria for active mobilization of mechanically ventilated critically ill adults. *Crit Care* 2014 Dec 4;18(6):658. doi: 10.1186/s13054-014-0658-y.

13. Rigotti NA, Munafo MR, Stead LF. Smoking cessation interventions for hospitalized smokers: A systematic review. *Arch Intern Med.* 2008;168(18):1950-1960.

14. Qasim H, Karim ZA, Rivera JO, et al. Impact of electronic cigarettes on the cardiovascular system. *J Am Heart Assoc.* 2017;6(9):1-14.

15. Veronovici1 NR, Lasiuk GC, Rempel1GR, et al. Discharge education to promote self-management following cardiovascular surgery: An integrative review. *Eur J Cardiovasc Nurs.* 2014, Vol. 13(1) 22-31.

16. Commodore-Mensah Y, Dennison-Himmelfarb CR. Patient education strategies for hospitalized cardiovascular patients a systematic review. *J Cardiovasc Nurs.* 2012;27(2):154-174.

17. Resources for patients. AACVPR website. https://www.aacvpr.org/Resources/Resources-for-Patients/Cardiac-Rehab-Patient-Resources Accessed June 20, 2018.

18. Seconds count. SCAI website. http://www.secondscount.org/Default.aspx. Accessed June 20, 2018.

19. Cardiosmart website. www.cardiosmart.org. Accessed June 20, 2018.

20. AARP. *Family Caregiving and Out-of-Pocket Costs: 2016 Report.* Washington, DC: AARP; 2016.

21. Drozda J Jr, Messer JV, Spertus J, et al. ACCF/AHA/AMA-PCPI 2011 performance measures for adults with coronary artery disease and hypertension: A report of the American College of Cardiology Foundation/American Heart Association and the American Medical Association–Physician Consortium for Performance Improvement. *J Am Coll Cardiol.* 2011;58:316-336.

22. ACVPR/ACCF/AHA 2010 update: Performance measures on cardiac rehabilitation for referral to cardiac rehabilitation/secondary prevention services. *J Cardiopulm Rehabil Prev.* 2010;30:279-288.

23. Thomas RJ, King M, Lui K, et al. AACVPR/ACC/AHA 2007 performance measures on cardiac rehabilitation for referral to and delivery of cardiac rehabilitation/secondary prevention

services. *J Cardiopulm Rehabil Prev.* 2007;27:260-290.

24. Mueller E, Savage PD, Schneider DJ, Howland LL, Ades PA. Effect of a computerized referral at hospital discharge on cardiac rehabilitation participation rates. *J Cardiopulm Rehabil Prev.* 2009;29:365-369.

25. Arena R, Williams M, Forman DE, et al. Increasing referral and participation rates to outpatient cardiac rehabilitation: The valuable role of healthcare professionals in the inpatient and home health settings: A science advisory from the American Heart Association. *Circulation.* 2012;125:1321-1329.

26. Titler MG, Pettit DM. Discharge readiness assessment. *J Cardiovasc Nurs.* 1995;9:64-74.

27. Mabire C, Coffey A, Weiss M. Readiness for hospital discharge scale for older people: psychometric testing and short form development with a three-country sample. *J Adv Nurs.* 2015;71(11):2686-2696.

28. Rotter T, Kinsman L, James E, et al. Clinical pathways: Effects on professional practice, patient outcomes, length of stay and hospital costs. *Cochrane Database Syst Rev.* 2010 17;(3):CD006632. doi:10.1002/14651858. CD006632.pub2

29. Edwardson SR. The consequences and opportunities of shortened lengths of stay for cardiovascular patients. *J Cardiovasc Nurs.* 1999;14:1-11.

30. Hamm LF, Sanderson BK, Ades PA, et al. Core competencies for cardiac rehabilitation/secondary prevention professionals: 2010 update: Position statement of the American Association of Cardiovascular and Pulmonary Rehabilitation. *J Cardiopulm Rehabil Prev.* 2011;31:2-10.

31. Joint Commission on Accreditation of Healthcare Organizations website. https://www.jointcommission.org/accreditation/ambulatory_healthcare.aspx. Accessed June 20, 2018.

32. Dolansky MA, Xu F, Zullo M, et al. Post-acute care services received by older adults following a cardiac event: A population-based analysis. *J Cardio Nurs*, 2010;25(4):342-249. PMID: 20539168

33. Dolansky MA, Zullo MD, Hassanein S, et al. Cardiac rehabilitation in skilled nursing facilities: A missed opportunity. *Heart & Lung.* 2012;41(2):115-124. PMID: 22054718.

34. Jurgens CY, Goodlin S, Dolansky MA (Co-chairs), et al. Heart failure management in skilled nursing facilities: A scientific statement from the American Heart Association and the Heart Failure Society of America. *Circulation.* 2015;4:263-269. doi:10.1161/HHHF.0000000000000005.

35. Anderson JA, Petersen NJ, Kistner C, Soltero ER, Willson P. Determining predictors of delayed recovery and the need for transitional cardiac rehabilitation after cardiac surgery. *J Am Acad Nurs Pract.* 2006;18:386-392.

36. Sansone GR, Alba A, Frengley JD. Analysis of FIM instrument scores for patients admitted to an inpatient cardiac rehabilitation program. *Arch Phys Med Rehabil.* 2002;83:506-512.

37. Alsara O, Reeves RK, Pyfferoen MD, et al. Inpatient rehabilitation outcomes for patients receiving left ventricular assist device. *Am J Phys Med Rehabil.* 2014;10:860-868.

38. Zullo M, Dolansky MA, Josephson R, et al. Older adults' attendance in cardiac rehabilitation: The impact of functional status and post-acute care after acute myocardial infarction in 63,092 Medicare beneficiaries. *J Cardiopulm Rehabil Prev.* 2018;38(1):17-23. doi: 10.1097/ HCR.0000000000000264

39. Kong KH, Kevorkian CG, Rossi CD. Functional outcomes of patients on a rehabilitation unit after open heart surgery. *J Cardiopulm Rehabil.* 1996;16:413-418.

40. Keith RA, Granger CV, Hamilton BB, Sherwin FS. The Functional Independence Measure: A new tool for rehabilitation. *Adv Clin Rehabil.* 1987;1:6-18.

41. Fiedler RC, Granger CV, Ottenbacher KJ. The uniform data system for medical rehabilitation: Report of first admissions for 1994. *Am J Phys Med Rehabil.* 1996;75:125-129.

42. Murtaugh C, Peng T, Totten A, et al. Complexity in geriatric home healthcare. *J Healthc Qual.* 2009;31(2):34-43.

43. Feinberg JL, Russell D, Mola A, at el. Developing an adapted cardiac rehabilitation training for home care clinicians: Patient perspectives, clinician knowledge, and curriculum overview. *J Cardiopulm Rehabil Prev.* 2017;37:404-411.

44. Dolansky MA, Zullo, MD, Boxer, RS. Initial efficacy of a cardiac rehabilitation transition program: Cardiac TRUST. *J Gerontol Nurs.* 2011;37(12):36-44. PMID: 22084960.

45. Freeman HP, Rodriguez RL. History and principles of patient navigation. *Cancer.* 2011;117(S15):3537-3540.

46. Ali-Faisal SF, Colella TJ, Medina-Jaudes N, et al. The effectiveness of patient navigation to improve healthcare utilization outcomes: A meta-analysis of randomized controlled trials. *Patient Educ Couns*. 2017;100(3):436-448. doi:10.1016/j.pec.2016.10.014.

47. DiPalo K, Patel K, Assafin M, et al. Implementation of a patient navigator program to reduce 30-day heart failure readmission rate. *Prog Cardiovasc Dis*. 2017;60(2):259-266.

48. Scott LB, Gravely S, Sexton TR, et al. Examining the effect of a patient navigation intervention on outpatient cardiac rehabilitation awareness and enrollment. *J Cardiopulm Rehabil Prev*. 2013;33(5):281-291.

49. Doran K, Sampson B, Status R, et al. Clinical pathways across tertiary and community care after an interventional cardiology procedure. *J Cardiovasc Nurs*. 1997;11(2):1-14.

Chapter 4

1. Fletcher GF, Ades PA, Kligfield P, et al. Exercise standards for testing and training: A scientific statement from the American Heart Association. *Circulation*. 2013;128(8):873-934.

2. Listerman J, Bittner V, Sanderson BK, Brown TM. Cardiac rehabilitation outcomes: Impact of comorbidities and age. *J Cardiopulm Rehabil Prev*. 2011;31:342-348

3. Sargent LA, Seyfer AE, Hollinger J, et al. The healing sternum: A comparison of osseous healing with wire versus rigid fixation. *Ann Thorac Surg*. 1991;52:490-494.

4. Losanoff JE, Jones JW, Richman BW. Primary closure of median sternotomy: techniques and principles. Cardiovasc Surg. 2002 Apr;10(2):102-10.

5. Gibbons RJ, Balady GJ, Bricker JT, et al. ACC/AHA 2002 guideline update for exercise testing: Summary article. *J Am Coll Cardiol*. 2002;40:1531-1540.

6. Myers J, Arena R, Franklin B, et al. Recommendations for clinical exercise laboratories: A scientific statement from the American Heart Association. *Circulation*. 2009;119:3144-3161.

7. American College of Sports Medicine. *ACSM Guidelines for Exercise Testing and Prescription*. 10th ed. Philadelphia: Lippincott Williams & Wilkins, 2017.

8. Fletcher GF, Balady GJ, Amsterdam EA, et al. Exercise standards for testing and training: A statement for healthcare professionals from the American Heart Association. *Circulation*. 2013 Aug 20;128(8):873-934

9. Wilke NA, Sheldahl LM, Dougherty SM, et al. Baltimore Therapeutic Equipment work simulator: Energy expenditure of work activities in cardiac patients. *Arch Phys Med Rehabil*. 1993;74:419-424.

10. Balady GJ, Arena R, Sietsema K, et al. Clinician's guide to cardiopulmonary exercise testing in adults. *Circulation*. 2010;122:191-225.

11. Keteyian SJ, Isaac D, Thadani U, et al. Safety of symptom-limited cardiopulmonary exercise testing in patients with chronic heart failure due to severe left ventricular systolic dysfunction. *Am Heart J*. 2009;158:S72-S77.

12. Physical Activity Readiness Questionnaire. Canadian Society for Exercise Physiology website. www.csep.ca/CMFiles/publications/parq/par-q.pdf. Published January, 2002. Accessed June 15, 2018.

13. Myers J, Forman DE, Balady GJ. Supervision of exercise testing by nonphysicians: A scientific statement from the American Heart Association. *Circulation*. 2014;130(12):1014-27.

14. Gibbons RJ, Balady GJ, Bricker JT, et al. ACC/AHA 2002 guideline update for exercise testing: Summary article. *Circulation*. 2002;106:1883-1892.

15. Maeder M, Wolber T, Atefy R, et al. A nomogram to select the optimal treadmill ramp protocol. *J Cardiopulm Rehabil*. 2006;26:16-23.

16. Arena R, Myers J, Williams MA, et al. Assessment of functional capacity in clinical and research settings: A scientific statement from the American Heart Association. *Circulation*. 2007;116:329-343.

17. Myers J, Buchanan N, Walsh D, et al. Comparison of the ramp versus standard exercise protocols. *J Am Coll Cardiol*. 1991;17:1334-1342.

18. Ades PA, Savage PD, Brawner CA, et al. Aerobic capacity in patients entering cardiac rehabilitation. *Circulation*. 2006;113(23):2706-12.

19. Myers J, Kaminsky LA, Lima R, et al. A reference equation for normal standards for $\dot{V}O_2max$: Analysis from the Fitness Registry and the Importance of Exercise National Database (FRIEND Registry). *Prog Cardiovasc Dis*. 2017;60(1):21-29.

20. Wasserman K, Hansen J, Sue D, et al. *Principles of Exercise Testing and Interpretation*. 5th ed. Philadelphia: Lippincott Williams & Wilkins, 2011.

21. Jones N. *Clinical Exercise Testing*. Philadelphia: Saunders, 1997.

22. Hansen JE, Sue DY, Wasserman K. Predicted values for clinical exercise testing. *Am Rev Respir Dis.* 1984;129:S49-S55.

23. Morris CK, Myers J, Froelicher VF, et al. Nomogram based on metabolic equivalents and age for assessing aerobic exercise capacity in men. *J Am Coll Cardiol.* 1993;22:175-182.

24. Cole CR, Blackstone EH, Pashkow FJ, et al. Heart-rate recovery immediately after exercise as a predictor of mortality. *N Engl J Med.* 1999;341:1351-1357.

25. Gauri AJ, Raxwal VK, Roux L, et al. Effects of chronotropic incompetence and beta-blocker use on the exercise treadmill test in men. *Am Heart J.* 2001;142:136-141.

26. Frolkis JP, Pothier CE, Blackstone EH, et al. Frequent ventricular ectopy after exercise as a predictor of death. *NEJM.* 2003;348:781-790.

27. Gaalema DE, Savage PD, Leadholm K, et al. Clinical and demographic trends in cardiac Rehabilitation: 1996-2015. J *Cardiopulm Rehabil Prev.* 2019;39(4):266-273. doi:10.1097/HCR.0000000000000390

28. Cheitlin MD, Armstrong WF, Aurigemma GP, et al. ACC/AHA/ASE 2003 guideline update for the clinical application of echocardiography. *Circulation.* 2003;108:1146-1162.

29. Kohli P, Gulati M. Exercise stress testing in women: Going back to the basics. *Circulation.* 2010;122:2570-2580.

30. Klocke FJ, Baird MG, Lorell BH, et al. ACC/AHA/ASNC guidelines for the clinical use of cardiac radionuclide imaging. *Circulation.* 2003;108:1404-1418.

31. American Thoracic Society statement: Guidelines for the six-minute walk test. *Am J Respir Crit Care Med.* 2002;166:111-117.

32. Verrill DE, Fox L, Moore JB, et al. Validity and reliability of the North Carolina 6-minute cycle test. *J Cardiopulm Rehabil* 2006; 26: 224-30

33. Ainsworth BE, Haskell WL, Herrmann SD, et al. 2011 Compendium of physical activities: A second update of codes and MET values. *Med Sci Sports Exerc,* 2011;43(8):1575-1581.

34. Myers J, Do D, Herbert W, et al. A nomogram to predict exercise capacity from a specific activity questionnaire and clinical data. *Am J Cardiol.* 1994;73:591-596.

35. Pereira MA, FitzGerald SJ, Gregg EW, et al. A collection of Physical Activity Questionnaires for health-related research. *Med Sci Sports Exerc.* 1997;29:S1-205.

36. Goldman L, Hashimoto B, Cook EF, et al. Comparative reproducibility and validity of systems for assessing cardiovascular functional class: Advantages of a new specific activity scale. *Circulation.* 1981;64:1227-1234.

37. Hlatky MA, Boineau RE, Higginbotham MB, et al. A brief self-administered questionnaire to determine functional capacity (the Duke Activity Status Index). *Am J Cardiol.* 1989;64:651-654.

38. Giné-Garriga M, Roqué-Fíguls M, Coll-Planas L, Sitjà-Rabert M, Salvà A. Physical exercise interventions for improving performance-based measures of physical function in community-dwelling, frail older adults: A systematic review and meta-analysis. *Arch Phys Med Rehabil.* 2014;95:753-769.

Chapter 5

1. Heran BS1, Chen JM, Ebrahim S, et al. Exercise-based cardiac rehabilitation for coronary heart disease. *Cochrane Database Syst Rev.* 2011;(7):CD001800. doi: 10.1002/14651858.CD001800.pub2

2. Gaalema DE, Savage PD, Leadholm K, et al. Clinical and demographic trends in cardiac rehabilitation: 1996-2015. J Cardiopulm Rehabil Prev. 2019 Jul;39(4):266-273. doi: 10.1097/HCR.0000000000000390.

3. Smith SC Jr, Benjamin EJ, Bonow RO, et al. AHA/ACC secondary prevention and risk reduction therapy for patients with coronary and other atherosclerotic vascular disease: 2011 update. *Circulation.* 2011;124:2458-2473.

4. Ades PA. Cardiac rehabilitation and secondary prevention of coronary heart disease. *New Engl J Med.* 2001 Sep 20;345(12):892-902.

5. DeBusk RF, Miller NH, Superko HR, et al. A case-management system for coronary risk factor modification after acute myocardial infarction. *Ann Intern Med.* 1994;120:721-729.

6. Gordon NF, English CD, Contractor AS, et al. Effectiveness of three models for comprehensive cardiovascular risk reduction. *Am J Cardiol.* 2002;89:1263-1268.

7. Haskell WL, Aldernam EL, Fair JM, et al. Effects of intensive multiple risk factor reduction on coronary atherosclerosis and clinical cardiac events in men and women with coronary artery disease. The Stanford Coronary Risk Intervention Project (SCRIP). *Circulation.* 1994;89:975-990.

8. Suaya JA, Shepard DS, Normand SL, Ades PA, Prottas J, Stason WB. Use of cardiac rehabilitation by Medicare beneficiaries after myocardial infarction or coronary bypass surgery. *Circulation.* 2007 Oct 9;116(15):1653-62. Epub 2007 Sep 24.

9. Fang J, Ayala C, Luncheon C, Ritchey M, Loustalot F. Use of outpatient cardiac rehabilitation among heart attack survivors—20 States and the District of Columbia, 2013 and Four States, 2015. *MMWR Morb Mortal Wkly Rep.* 2017;66(33):869-873. doi:10.15585/mmwr.mm6633a1

10. Beatty AL, Truong M, Schopfer DW, Shen H, Bachmann JM, Whooley MA. Geographic variation in cardiac rehabilitation participation in Medicare and Veterans Affairs Populations: Opportunity for improvement. *Circulation.* 2018;137(18):1899-1908. doi: 10.1161/CIRCU-LATIONAHA.117.029471.

11. Valencia HE, Savage PD, Ades PA. Cardiac rehabilitation participation in underserved populations: Minorities, low socioeconomic, and rural residents. *J Cardiopulm Rehabil Prev.* 2011;31(4):203-10. doi:10.1097/HCR.0b013e318220a7da

12. Taylor R, Brown A, Ebrahim S, et al. Exercise-based rehabilitation for patients with coronary heart disease: Systematic review and meta-analysis of randomized controlled trials. *Am J Med.* 2004;116:682-692.

13. Clark A, Hartling L, Vandermeer B, McAlister F. Meta-analysis: Secondary prevention programs for patients with coronary artery disease. *Ann Intern Med.* 2005;143:659-672.

14. Thomas RJ, King M, Lui K, Oldridge N, Piña Il. AACVPR/ACCF/AHA 2010 update: Performance measures on cardiac rehabilitation for referral to cardiac rehabilitation/secondary prevention services. *J Cardiopulm Rehabil Prev.* 2010;30:279-288.

15. Ades PA, Keteyian SJ, Wright JS, et al. Increasing cardiac rehabilitation participation from 20% to 70%: A road map from the Million Hearts Cardiac Rehabilitation Collaborative. *Mayo Clin Proc.* 2017;92(2):234-242. doi:10.1016/j.mayocp.2016.10.014.

16. Balady GJ, Williams MA, Ades PA, et al. Core components of cardiac rehabilitation/secondary prevention programs: 2007 update. *J Cardiopulm Rehabil Prev.* 2007;27:121-129.

17. Graham I, Atar D, Borch-Johnsen K, et al. European guidelines on cardiovascular disease prevention in clinical practice. Fourth Joint Task Force of the European Society of Cardiology and Societies on Cardiovascular Disease Prevention in Clinical Practice. Eur J Cardiovasc Prev Rehabil. 2007;14(suppl 2):S1-S113.

18. Ornish D, Scherwitz LW, Billings JH, et al. Intensive lifestyle changes for reversal of coronary heart disease. *JAMA.* 1998;280:2001-2007.

19. Schuler G, Hambrecht R, Schlierf G, et al. Regular physical exercise and low-fat diet: Effects on progression of coronary artery disease. *Circulation.* 1992 Jul;86(1):1-11.

20. Decision Memo for Cardiac Rehabilitation Programs (CAG-00089R). CMS website. https://www.medicare.gov/coverage/cardiac-rehabilitation-programs Published January, 2019. Accessed October 11, 201910/11/19.

21. Grace SL, Russell KL, Reid RD, et al., for the Cardiac Rehabilitation Care Continuity Through Automatic Referral Evaluation (CRCARE) investigators. Effect of cardiac rehabilitation referral strategies on utilization rates: A prospective, controlled study. *Arch Intern Med.* 2011;171:235-241.

22. Hamm LF, Sanderson BK, Ades PA, et al. Core competencies for cardiac rehabilitation/secondary prevention professionals: 2010 update: position statement of the American Association of Cardiovascular and Pulmonary Rehabilitation. *J Cardiopulm Rehabil Prev.* 2011;31:2-10.

23. Libby P, Ridker P, Hansson GK. Inflammation in atherosclerosis: From pathophysiology to practice. *J Am Coll Cardiol.* 2009;54:2129-2139.

24. Grundy SM. Metabolic syndrome: A multiplex cardiovascular risk factor. J Clin Endocrinol Metab. 2007;92:399-404.

25. Bovend'Eerdt TJH, Botell RE, Wade DT. Writing SMART rehabilitation goals and achieving goal attainment scaling: A practical guide. *Clin Rehabil.* 2009;23:352-361.

26. Williams MA. Exercise testing in cardiac rehabilitation. Exercise prescription and beyond. *Cardiol Clin.* 2001;19(3):415-31.

27. Franklin BA, Bonzheim K, Gordon S, Timmis GC. Safety of medically supervised outpatient cardiac rehabilitation exercise therapy: A 16-year follow-up. *Chest.* 1998;114(3):902-6.

28. Ades PA, Savage PD, Brawner CA, et al. Aerobic capacity in patients entering cardiac rehabilitation. *Circulation.* 2006;113(23):2706-12. Epub 2006 Jun 5.

29. O'Connor CM, Whelan DJ, Lee KL, et al. Efficacy and safety of exercise training in patients with chronic heart failure: HF-ACTION randomized controlled trial. *JAMA.* 2009;301:1439-1450.

30. Siscovick DS, Weiss NS, Fletcher RH, Lasky T. The incidence of primary cardiac arrest during vigorous exercise. N Engl J Med. 1984 Oct 4;311(14):874-7.

31. Pack QR, Mansour M, Barboza JS, et al. An early appointment to outpatient cardiac rehabilitation at hospital discharge improves attendance at orientation: A randomized, single-blind, controlled trial. *Circulation*. 2013 Jan 22;127(3):349-55. doi:10.1161/CIRCULATIONAHA.112.121996.

32. King M, Bittner V, Josephson R, Lui K, Thomas RJ, Williams MA. Medical director responsibilities for outpatient cardiac rehabilitation/ secondary prevention programs: 2012 update: A statement for health care professionals from the American Association of Cardiovascular and Pulmonary Rehabilitation and the American Heart Association. *Circulation*. 2012;126(21):2535-43. doi:10.1161/CIR.0b013e318277728c

33. Ades PA, Pashkow FJ, Fletcher G, Pina IL, Zohman LR, Nestor JR. A controlled trial of cardiac rehabilitation in the home setting using electrocardiographic and voice transtelephonic monitoring. *Am Heart J*. 2000;139(3):543-8.

34. Lounsbury P, Elokda AS, Bunning JM, Arena R, Gordon EE. The value of detecting asymptomatic signs of myocardial ischemia in patients with coronary artery disease in outpatient cardiac rehabilitation. *J Cardiovasc Nurs*. 2017 May/Jun;32(3):E1-E9. doi:10.1097/JCN.0000000000000380

35. Ades PA, Savage PD, Toth MJ, et al. High-calorie-expenditure exercise: A new approach to cardiac rehabilitation for overweight coronary patients. *Circulation*. 2009 26;119(20):2671-8. doi:10.1161/CIRCULATIONAHA.108.834184.

36. Forman DE, LaFond K, Panch T, Allsup K, Manning K, Sattelmair J. Utility and efficacy of a smartphone application to enhance the learning and behavior goals of traditional cardiac rehabilitation: A feasibility study. *J Cardiopulm Rehabil Prev*. 2014;34(5):327-34. doi:10.1097/HCR.0000000000000058

37. Schopfer DW, Krishnamurthi N, Shen H, Duvernoy CS, Forman DE, Whooley MA. Association of Veterans Health Administration home-based programs with access to and participation in cardiac rehabilitation. *JAMA Intern Med*. 201;178(5):715-717. doi:10.1001/jamainternmed.2017.8039.

38. Lear SA, Spinelli JJ, Linden W, et al. The Extensive Lifestyle Management Intervention (ELMI) after cardiac rehabilitation: A 4-year randomized controlled trial. *Am Heart J*. 2006;152(2):333-9.

39. Giannuzzi P, Temporelli PL, Marchioli R, et al. GOSPEL Investigators. Global secondary prevention strategies to limit event recurrence after myocardial infarction: Results of the GOSPEL study, a multicenter, randomized controlled trial from the Italian Cardiac Rehabilitation Network. *Arch Intern Med*. 2008;168(20):2194-204. doi:10.1001/archinte.168.20.2194

40. Giallauria F, Lucci R, D'Agostino M, et al. Two-year multicomprehensive secondary prevention program: Favorable effects on cardiovascular functional capacity and coronary risk profile after acute myocardial infarction. *J Cardiovasc Med*. 2009;10(10):772-80. doi:10.2459/JCM.0b013e32832d55fe

Chapter 6

1. Fletcher GF, Ades PA, Kligfield P, et al. Exercise standards for testing and training: A scientific statement from the American Heart Association. *Circulation*. 2013;128:873-934.

2. Haskell W, Lee I-M, Pate R, et al. Physical activity and public health: Updated recommendation for adults from the American College of Sports Medicine and the American Heart Association. *Circulation*. 2007;116:1081-1093.

3. *2018 Physical Activity Guidelines for Americans*. U.S. Department of Health and Human Services website. https://health.gov/paguidelines/second-edition/report. Published November 2019. Accessed October 29, 2019.

4. One in five adults meet overall physical activity guidelines. Centers for Disease Control and Prevention website. www.cdc.gov/media/releases/2013/p0502-physical-activity.html. Published May 2013. Accessed June 29, 2018.

5. Thompson PD, Buchner D, Pina IL, et al. AHA scientific statement: Exercise and physical activity in the prevention and treatment of atherosclerotic cardiovascular disease. *Circulation*. 2003;107:3109-3116.

6. Pate RR, Pratt M, Blair SN, et al. Physical activity and public health: A recommendation from the Centers for Disease Control and Prevention and the American College of Sports Medicine. *JAMA*. 1995;273:402-407.

7. U.S. Department of Health and Human Services. *Physical Activity and Health: A Report of the Surgeon General*. Atlanta: U.S. Department of Health and Human Services, Centers for Disease Control and Prevention, National Center for Chronic Disease Prevention and Health Promotion; 1996.

8. Myers J, McAuley P, Lavie C, Despres JP, Arena R, Kokkinos P. Physical activity and cardiorespiratory fitness as major markers of cardiovascular risk: Their independent and interwoven importance to health status. *Prog Cardiovasc Dis*. 2015;57:306-314.

9. Riebe D, Ehrman JK, Liguori G, Magal M, American College of Sports Medicine. *ACSM's Guidelines for Exercise Testing and Prescription*. 10th ed. Philadelphia: Wolters Kluwer; 2018.

10. Hambrecht R, Niebauer J, Marburger C, et al. Various intensities of leisure time physical activity in patients with coronary artery disease: Effects on cardiorespiratory fitness and progression of coronary atherosclerotic lesions. *J Am Coll Cardiol*. 1993;22:468-477.

11. Ayabe M, Brubaker PH, Dobrosielski D, et al. The physical activity patterns of cardiac rehabilitation program participants. *J Cardiopulm Rehabil*. 2004;24:80-86.

12. Savage PD, Brochu M, Scott P, et al. Low caloric expenditure in cardiac rehabilitation. *Am Heart J*. 2000;140:527-533.

13. Schairer JR, Keteyian SJ, Ehrman JK, et al. Leisure time physical activity of patients in maintenance cardiac rehabilitation. *J Cardiopulm Rehabil*. 2003;23:260-265.

14. Schairer JR, Kostelnik T, Proffitt SM, et al. Caloric expenditure during cardiac rehabilitation. *J Cardiopulm Rehabil*. 1998;18:290-294.

15. Ades PA, Savage PD, Harvey-Berino J. The treatment of obesity in cardiac rehabilitation. *J Cardiopulm Rehabil Prev*. 2010;30:289-298.

16. McConnell TR, Klinger TA, Gardner JK, et al. Cardiac rehabilitation without exercise tests for post-myocardial infarction and post-bypass surgery patients. *J Cardiopulm Rehabil*. 1998;18:458-463.

17. Ayabe M, Brubaker PH, Dobrosielski D, et al. Target step count for the secondary prevention of cardiovascular disease. *Circ J*. 2008;72:299-303.

18. Stevenson TG, Riggin K, Nagelkirk PR, et al. Physical activity habits of cardiac patients participating in an early outpatient rehabilitation program. *J Cardiopulm Rehabil Prev*. 2009;29:299-303.

19. Jones NL, Schneider PL, Kaminsky LA, et al. An assessment of the total amount of physical activity of patients participating in a phase III cardiac rehabilitation program. *J Cardiopulm Rehabil Prev*. 2007;27:81-85.

20. Ayabe M, Brubaker PH, Kumahara H, Kiyonaga A, Tanaka H, Aoki J. Self-monitoring moderate-vigorous physical activity versus steps/day is more effective in chronic disease exercise programs. *J Cardiopulm Rehabil Prev*. 2010;30:111-115.

21. Vogel J, Auinger A, Riedl R, Kindermann H, Helfert M. Helmuth Ocenasek. Digitally enhanced recovery: Investigating the use of digital self-tracking for monitoring leisure time physical activity of cardiovascular disease (CVD) patients undergoing cardiac rehabilitation. *PLoS ONE*. 2017;12:e0186261.

22. Williams M, Haskell W, Ades P, et al. Resistance training in individuals with and without cardiovascular disease: 2007 update: A scientific statement from the American Heart Association. *Circulation*. 2007;116:572-584.

23. Stewart KJ, Ratchford EV, Williams MA. Exercise for restoring health and preventing vascular disease. In: RS Blumenthal. JM Foody, ND Wong, eds. *Preventive Cardiology*. Philadelphia: Elsevier; 2011:541-551.

Chapter 7

1. U.S. Department of Health and Human Services and U.S. Department of Agriculture. *2015–2020 Dietary Guidelines for Americans*. 8th ed. Published 2015. http://health.gov/dietaryguidelines/2015/guidelines. Accessed 10/14/19

2. Eckel RH, Jakicic JM, Ard JD, et al. 2013 AHA/ACC Guideline on lifestyle management to reduce cardiovascular risk: A report of the American College of Cardiology/American Heart Association Task Force on Practice Guidelines. *Circulation*. 2013;129:S76-S99. doi:10.1161/01.cir.0000437740.48606.d1

3. Stone NJ, Robinson J, Lichtenstein AH, Bairey Merz CM. 2013 ACC/AHA Guideline on the treatment of blood cholesterol to reduce atherosclerotic cardiovascular risk in adults: A report of the American College of Cardiology/American Heart Association Task Force on Practice Guidelines. *Circulation*. 2013;63(25 Pt B):2889-934. doi:10.1161/01.cir.0000437738.63853.7a

4. Jensen MD, Ryan DH, Apovian CM, et al. AHA/ACC/TOS prevention guideline: 2013 AHA/ACC/TOS Guideline for the Management of Overweight and Obesity in Adults: A report of the American College of Cardiology/American Heart Association Task Force on Practice Guidelines and The Obesity Society. *Circulation*. 2013; 129(25 Suppl 2):S102-38. doi: 10.1161/01.cir.0000437739.71477.ee

5. Yancy CW, Jessup M, Bozkurt B, et al. 2013 ACCF/AHA Guideline for the management of heart failure: A report of the American College of Cardiology Foundation/American Heart Association Task Force on Practice Guidelines. *J Am Coll Cardiol*. 2013;62(16):e147-e239. doi:10.1016/j.jacc.2013.05.019

6. Jacobson TA, Ito MK, Maki KC, et al. National lipid association recommendations for patient-centered management of dyslipidemia: Full report. *J Clin Lipidol.* 2015;9(2) Part 1:129-169; Part 2:S1-S122.

7. Whelton PK, Carey RM, Aronow WS, et al. 2017 ACC/AHA/AAPA/ABC/ACPM-/AGS/APhA/ASH/ASPC/NMA/PCNA Guideline for the prevention, detection, evaluation, and management of high blood pressure in adults: A report of the American College of Cardiology/American Heart Association Task Force on Clinical Practice Guidelines. Hypertension. 2018 Jun; 71(6):1269-1324. Epub 2017 Nov 13.

8. Van Horn L, Carson J, Appel L, et al. Recommended dietary pattern to achieve adherence to the American Heart Association/American College of Cardiology (AHA/ACC) Guidelines: A scientific statement from the American Heart Association. *Circulation.* 2016;134(22):e505-e529. Epub 2016 Oct 27. doi:10.1161/CIR.0000000000000462

9. Moore C, Cunningham S. Social position, psychological stress and obesity: A systematic review. *J Acad Nutr Diet.* 2012;112(4):518-526.

10. Yang Q, Zhang Z, Gregg EW, Flanders W, Merritt R, Hu FB. Added Sugar Intake and CVD Mortality Among US Adults. *JAMA Intern Med.* 2014 174(4):516-524 doi:10.1001/jamainternmed.2013.13563

11. Howard BV, Wylie-Rosett J. Sugar and cardiovascular disease: A statement for healthcare professionals from the Committee on Nutrition of the Council on Nutrition, Physical Activity, and Metabolism of the American Heart Association. *Circulation.* 2002;106:523-527.

12. Kromhout D, Menotti A, Alberti-Fidanza A, et al. Comparative ecologic relationships of saturated fat, sucrose, food groups, and a Mediterranean food pattern score to 50-year coronary heart disease mortality rates among 16 cohorts of the Seven Countries Study. *Eur J Clin Nutr.* 2018 Aug;72(8):1103-1110. doi: 10.1038/s41430-018-0183-1.

13. Mellen PB, Walsh T, Herrington DM. Whole grain intake and cardiovascular disease: A meta-analysis. *Nutr Metab Cardiovasc Dis.* 2007;18(4):283-290.

14. Pereira MA. Dietary fiber and risk of CAD. A pooled Analysis of cohort studies. Arch Int Med. 2004;164:370-376.

15. U.S. Department of Health and Human Services and U.S. Department of Agriculture. What we eat in America. NHANES 2011–2012. Available at www. ars.usda.gov/SP2UserFiles/Place/80400530/pdf/1112/tables_1-40_2011-2012.pdf.

16. Rideout T, Harding S, Jones P, Fan M. Guar gum and similar soluble fibers in the regulation of cholesterol metabolism: Current understandings and future research priorities. *Vasc Health Risk Manag.* 2008;4(5):1023-1033.

17. Theuwisson E, Mensink RP. Water-soluble dietary fibers and cardiovascular disease. *Physiol Behav.* 2008:94:285-292.

18. Brown, L, Rosner B, Willett W, Sacks F. Cholesterol-lowering effects of dietary fiber: A meta-analysis *Am J Clin Nutr.* 1999;69(1):30-42.

19. Barclays AW, Petocz P, McMillan, et al. Glycemic index, glycemic load and chronic disease risk – A meta analysis of observational studies. *Am J Clin Nutr.* 2008; 87:627-37.

20. Calder, PC 2015 Functional Roles of Fatty Acids and Their Effects on Human Health. JPEN J Parenter Enteral Nutr. 2015; 39(suppl 1):18S-32S

21. van Bilsen M, Planavila A. Fatty acids and cardiac disease: Fuel carrying a message. *Acta Physiologica.* 211:476–490. doi: 10.1111/apha.12308

22. Vannice G, Rassmussen H. Position of the Academy of Nutrition and Dietetics: Dietary fatty acids for healthy adults. *J Acad Nutr Diet.* 2014;114:136-153.

23. Sacks FM, Lichtenstein AH, Wu JH, et al. Dietary fats and cardiovascular disease: A presidential advisory from the American Heart Association. *Circulation.* 2017. Jul 18;136(3):e1-e23. doi:CIR-0000000000000510.

24. Maki KC, Palacios OM, Bell M, et al. Use of supplemental long-chain omega-3 fatty acids and risk for cardiac death: An updated meta-analysis and review of research gaps. *J Clin Lipidol.* 2017;11(5):1152-1160.

25. Mozaffarian D. Dietary and policy priorities for cardiovascular disease, diabetes, and obesity. *Circulation.* 2016;133:187-225. doi:10.1161/CIRCULATIONAHA.115.018585

26. Wolfe RR, Cifelli AM, Kostas G, Kim I. Optimizing protein intake in adults: Interpretation and application of the recommended dietary allowance compared with the acceptable macronutrient distribution range. *Adv in Nutr.* 2015;8(2):266-275. doi:10.3945/an.116.013821

27. Rodriguez N. Introduction to Protein Summit 2.0: Continued exploration of the impact of high-quality protein on optimal health. *Am J Clin Nutr*. 2015;101(Suppl):1317S-9S.

28. Halton TL, Willett WC, Liu S, et al. Low-carbohydrate-diet score and the risk of coronary heart disease in women. *N Engl J Med*. 2006;355:1991-2002.

29. Schwingshackl L, Hoffmann G. Long-term effects of low-fat diets either low or high in protein on cardiovascular and metabolic risk factors:a systematic review and meta-analysis. *Nutr J*. 2013;12:48. doi:10.1186/1475-2891-12-48

30. Layman DK, Anthony TG, Rasmussen BB, et al. Defining meal requirements for protein to optimize metabolic roles of amino acids. *Am J Clin Nutr*. 2015;101(Suppl):1330S-8S.

31. Paddon-Jones D, Campbell WW, Jacques PF, et al. Protein and healthy aging. *Am J Clin Nutr*. 2015; 101(Suppl):1339S-45S.

32. Van Horn L, McCoin M, Kris-Etherton PM, et al. The evidence for dietary prevention and treatment of cardiovascular disease. *JADA*. 2008;108:287-331.

33. Mukamal KJ, Rimm EB. Alcohol's effects on risk for CHD. *Alcohol Res Health*. 2001;25:255-261.

34. Hanson C, Rutten EP, Woutes EF, Rennard S. Diet and vitamin D as risk factors for lung impairment and COPD. *Translational Research*. 2013;162(4):219-236.

35. Wang S, Melnyk JP, Tsao R, Marcone MF. How natural dietary antioxidants in fruits, vegetables and legumes promote vascular health. *Food Research International*. 2011;44(1):14-22.

36. Kanbay M, Bayram Y, Solak Y, Sanders PW. Dietary Potassium: A key mediator of the cardiovascular response to dietary sodium chloride. *J Am Soc Hypertens*. 2013;7(5):395-400. doi:10.1016/j.jash.2013.04.009

37. He FJ, MacGregor GA. Salt reduction lowers cardiovascular risk: Meta-analysis of outcome trials. *Lancet*. 2011;378:380–382.

38. Cobb LK, Appel LJ, Anderson CA. Strategies to reduce dietary sodium intake. Curr Treat Options Cardiovasc Med. 2012;14(4):425–434. doi:10.1007/s11936-012-0182-9

39. Pantsi W, Bester D, Esterhuyse A, Aboua G. Dietary antioxidant properties of vegetable oils and nuts: The race against cardiovascular disease progression. In: *Antioxidant-Antidiabetic Agents and Human Health*. Published: February 5th 2014. doi: 10.5772/57184. Accessed October 12, 2018

40. Pandey KB, Rizvi SI. Plant polyphenols as dietary antioxidants in human health and disease. *Ox Med Cell Longev*. 2009;2(5):270-278.

41. Clifton PM, Mano M, Duchateau GS, van der Knaap HCM, Trautwein EA. Dose-response effects of different plant sterol sources in fat spreads on serum lipids and C-reactive protein and on the kinetic behavior of serum plant sterols. *Eur J Clin Nutr*. 2008;62:968-977.

42. Ostlund R, Mcgill J, Zeng C, et al. Gastrointestinal absorption and plasma kinetics of soy delta phytosterols in humans. Am J Physiol End Metab. 2002; 282:E911-916.

43. Plat J, Mensink RP. Diets enriched with 2 different plant stanol esters on plasma ubiquinol-10 and fat-soluble antioxidant concentrations. *Metabolism*. 2001;50:520-529.

44. Mozaffarian D, Appel LJ, VanHorn L. Components of a cardioprotective diet: New insights. *Circulation*. 2011;123:2870-2891.

45. Bechthold A, Boeing H, Schwedhelm C, et al. Food groups and risk of coronary heart disease, stroke and heart failure: A systematic review and dose-response meta-analysis of prospective studies. Critical Reviews in Food Science and Nutrition. 2017;59(7):1071-1090 doi:10.1080/10408398.2017.1392288

46. Scalbert A, Johnson IT, Saltmarsh M. Polyphenols: Antioxidants and beyond. *Am J Clin Nutr*. 2005;81(1):215S-217S.

47. Koliaki C, Spinos T, Spinou M, Brinia ME, Mitsopoulou D, Katsilambros N. Defining the optimal dietary approach for safe, effective and sustainable weight loss in overweight and obese adults. *Healthcare (Basel)*. 2018;6(3). pii:E73. doi:10.3390/healthcare6030073.

48. Sabaté J, Wien M. Nuts, blood lipids and cardiovascular disease. *Asia Pac J Clin Nutr*. 2010;19(1):131-136.

49. Rimm EB, Appel LJ, Chiuve SE, et.al; American Heart Association Nutrition Committee of the Council on Lifestyle and Cardiometabolic Health; Council on Epidemiology and Prevention; Council on Cardiovascular Disease in the Young; Council on Cardiovascular and Stroke Nursing; and Council on Clinical Cardiology. Seafood long-chain n-3 polyunsaturated fatty acids and cardiovascular disease: a science advi-

sory from the American Heart Association. Circulation. 2018;138:e35–e47. DOI: 10.1161/CIR.0000000000000574.

50. Mozaffarin D. Fish and n-3 fatty acids for the prevention of fatal CAD and sudden cardiac death. *Am J Clin Nutr.* 2008;87(6):1991S-1996S.

51. O'Connor LE, Kim JE, Campbell WW. Total red meat intake of ≥0.5 servings/d does not negatively influence cardiovascular disease risk factors: A systemically searched meta-analysis of randomized controlled trials. *Am J Clin Nutr.* 2017;105(1):57-69. doi:10.3945/ajcn.116.142521

52. Pan A, Sun Q, Bernstein A, et al. Red meat consumption and mortality: Results from two prospective cohort studies. *Arch Intern Med.* 2012;172(7):555-563. doi:10.1001/archinternmed.2011.2287

53. Bernstein AM, Sun Q, Hu FB, et al. Major dietary protein sources and risk of coronary heart disease in women. *Circulation.* 2010;122(9):876–83.

54. Micha R, Michas G, Mozaffarian D. Unprocessed red and processed meats and risk of coronary artery disease and type 2 diabetes—An updated review of the evidence. *Curr Atheroscler Rep.* 2012;14(6):515-524. doi:10.1007/s11883-012-0282-8

55. Pan A. Red meat consumption and mortality: Results from two prospective cohort studies. 2012 *Arch Int Med.* 172(7): 555-63.

56. Menke A, Muntner P, FernaÅlndez-Real JM, Guallar E. The association of biomarkers of iron status with mortality in US adults. *Nutr Metab Cardiovasc Dis.* 2012 Sep;22(9):734-40. doi: 10.1016/j.numecd.2010.11.011. Epub 2011 Feb 16.

57. Maki KC, Van Elswyk ME, Alexander DD, Rains TM, Sohn EL, McNeill S. A meta-analysis of randomized controlled trials that compare the lipid effects of beef versus poultry and/or fish consumption. *J Clin Lipidol.* 2012;6:352-61.

58. Lorenzen JK, Jensen SK, Astrup A. Milk minerals modify the effect of fat intake on serum lipid profile: Results from an animal and a human short-term study. *Br J Nutr.* 2014;111:1412-1420.

59. Freeland-Graves JH and Nitzke S. Position of the Academy of Nutrition and Dietetics: Total diet approach to healthy eating. *J Acad Nutr Diet.* 2013;113(2):307-317.

60. Moore C, Cunningham S. Social position, psychological stress and obesity: A systematic review. *J Acad Nutr Diet.* 2012;112(4):518-526.

61. In Brief: Your guide to lowering your blood pressure with DASH. National Heart, Lung, and Blood Institute website. Pub: January 2006. www.nhlbi.nih.gov/files/docs/public/heart/dash_brief.pdf. Accessed October 18, 2018.

62. Estruch R, Ros E1, Salas-Salvadó J, et al. Primary prevention of cardiovascular disease with a Mediterranean diet supplemented with extra-virgin olive oil or nuts. *N Engl J Med.* 2018;378(25):e34. doi:10.1056/NEJMoa1800389.

63. Conlin PR, Erlinger TP, Rosner BA, et al. Effects of protein, monounsaturated fat, and carbohydrate intake on blood pressure and serum lipids: Results of the OmniHeart randomized trial. *JAMA.* 2005;294:2455-2464. doi:10.1001/jama.294.19.2455.

64. Esmaillzadeh WC, Kimiagar A, Mahrabi M, Azadbakht Y, Hu L, Willett FB. Fruit and vegetable intakes, C-reactive protein, and the metabolic syndrome. *Am J Clin Nutr.* 2006;84(6):1489-1497.

65. Djoussé L, Ho Y, Nguyen XT, et al. DASH score and subsequent risk of coronary artery disease: The findings from Million Veteran Program. *J Am Heart Assoc.* 2018;7(9):e008089. doi:10.1161/JAHA.117.008089

66. Appel L, Sacks FM, Carey VJ, et al. Effects of protein, monounsaturated fat, and carbohydrate intake on blood pressure and serum lipids: Results of the OmniHeart randomized trial. JAMA 2005;294 (19) 2455- 2464

67. Liese AD, Nichols M, Sun X, D'agostino RB, Haffner SM. Adherence to the DASH Diet is inversely associated with incidence of type 2 diabetes: The insulin resistance atherosclerosis study. *Diabetes Care.* 2009;32:1434-1436.

68. Singh RB. Effect of Indo-Mediterranean diet on progression of heart disease. *Lancet.* 2002;260:1455-1461.

69. deLorgeril M, et al. Mediterranean diet, traditional risk factors and rate of CV complications after MI. Circulation. 1999; 99:779-785.

70. Trichopoulou A, Costacou T, Bamia C, Trichopoulos D. Adherence to a Mediterranean diet and survival in a Greek population. *N Engl J Med.* 2003;348:2599–2608. doi:10.1056/NEJMoa025039.

71. Rees K, Hartley L, Flowers N, et al. "Mediterranean" dietary pattern for the primary prevention of cardiovascular disease. *Cochrane Database Syst Rev.* 2013;(8):CD009825. doi:10.1002/14651858.CD009825.pub2.

72. Then and now: How the Dietary Guidelines for Americans changed from 2010 to 2015. Academy of Nutrition and Dietetics website. www.eatrightpro.org/resource/news-center/in-practice/research-reports-and-studies/dgas-then-and-now. Published January 14, 2016. Accessed July 15, 2017

73. Key TJ, et al. Mortality in vegetarian and non-vegetarian 1998: A collaborative analysis of 8300 deaths among 76,000 men and women in 5 prospective studies. *Public Health Nutr.* 1998;1(1):33-41.

74. Farmer B, Larson BT, Fulgoni VL 3rd, Rainville AJ, Liepa GU. A vegetarian dietary pattern as a nutrient-dense approach to weight management: An analysis of the National Health and Nutrition Examination Survey 1999-2004. *J Am Diet Assoc.* 2011;111:819-827. doi:10.1016/j.jada.2011.03.012

75. Jian ZH, Chiang YC, Lung CC, et al. Vegetarian diet and cholesterol and TAG levels by gender. *Public Health Nutr.* 2015;18:721-726. doi:10.1017/S136898001400088

76. Shimazu, T, Kuriyama S, Hozawa A et al. Dietary patterns and CVD mortality in Japan: A prospective cohort study. *Inter J Epidemiol.* 2007;36(3):600-609.

77. Wilcox DC, et al. The Okinawan Diet: Health implications of a low calorie, nutrient dense, antioxidant rich dietary pattern low in glycemic load. *Am J Clin Nutr.* 2009;28 (suppl):5005-5165.

78. Lennon SL, DellaValle DM, Rodder SG, et.al. 2015 Evidence Analysis Library Evidence-Based Nutrition Practice Guideline for the Management of Hypertension in Adults. J Acad Nutr Diet. 2017 Sep;117(9):1445-1458.e17. doi: 10.1016/j.jand.2017.04.008. Epub 2017 Jun 1.

79. He J, Li J, MacGregor GA. Effect of longer term modest salt reduction on blood pressure: Cochrane systematic review and meta-analysis of randomized trials. *BMJ.* 2013;346:f1325.

80. He J, Gu D, Chen J, et al. Gender difference in blood pressure responses to dietary sodium intervention in the GenSalt study. *J Hypertens.* 2009;27:48-54.

81. Dinicolantonio, J, Niazi, A, Lavie, C, O'Keefe, J. Problems with the AHA Presidential Advisory advocating sodium restriction. *Amer J Hypertens.* 2013;26(10):1093.

82. Graudal N, Jurgens G, Baslund B, Alderman MH. Compared with usual sodium intake, low- and excessive-sodium diets are associated with increased mortality: a meta-analysis. *Am J Hypertens.* 2014;27(9):1129-1137. doi:10.1093/ajh/hpu028

83. Wang Y, Chen X. Between group differences in nutrition and health related psychosocial factors. *J Acad Nutr Diet.* 2012;112:486-498.

84. Whelton PK, Appel LJ, Sacco RL, et al. Sodium, blood pressure and cardiovascular disease. Further evidence supporting the AHA sodium reduction recommendations. *Circulation.* 2012;126:2880-2889.

85. Perez V, Chang ET; Sodium-to-potassium ratio and blood pressure, hypertension, and related factors. *Adv Nutr.* 2014;5(6):712-741. doi:10.3945/an.114.006783

86. Arnett DK, Blumenthal RS, Albert MA 2019 ACC/AHA Guideline on the Primary Prevention of Cardiovascular Disease. Am Coll Cardiol. 2019 Sep, 74 (10) e177-e232.

87. National Academies of Sciences, Engineering, and Medicine. Dietary Reference Intakes for Sodium and Potassium. Washington, DC; The National Academies Press; 2019.

88. Nissensohn M, Román-Viñas B, Sánchez-Villegas A, Piscopo S, Serra-Majem L. The effect of the Mediterranean diet on hypertension: A systematic review and meta-analysis. *J. Nutr. Educ. Behav.* 2016;48:42-53.

89. La Verde M, Mulè S, Zappalà G, et al. Higher adherence to the Mediterranean diet is inversely associated with having hypertension: Is low salt intake a mediating factor? *Int J Food Sci Nutr.* 2018;69(2):235-244. Epub July 14, 2017. doi:10.1080/09637486.2017.1350941

90. James PA, Oparil S, Carter BL, et al. 2014 Evidence-based guideline for the management of high blood pressure in adults: Report from the panel members appointed to the Eighth Joint National Committee (JNC 8). *JAMA.* 2014;311(5):507-520. doi:10.1001/jama.2013.284427

91. Potter JF, Beevers DG. Two possible mechanisms for alcohol associated hypertension. *Scand J Clin Lab Invest.* 1985;176:92-99.

92. Sesso HD, Cook NR, Buring JE, et al. Alcohol consumption and the risk of hypertension in women and men. *Hypertension.* 2008;51:1080-1087.

93. Rehm J, Room R, Monteiro M, et al. Alcohol as a risk factor for global burden of disease. *Eur Addict Res.* 2003;9:157-164.

94. EFSA Panel on Dietetic Products, Nutrition, and Allergies (NDA). Scientific opinion on the safety of caffeine. *EFSA Journal.* 2015;13(5):4102.

95. Pastors JG, Franz MJ. Effectiveness of medical nutrition therapy for diabetes. In: Franz, MJ, Evert AE. eds, *American Diabetes Association Guide to Nutrition Therapy in Diabetes.* Alexandria, VA: American Diabetes Association; 2013:1-18.

96. Bantle JP, Wylie-Rosett J, Albright AL, et al. American Diabetes Association. Nutrition recommendations and interventions for diabetes: Aposition statement of the American Diabetes Association. *Diabetes Care.* 2008;31(Suppl.1):S61-S78.

97. Wheeler ML, Dunbar SA, Jaacks LM, et al. Macronutrients, food groups, and eating patterns in the management of diabetes. *Diabetes Care.* 2012;35:434-445.

98. Norris SI, Lau J, Smith SJ, Schmid CH, Engelgau MM. Self-management education for adults with Type 2 diabetes. *Diabetes Care.* 2002;25(7):1159-1171.

99. Cramer JA. A systematic review of adherence with medications for diabetes. *Diabetes Care.* 2004;7(5):1218-1224.

100. Jannasch, F, Kroger J, Schulze MB. Dietary patterns and type 2 diabetes: A systematic literature review and meta-analysis of prospective studies. *J Nutr Epidemol.* 2017; 147:1174-82

101. American Diabetes Association. Standards of medical care in diabetes. *Diabetes Care.* 2013;36(Suppl):s11-s66.

102. Krebs JD, Parry-Strong A. Is there an optimal diet for patients with type 2 diabetes? Yes, the one that works for them! *British Journal DVD* 2013;13:60.

103. Barnard ND, Cohen J, Jenkins DJ, et al. A low-fat vegan diet and a conventional diabetes diet in the treatment of type 2 diabetes: A randomized, controlled, 74-wk clinical trial. *Am J Clin Nutr.* 2009;89:1588S-1596S.

104. Nilsson AC, Ostman EM, Holst JJ Björck. Including indigestible carbohydrates in the evening meal of healthy subjects improves glucose intolerance, lowers inflammatory markers and increases satiety after a subsequent standardized breakfast. *J Nutr.* 2008;138:732-739.

105. Ramini GV, Uber PA, Mehra MR. Chronic heart failure: Contemporary diagnosis and management. *May Clin Proc.* 2010;85:180-195.

106. Butler J, Papadimitriou L, Georgiopoulou V, Skopicki H, Dunbar S, Kalogeropoulos A. Comparing sodium intake strategies in heart failure: Rationale and design of the Prevent Adverse Outcomes in Heart Failure by Limiting Sodium (PROHIBIT) study. *Circ Heart Fail.* 2015;8(3), 636-645.

107. Doukky R, Avery E, Mangla A, et al. Impact of dietary sodium restriction on heart failure outcomes. *JACC Heart Fail.* 2016;4(1):24-35. doi:10.1016/j.jchf.2015.08.007

108. Arcand J, Mak S, Choleva M, et al. Adverse nutritional consequences of dietary sodium reduction in patients with heart failure. *Circulation.* 2011;124:A15807.

109. Rifal L, Hayden J, Pisano C, Silver M. Impact of DASH diet on endothelial function in HF patients. *Circulation.* 2013;128:A10406.

110. Hummel S, Seymour EM, Brook RD, et al. Low sodium DASH diet improves diastolic function and ventricular arterial coupling in hypertensive HF with preserved ejection fraction. *Circulation.* 2013;6:1165-1170.

111. Levitan E, Lewis CE, Tinker LF, et al. Mediterranean and DASH diet scores and mortality in women with heart failure. *Heart Failure.* 2013;6:1116-1123.

112. Kenchaiah S, Pocock SJ, Wang D, et al. Body Mass Index and prognosis in patients with chronic heart failure: Insights from the Candesartan in Heart failure: Assessment of Reduction in Mortality and Morbidity (CHARM) Program. *Circulation.* 2007;116:627-636.

113. Evangelista LS, Moser DK, Westlake C, Hamilton MA, Fonarow GC, Dracup K. Impact of obesity on quality of life and depression in patients with heart failure. *Eur J Heart Fail.* 2006;8:750-755.

114. Leidy HJ, Bossingham MJ, Mattes RD, Campbell WW. Increased dietary protein consumed at breakfast leads to initial and sustained feeling of fullness during energy restriction compared to other meal times. *Br J Nutr.* 2009;101(6):798-803.

115. Spahn JM, Lyon JMG, Alman JM, et al. The systematic review and methodology used to support 2010 Dietary Guidelines. *JADA.* 2010;111(4):520-523.

116. Hall KD, Sacks G, Chandramohan D, et al. Quantification of the effect of energy imbalance on body weight. *Lancet.* 2011;378: 826-837.

117. Boden WE, O'Rourke RA, Teo KK, et al. COURAGE Trial Research Group. Optimal medical therapy with or without PCI for stable coronary disease. *N Engl J Med.* 2007;356:1503-1516.

118. Thomas JG, Bond DS, Phelan S, Hill JO, Wing RR. Weight-loss maintenance for 10 years in the National Weight Control Registry. *Amer J Prev Med.* 2014;46(1)17-23.

119. VanWormer JJ, Boucher JL. Motivational interviewing and diet modification: A review of the evidence. *Diabetes Educator.* 2004;30(3):404-419.

120. Kristeller J, Wolever RQ. Mindfulness-based eating awareness training for treating binge eating disorder: The conceptual foundation. *Eating Disorders.* 2010;19(1):49-61.

121. Albers S. Mindful Eating Pledge website. eatq.com/wp-content/uploads/PledgetoEatMindfully.pdf. Published December 23, 2013. Accessed March 2, 2014.

122. Thompson C, Foster G. Dietary behaviors: Promoting healthy eating. In: Riekert KA, Ockene J, Pbert L, eds. *The Handbook of Health Behavior Change.* 4th ed. New York, NY, Springer Pub Co: 2014 139-154.

123. Thompson FE, Subar AF. Dietary assessment methodology. In: Coulston, AM, Boushey, C. *Nutrition in Prevention and Treatment of Disease.* San Diego: Academic Press; 2008:5-41.

124. Kristal AR, Kolar AS, Fisher JL, et al. Evaluation of web-based, self-administered, graphical food frequency questionnaire. *J Acad Nutr Diet.* 2014;114(4)613-621.

125. Collins KK, Aberegg ES. Dietary assessment: all tools are not created equal. Lecture presented at: American Association of Cardiovascular and Pulmonary Rehabilitation Annual Meeting; September 8, 2016; New Orleans, LA

126. Aberegg ES, Weiss R. Nutrition Assessment: Where We Stand and Where We Are Going. Lecture presented at: AACVPR Annual Meeting; October 6, 2017; Charleston, SC

127. Collins KK, Aberegg ES Dietary Assessment Tools: What's on the Horizon, Lecture presented at AACVPR Annual Meeting, September 19, 2019; Portland OR

128. Schneider JK, Wong-Anuchit C, Stallings D, Krieger, MM. Motivational interviewing and fruit/vegetable consumption in older adults. *Clin Nursing Res.* 2017;26(6)731-746.

129. Wasnick B. *Mindless Eating.* Bantam Dell Books New York, NY; 2007.

130. Tribole E, Resch E. *Intuitive Eating.* 3rd ed. St Martin's Griffen; New York, NY. 2012.

131. Drucker P. *Management Tasks, Responsibilities, Practices.* Harper & Row, New York, NY. 1973.

132. Brownell K. LEARN Program for Weight Management. American Health Pub. Dallas, TX 10th ed. 2004

133. Kostas G. The Cooper Clinic Solution to the Diet Revolution: Step Up to the Plate. Good Health Press, Dallas, TX; 2009.

134. Start Simple with MyPlate Toolkit for Professionals. https://www.choosemyplate.gov/resources/toolkits/StartSimpletoolkit 2019. Accessed October 21, 2019

135. de Melo Ghisi GL, Abdallah F, Grace SL, Thomas S, Oh P. A systematic review of patient education in cardiac patients: Do they increase knowledge and promote health behavior change? *Patient Educ Couns.* 2014;95(2)160-174.

136. McLaughlin G. SMOG grading: A new readability formula. *Journal of Reading.* 1969;12(8)639-646.

137. Sikand, G, Cole RE, Handu D, et al Clinical and cost benefits of medical nutrition therapy by registered dietitian nutritionists for management of dyslipidemia: A systematic review and meta-analysis. Journal of Clinical Lipidology, 2018 (12)5, 1113 - 11

138. Devries S, Agatston A, Aggarwal M, et al. A deficiency of nutrition education and practice in cardiology. *Amer J Med.* 2017;130(11):1298-1305.

139. Holmes AL, Sanderson B, Maisiak R, Brown A, Bittner V. Dietitian services are associated with improved patient outcomes and the MEDFICTS dietary assessment questionnaire is a suitable outcome measure in cardiac rehabilitation. *JAND.* 2005;105(10)1533-1540.

140. Luisi MLE, Biffi B, Gheri CF, et al. Efficacy of a nutritional education program to improve diet in patients attending a cardiac rehabilitation program: Outcomes of a one-year follow-up. *Intern Emerg Med.* 2015;10(6):671-676.

141. Cavallaro V, Dwyer J., Houser RF, et al. Influence of dietitian presence on outpatient cardiac rehabilitation nutrition services. *JAND.* 2004;104(4):611-614.

142. Find a Registered Dietitian Nutritionist. Academy of Nutrition and Dietetics website. www.eatright.org/find-an-expert. Published 2019. Accessed October 19.2019.

Chapter 8

1. Mazur JE. *Learning & Behavior*. Philadelphia, PA: Routledge; 2016.

2. Prochaska JO. Transtheoretical model of behavior change. In: Gellman MD, Turner JR, eds. *Encyclopedia of Behavioral Medicine*. New York: Springer; 2013.

3. Miller WR, Rollnick S. *Motivational Interviewing: Helping People Change*. New York, NY: Guilford Press; 2012.

4. McCracken L, ed. Mindfulness and Acceptance in Behavioral Medicine: Current Theory and Practice. Oakland, CA: New Harbinger Publications; 2011.

5. Taylor GH, Wilson SL, Sharp J. Medical, psychological, and sociodemographic factors associated with adherence to cardiac rehabilitation programs: A systematic review. *J Cardiovasc Nurs*. 2011;26(3):202-9.

6. Bickel WK, Jarmolowicz DP, Mueller ET, Koffarnus MN, Gatchalian KM. Excessive discounting of delayed reinforcers as a trans-disease process contributing to addiction and other disease-related vulnerabilities: emerging evidence. *Pharmacol Ther*. 2012;134(3):287-97.

7. Ades PA, Keteyian SJ, Wright JS, et al. Increasing cardiac rehabilitation participation from 20% to 70%: A road map from the Million Hearts Cardiac Rehabilitation Collaborative. *Mayo Clin Proc*. 2017;92, 234-242.

8. Beckie TM, Beckstead JW. Predicting cardiac rehabilitation attendance in a gender-tailored randomized clinical trial. J Cardiopul Rehabil Prev. 2010;30(3):147.

9. Colbert JD, Martin BJ, Haykowsky MJ, et al. Cardiac rehabilitation referral, attendance and mortality in women. Eur J Prev Cardiol. 2015 Aug;22(8):979-86.

10. Gaalema DE, Cutler AY, Higgins ST, Ades PA. Smoking and cardiac rehabilitation participation: Associations with referral, attendance and adherence. *Prev Med*. 2015;80:67-74.

11. Gaalema DE, Savage PD, Rengo JL, et al. Patient characteristics predictive of cardiac rehabilitation adherence. *J Cardiopul Rehabil Prev*. 2017;37(2):103-110.

12. Sun EY, Jadotte YT, Halperin W. Disparities in cardiac rehabilitation participation in the United States. *J Cardiopul Rehabil Prev*. 2017;37(1):2-10.

13. Rollnick S, Miller WR, Butler CC, Aloia MS. *Motivational Interviewing in Health Care: Helping Patients Change Behavior*. New York, NY: Guilford Press; 2008.

14. Balady GJ, Williams MA, Ades PA, et al. Core components of cardiac rehabilitation/secondary prevention programs: 2007 update: A scientific statement from the American Heart Association Exercise, Cardiac Rehabilitation, and Prevention Committee, the Council on Clinical Cardiology; the Councils on Cardiovascular Nursing, Epidemiology and Prevention, and Nutrition, Physical Activity, and Metabolism; and the American Association of Cardiovascular and Pulmonary Rehabilitation. *Circulation*. 2007;115(20):2675-82.

15. Li F, Harmer P, Cardinal BJ, et al. Built environment and 1-year change in weight and waist circumference in middle-aged and older adults: Portland Neighborhood Environment and Health Study. *Am J Epidemiol*. 2009;169(4):401-8.

16. Datar A, Nicosia N. Assessing social contagion in body mass index, overweight, and obesity using a natural experiment. *JAMA Pediatr*. 2018;172(3):239-46.

17. Kutner M, Greenberg E, Baer J. A First Look at the Literacy of America's Adults in the 21st Century. NCES 2006-470. National Center for Education Statistics. 2006. https://nces.ed.gov/naal/pdf/2006470.pdf. Accessed October 14, 2019.

18. Kutner M, Greenburg E, Jin Y, Paulsen C. The Health Literacy of America's Adults: Results from the 2003 National Assessment of Adult Literacy. NCES 2006-483. National Center for Education Statistics. 2006.

19. Cornett, S., "Assessing and Addressing Health Literacy" *OJIN: The Online Journal of Issues in Nursing*. 2009;14(3).

20. Order American Heart Association brochures. American Heart Association website. www.heart.org/en/health-topics/consumer-healthcare/order-american-heart-association-educational-brochures. Accessed October 1, 2018.

21. Making health communications programs work. National Cancer Institute website. www.cancer.gov/publications/health-communication/pinkbook.pdf. Published 2004. Accessed October 1, 2018.

22. Exercise: Stages of change (short form). University of Rhode Island, Cancer Prevention Research Center website. https://web.uri.edu/cprc/exercise-stages-of-change-short-form. Accessed October 1, 2018.

23. Marcus BH, Selby VC, Niaura RS, Rossi JS. Self-efficacy and the stages of exercise behavior change. *Res Q Exerc Sport*. 1992;63:60-66.

24. Weinberger AH, Mazure CM, Morlett A, McKee SA. Two decades of smoking cessation treatment research on smokers with depression: 1990–2010. *Nicotine & Tob Res*. 2012;15(6):1014-31.

25. Bovend'Eerdt TJ, Botell RE, Wade DT. Writing SMART rehabilitation goals and achieving goal attainment scaling: A practical guide. *Clin Rehabil*. 2009;23(4):352-61.

26. Bandura A. Health promotion by social cognitive means. *Health Educ Behav*. 2004;31(2):143-64.

27. Nevin JA. Resistance to extinction and behavioral momentum. *Behav Processes*. 2012;90(1):89-97.

28. Miller GF, Gupta S, Kropp JD, Grogan KA, Mathews A. The effects of pre-ordering and behavioral nudges on National School Lunch Program participants' food item selection. *Journal of Economic Psychology*. 2016;55:4-16.

29. Pierce WD, Cheney CD. *Behavior Analysis and Learning*. Psychology Press; 2013.

30. Burke LE, Wang J, Sevick MA. Self-monitoring in weight loss: a systematic review of the literature. *J Am Diet Assoc*. 2011;111(1):92-102.

31. Rachlin H. *The Science of Self-Control*. Cambridge, MA: Harvard University Press; 2000.

32. Sunstein, CR, Thaler, RH. *Nudge: Improving Decisions About Health, Wealth, and Happiness*. New York, NY: Springer; 2008.

33. Gaalema DE, Savage PD, Rengo JL, Cutler AY, Higgins ST, Ades PA. Financial incentives to promote cardiac rehabilitation participation and adherence among Medicaid patients. *Prev Med*. 2016;92:47-50.

34. Pack QR, Johnson LL, Barr LM, et al. Improving cardiac rehabilitation attendance and completion through quality improvement activities and a motivational program. *J Cardiopulm Rehabil Prev*. 2013;33(3):153-159.

35. Chaiton M, Diemert L, Cohen JE, et al. Estimating the number of quit attempts it takes to quit smoking successfully in a longitudinal cohort of smokers. *BMJ Open*. 2016;6:e011045. doi:10.1136/bmjopen-2016-011045

Chapter 9: Physical Inactivity Section

1. Fletcher GF, Ades PA, Kligfield P, et al. Exercise standards for testing and training: A scientific statement from the American Heart Association. *Circulation*. 2013;128:873-934.

2. Myers J. The new AHA/ACC guidelines on cardiovascular risk: When will fitness get the recognition it deserves? *Mayo Clin Proc*. 2014;89:722-726.

3. Fletcher GF, Landolfo C, Niebauer J, et al. Promoting physical activity and exercise. JACC Health Promotion Series. *J Amer Coll Cardiol*. 2018;72:1622-1629.

4. Wen CP, Wu X. Stressing harms of physical inactivity to promote exercise. *Lancet*. doi:10.1016/S0140-6736(12)60954-4, 2012

5. Gorczyca AM, Eaton CB, LaMonte MJ, et al. Change in physical activity and sitting time after myocardial infarction and mortality among postmenopausal women in the women's health initiative-observational study. *JAMA*. 2017;6:e005354.

6. Booth JN, Levitan EB, Brown TM, Farkouh ME, Safford MM. Effect of sustaining lifestyle modifications (nonsmoking, weight reduction, physical activity, and Mediterranean diet) after healing of myocardial infarction, percutaneous intervention, or coronary bypass (from the Reasons for Geographic and Racial Differences in Stroke Study). *Am J Cardiol*. 2014;113:1933-1940.

7. Haskell W, Lee I-M, Pate R, et al. Physical activity and public health: Updated recommendation for adults from the American College of Sports Medicine and the American Heart Association. *Circulation*. 2007;116:1081-1093.

8. *2018 Physical Activity Guidelines for Americans*. U.S. Department of Health and Human Services website. https://health.gov/paguidelines/second-edition/report. Published November 2018. Accessed July 7, 2018.

9. One in five adults meet overall physical activity guidelines. Centers for Disease Control and Prevention website. www.cdc.gov/media/releases/2013/p0502-physical-activity.html. Published May 2, 2013. Accessed June 29, 2018.

10. Thompson PD, Buchner D, Pina IL, et al. AHA scientific statement: Exercise and physical activity in the prevention and treatment of atherosclerotic cardiovascular disease. *Circulation*. 2003;107:3109-3116.

11. Hallal PC, Andersen LB, Bull FC, Guthold R, Haskell W, Ekelund U (for the Lancet Physical Activity Series Working Group). Global physical activity levels: Surveillance, progress, pitfalls, and prospects. *Lancet*. 2012;380:247-257.

12. Pate RR, Pratt M, Blair SN, et al. Physical activity and public health: A recommendation from the Centers for Disease Control and Prevention and the American College of Sports Medicine. *JAMA*. 1995;273:402-407.

13. U.S. Department of Health and Human Services. *Physical Activity and Health: A Report of the Surgeon General*. Atlanta: U.S. Department of Health and Human Services, Centers for Disease Control and Prevention, National Center for Chronic Disease Prevention and Health Promotion; 1996.

14. Prince S, Blanchard C, Grace S, Reid R. Objectively-measured sedentary time and its association with markers of cardiometabolic health and fitness among cardiac rehabilitation graduates. *Eur J Prev Cardiol*. 2016;23:818-25.

15. Gerber Y, Myers V, Goldbourt U, Benyamini Y, Scheinowitz M, Drory Y. Long-term trajectory of leisure time physical activity and survival after first myocardial infarction: A population-based cohort study. *Eur J Epidemiol*. 2011;26:109-16

16. Myers J, Prakash M, Froelicher V, et al. Exercise capacity and mortality among men referred for exercise testing. *NEJM*. 2002;346:793-801.

17. Blair SN, Kohl HW III, Paffenbarger RS Jr, et al. Physical fitness and all-cause mortality. A prospective study of healthy men and women. *JAMA*. 1989;262:2395-2401.

18. Myers J, McAuley P, Lavie C, Despres JP, Arena R, Kokkinos P. Physical activity and cardiorespiratory fitness as major markers of cardiovascular risk: Their independent and interwoven importance to health status. *Prog Cardiovasc Dis*. 2015;57:306-314.

19. Ross R, Blair S, Arena R, et al. Importance of assessing cardiorespiratory fitness in clinical practice: A case for fitness as a clinical vital sign. An American Heart Association scientific statement from the Committee on Physical Activity and the Council on Lifestyle and Cardiometabolic Health. *Circulation*. 2016;134:e653-e699.

20. Warren TY, Barry V, Hooker SP, Sui X, Church TS, Blair SN. Sedentary behaviors increase risk of cardiovascular disease mortality in men. *Med Sci Sports Exerc*. 2010;42:879-885.

21. Ekelund U, Steene-Johannessen J, Brown WJ, et al. Does physical activity attenuate, or even eliminate, the detrimental association of sitting time with mortality? A harmonised meta-analysis of data from more than 1 million men and women. *Lancet*. 2016;388 (10051):1302-10.

22. Katzmarzyk P, Church T, Craig C, et al. Sitting time and mortality from all causes, cardiovascular disease, and cancer. *Med Sci Sports Exerc*. 2009;41:998-1005.

23. Stamatakis E, Hamer M, Dunstan D. Screen-based entertainment time, all-cause mortality, and cardiovascular events: Population-based study with ongoing mortality and hospital events follow-up. *J Am Coll Cardiol*. 2011;57:292-299.

24. Matthews CE, George SM, Moore SC, et al. Amount of time spent in sedentary behaviors and cause-specific mortality in US adults. *Am J Clin Nutr*. 2012;95:437-445.

25. Swift DL, Lavie CJ, Johannsen NM, et al. Physical activity, cardiorespiratory fitness, and exercise training in primary and secondary coronary prevention. *Circ J*. 2013;77:281-92.

26. Lavie CJ, Kokkinos P, Ortega FB. Survival of the fittest - Promoting fitness throughout the life span. *Mayo Clin Proc*. 2017;92:1743-1745.

27. Lloyd-Jones D, Hong Y, Labarthe D, et al. Defining and setting national goals for cardiovascular health promotion and disease reduction: The American Heart Association's Strategic Impact Goal through 2020 and beyond. *Circulation*. 2010;121:586-613.

28. Biswas A, Oh PI, Faulkner GE, et al. Sedentary time and its association with risk for disease incidence, mortality, and hospitalization in adults: A systematic review and meta-analysis. *Ann Intern Med*. 2015;162:123-32.

29. Nocon M, Hiemann T, Müller-Riemenschneider F, Thalau F, Roll S, Willich SN. Association of physical activity with all-cause and cardiovascular mortality: A systematic review and meta-analysis. *Eur J Cardiovasc Prev Rehabil*. 2008;15:239-4.

30. Lee DC, Sui X, Artero EG, et al. Long-term effects of changes in cardiorespiratory fitness and body mass index on all-cause and cardiovascular disease mortality in men: The Aerobics Center Longitudinal Study. *Circulation*. 2011;124:2483-90.

31. Jiménez-Pavón D, Artero EG, Lee DC, et al. Cardiorespiratory fitness and risk of sudden cardiac death in men and women in the United States: A prospective evaluation from the Aerobics Center Longitudinal Study. *Mayo Clin Proc.* 2016;91:849-57.

32. Kokkinos P, Myers J, Pittaras A, et al. Exercise capacity and mortality in African-American and Caucasian men. *Circulation.* 2008;117: 614-622.

33. Myers J, Kokkinos P, Chan K, et al. Cardiorespiratory fitness and reclassification of risk for incidence of heart failure: The Veterans Exercise Testing Study. *Circulation: Heart Failure.* 2017PMID:28572213.

34. McAuley PA, Blaha MJ, Keteyian SJ, et al. Fitness, fatness, and mortality: The FIT (Henry Ford Exercise Testing) Project. *Am J Med.* 2016;129:960-965.

35. Ehrman JK, Brawner CA, Al-Mallah MH, Qureshi WT, Blaha MJ, Keteyian SJ. Cardiorespiratory fitness change and mortality risk among black and white patients: Henry Ford Exercise Testing (FIT) Project. *Am J Med.* 2017;130:1177-1183.

36. Shafiq A, Brawner CA, Aldred HA, et al. Prognostic value of cardiopulmonary exercise testing in heart failure with preserved ejection fraction. The Henry Ford HospITal CardioPulmonary EXercise Testing (FIT-CPX) project. *Am Heart J.* 2016;174:167-72.

37. Keteyian SJ, Leifer ES, Houston-Miller N, et al. Relation between volume of exercise and clinical outcomes in patients with heart failure. *J Am Coll Cardiol.* 2012;60:1899-905.

38. Swank AM, Horton J, Fleg JL, et al. Modest increase in peak $\dot{V}O_2$ is related to better clinical outcomes in chronic heart failure patients: Results from heart failure and a controlled trial to investigate outcomes of exercise training. *Circ Heart Fail.* 2012;5:579-85.

39. Warren JM, Ekelund U, Besson H, et al. Assessment of physical activity—A review of methodologies with reference to epidemiological research: A report of the exercise physiology section of the European Association of Cardiovascular Prevention and Rehabilitation. *Eur J Cardiovasc Prev Rehabil.* 2010;17:127-139.

40. Bravata DM, Smith-Spangler C, Sundaram V, et al. Using pedometers to increase physical activity and improve health: A systematic review. *JAMA.* 2007;298:2296-2304.

41. Mansi S, Milosavljevic S, Baxter GD, Tumilty S, Hendrick P. A systematic review of studies using pedometers as an intervention for musculoskeletal diseases. *BMC Musculoskelet Disord.* 2014:10;15:231.

42. Funk M, Taylor EL. Pedometer-based walking interventions for free-living adults with type 2 diabetes: A systematic review. *Curr Diabetes Rev.* 2013;9:462-71.

43. DeBusk RF, Stenestrand U, Sheehan M, Haskell WL. Training effects of long versus short bouts of exercise in healthy subjects. *Am J Cardiol.* 1990;65:1010-1013.

44. Riebe D, Ehrman JK, Liguori G, Maier M. *ACSM's Guidelines for Exercise Testing and Prescription.* 10th ed. Philadelphia: Lippincott Williams & Wilkins; 2018.

45. Balady GJ, Arena R, Sietsema K, et al. Clinician's guide to cardiopulmonary exercise testing in adults: a scientific statement from the American Heart Association. *Circulation.* 2010;122:191-225.

Chapter 9: Dyslipidemia Section

1. Cohen JC, Boerwinkle E, Mosley TH, Jr., Hobbs HH. Sequence variations in PCSK9, low LDL, and protection against coronary heart disease. *N Engl J Med.* 2006;354(12):1264-1272.

2. Lloyd-Jones DM, Morris PB, Ballantyne CM, et al. 2017 Focused update of the 2016 ACC expert consensus decision pathway on the role of non-statin therapies for LDL-cholesterol lowering in the management of atherosclerotic cardiovascular disease risk: A report of the American College of Cardiology Task Force on Expert Consensus Decision Pathways. *J Am Coll Cardiol.* 2017;70(14):1785-1822.

3. Grundy SM, Stone NJ, Bailey AL, et al. 2018 AHA/ACC/AACVPR/AAPA/ABC/ACPM/ADA/AGS/APhA/ASPC/NLA/PCNA guideline on the management of blood cholesterol: A report of the American College of Cardiology/American Heart Association Task Force on Clinical Practice Guidelines. *J Am Coll Cardiol.* 2019 Jun 25;73(24):3168-3209.\

4. Gardner CD, Fortmann SP, Krauss RM. Association of small low-density lipoprotein particles with the incidence of coronary artery disease in men and women. *JAMA.* 1996;276(11):875-881.

5. Carroll MD, Kit BK, Lacher DA, Shero ST, Mussolino ME. Trends in lipids and lipoproteins in US adults, 1988-2010. *JAMA.* 2012;308(15):1545-1554.

6. McClelland RL, Chung H, Detrano R, Post W, Kronmal RA. Distribution of coronary artery calcium by race, gender, and age: Results from the Multi-Ethnic Study of Atherosclerosis (MESA). *Circulation*. 2006;113(1):30-37.

7. O'Keefe JH, Jr., Cordain L, Harris WH, Moe RM, Vogel R. Optimal low-density lipoprotein is 50 to 70 mg/dl: lower is better and physiologically normal. *J Am Coll Cardiol*. Jun 2 2004;43(11):2142-2146.

8. Nissen SE, Nicholls SJ, Sipahi I, et al. Effect of very high-intensity statin therapy on regression of coronary atherosclerosis: the ASTEROID trial. *JAMA*. Apr 5 2006;295(13):1556-1565.

9. Ference BA, Ginsberg HN, Graham I, et al. Low-density lipoproteins cause atherosclerotic cardiovascular disease. 1. Evidence from genetic, epidemiologic, and clinical studies. A consensus statement from the European Atherosclerosis Society Consensus Panel. *Eur Heart J*. 2017;38(32):2459-2472.

10. Silverman MG, Ference BA, Im K, et al. Association between lowering LDL-C and cardiovascular risk reduction among different therapeutic interventions: A systematic review and meta-analysis. *JAMA*. 2016;316(12):1289-1297.

11. Goff DC, Jr., Lloyd-Jones DM, Bennett G, et al. 2013 ACC/AHA guideline on the assessment of cardiovascular risk: a report of the American College of Cardiology/American Heart Association Task Force on Practice Guidelines. *Circulation*. Jun 24 2014;129(25 Suppl 2):S49-73.

12. Marti-Carvajal AJ, Sola I, Lathyris D, Dayer M. Homocysteine-lowering interventions for preventing cardiovascular events. *Cochrane Database Syst Rev*. 2017;8:CD006612.

13. Eckel RH, Jakicic JM, Ard JD, et al. 2013 AHA/ACC guideline on lifestyle management to reduce cardiovascular risk: A report of the American College of Cardiology/American Heart Association Task Force on Practice Guidelines. *Circulation*. 2014;129(25 Suppl 2):S76-99.

14. Estruch R, Ros E, Salas-Salvado J, et al. Primary prevention of cardiovascular disease with a Mediterranean diet supplemented with extra-virgin olive oil or nuts. *N Engl J Med*. 2018;378(25):e34.

15. Heffron SP, Parikh A, Volodarskiy A, et al. Changes in lipid profile of obese patients following contemporary bariatric surgery: A meta-analysis. *Am J Med*. 2016;129(9):952-959.

16. Stone NJ, Robinson JG, Lichtenstein AH, et al. 2013 ACC/AHA guideline on the treatment of blood cholesterol to reduce atherosclerotic cardiovascular risk in adults: A report of the American College of Cardiology/American Heart Association Task Force on Practice Guidelines. *Circulation*. Jun 24 2014;129(25 Suppl 2):S1-45.

17. Thompson PD, Panza G, Zaleski A, Taylor B. Statin-associated side effects. *J Am Coll Cardiol*. 2016;67(20):2395-2410.

18. Rosenson RS, Baker S, Banach M, et al. Optimizing cholesterol treatment in patients with muscle complaints. *J Am Coll Cardiol*. 2017;70(10):1290-1301.

19. Cohen DE, Anania FA, Chalasani N, National Lipid Association Statin Safety Task Force Liver Expert Panel. An assessment of statin safety by hepatologists. *Am J Cardiol*. 2006;97(8A):77C-81C.

20. Muntner P, Colantonio LD, Cushman M, et al. Validation of the atherosclerotic cardiovascular disease pooled cohort risk equations. *JAMA*. 2014;311(14):1406-1415.

21. Cannon CP, Blazing MA, Giugliano RP, et al. Ezetimibe added to statin therapy after acute coronary syndromes. *N Engl J Med*. 2015;372(25):2387-2397.

22. Robinson JG, Farnier M, Krempf M, et al. Efficacy and safety of alirocumab in reducing lipids and cardiovascular events. *N Engl J Med*. 2015;372(16):1489-1499.

23. Giugliano RP, Pedersen TR, Park JG, et al. Clinical efficacy and safety of achieving very low LDL-cholesterol concentrations with the PCSK9 inhibitor evolocumab: A prespecified secondary analysis of the FOURIER trial. *Lancet*. 2017;390(10106):1962-1971.

24. Sabatine MS, Giugliano RP, Keech AC, et al. Evolocumab and clinical outcomes in patients with cardiovascular disease. *N Engl J Med*. 2017;376(18):1713-1722.

25. Schwartz GG, Steg PG, Szarek M, et al. Alirocumab and cardiovascular outcomes after acute coronary syndrome. *N Engl J Med*. 2018;379(22):2097-2107.

26. Kazi DS, Penko J, Coxson PG, et al. Updated cost-effectiveness analysis of PCSK9 inhibitors based on the results of the FOURIER Trial. *JAMA*. Aug 22 2017;318(8):748-750.

27. Tall AR, Rader DJ. Trials and tribulations of CETP inhibitors. *Circ Res*. 2018;122(1):106-112.

28. Investigators A-H, Boden WE, Probstfield JL, et al. Niacin in patients with low HDL cholesterol levels receiving intensive statin therapy. *N Engl J Med*. 2011;365(24):2255-2267.

29. Group HTC, Landray MJ, Haynes R, et al. Effects of extended-release niacin with laropiprant in high-risk patients. *N Engl J Med*. 2014;371(3):203-212.

30. Handelsman Y, Shapiro MD. Triglycerides, atherosclerosis, and cardiovascular outcome studies: Focus on omega-3 fatty acids. *Endocr Pract*. 2017;23(1):100-112.

31. Abdelhamid AS, Martin N, Bridges C, et al. Polyunsaturated fatty acids for the primary and secondary prevention of cardiovascular disease. *Cochrane Database Syst Rev*. Jul 18 2018;7:CD012345.

32. Miller M, Stone NJ, Ballantyne C, et al. Triglycerides and cardiovascular disease: A scientific statement from the American Heart Association. *Circulation*. 2011;123(20):2292-2333.Filippatos TD, Elisaf MS. Recommendations for severe hypertriglyceridemia treatment, are there new strategies? *Curr Vasc Pharmacol*. 2014;12(4):598-616.

33. Bhatt DL, Steg PG, Miller M, et al. Cardiovascular Risk Reduction with icosapent ethyl for hypertriglyceridemia. *N Engl J Med*. 2019 Jan 3; 380(1):11-22..

34. Kataoka Y, St John J, Wolski K, et al. Atheroma progression in hyporesponders to statin therapy. *Arterioscler Thromb Vasc Biol*. 2015;35(4):990-995.

Chapter 9: Diabetes Section

1. 2017 National diabetes statistics report, 2017. Centers for Disease Control and Prevention, March 6, 2018. www.cdc.gov/diabetes/data/statistics-report/index.html. Accessed October 15, 2019.

2. Sacks FM. Lipid-lowering therapy in acute coronary syndromes. *JAMA*. 2001;285:1758-1760.

3. Colberg SR, Albright AL, Blissmer BJ, et al. American College of Sports Medicine and the American Diabetes Association joint position statement. Exercise and type 2 diabetes. *Med Sci Sports Exerc*. 2010;42:2282-2303.

4. Knowler WC, Barrett-Connor E, Fowler SE, et al. Reduction in the incidence of type 2 diabetes with lifestyle intervention or metformin. *NEJM*. 2002;346:393-403.

5. Kokkinos P, Myers J, Nylen E, et al. Exercise capacity and all-cause mortality in African American and Caucasian men with type 2 diabetes. *Diabetes Care*. 2009;32:623-628.

6. Gill JM. Physical activity, cardiorespiratory fitness and insulin resistance: A short update. *Curr Opin Lipidol*. 2007;18:47-52.

7. Horowitz JF. Exercise-induced alterations in muscle lipid metabolism improve insulin sensitivity. *Exerc Sport Sci Rev*. 2007;35:192-196.

8. Colberg SR, Sigal RJ, Yardley JE, et al. Physical activity/exercise and diabetes: A position statement of the American Diabetes Association. *Diabetes Care*. 2016;39:2065-2079.

9. Riddell MC, Gallen IW, Smart CE, et al. Exercise management in type 1 diabetes: A consensus statement. *Lancet Diab Endocrinol*. 2017;5:377–390.

10. Garber CE, Blissmer B, Deschenes MR, et al. American College of Sports Medicine position stand. Quantity and quality of exercise for developing and maintaining cardiorespiratory, musculoskeletal, and neuromotor fitness in apparently healthy adults: Guidance for prescribing exercise. *Med Sci Sports Exerc*. 2011;43:1334-1359.

11. Pinzur MS, Slovenkai MP, Trepman E, et al. Guidelines for diabetic foot care. *Foot Ankle Int*. 2005;26:113-119.

12. American Diabetes Association. 10. Microvascular complications and foot care: Standards of medical care in diabetes—2018. *Diab Care*. 2018;41:S105-S118.

13. Lopez-Jimenez F, Kramer VC, Masters B, et al. Recommendations for managing patients with diabetes mellitus in cardiopulmonary rehabilitation. An American Association of Cardiovascular and Pulmonary Rehabilitation statement. *J Cardiopulm Rehabil Prev*. 2012;32:101-112.

14. American Diabetes Association. 4. Lifestyle management: Standards of medical care in diabetes—2018. *Diab Care*. 2018;41:S38-S50.

Chapter 9: Tobacco Use Section

1. Pack QR, Bauldoff G, Lichtman SW, et al. Prioritization, development, and validation of American Association of Cardiovascular and Pulmonary Rehabilitation performance measures. *J Cardiopulm Rehabil Prev*. 2018;38(4):208-214.

2. Fiore MC, Jaen CR, Baker TB, et al. Treating Tobacco Use and Dependence: 2008 Update.. Clinical Practice Guideline. Rockville, MD: U.S. Department of Health and Human Services. Public Health Service. May 2008.

3. Fiore MC, Baker TB. Clinical practice. Treating smokers in the health care setting. *N Engl J Med.* 2011;365(13):1222-1231.

4. Prochaska JJ, Benowitz NL. Smoking cessation and the cardiovascular patient. *Curr Opin Cardiol.* 2015;30(5):506-511.

5. Mola A, Lloyd MM, Villegas-Pantoja MA. A mixed method review of tobacco cessation for the cardiopulmonary rehabilitation clinician. *J Cardiopulm Rehabil Prev.* 2017;37(3):160-174.

6. US Department of Health and Human Services. *The Health Consequences of Smoking-50 Years of Progress: A Report of the Surgeon General.* Atlanta, GA. U.S. Department of Health and Human Services, Centers for Disease Control and Prevention, National Center for Chronic Disease Prevention and Health Promotion, Office of Smoking and Health; 2014.

7. Pirie K, Peto R, Reeves GK, Green J, Beral V, Million Women Study Collaborators. The 21st century hazards of smoking and benefits of stopping: A prospective study of one million women in the UK. *Lancet.* 2013;381(9861):133-141.

8. Critchley JA, Capewell S. Mortality risk reduction associated with smoking cessation in patients with coronary heart disease: A systematic review. *JAMA.* 2003;290(1):86-97.

9. Colivicchi F, Mocini D, Tubaro M, Aiello A, Clavario P, Santini M. Effect of smoking relapse on outcome after acute coronary syndromes. *Am J Cardiol.* 2011;108(6):804-808.

10. Rallidis LS, Hamodraka ES, Foulidis VO, Pavlakis GP. Persistent smokers after myocardial infarction: A group that requires special attention. *Int J Cardiol.* 2005;100(2):241-245.

11. Benowitz NL. Nicotine addiction. *N Engl J Med.* 2010;362(24):2295-2303.

12. Lloyd A, Steele L, Fotheringham J, et al. Pronounced increase in risk of acute ST-segment elevation myocardial infarction in younger smokers. *Heart.* 2017;103(8):586-591.

13. Pipe AL, Papadakis S, Reid RD. The role of smoking cessation in the prevention of coronary artery disease. *Current atherosclerosis reports.* Mar 2010;12(2):145-150.

14. Fiore MC. Tobacco control in the Obama era—Substantial progress, remaining challenges. *N Engl J Med.* 2016;375(15):1410-1412.

15. Gaalema DE, Cutler AY, Higgins ST, Ades PA. Smoking and cardiac rehabilitation participation: Associations with referral, attendance and adherence. *Prev Med.* 2015; Nov; 80:67-74.

16. Sochor O, Lennon RJ, Rodriguez-Escudero JP, et al. Trends and predictors of smoking cessation after percutaneous coronary intervention (from Olmsted County, Minnesota, 1999 to 2010). *Am J Cardiol.* 2015;115(4):405-410.

17. Auer R, Gencer B, Tango R, et al. Uptake and efficacy of a systematic intensive smoking cessation intervention using motivational interviewing for smokers hospitalised for an acute coronary syndrome: A multicentre before-after study with parallel group comparisons. *BMJ Open.* 2016;6(9):e011520.

18. Riley H, Headley S, Winter C, et al. Effect of smoking status on exercise perception and intentions for cardiac rehabilitation enrollment among patients hospitalized with an acute cardiac condition. *J Cardiopulm Rehabil Prev.* 2018 Sep;38(5):286-290.

19. Berndt NC, Bolman C, de Vries H, Segaar D, van Boven I, Lechner L. Smoking cessation treatment practices: Recommendations for improved adoption on cardiology wards. *J Cardiovasc Nurs.* 2013;28(1):35-47.

20. Bock BC, Becker BM, Partridge R, Niaura R. Are emergency chest pain patients ready to quit smoking? *Preventive cardiology.* Spring 2007;10(2):76-82.

21. Lynch KL, Twesten JE, Stern A, Augustson EM. Level of alcohol consumption and successful smoking cessation. *Nicotine Tob Res.* 2019 Jul 17;21(8):1058-1064.

22. Stockwell T, Zhao J, Panwar S, Roemer A, Naimi T, Chikritzhs T. Do "moderate" drinkers have reduced mortality risk? A systematic review and Meta-analysis of alcohol consumption and all-cause mortality. *J Stud Alcohol Drugs.* 2016;77(2):185-198.

23. Mukamal KJ, Clowry CM, Murray MM, et al. Moderate alcohol consumption and chronic disease: The case for a long-term trial. *Alcohol Clin Exp Res.* 2016;40(11):2283-2291.

24. Ewing JA. Detecting alcoholism. The CAGE questionnaire. *JAMA.* 1984;252(14):1905-1907.

25. Windle SB, Dehghani P, Roy N, et al. Smoking abstinence 1 year after acute coronary syndrome: Follow-up from a randomized controlled trial of varenicline in patients admitted to hospital. *CMAJ.* 2018;190(12):E347-E354.

26. Rigotti NA, Clair C, Munafo MR, Stead LF. Interventions for smoking cessation in hospitalised patients. *Cochrane Database Syst Rev.* 2012(5):CD001837.

27. Pack QR, Mansour M, Barboza JS, et al. An early appointment to outpatient cardiac rehabilitation at hospital discharge improves attendance at orientation: A randomized, single-blind, controlled trial. *Circulation*. 2013;127(3):349-355.

28. Taylor G, McNeill A, Girling A, Farley A, Lindson-Hawley N, Aveyard P. Change in mental health after smoking cessation: Systematic review and meta-analysis. *BMJ*. 2014;348:g1151.

29. Abrams DB, Graham AL, Levy DT, Mabry PL, Orleans CT. Boosting population quits through evidence-based cessation treatment and policy. *Am J Prev Med*. Mar 2010;38(3 Suppl):S351-363.

30. Carlsson R, Lindberg G, Westin L, Israelsson B. Influence of coronary nursing management follow up on lifestyle after acute myocardial infarction. *Heart*. 1997;77(3):256-259.

31. Joseph AM, Norman SM, Ferry LH, et al. The safety of transdermal nicotine as an aid to smoking cessation in patients with cardiac disease. *N Engl J Med*. 1996;335(24):1792-1798.

32. Woolf KJ, Zabad MN, Post JM, McNitt S, Williams GC, Bisognano JD. Effect of nicotine replacement therapy on cardiovascular outcomes after acute coronary syndromes. *Am J Cardiol*. 2012;110(7):968-970.

33. Ortega F, Vellisco A, Marquez E, et al. Effectiveness of a cognitive orientation program with and without nicotine replacement therapy in stopping smoking in hospitalised patients. *Arch Bronconeumol*. 2011;47(1):3-9.

34. Benowitz NL, Pipe A, West R, et al. Cardiovascular safety of varenicline, bupropion, and nicotine patch in smokers: A randomized clinical trial. *JAMA Intern Med*. 2018;178(5):622-631.

35. Anthenelli RM, Benowitz NL, West R, et al. Neuropsychiatric safety and efficacy of varenicline, bupropion, and nicotine patch in smokers with and without psychiatric disorders (EAGLES): A double-blind, randomised, placebo-controlled clinical trial. *Lancet*. 2016;387(10037):2507-2520.

36. Ebbert JO, Hughes JR, West RJ, et al. Effect of varenicline on smoking cessation through smoking reduction: A randomized clinical trial. *JAMA*. 2015;313(7):687-694.

37. Schnoll RA, Goelz PM, Veluz-Wilkins A, et al. Long-term nicotine replacement therapy: A randomized clinical trial. *JAMA Intern Med*. Apr 2015;175(4):504-511.

38. Bhatnagar A, Whitsel LP, Ribisl KM, et al. Electronic cigarettes: A policy statement from the American Heart Association. *Circulation*. 2014;130(16):1418-1436.

Chapter 9: Hypertension Section

1. Pack QR, Bauldoff G, Lichtman SW, et al. Prioritization, development, and validation of American Association of Cardiovascular and Pulmonary Rehabilitation performance measures. *J Cardiopulm Rehabil Prev*. Jul 2018;38(4):208-214.

2. Whelton PK, Carey RM, Aronow WS, et al. 2017 ACC/AHA/AAPA/ABC/ACPM/AGS/APhA/ASH/ASPC/NMA/PCNA Guideline for the prevention, detection, evaluation, and management of high blood pressure in adults: A report of the American College of Cardiology/American Heart Association Task Force on Clinical Practice Guidelines. *Hypertension*. 2018;71(6):e13-e115.

3. Group SR, Wright JT, Jr., Williamson JD, et al. A randomized trial of intensive versus standard blood-pressure control. *N Engl J Med*. 2015;373(22):2103-2116.

4. Abbasi J. Medical students fall short on blood pressure check challenge. *JAMA*. 2017;318(11):991-992.

5. Pickering TG, Hall JE, Appel LJ, et al. Recommendations for blood pressure measurement in humans and experimental animals: Part 1: Blood pressure measurement in humans: A statement for professionals from the Subcommittee of Professional and Public Education of the American Heart Association Council on High Blood Pressure Research. *Circulation*. 2005;111(5):697-716.

6. Kang YY, Li Y, Huang QF, et al. Accuracy of home versus ambulatory blood pressure monitoring in the diagnosis of white-coat and masked hypertension. *J Hypertens*. 2015;33(8):1580-1587.

7. Kario K, Saito I, Kushiro T, et al. Morning home blood pressure is a strong predictor of coronary artery disease: The HONEST Study. *J Am Coll Cardiol*. 2016;67(13):1519-1527.

8. McManus RJ, Mant J, Haque MS, et al. Effect of self-monitoring and medication self-titration on systolic blood pressure in hypertensive patients at high risk of cardiovascular disease: the TASMIN-SR randomized clinical trial. *JAMA*. Aug 27 2014;312(8):799-808.

9. Barochiner J, Aparicio LS, Alfie J, et al. Alerting Reaction in office blood pressure and target organ damage: An innocent phenomenon? *Curr Hypertens Rev*. 2017;13(2):104-108.

10. Rizzoni D. Masked hypertension: How to identify and when to treat? *High Blood Press & Cardiovasc Prev*. 2016;23(3):181-186.

11. de la Sierra A, Banegas JR, Vinyoles E, et al. Prevalence of masked hypertension in untreated and treated patients with office blood pressure below 130/80 mm Hg. *Circulation.* 2018;137(24):2651-2653.

12. Tientcheu D, Ayers C, Das SR, et al. Target organ complications and cardiovascular events associated with masked hypertension and white-coat hypertension: Analysis from the Dallas Heart Study. *J Am Coll Cardiol.* 2015;66(20):2159-2169.

13. Blumenthal JA, Sherwood A, Smith PJ, et al. Lifestyle modification for resistant hypertension: The TRIUMPH randomized clinical trial. *Am Heart J.* 2015;170(5):986-994 e985.

14. Aronow WS, Fleg JL, Pepine CJ, et al. ACCF/AHA 2011 expert consensus document on hypertension in the elderly: A report of the American College of Cardiology Foundation Task Force on Clinical Expert Consensus Documents. *Circulation.* 2011;123(21):2434-2506.

15. Dimeo F, Pagonas N, Seibert F, Arndt R, Zidek W, Westhoff TH. Aerobic exercise reduces blood pressure in resistant hypertension. *Hypertension.* Sep 2012;60(3):653-658.

16. Appel LJ, Moore TJ, Obarzanek E, et al. A clinical trial of the effects of dietary patterns on blood pressure. DASH Collaborative Research Group. *New Engl J Med.* 1997;336(16):1117-1124.

17. Sacks FM, Svetkey LP, Vollmer WM, et al. Effects on blood pressure of reduced dietary sodium and the Dietary Approaches to Stop Hypertension (DASH) diet. DASH-Sodium Collaborative Research Group. *New Engl J Med.* 2001;344(1):3-10.

18. Bray GA, Vollmer WM, Sacks FM, et al. A further subgroup analysis of the effects of the DASH diet and three dietary sodium levels on blood pressure: Results of the DASH-Sodium Trial. *Am J Cardiol.* 2004;94(2):222-227.

19. Moore LV, Thompson FE. Adults meeting fruit and vegetable intake recommendations - United States, 2013. *MMWR.* 2015;64(26):709-713.

20. Eckel RH, Jakicic JM, Ard JD, et al. 2013 AHA/ACC guideline on lifestyle management to reduce cardiovascular risk: A report of the American College of Cardiology/American Heart Association Task Force on Practice Guidelines. *Circulation.* 2014;129(25 Suppl 2):S76-99.

21. Adrogue HJ, Madias NE. Sodium and potassium in the pathogenesis of hypertension. *N Engl J Med.* 2007;356(19):1966-1978.

22. Calhoun DA, Jones D, Textor S, et al. Resistant hypertension: Diagnosis, evaluation, and treatment: A scientific statement from the American Heart Association Professional Education Committee of the Council for High Blood Pressure Research. *Circulation.* 2008;117(25):e510-526.

23. Williams B, MacDonald TM, Morant S, et al. Spironolactone versus placebo, bisoprolol, and doxazosin to determine the optimal treatment for drug-resistant hypertension (PATHWAY-2): A randomised, double-blind, crossover trial. *Lancet.* 2015;386(10008):2059-2068.

Chapter 9: Overweight and Obesity Section

1. Go AS, Mozaffarian D, Roger VL, et al. Executive summary: Heart disease and stroke statistics—2014 update: A report from the American Heart Association. *Circulation.* 2014;129:399-410.

2. Yatsuya H, Li Y, Hilawe EH, et al. Global trend in overweight and obesity and its association with cardiovascular disease incidence. *Circ J.* 2014;78:2807-2818

3. Hales CM, Carroll MD, Fryar CD, Ogden CL. Prevalence of obesity among adults and youth: United States, 2015–2016. *NCHS data brief.* 2017;(288)1-8.

4. Anonymous. National Center for Health Statistics. National Health and Nutrition Examination Survey 2015-2016. https://wwwn.cdc.gov/NCHS/NHANES/ContinuousNhanes/Default.aspx?Beginyear=2015.

5. Klein S, Burke LE, Bray GA, et al. Clinical implications of obesity with specific focus on cardiovascular disease: A statement for professionals from the American Heart Association Council on Nutrition, Physical Activity, and Metabolism: Endorsed by the American College of Cardiology Foundation. *Circulation.* 2004;110:2952-2967.

6. Whitlock G, Lewington S, Sherliker P, et al. Body-mass index and cause-specific mortality in 900 000 adults: Collaborative analyses of 57 prospective studies. *Lancet.* 2009;373:1083-1096.

7. Heinl RE, Dhindsa DS, Mahlof EN, et al. Comprehensive cardiovascular risk reduction and cardiac rehabilitation in diabetes and the metabolic syndrome. *Can J Cardiol.* 2016;32:S349-S357.

8. Lyon CJ, Law RE, Hsueh WA. Minireview: Adiposity, inflammation, and atherogenesis. *Endocrinology.* 2003;144:2195-2200.

9. Poirier P, Giles TD, Bray GA, et al. Obesity and cardiovascular disease: Pathophysiology, evaluation, and effect of weight loss. *Arterioscler Thromb Vasc Biol.* 2006;26:968-976.

10. Lavie CJ, Milani RV. Effects of cardiac rehabilitation, exercise training, and weight reduction on exercise capacity, coronary risk factors, behavioral characteristics, and quality of life in obese coronary patients. *Am J Cardiol.* 1997;79:397-401.

11. Bader DS, Maguire TE, Spahn CM, O'Malley CJ, Balady GJ. Clinical profile and outcomes of obese patients in cardiac rehabilitation stratified according to national heart, lung, and blood institute criteria. *J Cardiopulm Rehabil.* 2001;21:210-217.

12. Gomadam PS, Douglas CJ, Sacrinty MT, Brady MM, Paladenech CC, Robinson KC. Degree and direction of change of body weight in cardiac rehabilitation and impact on exercise capacity and cardiac risk factors. *Am J Cardiol.* 2016;117:580-584.

13. Zullo MD, Jackson LW, Whalen CC, Dolansky MA. Evaluation of the recommended core components of cardiac rehabilitation practice: An opportunity for quality improvement. *J Cardiopulm Rehabil Prev.* 2012;32:32-40.

14. Brochu M, Poehlman ET, Ades PA. Obesity, body fat distribution, and coronary artery disease. *J Cardiopulm Rehabil.* 2000;20:96-108.

15. Jensen MD, Ryan DH, Apovian CM, et al. 2013 AHA/ACC/TOS guideline for the management of overweight and obesity in adults: A report of the American College of Cardiology/American Heart Association task force on practice guidelines and the obesity society. *J Am Coll Cardiol.* 2014;63:2985-3023.

16. Brochu M, Poehlman ET, Savage P, Fragnoli-Munn K, Ross S, Ades PA. Modest effects of exercise training alone on coronary risk factors and body composition in coronary patients. *J Cardiopulm Rehabil.* 2000;20:180-188.

17. Milani RV, Lavie CJ. Prevalence and profile of metabolic syndrome in patients following acute coronary events and effects of therapeutic lifestyle change with cardiac rehabilitation. *Am J Cardiol.* 2003;92:50-54.

18. Eilat-Adar S, Eldar M, Goldbourt U. Association of intentional changes in body weight with coronary heart disease event rates in overweight subjects who have an additional coronary risk factor. *Am J Epidemiol.* 2005;161:352-358.

19. Sierra-Johnson J, Romero-Corral A, Somers VK, et al. Prognostic importance of weight loss in patients with coronary heart disease regardless of initial body mass index. *Eur J Cardiovasc Prev Rehabil.* 2008;15:336-340.

20. Ades PA, Savage PD, Toth MJ, et al. High-calorie-expenditure exercise: A new approach to cardiac rehabilitation for overweight coronary patients. *Circulation.* 2009;119:2671-2678.

21. Berk KA, Oudshoorn TP, Verhoeven AJM, et al. Diet-induced weight loss and markers of endothelial dysfunction and inflammation in treated patients with type 2 diabetes. *Clin Nutr ESPEN.* 2016;15:101-106.

22. Keating FK, Schneider DJ, Savage PD, et al. Effect of exercise training and weight loss on platelet reactivity in overweight patients with coronary artery disease. *J Cardiopulm Rehabil Prev.* 2013;33:371-377.

23. Pope L, Harvey-Berino J, Savage P, Bunn J, Ludlow M, Oldridge N, Ades P. The impact of high-calorie-expenditure exercise on quality of life in older adults with coronary heart disease. *J Aging Phys Act.* 2011;19:99-116.

24. Seidell JC, Flegal KM. Assessing obesity: Classification and epidemiology. *Br Med Bull.* 1997;53:238-252.

25. Executive summary of the third report of the national cholesterol education program (NCEP) expert panel on detection, evaluation, and treatment of high blood cholesterol in adults (adult treatment panel iii). *JAMA.* 2001;285:2486-2497.

26. About metabolic syndrome. 2016. http://www.heart.org/HEARTORG/Conditions/More/MetabolicSyndrome/About-Metabolic-Syndrome_UCM_301920_Article.jsp#.WvWhSO-UtNA

27. Savage PD, Banzer JA, Balady GJ, Ades PA. Prevalence of metabolic syndrome in cardiac rehabilitation/secondary prevention programs. *Am Heart J.* 2005;149:627-631.

28. Ford ES, Giles WH, Dietz WH. Prevalence of the metabolic syndrome among us adults: Findings from the third National Health and Nutrition Examination Survey. *JAMA.* 2002;287:356-359.

29. Rana JS, Mukamal KJ, Morgan JP, Muller JE, Mittleman MA. Obesity and the risk of death after acute myocardial infarction. *Am Heart J.* 2004;147:841-846.

30. Wolk R, Berger P, Lennon RJ, Brilakis ES, Somers VK. Body mass index: A risk factor for unstable angina and myocardial infarction in patients with angiographically confirmed coronary artery disease. *Circulation.* 2003;108:2206-2211.

31. Wilson PW, D'Agostino RB, Sullivan L, Parise H, Kannel WB. Overweight and obesity as determinants of cardiovascular risk: The framingham experience. *Arch Intern Med*. 2002;162:1867-1872.

32. Schwartz GG, Olsson AG, Szarek M, Sasiela WJ. Relation of characteristics of metabolic syndrome to short-term prognosis and effects of intensive statin therapy after acute coronary syndrome: An analysis of the myocardial ischemia reduction with aggressive cholesterol lowering (miracl) trial. *Diabetes Care*. 2005;28:2508-2513.

33. Levantesi G, Macchia A, Marfisi R, et al. Metabolic syndrome and risk of cardiovascular events after myocardial infarction. *J Am Coll Cardiol*. 2005;46:277-283.

34. Daly CA, Hildebrandt P, Bertrand M, et al. Adverse prognosis associated with the metabolic syndrome in established coronary artery disease: Data from the EUROPA trial. *Heart*. 2007;93:1406-1411.

35. Romero-Corral A, Montori VM, Somers VK, et al. Association of bodyweight with total mortality and with cardiovascular events in coronary artery disease: A systematic review of cohort studies. *Lancet*. 2006;368:666-678.

36. Medina-Inojosa JR, Somers VK, Thomas RJ, et al. Association between adiposity and lean mass with long-term cardiovascular events in patients with coronary artery disease: No paradox. *J Am Heart Assoc*. 2018;7.

37. Lamonte MJ, Ainsworth BE. Quantifying energy expenditure and physical activity in the context of dose response. *Med Sci Sports Exerc*. 2001;33:S370-378; discussion S419-320.

38. Prochaska JO, DiClemente CC. Stages and processes of self-change of smoking: Toward an integrative model of change. *J Consult Clin Psychol*. 1983;51:390-395.

39. Ades PA, Savage PD, Harvey-Berino J. The treatment of obesity in cardiac rehabilitation. *J Cardiopulm Rehabil Prev*. 2010;30:289-298.

40. Harvey-Berino J. Weight loss in the clinical setting: Applications for cardiac rehabilitation. *Coron Artery Dis*. 1998;9:795-798.

41. Savage PD, Lee M, Harvey-Berino J, Brochu M, Ades PA. Weight reduction in the cardiac rehabilitation setting. *J Cardiopulm Rehabil*. 2002;22:154-160.

42. Wadden TA, Butryn ML, Wilson C. Lifestyle modification for the management of obesity. *Gastroenterology*. 2007;132:2226-2238.

43. Lichtenstein AH, Appel LJ, Brands M, et al. Summary of American Heart Aassociation diet and lifestyle recommendations revision 2006. *Arterioscler Thromb Vasc Biol*. 2006;26:2186-2191.

44. Noren E, Forssell H. Very low calorie diet without aspartame in obese subjects: Improved metabolic control after 4 weeks treatment. *Nutr J*. 2014;13:77.

45. Widmer RJ, Allison TG, Lerman LO, Lerman A. Digital health intervention as an adjunct to cardiac rehabilitation reduces cardiovascular risk factors and rehospitalizations. *J Cardiovasc Transl Res*. 2015;8:283-292.

46. Widmer RJ, Allison TG, Lennon R, Lopez-Jimenez F, Lerman LO, Lerman A. Digital health intervention during cardiac rehabilitation: A randomized controlled trial. *Am Heart J*. 2017;188:65-72.

47. Patel MS, Asch DA, Rosin R, et al. Framing financial incentives to increase physical activity among overweight and obese adults: A randomized, controlled trial. *Ann Intern Med*. 2016;164:385-394.

48. Ornish D, Brown SE, Scherwitz LW, et al. Can lifestyle changes reverse coronary heart disease? The lifestyle heart trial. *Lancet*. 1990;336:129-133.

49. de Lorgeril M, Salen P, Martin JL, Monjaud I, Delaye J, Mamelle N. Mediterranean diet, traditional risk factors, and the rate of cardiovascular complications after myocardial infarction: Final report of the lyon diet heart study. *Circulation*. 1999;99:779-785

50. Dansinger ML, Gleason JA, Griffith JL, Selker HP, Schaefer EJ. Comparison of the Atkins, Ornish, Weight Watchers, and zone diets for weight loss and heart disease risk reduction: A randomized trial. *JAMA*. 2005;293:43-53.

51. de Lorgeril M. Mediterranean diet and cardiovascular disease: Historical perspective and latest evidence. *Curr Atheroscler Rep*. 2013;15:370

52. Embree GG, Samuel-Hodge CD, Johnston LF, et al. Successful long-term weight loss among participants with diabetes receiving an intervention promoting an adapted Mediterranean-style dietary pattern: The heart healthy lenoir project. *BMJ Open Diabetes Res Care*. 2017;5:e000339.

53. Noakes M, Keogh JB, Foster PR, Clifton PM. Effect of an energy-restricted, high-protein, low-fat diet relative to a conventional high-carbohydrate, low-fat diet on weight loss, body composition, nutritional status, and markers of cardiovascular health in obese women. *Am J Clin Nutr*. 2005;81:1298-1306.

54. Claessens M, van Baak MA, Monsheimer S, Saris WH. The effect of a low-fat, high-protein or high-carbohydrate ad libitum diet on weight loss maintenance and metabolic risk factors. *Int J Obes (Lond)*. 2009;33:296-304.

55. Gardner CD, Kiazand A, Alhassan S, et al. Comparison of the Atkins, Zone, Ornish, and LEARN diets for change in weight and related risk factors among overweight premenopausal women: The a to z weight loss study: A randomized trial. *JAMA*. 2007;297:969-977.

56. Mertens DJ, Kavanagh T, Campbell RB, Shephard RJ. Exercise without dietary restriction as a means to long-term fat loss in the obese cardiac patient. *J Sports Med Phys Fitness*. 1998;38:310-316.

57. Savage PD, Brochu M, Poehlman ET, Ades PA. Reduction in obesity and coronary risk factors after high caloric exercise training in overweight coronary patients. *Am Heart J*. 2003;146:317-323.

58. Donnelly JE, Blair SN, Jakicic JM, Manore MM, Rankin JW, Smith BK. American College of Sports Medicine position stand. Appropriate physical activity intervention strategies for weight loss and prevention of weight regain for adults. *Med Sci Sports Exerc*. 2009;41:459-471.

59. Swain DP, Franklin BA. Is there a threshold intensity for aerobic training in cardiac patients? *Med Sci Sports Exerc*. 2002;34:1071-1075.

60. Hamm LF, Kavanagh T, Campbell RB, et al. Timeline for peak improvements during 52 weeks of outpatient cardiac rehabilitation. *J Cardiopulm Rehabil*. 2004;24:374-380; quiz 381-372.

61. Zeni AI, Hoffman MD, Clifford PS. Energy expenditure with indoor exercise machines. *JAMA*. 1996;275:1424-1427.

62. 2008 Physical Activity Guidelines for Americans. https://health.gov/paguidelines/2008/pdf/paguide.pdf.

63. Levine JA. Nonexercise activity thermogenesis—liberating the life-force. *J Intern Med*. 2007;262:273-287.

64. Saint-Maurice PF, Troiano RP, Matthews CE, Kraus WE. Moderate-to-vigorous physical activity and all-cause mortality: Do bouts matter? *J Am Heart Assoc*. 2018;7.

65. Riebe D, Ehrman JK, Liguori G, Magal M. *ACSM's Guidelines for Exercise Testing and Prescription*. 10th edition. Philadelphia: Wolters Kluwer Health, Lippincott Williams & Wilkins.

66. Healy GN, Dunstan DW, Salmon J, et al. Breaks in sedentary time: Beneficial associations with metabolic risk. *Diabetes Care*. 2008;31:661-666.

Chapter 9: Psychosocial Considerations Section

1. Kolman L, Shin N-M, Krishnan SM, et al. Psychological distress in CR participants. *J Cardiopulm Rehabil Prev*. 2011;31(2):81-86.

2. Balady GJ, Ades PA, Bittner VA, et al. Referral, enrollment, and delivery of CR/secondary prevention programs at clinical centers and beyond: a presidential advisory from the American Heart Association. *Circulation*. 2011;124(25):2951-2960.

3. Suaya JA, Stason WB, Ades PA, Normand S-LT, Shepard DS. CR and survival in older coronary patients. *J Am Coll Cardiol*. 2009;54(1):25-33.

4. Hamm LF, Sanderson BK, Ades PA, et al. Core competencies for CR/secondary prevention professionals: 2010 update position statement of the American Association of Cardiovascular and Pulmonary Rehabilitation. *J Cardiopulm Rehabil Prev*. 2011;31(1):2-10.

5. Whalley B, Thompson DR, Taylor RS. Psychological interventions for coronary heart disease: Cochrane systematic review and meta-analysis. *Int J Behav Med*. 2014;21(1):109-121.

6. Richards SH, Anderson L, Jenkinson CE, et al. Psychological interventions for coronary heart disease. *Cochrane Database of Syst Rev*. 2017;(4). Cochrane AN: CD002902. Date of Electronic Publication: 2017 Apr 28.

7. Orth-Gomér K, Schneiderman N, Wang H-X, Walldin C, Blom M, Jernberg T. Stress reduction prolongs life in women with coronary disease: the Stockholm Women's Intervention Trial for Coronary Heart Disease (SWITCHD). *Circulation Cardiovascular Quality And Outcomes*. 2009;2(1):25-32. doi:10.1161/CIRCOUTCOMES.108.812859.

8. Blumenthal JA, Sherwood A, Smith PJ, et al. Enhancing CR with stress management training: A randomized clinical efficacy trial. *Circulation*. 2016; 133(14):1341-1350. doi:10.1161/CIRCULATIONAHA.115.018926.

9. Gulliksson M, Burell G, Vessby B, Lundin L, Toss H, Svärdsudd K. Randomized controlled trial of cognitive behavioral therapy vs standard treatment to prevent recurrent cardiovascular events in patients with coronary heart disease: Secondary Prevention in Uppsala Primary Health Care project (SUPRIM). *Arch Intern Med*. 2011;171(2):134-140.

10. Van Melle JP, De Jonge P, Honig A, et al. Effects of antidepressant treatment following myocardial infarction. *Br J Psychiatry*. 2007;190(6):460-466.

11. O'Connor CM, Jiang W, Kuchibhatla M, et al. Safety and efficacy of sertraline for depression in patients with heart failure: Results of the SAD-HART-CHF (Sertraline Against Depression and Heart Disease in Chronic Heart Failure) trial. *J Am Coll Cardiol*. 2010;56(9):692-699.

12. Angermann CE, Gelbrich G, Störk S, et al. Effect of escitalopram on all-cause mortality and hospitalization in patients with heart failure and depression: The MOOD-HF randomized clinical trial. *JAMA*. 2016;315(24):2683-2693.

13. Glassman AH, O'connor CM, Califf RM, et al. Sertraline treatment of major depression in patients with acute MI or unstable angina. *JAMA*. 2002;288(6):701-709.

14. Kim J-M, Stewart R, Lee Y-S, et al. Effect of escitalopram vs placebo treatment for depression on long-term cardiac outcomes in patients with acute coronary syndrome: A randomized clinical trial. *JAMA*. 2018;320(4):350-358.

15. American Psychiatric Association. *Diagnostic and Statistical Manual of Mental Disorders*. 4th ed. *Washington, DC:* American Psychiatric Association; 2000.

16. American Psychiatric Association. *Diagnostic and Statistical Manual of Mental Disorders (DSM-5)*. American Psychiatric Association: Washington, DC; 2013.

17. Lavie CJ, Menezes AR, De Schutter A, Milani RV, Blumenthal JA. Impact of CR and exercise training on psychological risk factors and subsequent prognosis in patients with cardiovascular disease. *Can J Cardiol*. 2016;32(10):S365-S373.

18. Blumenthal JA, Carney RM, Doering LV, et al. Depression as a risk factor for poor prognosis among patients with acute coronary syndrome: Systematic review and recommendations. *Circulation*. 2014;129:1350-1369.

19. Lichtman JH, Froelicher ES, Blumenthal JA, et al. Depression as a risk factor for poor prognosis among patients with acute coronary syndrome: Systematic review and recommendations. *Circulation*. 2014; 129(12):1350-69.:CIR. 0000000000000019

20. Gathright EC, Goldstein CM, Josephson RA, Hughes JW. Depression increases the risk of mortality in patients with heart failure: A meta-analysis. *J Psychosom Res*. 2017;94:82-89.

21. Ziegelstein RC, Fauerbach JA, Stevens SS, Romanelli J, Richter DP, Bush DE. Patients with depression are less likely to follow recommendations to reduce cardiac risk during recovery from a myocardial infarction. *Arch Intern Med*. 2000;160(12):1818-1823.

22. Gathright EC, Dolansky MA, Gunstad J, et al. The impact of medication nonadherence on the relationship between mortality risk and depression in heart failure. *Health Psychol*. 2017;36(9):839.

23. Jaarsma T, van der Wal MH, Lesman-Leegte I, et al. Effect of moderate or intensive disease management program on outcome in patients with heart failure: Coordinating Study Evaluating Outcomes of Advising and Counseling in Heart Failure (COACH). *Arch Intern Med*. 2008;168(3):316-324.

24. Casey E, Hughes JW, Waechter D, Josephson R, Rosneck J. Depression predicts failure to complete phase-II CR. *J Behav Med*. 2008;31(5):421-431.

25. Resurrección DM, Motrico E, Rubio-Valera M, Mora-Pardo JA, Moreno-Peral P. Reasons for dropout from CR programs in women: A qualitative study. *PloS One*. 2018;13(7):e0200636.

26. Lichtman JH, Bigger Jr JT, Blumenthal JA, et al. Depression and coronary heart disease: Recommendations for screening, referral, and treatment: A science advisory from the American Heart Association Prevention Committee of the Council on Cardiovascular Nursing, Council on Clinical Cardiology, Council on Epidemiology and Prevention, and Interdisciplinary Council on Quality of Care and Outcomes Research: Endorsed by the American Psychiatric Association. *Focus*. 2009;7(3):406-413.

27. Williams RB. Loneliness and social isolation and increased risk of coronary heart disease and stroke: Clinical implications. *Heart*. 2016;102(24).

28. Williams RB, Barefoot JC, Califf RM, et al. Prognostic importance of social and economic resources among medically treated patients with angiographically documented coronary artery disease. *JAMA*. 1992;267(4):520-524.

29. Masi CM, Chen H-Y, Hawkley LC, Cacioppo JT. A meta-analysis of interventions to reduce loneliness. *Pers Soc Psychol Rev*. 2011;15(3):219-266.

30. Thomas RJ, King M, Lui K, et al. AACVPR/ACC/AHA 2007 Performance Measures on Cardiac Rehabilitation for Referral to and Delivery of Cardiac Rehabilitation/Secondary Prevention ServicesEndorsed by the American College of Chest Physicians, American College of Sports Medicine, American Physical Therapy Association, Canadian Association of Cardiac Rehabilitation, European Association for Cardiovascular Prevention and Rehabilitation, InterAmerican Heart Foundation, National Association of Clinical Nurse Specialists, Preventive Cardiovascular Nurses Association, and the Society of Thoracic Surgeons. Journal of the American College of Cardiology. 2007; 50(14):1400–1433. [PubMed: 17903645]

31. Medicare Improvements for Patients and Providers Act of 2008. Pub L No 110–275, 122 Stat 2494. As updated by Related Change Request (CR) #: 6850 effective January 1, 2010. Retrieved 10.21.2019 from: https://www.govinfo.gov/app/details/PLAW-110publ275

32. Mitchell PH, Powell L, Blumenthal J, et al. A short social support measure for patients recovering from myocardial infarction: The ENRICHD Social Support Inventory. *J Cardiopulm Rehabil Prev.* 2003;23(6):398-403.

33. Blumenthal JA, Sherwood A, Rogers SD, et al. Understanding prognostic benefits of exercise and antidepressant therapy for persons with depression and heart disease: The UPBEAT study—rationale, design, and methodological issues. *Clinical Trials.* 2007;4(5):548-559.

34. Lespérance F, Frasure-Smith N, Koszycki D, et al. Effects of citalopram and interpersonal psychotherapy on depression in patients with coronary artery disease: The Canadian Cardiac Randomized Evaluation of Antidepressant and Psychotherapy Efficacy (CREATE) trial. *JAMA.* 2007;297(4):367-379.

35. Milani RV, Lavie CJ, Mehra MR, Ventura HO. Impact of exercise training and depression on survival in heart failure due to coronary heart disease. *Am J Cardiol.* 2011;107(1):64-68.

36. Josephson EA, Casey EC, Waechter D, Rosneck J, Hughes JW. Gender and depression symptoms in CR: Women initially exhibit higher depression scores but experience more improvement. *J Cardiopulm Rehabil Prev.* 2006;26(3):160-163.

37. Barbour KA, Blumenthal JA. Exercise training and depression in older adults. *Neurobiol Aging.* 2005;26(1):119-123.

38. Blumenthal JA, Babyak MA, O'Connor C, et al. Effects of exercise training on depressive symptoms in patients with chronic heart failure: The HF-ACTION randomized trial. *JAMA.* 2012;308(5):465-474.

39. Blumenthal JA, Sherwood A, Babyak MA, et al. Exercise and pharmacological treatment of depressive symptoms in patients with coronary heart disease: Results from the UPBEAT (Understanding the Prognostic Benefits of Exercise and Antidepressant Therapy) study. *J Am Coll Cardiol.* 2012;60(12):1053-1063.

40. Brosse AL, Sheets ES, Lett HS, Blumenthal JA. Exercise and the treatment of clinical depression in adults. *Sports Med.* 2002;32(12):741-760.

41. Dracup K, Bryan-Brown CW. An open door policy in ICU. *Am J Crit Care.* 1992;1(2):16.

42. Hughes JW, Bon-Wilson A, Kent Eichenauer P, Feltz G. Behavioral medicine for patients with heart disease—The case of depression and CR. *US Cardiology.* 2010;7:55-60.

43. Hollon SD, DeRubeis RJ, Shelton RC, Weiss B. The emperor's new drugs: Effect size and moderation effects. 2002;5(1): No Pagination Specified Article 28.

44. Kirsch I, Deacon BJ, Huedo-Medina TB, Scoboria A, Moore TJ, Johnson BT. Initial severity and antidepressant benefits: A meta-analysis of data submitted to the Food and Drug Administration. *PLoS Med.* 2008;5(2):e45.

45. Kirsch I. Yes, there is a placebo effect, but is there a powerful antidepressant drug effect? *Prevention & Treatment.* 2002;5(1):22i.

46. Kirsch I, Scoboria A, Moore TJ. Antidepressants and placebos: secrets, revelations, and unanswered questions. 2002; 5(1): No Pagination Specified Article 28.

47. Kirsch I, Sapirstein G. Listening to Prozac but hearing placebo: A meta-analysis of antidepressant medication. American Psychological Association; 1998.

48. Lacasse JR, Leo J. Antidepressants and the chemical imbalance theory of depression. *The Behavior Therapist.* 2015;38(7).

49. Lacasse JR, Leo J. Serotonin and depression: a disconnect between the advertisements and the scientific literature. *PLoS Med.* 2005;2(12):e392.

50. Möller H-J, Bitter I, Bobes J, Fountoulakis K, Höschl C, Kasper S. Position statement of the European Psychiatric Association (EPA) on the value of antidepressants in the treatment of unipolar depression. *Eur Psychiatry.* 2012;27(2):114-128.

51. Fihn SD, Gardin JM, Abrams J, et al. 2012 ACCF/AHA/ACP/AATS/PCNA/SCAI/STS

guideline for the diagnosis and management of patients with stable ischemic heart disease: A report of the American College of Cardiology Foundation/American Heart Association task force on practice guidelines, and the American College of Physicians, American Association for Thoracic Surgery, Preventive Cardiovascular Nurses Association, Society for Cardiovascular Angiography and Interventions, and Society of Thoracic Surgeons. *J Am Coll Cardiol.* 2012;60(24):e44-e164.

Chapter 9: Environmental Considerations Section

1. Cosselman KE, Navas-Acien A, Kaufman JD. Environmental factors in cardiovascular disease. *Nat Rev Cardiol.* 2015;12:627.

2. Bhatnagar A. Environmental determinants of cardiovascular disease. *Circ Res.* 2017;121(2):162. doi:10.1161/CIRCRESAHA.117.306458

3. Van Eeden S, Leipsic J, Paul Man SF, Sin DD. The relationship between lung inflammation and cardiovascular disease. *Am J Respir Crit Care Med.* 2012;186(1):11-16. doi:10.1164/rccm.201203-0455PP

4. Brook RD. Air pollution and cardiovascular disease: A statement for healthcare professionals From the expert panel on population and prevention science of the American Heart Association. *Circulation.* 2004;109(21):2655-2671. doi:10.1161/01.CIR.0000128587.30041.C8

5. Franklin BA, Brook R, Arden Pope C. Air pollution and cardiovascular disease. *Curr Probl Cardiol.* 2015;40(5):207-238. doi:10.1016/j.cpcardiol.2015.01.003

6. Münzel T, Sørensen M, Gori T, et al. Environmental stressors and cardio-metabolic disease: Part I-epidemiologic evidence supporting a role for noise and air pollution and effects of mitigation strategies. *Eur Heart J.* 2017;38(8):550-556. doi:10.1093/eurheartj/ehw269

7. Mustafić H, Jabre P, Caussin C, et al. Main air pollutants and myocardial infarction: A systematic review and meta-analysis. *JAMA.* 2012;307(7):713. doi:10.1001/jama.2012.126

8. World Health Organization. Ambient (outdoor) air quality and health. World Health Organization. www.who.int/news-room/fact-sheets/detail/ambient-(outdoor)-air-quality-and-health. Published 2018. Accessed June 14, 2018.

9. Brook RD, Newby DE, Rajagopalan S. Air pollution and cardiometabolic disease: An update and call for clinical trials. *Am J Hypertens.* 2018;31(1):1-10. doi:10.1093/ajh/hpx109

10. Kelly FJ, Fussell JC. Air pollution and public health: Emerging hazards and improved understanding of risk. *Environ Geochem Health.* 2015;37(4):631-649. doi:10.1007/s10653-015-9720-1

11. Lelieveld J, Evans JS, Fnais M, Giannadaki D, Pozzer A. The contribution of outdoor air pollution sources to premature mortality on a global scale. *Nature.* 2015;525(7569):367-371. doi:10.1038/nature15371

12. Newell K, Kartsonaki C, Lam KBH, Kurmi OP. Cardiorespiratory health effects of particulate ambient air pollution exposure in low-income and middle-income countries: A systematic review and meta-analysis. *Lancet Planet Health.* 2017;1(9):e368-e380. doi:10.1016/S2542-5196(17)30166-3

13. Requia WJ, Adams MD, Arain A, Papatheodorou S, Koutrakis P, Mahmoud M. Global association of air pollution and cardiorespiratory diseases: A systematic review, meta-analysis, and investigation of modifier variables. *Am J Public Health.* 2018;108(S2):S123-S130. doi:10.2105/AJPH.2017.303839

14. Gakidou E, Afshin A, Abajobir AA, et al. Global, regional, and national comparative risk assessment of 84 behavioural, environmental and occupational, and metabolic risks or clusters of risks, 1990-2016: A systematic analysis for the Global Burden of Disease Study 2016. *Lancet.* 2017;390(10100):1345-1422. doi:10.1016/S0140-6736(17)32366-8

15. Lipfert FW. A critical review of the ESCAPE project for estimating long-term health effects of air pollution. *Environ Int.* 2017;99:87-96. doi:10.1016/j.envint.2016.11.028

16. Argacha JF, Bourdrel T, van de Borne P. Ecology of the cardiovascular system: A focus on air-related environmental factors. *Trends Cardiovasc Med.* 2018;28(2):112-126. doi:10.1016/j.tcm.2017.07.013

17. Bourdrel T, Bind M-A, Béjot Y, Morel O, Argacha J-F. Cardiovascular effects of air pollution. *Arch Cardiovasc Dis.* 2017;110(11):634-642. doi:10.1016/j.acvd.2017.05.003

18. Asikainen A, Carrer P, Kephalopoulos S, Fernandes Ede O, Wargocki P, Hänninen O. Reducing burden of disease from residential indoor air exposures in Europe (HEALTHVENT project). *Environ Health.* 2016;15(S1). doi:10.1186/s12940-016-0101-8

19. Newby DE, Mannucci PM, Tell GS, et al. Expert position paper on air pollution and cardiovascular disease. *Eur Heart J.* 2015;36(2):83-93b. doi:10.1093/eurheartj/ehu458

20. Achilleos S, Kioumourtzoglou M-A, Wu C-D, Schwartz JD, Koutrakis P, Papatheodorou SI. Acute effects of fine particulate matter constituents on mortality: A systematic review and meta-regression analysis. *Environ Int.* 2017;109:89-100. doi:10.1016/j.envint.2017.09.010

21. Gold DR, Mittleman MA. New insights into pollution and the cardiovascular system: 2010 to 2012. *Circulation.* 2013;127(18):1903-1913. doi:10.1161/CIRCULATIONAHA.111.064337

22. Kim H, Kim J, Kim S, et al. Cardiovascular effects of long-term exposure to air pollution: A population-based study with 900 845 person-years of follow-up. *JAMA.* 2017;6(11):e007170. doi:10.1161/JAHA.117.007170

23. Du Y, Xu X, Chu M, Guo Y, Wang J. Air particulate matter and cardiovascular disease: The epidemiological, biomedical and clinical evidence. *J Thorac Dis.* 2015;8(1):E8-E19.

24. Hoek G, Krishnan RM, Beelen R, et al. Long-term air pollution exposure and cardio- respiratory mortality: A review. *Environ Health.* 2013;12(1). doi:10.1186/1476-069X-12-43

25. Abatzoglou JT, Williams AP. Impact of anthropogenic climate change on wildfire across western US forests. *Proc Natl Acad Sci.* 2016;113(42):11770-11775. doi:10.1073/pnas.1607171113

26. Pechony O, Shindell DT. Driving forces of global wildfires over the past millennium and the forthcoming century. *Proc Natl Acad Sci.* 2010;107(45):19167-19170. doi:10.1073/pnas.1003669107

27. Laden F, Neas LM, Dockery DW, Schwartz J. Association of fine particulate matter from different sources with daily mortality in six U.S. cities. *Environ Health Perspect.* 2000;108(10):941-947.

28. Brook RD, Rajagopalan S, Pope CA, et al. Particulate matter air pollution and cardiovascular disease: An update to the scientific statement from the American Heart Association. *Circulation.* 2010;121(21):2331-2378. doi:10.1161/CIR.0b013e3181dbece1

29. van der Zee SC, Fischer PH, Hoek G. Air pollution in perspective: Health risks of air pollution expressed in equivalent numbers of passively smoked cigarettes. *Environ Res.* 2016;148:475-483. doi:10.1016/j.envres.2016.04.001

30. Gan WQ, Davies HW, Koehoorn M, Brauer M. Association of long-term exposure to community noise and traffic-related air pollution with coronary heart disease mortality. *Am J Epidemiol.* 2012;175(9):898-906. doi:10.1093/aje/kwr424

31. Hooper LG, Kaufman JD. Ambient air pollution and clinical implications for susceptible populations. *Ann Am Thoracic Soc.* 2018;15(Supplement 2):S64-S68. doi:10.1513/AnnalsATS.201707-574MG

32. Nawrot TS, Perez L, Künzli N, Munters E, Nemery B. Public health importance of triggers of myocardial infarction: A comparative risk assessment. *Lancet.* 2011;377(9767):732-740. doi:10.1016/S0140-6736(10)62296-9

33. Pope CA, Burnett RT, Krewski D, et al. Cardiovascular mortality and exposure to airborne fine particulate matter and cigarette smoke: Shape of the exposure-response relationship. *Circulation.* 2009;120(11):941-948. doi:10.1161/CIRCULATIONAHA.109.857888

34. Rajagopalan S, Brook RD. Air pollution and type 2 diabetes: Mechanistic insights. *Diabetes.* 2012;61(12):3037-3045. doi:10.2337/db12-0190

35. Shah AS, Langrish JP, Nair H, et al. Global association of air pollution and heart failure: A systematic review and meta-analysis. *Lancet.* 2013;382(9897):1039-1048. doi:10.1016/S0140-6736(13)60898-3

36. Song X, Liu Y, Hu Y, et al. Short-term exposure to air pollution and cardiac arrhythmia: A meta-analysis and systematic review. *Int J Environ Res Public Health.* 2016;13(7):642. doi:10.3390/ijerph13070642

37. Cakmak S, Dales R, Leech J, Liu L. The influence of air pollution on cardiovascular and pulmonary function and exercise capacity: Canadian Health Measures Survey (CHMS). *Environ Res.* 2011;111(8):1309-1312. doi:10.1016/j.envres.2011.09.016

38. Li J, Sun S, Tang R, et al. Major air pollutants and risk of COPD exacerbations: A systematic review and meta-analysis. *International Journal of Chronic Obstructive Pulmonary Disease.* 2016;11:3079-3091. doi:10.2147/COPD.S122282

39. Guarnieri M, Balmes JR. Outdoor air pollution and asthma. *Lancet.* 2014;383(9928):1581-1592. doi:10.1016/S0140-6736(14)60617-6

40. Gan WQ, Tamburic L, Davies HW, Demers PA, Koehoorn M, Brauer M. Changes in residential proximity to road traffic and the risk of death from coronary heart disease. *Epidemiology.* 2010;21(5):642-649. doi:10.1097/EDE.0b013e3181e89f19

41. Hart JE, Rimm EB, Rexrode KM, Laden F. Changes in traffic exposure and the risk of incident myocardial infarction and all-cause

mortality: *Epidemiology.* 2013;24(5):734-742. doi:10.1097/EDE.0b013e31829d5dae

42. Hart JE, Chiuve SE, Laden F, Albert CM. Roadway proximity and risk of sudden cardiac death in women. *Circulation.* 2014;130(17):1474-1482. doi:10.1161/CIRCULATIONAHA.114.011489

43. Hoek G, Brunekreef B, Goldbohm S, Fischer P, van den Brandt PA. Association between mortality and indicators of traffic-related air pollution in the Netherlands: A cohort study. *Lancet.* 2002;360(9341):1203-1209. doi:10.1016/S0140-6736(02)11280-3

44. Kaufman JD, Spalt EW, Curl CL, et al. Advances in understanding air pollution and CVD. *Glob Heart.* 2016;11(3):343-352. doi:10.1016/j.gheart.2016.07.004

45. Aslibekyan S, Claas SA, Arnett DK. Clinical applications of epigenetics in cardiovascular disease: The long road ahead. *Transl Res.* 2015;165(1):143-153. doi:10.1016/j.trsl.2014.04.004

46. Nilsson EE, Skinner MK. Environmentally induced epigenetic transgenerational inheritance of disease susceptibility. *Transl Res.* 2015;165(1):12-17. doi:10.1016/j.trsl.2014.02.003

47. Chen H, Burnett RT, Kwong JC, et al. Risk of incident diabetes in relation to long-term exposure to fine particulate matter in Ontario, Canada. *Environ Health Perspect.* 2013;121(7):804-810. doi:10.1289/ehp.1205958

48. Kampfrath T, Maiseyeu A, Ying Z, et al. Chronic fine particulate matter exposure induces systemic vascular dysfunction via NADPH oxidase and TLR4 pathways. *Circ Res.* 2011;108(6):716-726. doi:10.1161/CIRCRESAHA.110.237560

49. Zheng Z, Xu X, Zhang X, et al. Exposure to ambient particulate matter induces a NASH-like phenotype and impairs hepatic glucose metabolism in an animal model. *J Hepatol.* 2013;58(1):148-154. doi:10.1016/j.jhep.2012.08.009

50. Jerrett M, McConnell R, Wolch J, et al. Traffic-related air pollution and obesity formation in children: A longitudinal, multilevel analysis. *Environ Health.* 2014;13:49. doi:10.1186/1476-069X-13-49

51. Wang Y, Eliot MN, Kuchel GA, et al. Long-term exposure to ambient air pollution and serum leptin in older adults: Results from the MOBILIZE Boston Study. *J Occup Environ Med.* 2014;56(9):e73-e77. doi:10.1097/JOM.0000000000000253

52. Gold DR. Vulnerability to cardiovascular effects of air pollution in people with diabetes. *Curr Diab Rep.* 2008;8(5):333-335. doi:10.1007/s11892-008-0058-2

53. Lamas GA, Navas-Acien A, Mark DB, Lee KL. Heavy metals, cardiovascular disease, and the unexpected benefits of chelation therapy. *J Amer Coll Cardiol.* 2016;67(20):2411-2418. doi:10.1016/j.jacc.2016.02.066

54. Nigra AE, Ruiz-Hernandez A, Redon J, Navas-Acien A, Tellez-Plaza M. Environmental metals and cardiovascular disease in adults: A systematic review beyond lead and cadmium. *Curr Environ Health Rep.* 2016;3(4):416-433. doi:10.1007/s40572-016-0117-9

55. Solenkova NV, Newman JD, Berger JS, Thurston G, Hochman JS, Lamas GA. Metal pollutants and cardiovascular disease: Mechanisms and consequences of exposure. *Am Heart J.* 2014;168(6):812-822. doi:10.1016/j.ahj.2014.07.007

56. Agency for Toxic Substances and Disease Registry. ATSDR's substance priority list. www.atsdr.cdc.gov/spl/index.html. Published October 3, 2017. Accessed July 5, 2018.

57. Gambelunghe A, Sallsten G, Borné Y, et al. Low-level exposure to lead, blood pressure, and hypertension in a population-based cohort. *Environ Res.* 2016;149:157-163. doi:10.1016/j.envres.2016.05.015

58. Giles LV, Barn P, Künzli N, et al. From good intentions to proven interventions: Effectiveness of actions to reduce the health impacts of air pollution. *Environ Health Perspect.* 2010;119(1):29-36. doi:10.1289/ehp.1002246

59. Lissåker CTK, Talbott EO, Kan H, Xu X. Status and determinants of individual actions to reduce health impacts of air pollution in US adults. *Arch Environ Occup Health.* 2016;71(1):43-48. doi:10.1080/19338244.2014.988673

60. Morishita M, Thompson KC, Brook RD. Understanding air pollution and cardiovascular diseases: Is it preventable? *Curr Cardiovasc Risk Rep.* 2015;9(6). doi:10.1007/s12170-015-0458-1

61. Giles LV, Koehle MS. The health effects of exercising in air pollution. *Sports Med.* 2014;44(2):223-249. doi:10.1007/s40279-013-0108-z

62. Alves AJ, Viana JL, Cavalcante SL, et al. Physical activity in primary and secondary prevention of cardiovascular disease: Overview updated. *World J Cardiol.* 2016;8(10):575-583. doi:10.4330/wjc.v8.i10.575

63. Giannuzzi P, Mezzani A, Saner H, et al. Physical activity for primary and secondary prevention. Position paper of the Working Group on Cardiac Rehabilitation and Exercise Physiology of the European Society of Cardiology. *Eur J Cardiovasc Prev Rehab.* 2003;10(5):319-327. doi:10.1097/01.hjr.0000086303.28200.50

64. Durstine JL, Gordon B, Wang Z, Luo X. Chronic disease and the link to physical activity. *J Sport Health Sci.* 2013;2(1):3-11. doi:10.1016/j.jshs.2012.07.009

65. Tainio M, de Nazelle AJ, Götschi T, et al. Can air pollution negate the health benefits of cycling and walking? *Prev Med.* 2016;87:233-236. doi:10.1016/j.ypmed.2016.02.002

66. Woodward A, Samet J. Active transport: Exercise trumps air pollution, almost always. *Prev Med.* 2016;87:237-238. doi:10.1016/j.ypmed.2016.03.027

67. Giorgini P, Rubenfire M, Bard RL, Jackson EA, Ferri C, Brook RD. Air pollution and exercise: A review of the cardiovascular implications for health care professionals. *J Cardiopulm Rehab Prev.* 2016;36(2):84. doi:10.1097/HCR.0000000000000139

Chapter 10: CR for Patients With CVD Section

1. Thomas RJ, Balady G, Banka G, et al. 2018 ACC/AHA clinical performance and quality measures for cardiac rehabilitation: A report of the American College of Cardiology/American Heart Association Task Force on Performance Measures. *J Am Coll Cardiol* 2018;71(16):1814-37.

2. Balady GJ, Williams MA, Ades PA, et al. Core components of cardiac rehabilitation/secondary prevention programs: 2007 update: A scientific statement from the American Heart Association Exercise, Cardiac Rehabilitation, and Prevention Committee, the Council on Clinical Cardiology; the Councils on Cardiovascular Nursing, Epidemiology and Prevention, and Nutrition, Physical Activity, and Metabolism; and the American Association of Cardiovascular and Pulmonary Rehabilitation. *J Cardiopulm Rehabil Prev.* 2007;27(3):121-9.

3. Hamm LF, Sanderson BK, Ades PA, et al. Core competencies for cardiac rehabilitation/secondary prevention professionals: 2010 update: Position statement of the American Association of Cardiovascular and Pulmonary Rehabilitation. *J Cardiopulm Rehabil Prev.* 2011;31(1):2-10.

4. Benjamin EJ, Blaha MJ, Chiuve SE, et al. Heart disease and stroke statistics-2017 update: A report from the American Heart Association. *Circulation.* 2017;135(10):e146-e603.

5. Cardiac Rehabilitation and Intensive Cardiac Rehabilitation – JA6850. Secondary Cardiac Rehabilitation and Intensive Cardiac Rehabilitation – JA6850. Centers for Medicare & Medicaid website. www.cms.gov/Medicare/Medicare-Contracting/ContractorLearningResources/downloads/JA6850.pdf. Published March 21, 2010. Accessed October 23, 2019.

6. Lawler PR, Filion KB, Eisenberg MJ. Efficacy of exercise-based cardiac rehabilitation post-myocardial infarction: A systematic review and meta-analysis of randomized controlled trials. *Am Heart J.* 2011;162(4):571-84.

7. Goel K, Lennon RJ, Tilbury RT, Squires RW, Thomas RJ. Impact of cardiac rehabilitation on mortality and cardiovascular events after percutaneous coronary intervention in the community. *Circulation.* 2011;123(21):2344-52.

8. Pack QR, Goel K, Lahr BD, et al. Participation in cardiac rehabilitation and survival after coronary artery bypass graft surgery: A community-based study. *Circulation.* 2013;128(6):590-7.

9. Suaya JA, Stason WB, Ades PA, Normand SL, Shepard DS. Cardiac rehabilitation and survival in older coronary patients. *J Am Coll Cardiol.* 2009;54(1):25-33.

10. Hammill BG, Curtis LH, Schulman KA, Whellan DJ. Relationship between cardiac rehabilitation and long-term risks of death and myocardial infarction among elderly Medicare beneficiaries. *Circulation.* 2010;121(1):63-70.

11. Shepherd CW, While AE. Cardiac rehabilitation and quality of life: A systematic review. *Int J Nurs Stud.* 2012;49(6):755-71.

12. Dunlay SM, Pack QR, Thomas RJ, Killian JM, Roger VL. Participation in cardiac rehabilitation, readmissions, and death after acute myocardial infarction. *Am J Med.* 2014;127(6):538-46.

13. Lamberti M, Ratti G, Gerardi D, et al. Work-related outcome after acute coronary syndrome: Implications of complex cardiac rehabilitation in occupational medicine. *Int J Occup Med Environ Health.* 2016;29(4):649-57.

14. Dugmore LD, Tipson RJ, Phillips MH, et al. Changes in cardiorespiratory fitness, psychological wellbeing, quality of life, and vocational status following a 12 month cardiac exercise rehabilitation programme. *Heart.* 1999;81(4):359-66.

15. Hillis LD, Smith PK, Anderson JL, et al. 2011 ACCF/AHA guideline for coronary artery bypass graft surgery. A report of the American College of Cardiology Foundation/American Heart Association Task Force on Practice Guidelines. *J Am Coll Cardiol*. 2011;58(24):e123-210.

16. Levine GN, Bates ER, Blankenship JC, et al. 2011 ACCF/AHA/SCAI Guideline for percutaneous coronary intervention. A report of the American College of Cardiology Foundation/American Heart Association Task Force on Practice Guidelines and the Society for Cardiovascular Angiography and Interventions. *J Am Coll Cardiol*. 2011;58(24):e44-122.

17. Smith SC, Jr., Benjamin EJ, Bonow RO, et al. AHA/ACCF Secondary prevention and risk reduction therapy for patients with coronary and other atherosclerotic vascular disease: 2011 update: A guideline from the American Heart Association and American College of Cardiology Foundation. *Circulation*. 2011;124(22):2458-73.

18. O'Gara PT, Kushner FG, Ascheim DD, et al. 2013 ACCF/AHA guideline for the management of ST-elevation myocardial infarction: A report of the American College of Cardiology Foundation/American Heart Association Task Force on Practice Guidelines. *Circulation*. 2013;127(4):e362-425.

19. Amsterdam EA, Wenger NK, Brindis RG, et al. 2014 AHA/ACC Guideline for the management of patients with non-ST-elevation acute coronary syndromes: A report of the American College of Cardiology/American Heart Association Task Force on Practice Guidelines. *J Am Coll Cardiol*. 2014;64(24):e139-e228.

20. Suaya JA, Shepard DS, Normand SL, Ades PA, Prottas J, Stason WB. Use of cardiac rehabilitation by Medicare beneficiaries after myocardial infarction or coronary bypass surgery. *Circulation*. 2007;116(15):1653-62.

21. Aragam KG, Dai D, Neely ML, et al. Gaps in referral to cardiac rehabilitation of patients undergoing percutaneous coronary intervention in the United States. *J Am Coll Cardiol*. 2015;65(19):2079-88.

22. Grace SL, Russell KL, Reid RD, et al. Effect of cardiac rehabilitation referral strategies on utilization rates: A prospective, controlled study. *Arch Intern Med*. 2011;171(3):235-41.

23. Ades PA, Keteyian SJ, Wright JS, et al. Increasing cardiac rehabilitation participation From 20% to 70%: A road map from the Million Hearts Cardiac Rehabilitation Collaborative. *Mayo Clin Proc*. 2017;92(2):234-42.

24. Russell KL, Holloway TM, Brum M, Caruso V, Chessex C, Grace SL. Cardiac rehabilitation wait times: Effect on enrollment. *J Cardiopulm Rehabil Prev*. 2011;31(6):373-7.

25. Marzolini S, Blanchard C, Alter DA, Grace SL, Oh PI. Delays in referral and enrollment are associated with mitigated benefits of cardiac rehabilitation after coronary artery bypass surgery. *Circ Cardiovasc Qual Outcomes*. 2015;8(6):608-20.

26. Bhatt DL. Percutaneous coronary intervention in 2018. JAMA 2018;319(20):2127-28.

27. Jneid H, Addison D, Bhatt DL, et al. 2017 AHA/ACC clinical performance and quality measures for adults with ST-elevation and non–ST-elevation myocardial infarction: a report of the American College of Cardiology/American Heart Association Task Force on Performance Measures. J Am Coll Cardiol. 2017; 70(16):2048-2090.

28. Head SJ, Milojevic M, Daemen J, et al. Mortality after coronary artery bypass grafting versus percutaneous coronary intervention with stenting for coronary artery disease: A pooled analysis of individual patient data. *Lancet*. 2018;391(10124):939-48.

29. Fletcher GF, Ades PA, Kligfield P, et al. Exercise standards for testing and training: A scientific statement from the American Heart Association. *Circulation*. 2013;128(8):873-934.

30. Riebe D, Ehrman JK, Liguori G, Maier M. *ACSM's Guidelines for Exercise Testing and Prescription*. 10th ed. Philadelphia: Lippincott Williams & Wilkins; 2018.

31. Pack QR, Dudycha KJ, Roschen KP, Thomas RJ, Squires RW. Safety of early enrollment into outpatient cardiac rehabilitation after open heart surgery. *Am J Cardiol*. 2015;115(4):548-52.

32. Haykowsky M, Scott J, Esch B, et al. A meta-analysis of the effects of exercise training on left ventricular remodeling following myocardial infarction: Start early and go longer for greatest exercise benefits on remodeling. *Trials*. 2011;12:92.

33. Kavanagh T, Mertens DJ, Hamm LF, et al. Prediction of long-term prognosis in 12 169 men referred for cardiac rehabilitation. *Circulation*. 2002;106(6):666-71.

34. De Schutter A, Kachur S, Lavie CJ, et al. Cardiac rehabilitation fitness changes and subsequent survival. *Eur Heart J Qual Care Clin Outcomes*. 2018;4(3):173-79.

35. Hannan AL, Hing W, Simas V, et al. High-intensity interval training versus moderate-intensity continuous training within cardiac rehabilitation: A systematic review and meta-analysis. *Open Access J Sports Med.* 2018;9:1-17.

36. Andries G, Khera S, Timmermans RF, et al. Complete versus culprit only revascularization in ST-elevation myocardial infarction—A perspective on recent trials and recommendations. *J Thorac Dis.* 2017 Jul; 9(7): 2159–2167.

37. Boden WE, O'Rourke RA, Teo KK, et al. Optimal medical therapy with or without PCI for stable coronary disease. *N Engl J Med.* 2007;356(15):1503-16.

38. Rechcinski T, Kalowski M, Kasprzak JD, Trzos E, Kurpesa M. Beneficial effects of cardiac rehabilitation in patients with incomplete revascularization after primary coronary angioplasty. *Eur J Phys Rehabil Med.* 2013;49(6):785-91.

39. Waldo SW, Gokhale M, O'Donnell CI, et al. Temporal trends in coronary angiography and percutaneous coronary intervention: Insights from the VA clinical assessment, reporting, and tracking program. *JACC Cardiovasc Interv.* 2018;11(9):879-88.

40. Katijjahbe MA, Granger CL, Denehy L, et al. Standard restrictive sternal precautions and modified sternal precautions had similar effects in people after cardiac surgery via median sternotomy ('SMART' Trial): A randomised trial. *J Physiother.* 2018;64(2):97-106.

41. Cahalin LP, Lapier TK, Shaw DK. Sternal precautions: Is it time for change? Precautions versus restrictions - A review of literature and recommendations for revision. *Cardiopulm Phys Ther J.* 2011;22(1):5-15.

42. Cahalin LP, Saponaro CM, Zuckerman JL, Krumpelbeck M, Keliher C. A cardiothoracic surgeons perspective on sternal precautions: Implications for rehabilitation professionals. *Chest.* 2009;136 (4):98S.

43. Balachandran S, Lee A, Royse A, Denehy L, El-Ansary D. Upper limb exercise prescription following cardiac surgery via median sternotomy: A web survey. *J Cardiopulm Rehabil Prev.* 2014;34(6):390-5.

44. Adams J, Cline MJ, Hubbard M, McCullough T, Hartman J. A new paradigm for post-cardiac event resistance exercise guidelines. *Am J Cardiol.* 2006;97(2):281-6.

45. Sturgess T DL, Tully E, El-Ansary D. A pilot thoracic exercise programme reduces early (0–6 weeks) sternal pain following open heart surgery. *Int J Ther Rehabil.* 2014;21:110-17.

46. Bessissow A, Khan J, Devereaux PJ, Alvarez-Garcia J, Alonso-Coello P. Postoperative atrial fibrillation in non-cardiac and cardiac surgery: An overview. *J Thromb Haemost.* 2015;13 Suppl 1:S304-12.

Chapter 10: Heart Valve Replacement and Repair Surgery Section

1. Clavel MA, Iung B and Pibarot P. A nationwide contemporary epidemiological portrait of valvular heart diseases. *Heart.* 2017;103:1660-1662.

2. Nkomo VT, Gardin JM, Skelton TN, Gottdiener JS, Scott CG, Enriquez-Sarano M. Burden of valvular heart diseases: A population-based study. *Lancet.* 2006;368:1005-11.

3. Go AS, Mozaffarian D, Roger VL, et al. Heart disease and stroke statistics—2013 update: A report from the American Heart Association. *Circulation.* 2013;127:e6-e245.

4. Kodali SK, Williams MR, Smith CR, et al. Two-year outcomes after transcatheter or surgical aortic-valve replacement. *N Engl J Med.* 2012;366:1686-95.

5. Smith CR, Leon MB, Mack MJ, et al. Transcatheter versus surgical aortic-valve replacement in high-risk patients. *N Engl J Med.* 2011;364:2187-98.

6. Ak A, Porokhovnikov I, Kuethe F, Schulze PC, Noutsias M, Schlattmann P. Transcatheter vs. surgical aortic valve replacement and medical treatment: Systematic review and meta-analysis of randomized and non-randomized trials. *Herz.* 2018;43:325-337.

7. Feldman T, Foster E, Glower DD, et al. Percutaneous repair or surgery for mitral regurgitation. *N Engl J Med.* 2011;364:1395-406.

8. D'Ascenzo F, Moretti C, Marra WG, et al. Meta-analysis of the usefulness of Mitraclip in patients with functional mitral regurgitation. *Am J Cardiol.* 2015;116:325-31.

9. Thomas RJ, King M, Lui K, Oldridge N, Pina IL, Spertus J. AACVPR/ACCF/AHA 2010 update: Performance measures on cardiac rehabilitation for referral to cardiac rehabilitation/secondary prevention services endorsed by the American College of Chest Physicians, the American College of Sports Medicine, the American Physical Therapy Association, the Canadian Association of Cardiac Rehabilitation,

the Clinical Exercise Physiology Association, the European Association for Cardiovascular Prevention and Rehabilitation, the Inter-American Heart Foundation, the National Association of Clinical Nurse Specialists, the Preventive Cardiovascular Nurses Association, and the Society of Thoracic Surgeons. *J Am Coll Cardiol.* 2010;56:1159-67.

10. Balady GJ, Williams MA, Ades PA, et al. Core components of cardiac rehabilitation/secondary prevention programs: 2007 update: A scientific statement from the American Heart Association Exercise, Cardiac Rehabilitation, and Prevention Committee, the Council on Clinical Cardiology; the Councils on Cardiovascular Nursing, Epidemiology and Prevention, and Nutrition, Physical Activity, and Metabolism; and the American Association of Cardiovascular and Pulmonary Rehabilitation. *Circulation.* 2007;115:2675-82.

11. Piepoli MF, Corra U, Benzer W, et al. Secondary prevention through cardiac rehabilitation: From knowledge to implementation. A position paper from the Cardiac Rehabilitation Section of the European Association of Cardiovascular Prevention and Rehabilitation. *Eur J Cardiovasc Prev Rehabil.* 2010;17:1-17.

12. Dodson JA, Wang Y, Desai MM, et al. Outcomes for mitral valve surgery among Medicare fee-for-service beneficiaries, 1999 to 2008. *Circ Cardiovasc Qual Outcomes.* 2012;5:298-307.

13. Baumgartner H, Falk V, Bax JJ, et al. 2017 ESC/EACTSgGuidelines for the management of valvular heart disease. *Eur Heart J.* 2017;38:2739-2791.

14. Nishimura RA, Otto CM, Bonow RO, et al. 2017 AHA/ACC focused update of the 2014 AHA/ACC guideline for the management of patients with valvular heart disease: A report of the American College of Cardiology/American Heart Association Task Force on Clinical Practice Guidelines. *J Am Coll Cardiol.* 2017;70:252-289.

15. Sordelli C, Severino S, Ascione L, Coppolino P, Caso P. Echocardiographic assessment of heart valve prostheses. *J Cardiovasc Echogr.* 2014;24:103-113.

16. Pibarot P, Dumesnil JG. Prosthetic heart valves: Selection of the optimal prosthesis and long-term management. *Circulation.* 2009;119:1034-48.

17. Smolka G, and Wojakowski, W. Paravalvular leak – Important complication after implantation of prosthetic valve. *e-journal of Cardiology Practice.* 2010;9. https://www.escardio.org/Journals/E-Journal-of-Cardiology-Practice

18. You SC, Shim CY, Hong GR, et al. Incidence, predictors, and clinical outcomes of postoperative cardiac tamponade in patients undergoing heart valve surgery. *PloS One.* 2016;11:e0165754.

19. Sibilitz KL, Berg SK, Thygesen LC, et al. High readmission rate after heart valve surgery: A nationwide cohort study. *Int J Cardiol.* 2015;189:96-104.

20. Danielsen SO, Moons P, Sandven I, et al. Thirty-day readmissions in surgical and transcatheter aortic valve replacement: A systematic review and meta-analysis. *Int J Cardiol.* 2018;268:85-91.

21. Borregaard et al. Sociodemographic-, clinical- and patient-reported outcomes and readmission after heart valve surgery. *J Heart Valve Disease, accepted for publication.* 2018; 27(1):78-86.

22. Borregaard B, Ekholm O, Riber L, Sorensen J, et al. Patient-reported outcomes after aortic and mitral valve surgery - Results from the DenHeart Study. *Eur J Cardiovasc Nurs.* 2018;17:246-254.

23. Lie I, Danielsen SO, Tonnessen T, et al. Determining the impact of 24/7 phone support on hospital readmissions after aortic valve replacement surgery (the AVRre study): Study protocol for a randomised controlled trial. *Trials.* 2017;18:246.

24. Borregaard B, Riber L, Ekholm O, et al. Effect of early, individualised and intensified follow-up after open heart valve surgery on unplanned cardiac hospital readmissions and all-cause mortality.. In J Cardiol. 2019;289:30-36.

25. Lowres N, Mulcahy G, Jin K, Gallagher R, Neubeck L, Freedman B. Incidence of postoperative atrial fibrillation recurrence in patients discharged in sinus rhythm after cardiac surgery: A systematic review and meta-analysis. *Interact Cardiovasc Thorac Surg.* 2018;26(3):504-511.

26. Hansen TB, Zwisler AD, Berg SK, et al. Exercise-based cardiac rehabilitation after heart valve surgery: Cost analysis of healthcare use and sick leave. *Open Heart.* 2015;2:e000288.

27. Lund K, Sibilitz KL, Berg SK, Thygesen LC, Taylor RS, Zwisler AD. Physical activity increases survival after heart valve surgery. *Heart.* 2016;102:1388-95.

28. Ribeiro GS, Melo RD, Deresz LF, Dal Lago P, Pontes MR, Karsten M. Cardiac rehabilitation programme after transcatheter aortic valve implantation versus surgical aortic valve replacement: Systematic review and meta-analysis. *Eur J Prev Cardiol.* 2017;24:688-697.

29. Sibilitz KL, Berg SK, Rasmussen TB, et al. Cardiac rehabilitation increases physical capacity but not mental health after heart valve surgery: A randomised clinical trial. *Heart*. 2016;102:1995-2003.

30. Sibilitz KL, Berg SK, Tang LH, et al. Exercise-based cardiac rehabilitation for adults after heart valve surgery. *Cochrane Database Syst Rev*. 2016;3:Cd010876.

31. Anderson L, Taylor RS. Cardiac rehabilitation for people with heart disease: An overview of Cochrane systematic reviews. *Cochrane Database Syst Rev*. 2014;12:Cd011273.

32. Williams MA, Haskell WL, Ades PA, et al. Resistance exercise in individuals with and without cardiovascular disease: 2007 update: A scientific statement from the American Heart Association Council on Clinical Cardiology and Council on Nutrition, Physical Activity, and Metabolism. *Circulation*. 2007;116:572-84.

33. Hamm LF, Sanderson BK, Ades PA, et al. Core competencies for cardiac rehabilitation/secondary prevention professionals: 2010 update: Position statement of the American Association of Cardiovascular and Pulmonary Rehabilitation. *J Cardiopulm Rehabil Prev*. 2011;31:2-10.

34. Piepoli MF, Corra U, Adamopoulos S, et al. Secondary prevention in the clinical management of patients with cardiovascular diseases. Core components, standards and outcome measures for referral and delivery: A policy statement from the cardiac rehabilitation section of the European Association for Cardiovascular Prevention & Rehabilitation. Endorsed by the Committee for Practice Guidelines of the European Society of Cardiology. *Eur J Prev Cardiol*. 2014;21:664-81.

35. Cahalin LP, Lapier TK, Shaw DK. Sternal precautions: Is it time for change? Precautions versus restrictions - A review of literature and recommendations for revision. *Cardiopulm Phys Ther J*. 2011;22:5-15.

36. Katijjahbe MA, Granger CL, Denehy L. Standard restrictive sternal precautions and modified sternal precautions had similar effects in people after cardiac surgery via median sternotomy ('SMART' Trial): A randomised trial. *J Physiother*. 2018;64:97-106.

37. Berg SK, Zwisler AD, Pedersen BD, Haase K, Sibilitz KL. Patient experiences of recovery after heart valve replacement: Suffering weakness, struggling to resume normality. *BMC Nurs*. 2013;12:23.

38. Lapum J, Angus JE, Peter E, Watt-Watson J. Patients' discharge experiences: Returning home after open-heart surgery. *Heart Lung*. 2011;40:226-35.

Chapter 10: Dysrhythmias Section

1. Galante A, Pietroiusti A, Cavazzini C, et al. Incidence and risk factors associated with cardiac arrhythmias during rehabilitation after coronary artery bypass surgery. *Arch Phys Med Rehabil*. 2000;81(7):947-952. doi:10.1053/apmr.2000.5587

2. O'Connor CM, Whellan DJ, Lee KL, et al. Efficacy and safety of exercise training in patients with chronic heart failure. *JAMA*. 2009;301(14):1439-1450. doi:10.1001/jama.2009.454

3. Beatty AL, Truong M, Schopfer DW, Shen H, Bachmann JM, Whooley MA. Geographic variation in cardiac rehabilitation participation in Medicare and Veterans Affairs populations: Opportunity for improvement. *Circulation*. 2018;137(18):1899-1908. doi:10.1161/CIRCULATIONAHA.117.029471

4. Van Camp SP. Cardiovascular complications of outpatient cardiac rehabilitation programs. *JAMA*. 1986;256(9):1160. doi:10.1001/jama.1986.03380090100025

5. Digenio AG, Sim JG, Dowdeswell RJ, Morris R. Exercise-related cardiac arrest in cardiac rehabilitation. The Johannesburg experience. *S Afr Med J*. 1991;79(4):188-191.

6. Vongvanich P, Paul-Labrador MJ, Merz CN. Safety of medically supervised exercise in a cardiac rehabilitation center. *Am J Cardiol*. 1996;77(15):1383-1385.

7. Franklin BA, Bonzheim K, Gordon S, Timmis GC. Safety of medically supervised outpatient cardiac rehabilitation exercise therapy. *Chest*. 1998;114(3):902-906. doi:10.1378/chest.114.3.902

8. January CT, Wann LS, Alpert JS, et al. 2014 AHA/ACC/HRS guideline for the management of patients with atrial fibrillation: A report of the American College of Cardiology/American Heart Association task force on practice guidelines and the Heart Rhythm Society. *Circulation*. 2014;130(23):e199-e267. doi:10.1161/CIR.0000000000000041

9. Mozaffarian D, Furberg CD, Psaty BM, Siscovick D. Physical activity and incidence of atrial fibrillation in older adults: The Cardiovascular Health Study. *Circulation*. 2008;118(8):800-807. doi:10.1161/CIRCULATIONAHA.108.785626

10. Abdulla J, Nielsen JR. Is the risk of atrial fibrillation higher in athletes than in the general population? A systematic review and meta-analysis. *Europace*. 2009;11(9):1156-1159. doi:10.1093/europace/eup197

11. Mont L, Elosua R, Brugada J. Endurance sport practice as a risk factor for atrial fibrillation and atrial flutter. *Europace*. 2009;11(1):11-17. doi:10.1093/europace/eun289

12. Plisiene J, Blumberg A, Haager G, et al. Moderate physical exercise: A simplified approach for ventricular rate control in older patients with atrial fibrillation. *Clin Res Cardiol*. 2008;97(11):820-826. doi:10.1007/s00392-008-0692-3.

13. Mertens DJ. Exercise training for patients with chronic atrial fibrillation. *J Cardiopulm Rehabil*. 2006;26(1):30-31. http://eutils.ncbi.nlm.nih.gov/entrez/eutils/elink.fcgi?dbfrom=pubmed&id=16617224&retmode=ref&cmd=prlinks. Accessed October 23, 2019.

14. Malmo V, Nes BM, Amundsen BH, et al. Aerobic interval training reduces the burden of atrial fibrillation in the short term: A randomized trial. *Circulation*. 2016;133(5):466-473. doi:10.1161/CIRCULATIONAHA.115.018220

15. Risom SS, Zwisler A-D, Johansen PP, et al. Exercise-based cardiac rehabilitation for adults with atrial fibrillation. *Cochrane Database Syst Rev*. 2017;2(1):CD011197. doi:10.1002/14651858.CD011197.pub2

16. Dell'Orto S, Valli P, Greco EM. Sensors for rate responsive pacing. *Indian Pacing Electrophysiol J*. 2004;4(3):137-145.

17. Palmisano P, Aspromonte V, Ammendola E, et al. Effect of fixed-rate vs. rate-RESPONSIve pacing on exercise capacity in patients with permanent, refractory atrial fibrillation and left ventricular dysfunction treated with atrioventricular junction aBLation and bivEntricular pacing (RESPONSIBLE): A prospective, multicentre, randomized, single-blind study. *Europace*. 2017;19(3):414-420. doi:10.1093/europace/euw035

18. Caloian B, Sitar-Taut AV, Gusetu GN, Pop D, Zdrenghea DT. The influence of cardiac pacemaker programming modes on exercise capacity. *In Vivo*. 2018;32(2):419-424. doi:10.21873/invivo.11256

19. Gierula J, Paton MF, Lowry JE, et al. Rate-response programming tailored to the force-frequency relationship improves exercise tolerance in chronic heart failure. *JACC Heart Fail*. 2018;6(2):105-113. doi:10.1016/j.jchf.2017.09.018

20. Riebe D, Ehrman JK, Liguori G, Maier M. *ACSM's Guidelines for Exercise Testing and Prescription*. 10th ed. Philadelphia: Lippincott Williams & Wilkins; 2018.

21. Isaksen K, Morken IM, Munk PS, Larsen AI. Exercise training and cardiac rehabilitation in patients with implantable cardioverter defibrillators: A review of current literature focusing on safety, effects of exercise training, and the psychological impact of programme participation. *Eur J Prev Cardiol*. 2012;19(4):804-812.

22. Piccini JP, Hellkamp AS, Whellan DJ, et al. Exercise training and implantable cardioverter-defibrillator shocks in patients with heart failure: Results from HF-ACTION (Heart Failure and A Controlled Trial Investigating Outcomes of Exercise TraiNing). *JACC Heart Fail*. 2013;1(2):142-148. doi:10.1016/j.jchf.2013.01.005

23. Dougherty CM, Glenny RW, Burr RL, Flo GL, Kudenchuk PJ. Prospective randomized trial of moderately strenuous aerobic exercise after an implantable cardioverter defibrillator. *Circulation*. 2015;131(21):1835-1842. doi:10.1161/CIRCULATIONAHA.114.014444

24. Alswyan AH, Liberato ACS, Dougherty CM. A systematic review of exercise training in patients with cardiac implantable devices. *J Cardiopulm Rehabil Prev*. 2018;38(2):70-84. doi:10.1097/HCR.0000000000000289

25. Zipes DP, Link MS, Ackerman MJ, et al. Eligibility and disqualification recommendations for competitive athletes with cardiovascular abnormalities: Task Force 9: Arrhythmias and conduction defects: A scientific statement from the American Heart Association and American College of Cardiology. *Circulation*. 2015;132(22):e315-e325. doi:10.1161/CIR.0000000000000245

26. Philippon F. Cardiac resynchronization therapy: Device-based medicine for heart failure. *J Card Surg*. 2004;19(3):270-274. doi:10.1111/j.0886-0440.2004.04081.x

27. Abraham WT, Fisher WG, Smith AL, et al. Cardiac resynchronization in chronic heart failure. *N Engl J Med*. 2002;346(24):1845-1853. doi:10.1056/NEJMoa013168

28. Ennezat P-V, Gal B, Kouakam C, et al. Cardiac resynchronisation therapy reduces functional mitral regurgitation during dynamic exercise in patients with chronic heart failure: An acute echocardiographic study. *Heart*. 2006;92(8):1091-1095. doi:10.1136/hrt.2005.071654

29. Seifert M, Schlegl M, Hoersch W, et al. Functional capacity and changes in the neurohormonal and cytokine status after long-term CRT in heart failure patients. *Int J Cardiol*. 2007;121(1):68-73. doi:10.1016/j.ijcard.2007.04.069.

30. Sitges M, Vidal B, Delgado V, et al. Long-term effect of cardiac resynchronization therapy on functional mitral valve regurgitation. *Am J Cardiol*. 2009;104(3):383-388. doi:10.1016/j.amjcard.2009.03.060

31. Seidl K, Rameken M, Vater M, Senges J. Cardiac resynchronization therapy in patients with chronic heart failure: Pathophysiology and current experience. *Am J Cardiovasc Drugs*. 2002;2(4):219-226.

32. De Marco T, Wolfel E, Feldman AM, et al. Impact of cardiac resynchronization therapy on exercise performance, functional capacity, and quality of life in systolic heart failure with QRS prolongation: COMPANION trial sub-study. *J Card Fail*. 2008;14(1):9-18. doi:10.1016/j.cardfail.2007.08.003

33. Hoth KF, Nash J, Poppas A, Ellison KE, Paul RH, Cohen RA. Effects of cardiac resynchronization therapy on health-related quality of life in older adults with heart failure. *Clin Interv Aging*. 2008;3(3):553-560.

34. Chen S, Yin Y, Krucoff MW. Effect of cardiac resynchronization therapy and implantable cardioverter defibrillator on quality of life in patients with heart failure: A meta-analysis. *Europace*. 2012;14(11):1602-1607. doi:10.1093/europace/eus168

35. Chen S, Ling Z, Kiuchi MG, Yin Y, Krucoff MW. The efficacy and safety of cardiac resynchronization therapy combined with implantable cardioverter defibrillator for heart failure: A meta-analysis of 5674 patients. *Europace*. 2013;15(7):992-1001. doi:10.1093/europace/eus419

36. Cleland JG, Abraham WT, Linde C, et al. An individual patient meta-analysis of five randomized trials assessing the effects of cardiac resynchronization therapy on morbidity and mortality in patients with symptomatic heart failure. *Eur Heart J*. 2013;34(46):3547-3556. doi:10.1093/eurheartj/eht290

37. Brugada J, Delnoy PP, Brachmann J, et al. Contractility sensor-guided optimization of cardiac resynchronization therapy: Results from the RESPOND-CRT trial. *Eur Heart J*. 2017;38(10):730-738. doi:10.1093/eurheartj/ehw526

38. Whinnett ZI, Sohaib SMA, Mason M, et al. Multicenter randomized controlled crossover trial comparing hemodynamic optimization against echocardiographic optimization of AV and VV delay of cardiac resynchronization therapy: The BRAVO trial. *JACC Cardiovasc Imaging*. May 2018. doi:10.1016/j.jcmg.2018.02.014

39. Conraads VMA, Vanderheyden M, Paelinck B, et al. The effect of endurance training on exercise capacity following cardiac resynchronization therapy in chronic heart failure patients: A pilot trial. *Eur J Cardiovasc Prev Rehabil*. 2007;14(1):99-106. doi:10.1097/HJR.0b013e32801164b3

40. Patwala AY, Woods PR, Sharp L, Goldspink DF, Tan LB, Wright DJ. Maximizing patient benefit from cardiac resynchronization therapy with the addition of structured exercise training: A randomized controlled study. *J Am Coll Cardiol*. 2009;53(25):2332-2339. doi:10.1016/j.jacc.2009.02.063

41. Kelly TM. Exercise testing and training of patients with malignant ventricular arrhythmias. *Med Sci Sports Exerc*. 1996;28(1):53-61.

42. Pashkow FJ, Schweikert RA, Wilkoff BL. Exercise testing and training in patients with malignant arrhythmias. *Exerc Sport Sci Rev*. 1997;25:235-269.

43. Mann D, Zipes D, Libby P, Bonow R. Atrial fibrillation: Clinical features, mechanisms and management. In: *Braunwald's Heart Disease: A Textbook of Cardiovascular Medicine*. 10th ed. New York: Elsevier; 2015: 800-801.

44. January CT, Wann LS, Alpert JS, et al. 2014 AHA/ACC/HRS guideline for the management of patients with atrial fibrillation: A report of the American College of Cardiology/American Heart Association Task Force on Practice Guidelines and the Heart Rhythm Society. *Circulation*. 2014; 130:e199.

45. Keteyian SJ, Ehrman JK, Fuller B, Pack QR. Exercise testing and exercise rehabilitation for patients with atrial fibrillation. *J Cardiopulm Rehabil Prev*. 2019 Mar;39(2):65-72. doi:10.1097/HCR.0000000000000423

46. Myrstad M, Malmo V, Ulimoen SR, Tveit A, Loennechen JP. Exercise in individuals with atrial fibrillation. *Clin Res Cardiol*. 2019 Apr;108(4):347-354. doi: 10.1007/s00392-018-1361-9

47. Beaser AD, Cifu AS. Management of patients with atrial fibrillation. *JAMA*. 2019;321(11):1100-1101. doi:10.1001/jama.2019.1264

48. Ades PA, Savage PD, Toth MJ, et al. High-calorie-expenditure exercise: A new approach to cardiac rehabilitation for overweight coronary patients. *Circulation*. 2009 May 26;119(20):2671-8. doi:10.1161/CIRCULATIONAHA.108.834184

49. Taylor RS, Dalal H, Jolly K, et al. Home-based versus centre-based cardiac rehabilitation. The Cochrane database of systematic reviews. 2015;(8):CD007130. doi:10.1002/14651858.CD007130.pub3.

50. January CT, Wann LS, Calkins H, et al. 2019 AHA/ACC/HRS Focused Update of the 2014 AHA/ACC/HRS Guideline for the Management of Patients With Atrial Fibrillation: A Report of the American College of Cardiology/American Heart Association Task Force on Clinical Practice Guidelines and the Heart Rhythm Society in Collaboration With the Society of Thoracic Surgeons. Circulation. 2019 Jul 9;140(2):e125-e151. doi: 10.1161/CIR.0000000000000665.

Chapter 10: Heart Failure and Left Ventricular Assist Devices Section

1. Benjamin EJ, Virani SS, Callaway CW, et al. Heart disease and stroke statistics-2018 update: A report from the American Heart Association. *Circulation*. 2018;137:e67-e492.

2. Yancy CW, Jessup M, Bozkurt B, et al. 2017 ACC/AHA/HFSA focused update of the 2013 ACCF/AHA guideline for the management of heart failure: A report of the American College of Cardiology/American Heart Association Task Force on Clinical Practice Guidelines and the Heart Failure Society of America. *Circulation*. 2017;136:e137-e161.

3. Jessup M, Abraham WT, Casey DE, et al. Focused update: ACCF/AHA guidelines for the diagnosis and management of heart failure in adults. *Circulation*. 2009;119:1977-2016.

4. Rector TS, Kubo SH, Cohn JN. Patients' self-assessment of their congestive heart failure. Part 2: Content, reliability and validity of a new measure, The Minnesota Living with Heart Failure Questionnaire. *Heart Fail*. 1987;3:198-209.

5. Green CP, Porter CB, Bresnahan DR, Spertus JA. Development and evaluation of the Kansas City Cardiomyopathy Questionnaire: A new health status measure for heart failure. *J Am Coll Cardiol*. 2000;35:1245-1255.

6. Ware JE, Sherbourne CD. The MOS 36-item short-form health survey (SF-36): Conceptual framework and item selection. *Med Care*. 1992;30:42-49.

7. Ades PA, Keteyian SJ, Balady GJ, et al. Cardiac rehabilitation exercise and self-care for chronic heart failure. *JACC Heart Fail*. 2013;1:540-7.

8. Taylor RS, Sagar VA, Davies EJ, et al. Exercise-based rehabilitation for heart failure. *Cochrane Database Syst Rev*. 2014;(4):CD003331.

9. Reeves GR, Whellan DJ, O'Connor CM, et al. A novel rehabilitation intervention for older patients with acute decompensated heart failure: The REHAB-HF Pilot Study. *JACC Heart Fail*. 2017;5(5):359-366. doi: 10.1016/j.jchf.2016.12.019

10. Thomas RJ, Beatty AL, Beckie TM, et al. Home-based cardiac rehabilitation: An AACVPR/ACCF/AHA scientific statement. *J Am Coll Cardiol*. 2018;71:1814-1837.

11. Keteyian SJ, Marks CRC, Brawner CA, et al. Responses to arm exercise in patients with compensated heart failure. *J Cardiopulm Rehabil*. 1996;16:366-371.

12. Kitzman DW, Little WC, Brubaker PH, et al. Pathophysiological characterization of isolated diastolic heart failure in comparison to systolic heart failure. *JAMA*. 2002;288:2144-2150.

13. Wilson JR, Martin JL, Schwartz D, et al. Exercise intolerance in patients with chronic heart failure: Role of impaired nutritive flow to skeletal muscle. *Circulation*. 1984;69:1079-1087.

14. Mancini D, Walter G, Reicheck N, et al. Contribution of skeletal muscle atrophy to exercise intolerance and altered muscle metabolism in heart failure. *Circulation*. 1992;85:1364-1373.

15. Adams V, Jiang H, Yu J, et al. Apoptosis in skeletal muscle myocytes of patients with chronic heart failure is associated with exercise intolerance. *J Am Coll Cardiol*. 1999;33:959-965.

16. Piepoli M, Kaczmerik A, Francis D, et al. Reduced peripheral skeletal muscle mass and abnormal reflex physiology in chronic heart failure. *Circulation*. 2006;114:126-134.

17. Olson TP, Snyder EM, Johnson BD. Exercise-disordered breathing in chronic heart failure. *Exerc Sport Sci Rev*. 2006;34:194-201.

18. Haykowsky MJ, Tomczak CR, Scott JM, Paterson DI, Kitzman DW. Determinants of exercise intolerance in patients with heart failure and reduced or preserved ejection fraction. *J Appl Physiol*. 2015;119:739-44.

19. Haykowsky MJ, Kitzman DW. Exercise physiology in heart failure and preserved ejection fraction. *Heart Fail Clin*. 2014;10:445–452.

20. Duscha BD, Schulz PC, Robbins JL, Forman DE. Implications of chronic heart failure on peripheral vasculature and skeletal muscle before and after exercise training. *Heart Fail Rev.* 2008;13:21-27.

21. Keteyian SJ, Brawner CA, Pina IL. Role and benefits of exercise in the management of patients with heart failure. *Heart Fail Rev.* 2010;15:523-530.

22. Keteyian SJ. Exercise training in congestive heart failure: Risks and benefits. *Prog Cardiovasc Dis.* 2011;53:419-428.

23. O'Connor CM, Whellan DJ, Lee KL, et al. Efficacy and safety of exercise training in patients with chronic heart failure. *JAMA.* 2009;301:1439-1450.

24. Wisloff U, Stoylen A, Loennechen JP, et al. Superior cardiovascular effect of aerobic interval training versus moderate continuous training in heart failure patients: A randomized study. *Circulation.* 2007;115:3086-3094.

25. Ellingsen Ø, Halle M, Conraads V, et al. High-intensity interval training in patients with heart failure with reduced ejection fraction. *Circulation.* 2017;135:839-849.

26. Tabet JY, Meurin P, Beauvais F, et al. Absence of exercise capacity improvement after exercise training program a strong prognostic factor in patients with chronic heart failure. *Circ Heart Fail.* 2008;1:220-226.

27. Taylor RS, Walker S, Smart NA, et al. Impact of exercise-based rehabilitation in patients with heart failure (ExTraMATCH II) on mortality and hospitalization: An individual-patient data meta-analysis of randomized trials. *Eur J Heart Failure.* 2018;20:1735-1743

28. Keteyian SJ, Leifer ES, Houston-Miller N, et al. Relation between volume of exercise and clinical outcomes in patients with heart failure. *J Am Coll Cardiol.* 2012;60:1899-905.

29. Flynn KE, Pina IL, Whellan DJ, et al. Effects of exercise training on health status in patients with chronic heart failure. *JAMA.* 2009;301:1451-1459.

30. Squires RW, Kaminsky LA, Porcari JP, Ruff JE, Savage PD, Williams MA. Progression of exercise training in early outpatient cardiac rehabilitation: An official statement from the American Association of Cardiovascular and Pulmonary Rehabilitation. *J Cardiopulm Rehabil Prev.* 2018;38:139-146.

31. Riebe D, Ehrman JK, Liguori G, Maier M. *ACSM's Guidelines for Exercise Testing and Prescription.* 10th ed. Philadelphia: Lippincott Williams & Wilkins; 2018.

32. Keteyian SJ, Issac D, Thadani U, et al. Safety of symptom-limited cardiopulmonary exercise testing in patients with chronic heart failure due to left ventricular systolic dysfunction. *Am Heart J.* 2009;158:S72-S77.

33. Keteyian SJ, Ehrman JK, Fuller B, Pack, QR. Exercise testing and exercise rehabilitation in patients with atrial fibrillation. *J Cardiopulm Rehabil Prev.* 2019; 39:65-72.

34. McKelvie RS, McCarthy N, Tomlinson C, et al. Comparision of hemodynamic responses to cycling and resistance exercise in congestive heart failure secondary to ischemic cardiomyopathy. *Am J Cardiol.* 1995;76:977-979.

35. Feiereisen P, Delagardelle C, Vaillant M, et al. Is strength training the more efficient training modality in chronic heart failure? *Med Sci Sports Exerc.* 2007;39:1910-1917.

36. Pu C, Johnson MT, Forman DE, et al. Randomized trial of progressive resistance training to counteract the myopathy of chronic heart failure. *J Appl Physiol.* 2001;90:2341-2350.

37. Palevo G, Keteyian SJ, Kang M, et al. Resistance exercise training improves heart function and physical fitness in stable patients with heart failure. *J Cardiopulm Rehabil.* 2009;29:294-298.

38. Braith RW, Beck DT. Resistance exercise: Training adaptations and developing a safe exercise prescription. *Heart Fail Rev.* 2008;13:69-79.

39. Delagardelle C, Feiereisen P, Autier P, et al. Strength/endurance training versus endurance training in congestive heart failure. *Med Sci Sports Exerc.* 2002;34:1868-1872.

40. Williams MA, Haskell WL, Ades PA, et al. Resistance exercise in individuals with and without cardiovascular disease. *Circulation.* 2007;116:572-584.

41. Pack QR and Riley H. General interview and examination skills. In: Ehrman JE, Keteyian SJ, Gordon PM, Visich PS, eds. *Clinical Exercise Physiology.* 4th ed. Champaign, IL: Human Kinetics; 2018:45-59.

42. Rose EA, Gelijns AC, Moskowitz AJ, et al. Long-term use of a left ventricular assist device for end-stage heart failure. *N Engl J Med.* 2001;345:1435-1443.

43. Kirklin JK, Pagani FD, Kormos RL, et al. Eighth annual INTERMACS report: Special focus on framing the impact of adverse events. *J Heart Lung Transplant*. 2017;36:1080-1086.

44. Griffith BP, Kormos RL, Borovetz HS, et al. HeartMate II left ventricular assist system: From concept to first clinical use. *Ann Thorac Surg*. 2001;71:S116-120; discussion S114-116.

45. Lietz K, Long JW, Kfoury AG, et al. Outcomes of left ventricular assist device implantation as destination therapy in the post-REMATCH era - Implications for patient selection. *Circulation*. 2007;116:497-505.

46. Alsara O, Perez-Terzic C, Squires RW, et al. Is exercise training safe and beneficial in patients receiving left ventricular assist device therapy? *J Cardiopulm Rehabil Prev*. 2014;34:233-240.

47. Grosman-Rimon L, Lalonde SD, Sieh N, et al. Exercise rehabilitation in ventricular assist device recipients: A meta-analysis of effects on physiological and clinical outcomes. *Heart Fail Rev*. 2018.

48. Mahfood Haddad T, Saurav A, Smer A, et al. Cardiac rehabilitation in patients with left ventricular assist device: A systematic review and meta-analysis. *J Cardiopulm Rehabil Prev*. 2017;37:390-396.

49. Kerrigan DJ, Williams CT, Ehrman JK, et al. Cardiac rehabilitation improves functional capacity and patient-reported health status in patients with continuous-flow left ventricular assist devices: The Rehab-VAD randomized controlled trial. *JACC Heart Fail*. 2014;2:653-659.

50. Slaughter MS, Rogers JG, Milano CA, et al. Advanced heart failure treated with continuous-flow left ventricular assist device. *N Engl J Med*. 2009;361:2241-2251.

51. Brassard P, Jensen AS, Nordsborg N, et al. Central and peripheral blood flow during exercise with a continuous-flow left ventricular assist device: Constant versus increasing pump speed: A pilot study. *Circ Heart Fail*. 2011;4:554-560.

52. Jung MH, Hansen PB, Sander K, et al. Effect of increasing pump speed during exercise on peak oxygen uptake in heart failure patients supported with a continuous-flow left ventricular assist device. A double-blind randomized study. *Eur J Heart Fail*. 2014;16:403-408.

53. Jakovljevic DG, George RS, Nunan D, et al. The impact of acute reduction of continuous-flow left ventricular assist device support on cardiac and exercise performance. *Heart*. 2010;96:1390-1395.

54. Dunlay SM, Allison TG, Pereira NL. Changes in cardiopulmonary exercise testing parameters following continuous flow left ventricular assist device implantation and heart transplantation. *J Cardiac Fail*. 2014;20:548-554.

55. Allen JG, Weiss ES, Schaffer JM, et al. Quality of life and functional status in patients surviving 12 months after left ventricular assist device implantation. *J Heart Lung Transplant*. 2010;29:278-285.

56. Pagani FD, Miller LW, Russell SD, et al. Extended mechanical circulatory support with a continuous-flow rotary left ventricular assist device. *J Am Coll Cardiol*. 2009;54:312-321.

57. Miller LW, Pagani FD, Russell SD, et al. Use of a continuous-flow device in patients awaiting heart transplantation. *N Engl J Med*. 2007;357:885-896.

58. Laoutaris ID, Vasiliadis IK, Dritsas A, et al. High plasma adiponectin is related to low functional capacity in patients with chronic heart failure. *Int J Cardiol*. 2010;144:230-231.

59. Hayes K, Leet AS, Bradley SJ, Holland AE. Effects of exercise training on exercise capacity and quality of life in patients with a left ventricular assist device: A preliminary randomized controlled trial. *J Heart Lung Transplant*. 2012;31:729-734.

60. Kerrigan DJ, Williams CT, Ehrman JK, et al. Muscular strength and cardiorespiratory fitness are associated with health status in patients with recently implanted continuous-flow LVADs. *J Cardiopulm Rehabil Prev*. 2013;33:396-400.

61. Bachmann JM, Duncan MS, Shah AS, et al. Association of cardiac rehabilitation with decreased hospitalizations and mortality after ventricular assist device implantation. *JACC Heart Fail*. 2018;6:130-139.

62. Drazner MH. A new left ventricular assist device - Better, but still not ideal. *N Engl J Med*. 2018;378:1442-1443.

63. Marko C, Danzinger G, Kaferback M, et al. Safety and efficacy of cardiac rehabilitation for patients with continuous flow left ventricular assist devices. *Eur J Prev Cardiol*. 2015;22:1378-1384.

64. Kerrigan DJ, Williams CT, Brawner CA, et al. Heart rate and V O2 concordance in continuous-flow left ventricular assist devices. *Med Sci Sports Exerc*. 2016;48:363-367.

65. Robertson J, Long B, Koyfman A. The emergency management of ventricular assist devices. *Am J Emerg Med.* 2016;34:1294-1301.

66. DeVore AD, Patel PA, Patel CB. Medical Management of Patients With a Left Ventricular Assist Device for the Non-Left Ventricular Assist Device Specialist. *JACC Heart Fail.* 2017;5:621-631.

67. Taylor RS, Walker S, Smart NA, et al. Impact of exercise rehabilitation on exercise capacity and quality-of-life in heart failure: Individual participant meta-analysis. J Am Coll Cardiol. 2019;73(12):1430-1443.

Chapter 10: Heart Transplantation Section

1. Lund LH, Edwards LB, Kucheryavaya AY, et al. The registry of the International Society for Heart and Lung Transplantation: Thirty-second official adult heart transplant report—2015; focus theme: Early graft failure. *J Heart Lung Transplant.* 2015;34:1244-1254.

2. Lund LH, Khush KK, Cherikh WS, et al. The registry of the International Society for Heart and Lung Transplantation: Thirty-fourth adult heart transplant report—2017; focus theme: Allograft ischemic time. *J Heart Lung Transplant.* 2017;36:1037-1046.

3. Rossano JW, Cherikh WS, Chambers DC, et al. The registry of the International Society for Heart and Lung Transplantation: Twentieth pediatric heart transplant report—2017; focus theme: Allograft ischemic time. *J Heart Lung Transplant.* 2017;36:1060-1069.

4. Stehlik J, Stevenson LW, Edwards LB, et al. Organ allocation around the world: Insights from the ISHLT International Registry for Heart and Lung Transplantation. *J Heart Lung Transplant.* 2014;33:975-984.

5. Squires RW. Cardiac rehabilitation issues for heart transplantation patients. *J Cardiopulmonary Rehabil.* 1990;10:159-168.

6. Slaughter MS, Pagani FD, Rogers JG, et al. Clinical management of continuous-flow left ventricular assist devices in advanced heart failure. *J Heart Lung Transplant.* 2010; 29:S1-S39.

7. Kirklin JK, Naftel DC, Pagani FD, et al. Long-term mechanical circulatory support (destination therapy): On track to compete with heart transplantation? J *Thoracic Cardiovasc Surg.* 2012;144:584-603.

8. Kobashigawa J, Zuckermann A, Macdonald P, et al. Report from a consensus conference on primary graft dysfunction after cardiac transplantation. *J Heart Lung Transplant.* 2014;33:327-340.

9. Lindenfield J, Miller GG, Shakar SF et al. Drug therapy in heart transplant recipients: Part 1: Cardiac rejection and immunosuppressive drugs. *Circulation.* 2004;110:3734-3740.

10. Weis M, von Scheidt W. Cardiac allograft vasculopathy: A review. *Circulation.* 1997;96:2069-2077

11. Taylor DO, Edwards LB, Boucek MM, et al. The registry of the International Society for Heart and Lung Transplantation: Twenty-first official adult heart transplant report-2004. *J Heart Lung Transplant.* 2004;23:796-803.

12. Lund LH, Edwards LB, Kucherayavaya AY, et al. The registry of the International Society for Heart and Lung Transplantation: Thirty-first official adult heart transplant report—2014; Focus theme: Retransplantation. *J Heart Lung Transplant.* 2014;33:996-1008.

13. Stapleton DD, Mehra MR, Dumas D, et al. Lipid-lowering therapy and long-term survival in heart transplantation. *Am J Cardiol.* 1997; 80:802-804.

14. Wu AH, Ballantyne CM, Short BC, et al. Statin use and risks of death or fatal rejection in the heart transplant lipid registry. *Am J Cardiol.* 2005; 95:367-372.

15. Jenkins GH, Grieve LA, Yacoub MH, Singer DRJ. Effect of simvastatin on ejection fraction in cardiac transplant recipients. *Am J Cardiol.* 1996; 78:1453-1456.

16. Lindenfeld J, Page II RL, Zolty R, et al. Drug therapy in the heart transplant recipient part III: Common medical problems. *Circulation.* 2005;111:113-117.

17. Squires RW, Leung TC, Cyr NS, et al. Partial normalization of the heart rate response to exercise after cardiac transplantation: Frequency and relationship to exercise capacity. *Mayo Clin Proc.* 2002;77:1295-1300.

18. Wenke K, Meiser B, Thiery J, et al. Simvastatin reduces graft vessel disease and mortality after heart transplantation: A four-year randomized trial. *Circulation.* 1997;96:1398-1402.

19. Squires RW. Transplant. In: Pashkow FJ, Dafoe WA, eds. *Clinical Cardiac Rehabilitation: A Cardiologist's Guide.* 2nd ed. Baltimore: Williams & Wilkins; 1999:175-191.

20. Keteyian SJ, Brawner C. Cardiac transplant. In: American College of Sports Medicine. *ACSM's Exercise Management for Persons With Chronic Diseases and Disabilities.* Champaign, IL: Human Kinetics; 1997:54-58.

21. Kao AC, Van Trigt P, Shaeffer-McCall GS, et al. Central and peripheral limitations to upright exercise in untrained cardiac transplant recipients. *Circulation.* 1994;89:2605-2615.

22. Pope SE, Stinson EB, Daughters GT, et al. Exercise response of the denervated heart in long-term cardiac transplant recipients. *Am J Cardiol.* 1980; 46:213-218.

23. Stratton JR, Kemp GJ, Daly RC, et al. Effects of cardiac transplantation on bioenergetic abnormalities of skeletal muscle in congestive heart failure. *Circulation.* 1994;89:1624-1631.

24. Lampert E, Mettauer B, Hoppeler H, et al. Structure of skeletal muscle in heart transplant recipients. J Am Coll Cardiol 1996;28:980-984.

25. Brubaker PH, Brozena SC, Morley DL, et al. Exercise-induced ventilatory abnormalities in orthotopic heart transplant patients. *J Heart Lung Transplant.* 1997;16:1011-1017.

26. Squires RW, Hoffman CJ, James GA, et al. Arterial oxygen saturation during graded exercise testing after cardiac transplantation. *J Cardiopulmonary Rehabil.* 1998;18:348.

27. Ehrman JK, Keteyian SJ, Levine AB, et al. Exercise stress tests after cardiac transplantation. *Am J Cardiol.* 1993;71:1372-1373.

28. Mettauer B, Zhao QM, Epailly E, et al. VO(2) kinetics reveal a central limitation at the onset of subthreshold exercise in heart transplant recipients. *J Appl Physiol.* 2000;88:1228-1238.

29. Richard R, Verdier JC, Duvallet A, et al. Chronotropic competence in endurance trained heart transplant recipients: Heart rate is not a limiting factor for exercise capacity. *J Am Coll Cardiol.* 1999; 33:192-197.

30. Pokan R, Von Duvillard SP, Ludwig J, et al. Effect of high-volume and –intensity endurance training in heart transplant recipients. *Med Sci Sports Exerc.* 2004;36:2011-2016.

31. Haykowski MJ, Halle M, Baggish A. Upper limits of aerobic power and performance in heart transplant recipients: Legacy effect of prior endurance training. *Circulation.* 2018; 137:650-652.

32. Kaye DM, Esler M, Kingwell B, et al. Functional and neurochemical evidence for partial cardiac sympathetic reinnervation after cardiac transplantation in humans. *Circulation.* 1993;88:1110-1118.

33. Daida H, Squires RW, Allison TG, et al. Sequential assessment of exercise tolerance in heart transplantation compared with coronary artery bypass surgery after phase II cardiac rehabilitation. *Am J Cardiol.* 1996;77:696-700.

34. Scott CD, Dark JH, McComb JM. Evolution of the chronotropic response to exercise after cardiac transplantation. *Am J Cardiol.* 1995;76:1292-1296.

35. Marconi C, Marzorati M, Fiocchi R, et al. Age-related heart rate response to exercise in heart transplant recipients. Functional significance. *Pflugers Arch.* 2002;443:698-706.

36. Ville NS, Mercier B, Hayot M, et al. Effects of an enhanced heart rate reserve on aerobic performance in patients with a heart transplant. *Am J Phys Med Rehabil.* 2002; 81:584-589.

37. Nytroen K, Gullestad L. Effect of exercise in heart transplant recipients. *Am J Transplant.* 2013;13:527.

38. Keteyian SJ, Brawner C. Cardiac transplant. In: *American College of Sports Medicine. ACSM's Exercise Management for Persons with Chronic Diseases and Disabilities.* 2nd ed. Champaign, IL: Human Kinetics; 2003:70-75.

39. Kavanagh T. Physical training in heart transplant recipients. *J Cardiovasc Risk.* 1996;3:154-159.

40. Gibbons RJ, Balady GJ, Beasley JW, et al. ACC/AHA guidelines for exercise testing: A report of the American College of Cardiology/American Heart Association task force on practice guidelines (committee on exercise testing). *J Am Coll Cardiol.* 1997; 30:260-315.

41. Squires RW, Arthur PA, Gau GT, et al. Exercise after cardiac transplantation: A report of two cases. *J Cardiopulmonary Rehabil.* 1983; 3:570-574.

42. Didsbury M, McGee RG, Tong A, et al. Exercise training in solid organ transplant recipients: A systematic review and meta-analysis. *Transplantation.* 2013;95:679-687.

43. Kavanagh T, Yacoub MH, Mertens DJ, et al. Cardiorespiratory responses to exercise training after orthotopic cardiac transplantation. *Circulation.* 1988;77:162-171.

44. Kavanagh T, Yacoub MH, Mertens DJ, et al. Exercise rehabilitation after heterotopic cardiac transplantation. *J Cardiopulmonary Rehabil.* 1989;9:303-310.

45. Kobashigawa JA, Leaf DA, Lee N, et al. A controlled trial of exercise rehabilitation after heart transplantation. *N Engl J Med.* 1999;340:272-277.

46. Doll CH, Snoer M, Christensen S, et al. Effect of high-intensity training versus moderate training on peak oxygen uptake and chronotropic response in heart transplant recipients: A randomized crossover trial. *Am J Transplant 2014;* 14:2391-2399.

47. Squires RW. Exercise therapy for cardiac transplant recipients. *Prog Cardiovasc Dis.* 2011;53:429-436.

48. Horber FF, Scheidegger JR, Grunig BF, et al. Evidence that prednisone-induced myopathy is reversed by physical training. *J Clin Endocrinol Metab.* 1985;61:83-88.

49. Braith RW, Mills RM, Welsch MA, et al. Resistance exercise training restores bone mineral density in heart transplant recipients. *J Am Coll Cardiol.* 1996;28:1471-1477.

50. Rosenbaum AN, Kremers WK, Schirger JA, et al. Association between early cardiac rehabilitation and long-term survival in cardiac transplant recipients. *Mayo Clin Proc.* 2016;91:149-156.

51. Nytroen K, Rustad LA, Erikstad I, et al. Effect of high-intensity interval training on progression of cardiac allograft vasculopathy. *J Heart Lung Transplant.* 2013;32:1073-1080.

52. Bachman JM, Shah AS, Duncan MS, et al. Cardiac rehabilitation and readmissions after heart transplantation. *J Heart Lung Transplant.* 2018;37:467-476.

53. Mancini DM, Eisen H, Kussmaul W, et al. Value of peak exercise oxygen consumption for optimal timing of cardiac transplantation in ambulatory patients with heart failure. *Circulation.* 1991;83:778-786.

54. McGregor CGA. Cardiac transplantation: Surgical considerations and early postoperative management. *Mayo Clin Proc.* 1992;67:577-585.

55. Keteyian SJ, Brawner C. Cardiac transplant. In: American College of Sports Medicine. *ACSM's Exercise Management for Persons With Chronic Diseases and Disabilities.* Champaign, IL: Human Kinetics; 1997:54-58.

Chapter 10: Peripheral Artery Disease Section

1. Hiatt WR, Goldstone J, Smith SC, Jr., et al. Atherosclerotic peripheral vascular disease symposium ii: Nomenclature for vascular diseases. *Circulation.* 2008;118(25): 2826-2829.

2. Hirsch AT, Criqui MH, Treat-Jacobson D, et al. Peripheral arterial disease detection, awareness, and treatment in primary care. *JAMA.* 2001;286(11): 1317-1324.

3. Kim ES, Wattanakit K, Gornik HL. Using the ankle-brachial index to diagnose peripheral artery disease and assess cardiovascular risk. *Cleve Clin J Med.* 2012;79(9): 651-661.

4. Murabito JM, D'Agostino RB, Silbershatz H, et al. Intermittent claudication. A risk profile from the framingham heart study. *Circulation* 1997;96(1): 44-49.

5. Meijer WT, Grobbee DE, Hunink MG, et al. Determinants of peripheral arterial disease in the elderly: The rotterdam study. *Arch Intern Med.* 2000;160(19):2934-2938.

6. Selvin E, Erlinger TP. Prevalence of and risk factors for peripheral arterial disease in the United States: Results from the National Health and Nutrition Examination Survey, 1999-2000. *Circulation.* 2004;110(6): 738-743.

7. Criqui MH, Aboyans V. Epidemiology of peripheral artery disease. *Circ Res.* 2015;116(9):1509-1526.

8. McDermott MM, Guralnik JM, Tian L, et al. Baseline functional performance predicts the rate of mobility loss in persons with peripheral arterial disease. *J Am Coll Cardiol.* 2007;50(10): 974-982.

9. Regensteiner JG, Hiatt WR, Coll JR, et al. The impact of peripheral arterial disease on health-related quality of life in the peripheral arterial disease awareness, risk, and treatment: New resources for survival (partners) program. *Vasc Med.* 2008;13(1): 15-24.

10. Steg PG, Bhatt DL, Wilson PW, et al. One-year cardiovascular event rates in outpatients with atherothrombosis. *JAMA.* 2007;297(11):1197-1206.

11. Creager MA, Libby P. Peripheral artery diseases. In: Mann DL, Zipes DP, Libby P, Bonow RO and Braunwald E, eds. *Braunwald's Heart Disease: A Textbook of Cardiovascular Medicine.* 10th ed. Philadelphia, PA: Elsevier; 2015.

12. Norgren L, Hiatt WR, Dormandy JA, et al. Inter-society consensus for the management of peripheral arterial disease (tasc ii). *J Vasc Surg.* 2007;45 SupplS:S5-67.

13. Aboyans V, Criqui MH, Abraham P, et al. Measurement and interpretation of the ankle-brachial index: A scientific statement from the american heart association. *Circulation.* 2012;126(24): 2890-2909.

14. Weinberg I, Giri J, Calfon MA, et al. Anatomic correlates of supra-normal ankle brachial indices. *Catheter Cardiovasc Interv.* 2013; 81(6): 1025-1030.

15. Vincent DG, Salles-Cunha SX, Bernhard VM, et al. Noninvasive assessment of toe systolic pressures with special reference to diabetes mellitus. *J Cardiovasc Surg (Torino).* 1983;24(1): 22-28.

16. Covic A, Kanbay M, Voroneanu L, et al. Vascular calcification in chronic kidney disease. *Clin Sci (Lond).* 2010;119(3):111-121.

17. Aday AW, Kinlay S, Gerhard-Herman MD. Comparison of different exercise ankle pressure indices in the diagnosis of peripheral artery disease. *Vasc Med.* 2018;23(6):541-548.

18. Raines JK, Darling RC, Buth J, et al. Vascular laboratory criteria for the management of peripheral vascular disease of the lower extremities. *Surgery.* 1976;79(1): 21-29.

19. Eslahpazir BA, Allemang MT, Lakin RO, et al. Pulse volume recording does not enhance segmental pressure readings for peripheral arterial disease stratification. *Ann Vasc Surg.* 2014;28(1):18-27.

20. Yamada T, Ohta T, Ishibashi H, et al. Clinical reliability and utility of skin perfusion pressure measurement in ischemic limbs—comparison with other noninvasive diagnostic methods. *J Vasc Surg.* 2008;47(2):318-323.

21. Abraham P, Colas-Ribas C, Signolet I, et al. Transcutaneous exercise oximetry for patients with claudication—a retrospective review of approximately 5,000 consecutive tests over 15 years. *Circ J.* 2018; 82(4):1161-1167.

22. Gerhard-Herman MD, Gornik HL, Barrett C, et al. 2016 AHA/ACC guideline on the management of patients with lower extremity peripheral artery disease: A report of the American College of Cardiology/American Heart Association Task Force on Clinical Practice Guidelines. *Circulation.* 2017;135(12):e726-e779.

23. Hiatt W, Nawaz D, Regensteiner J, et al. The evaluation of exercise performance in patients with peripheral vascular disease. *J Cardiopulm Rehabil.* 1988;12:525-532.

24. Gardner AW, Skinner JS, Cantwell BW, et al. Progressive vs single-stage treadmill tests for evaluation of claudication. *Med Sci Sports Exerc.* 1991;23(4):402-408.

25. Treat-Jacobson D, Bronas UG, Leon AS. Efficacy of arm-ergometry versus treadmill exercise training to improve walking distance in patients with claudication. *Vasc Med* 2009;14(3):203-213.

26. Naughton J, Balke B, Nagle F. Refinements in method of evaluation and physical conditioning before and after myocardial infarction. *Am J Cardiol* 1964; 14: 837-843.

27. Cooper CB, Dolezal BA, Durstine JL, et al. Chronic conditions very strongly associated with tobacco. In: Moore GE, Durstine JL and Painter PL, eds. *Acsm's Exercise Management for Persons With Chronic Disease and Disabilities.* 4th ed. Champaign, IL: Human Kinetics; 2016:95-113.

28. ATS Committee on Proficiency Standards for Clinical Pulmonary Function Laboratories. ATS statement: Guidelines for the six-minute walk test. *Am J Respir Crit Care Med.* 2002; 166(1): 111-117.

29. Montgomery PS, Gardner AW. The clinical utility of a six-minute walk test in peripheral arterial occlusive disease patients. *J Am Geriatr Soc.* 1998;46(6):706-711.

30. Guralnik JM, Simonsick EM, Ferrucci L, et al. A short physical performance battery assessing lower extremity function: Association with self-reported disability and prediction of mortality and nursing home admission. *J Gerontol.* 1994;49(2):M85-94.

31. McDermott MM, Guralnik JM, Criqui MH, et al. Unsupervised exercise and mobility loss in peripheral artery disease: A randomized controlled trial. *J Am Heart Assoc.* 2015;4(5).

32. Podsiadlo D and Richardson S. The timed "up & go": A test of basic functional mobility for frail elderly persons. *J Am Geriatr Soc.* 1991; 39(2): 142-148.

33. Steffen TM, Hacker TA, Mollinger L. Age- and gender-related test performance in community-dwelling elderly people: Six-Minute Walk Test, Berg Balance Scale, Timed Up & Go Test, and gait speeds. *Phys Ther.* 2002;82(2):128-137.

34. Mays RJ, Casserly IP, Kohrt WM, et al. Assessment of functional status and quality of life in claudication. *J Vasc Surg* 2011; 53(5): 1410-1421.

35. Ware JE, Sherbourne CD, Davies AR. Developing and Testing the MOS 20-Item Short-Form Health Survey A General Population Application Published in: Measuring Functioning and Well-Being: The Medical Outcomes Study Approach / edited by Anita L. Stewart and John E. Ware, Jr., (Durham, N.C.: Duke University Press, 1992), Chapter 16, p. 277-290

36. Ware Jr JE. SF-36 health survey update. Spine (Phila Pa 1976). 2000;25(24):3130-3139. \

37. Cella D, Riley W, Stone A, et al. The Patient-Reported Outcomes Measurement Information System (PROMIS) developed and tested its first wave of adult self-reported health outcome item banks: 2005-2008. *J Clin Epidemiol* 2010;63(11):1179-1194.

38. Regensteiner JG, Steiner JF, Panzer RJ, et al. Evaluation of walking impairment by questionniare in patients with peripheral artery disease. *J Vasc Med Biol.* 1990;2:142-152.

39. Treat-Jacobson D, Lindquist RA, Witt DR, et al. The PADQOL: Development and validation of a PAD-specific quality of life questionnaire. *Vasc Med.* 2012;17(6):405-415.

40. Spertus J, Jones P, Poler S, et al. The peripheral artery questionnaire: A new disease-specific health status measure for patients with peripheral arterial disease. *Am Heart J* 2004; 147(2): 301-308.

41. Parmenter BJ, Dieberg G, Smart NA. Exercise training for management of peripheral arterial disease: A systematic review and meta-analysis. *Sports Med.* 2015; 45(2): 231-244.

42. Lane R, Ellis B, Watson L, et al. Exercise for intermittent claudication. *Cochrane Database Syst Rev.* 2014;7:CD000990.

43. Jensen TS, Chin J, Ashby L, et al. Decision memo: National coverage determination for supervised exercise therapy (SET) for symptomatic peripheral artery disease (PAD) (CAG-00449N). *The Centers for Medicare & Medicaid Services.* https://www.cms.gov/medicare-coverage-database/details/nca-decision-memo.aspx?NCAId=287. Published May 25 2017. Accessed October 23, 2019.

44. Garber CE, Blissmer B, Deschenes MR, et al. American College of Sports Medicine position stand. Quantity and quality of exercise for developing and maintaining cardiorespiratory, musculoskeletal, and neuromotor fitness in apparently healthy adults: Guidance for prescribing exercise. *Med Sci Sports Exerc.* 2011;43(7):1334-1359.

45. Degischer S, Labs KH, Hochstrasser J, et al. Physical training for intermittent claudication: A comparison of structured rehabilitation versus home-based training. *Vasc Med.* 2002;7(2):109-115.

46. Regensteiner JG, Meyer TJ, Krupski WC, et al. Hospital vs home-based exercise rehabilitation for patients with peripheral arterial occlusive disease. *Angiology.* 1997; 48(4): 291-300.

47. Kakkos SK, Geroulakos G, Nicolaides AN. Improvement of the walking ability in intermittent claudication due to superficial femoral artery occlusion with supervised exercise and pneumatic foot and calf compression: A randomised controlled trial. *Eur J Vasc Endovasc Surg.* 2005;30(2):164-175.

48. Allen JD, Stabler T, Kenjale A, et al. Plasma nitrite flux predicts exercise performance in peripheral arterial disease after 3 months of exercise training. *Free Radic Biol Med.* 2010;49(6):1138-1144.

49. Mays RJ, Hiatt WR, Casserly IP, et al. Community-based walking exercise for peripheral artery disease: An exploratory pilot study. *Vasc Med.* 2015;20(4):339-347.

50. McDermott MM, Liu K, Guralnik JM, et al. Home-based walking exercise intervention in peripheral artery disease: A randomized clinical trial. *JAMA* 2013; 310(1): 57-65.

51. Gardner AW, Parker DE, Montgomery PS, et al. Step-monitored home exercise improves ambulation, vascular function, and inflammation in symptomatic patients with peripheral artery disease: A randomized controlled trial. *J Am Heart Assoc.* 2014;3(5):e001107.

52. Zwierska I, Walker RD, Choksy SA, et al. Upper- vs lower-limb aerobic exercise rehabilitation in patients with symptomatic peripheral arterial disease: A randomized controlled trial. *J Vasc Surg.* 2005;42(6):1122-1130.

53. Tew G, Nawaz S, Zwierska I, et al. Limb-specific and cross-transfer effects of arm-crank exercise training in patients with symptomatic peripheral arterial disease. *Clin Sci.* 2009;117(12):405-413.

54. Parmenter BJ, Raymond J, Dinnen P, et al. High-intensity progressive resistance training improves flat-ground walking in older adults with symptomatic peripheral arterial disease. *J Am Geriatr Soc* 2013; 61(11): 1964-1970.

55. McDermott MM, Ades P, Guralnik JM, et al. Treadmill exercise and resistance training in patients with peripheral arterial disease with and without intermittent claudication: A randomized controlled trial. *JAMA*. 2009;301(2):165-174.

56. Hood SC, Moher D, Barber GG. Management of intermittent claudication with pentoxifylline: Meta-analysis of randomized controlled trials. *CMAJ*. 1996;155(8):1053-1059.

57. Girolami B, Bernardi E, Prins MH, et al. Treatment of intermittent claudication with physical training, smoking cessation, pentoxifylline, or nafronyl: A meta-analysis. *Arch Intern Med*. 1999;159(4):337-345.

58. Full prescribing information: Pletal (cilostazol). FDA website. https://www.accessdata.fda.gov/drugsatfda_docs/label/2017/020863s024lbl.pdf. Revised May, 2017. Accessed October 23, 2019.

59. Bedenis R, Stewart M, Cleanthis M, et al. Cilostazol for intermittent claudication. *Cochrane Database Syst Rev*. 2014;(10):CD003748.

60. Pande RL, Hiatt WR, Zhang P, et al. A pooled analysis of the durability and predictors of treatment response of cilostazol in patients with intermittent claudication. *Vasc Med*. 2010;15(3):181-188.

61. Packer M, Carver JR, Rodeheffer RJ, et al. Effect of oral milrinone on mortality in severe chronic heart failure. The promise study research group. *N Engl J Med*. 1991;325(21):1468-1475.

62. Chi YW, Lavie CJ, Milani RV, et al. Safety and efficacy of cilostazol in the management of intermittent claudication. *Vasc Health Risk Manag*. 2008;4(6):1197-1203.

63. Gornik HL and Creager MA. Medical treatment of peripheral artery disease. In: Creager MA, Beckman JA and Loscalzo J, eds. *Vascular Medicine: A Companion to Braunwald's Heart Disease*. 2nd ed. Philadelphia, PA: Elsevier; 2013:242-258.

64. Murphy TP, Cutlip DE, Regensteiner JG, et al. Supervised exercise versus primary stenting for claudication resulting from aortoiliac peripheral artery disease: Six-month outcomes from the Claudication: Exercise Versus Endoluminal Revascularization (CLEVER) study. *Circulation* 2011.

65. Murphy TP, Cutlip DE, Regensteiner JG, et al. Supervised exercise versus primary stenting for claudication resulting from aortoiliac peripheral artery disease: Six-month outcomes from the Claudication: Exercise Versus Endoluminal Revascularization (CLEVER) study. *Circulation*. 2012;125(1):130-139.

66. Murphy TP, Cutlip DE, Regensteiner JG, et al. Supervised exercise, stent revascularization, or medical therapy for claudication due to aortoiliac peripheral artery disease: The CLEVER study. *J Am Coll Cardiol*. 2015;65(10):999-1009.

67. Treat-Jacobson D, McDermott MM, Beckman JA, Burt MS, Creager MA, Ehrman JK, Gardner AW, Mays RJ, Regensteiner JG, Salisbury DL, Schorr EN, Walsh ME, American Heart Association Council on Peripheral Vascular Disease. (2019) Implementation of Supervised Exercise Therapy for Patients with Symptomatic Peripheral Artery Disease. Circulation e-pub ahead of print 26 August 2019. PMID: 31446770.

Chapter 10: Chronic Lung Disease Section

1. Fabbri LM, Luppi F, Beghe B, Rabe KF. Complex comorbidities of COPD. *Eur Respir J*. 2008;31(1):204-12.

2. Roversi S, Roversi P, Spadafora G, Rossi R, Fabgri LM. Coronary artery disease concomitant with chronic obstructive pulmonary disease. *Eur J Clin Invest*. 2014;44(1):93-102.

3. Mota IL, Sousa ACS, Almeida MLD, Ferreira EJP, et al. Coronary lesions in patients with COPD (GOLD stages I-III) and suspected or confirmed coronary arterial disease. *Int J COPD*. 2018;13:1999-2006.

4. Ko FWS, Yan BP, Lam Y, Chu JHY, Chan J-P, Hui DSC. Undiagnosed airflow limitation is common in patients with coronary artery disease and associated with cardiac stress. *Respirology*. 2016;21(1):137-142.

5. Chen W, Thomas J, Sadatsafavi M, Fitzgerald JM. Risk of cardiovascular comorbidity in patients with chronic obstructive pulmonary disease: A systematic review and meta-analysis. *Lancet Respir med*. 2015;3(8):631-639.

6. Montserrat-Capdevila J, Seminario MA, Godoy P, et al. Prevalence of chronic obstructive pulmonary disease (COPD) not diagnosed in a population with cardiovascular risk factors. *Med Clin (Barc)*. 2018;Pii:S0025-7753(18)30061-7. doi:10.1016/j.medcli.2017.12.018 [Epub ahead of print]

7. Martinez FJ, Taczek AE, Seifer FD, et al. Development and initial validation of a self-scored population screener questionnaire (COPD-PS). *J COPD*. 2008;5:85-95.

8. Yawn BP, Mapel DW, Mannino DM, et al. Development of the lung function questionnaire (LFQ) to identify airflow obstruction. *Int J COPD.* 2010;5:1-10.

9. Ruppel GL, Carlin BW, Hart M, Doherty DE. Office spirometry in primary care for the diagnosis and management of COPD: National Lung Health Education Program Update. *Respir Care.* 2018;63(2):242-252.

10. Bossone E, D'Andrea A, D'Alto, et al. Echocardiography in pulmonary arterial hypertension: from diagnosis to prognosis. *J Am Soc Echocardiogr.* 2013;26:1-14.

11. Arena R, Sietsema KE. Cardiopulmonary exercise testing in the clinical evaluation of patients with heart and lung disease. *Circulation.* 2011;123:668-690.

12. Holland AE, Spruit MA, Troosters T, et al. An official European Respiratory Society/American Thoracic Society technical standard: Field walking tests in chronic respiratory disease. *Eur Respir J.* 2014;44:15428-1446.

13. Postma DS, Rabe KF. The asthma-COPD syndrome. *N Engl J Med.* 2015;373:1241-1249.

14. Khaled A, Stoller JK. A review of long-term oxygen therapy in chronic obstructive pulmonary disease. *Clin Pulm Med.* 2018;25(1):1-6.

15. Ries AL, Bauldoff GS, Carlin BW, et al. Pulmonary rehabilitation: Joint ACCP/AACVPR evidence-based clinical practice guidelines. *Chest.* 2007;131(5 suppl):2s-42S.

16. Spruit MA, Singh SJ, Garvey C, et al. ATS/ERS Task Force on Pulmonary Rehabilitation. An official American Thoracic Society/European Respiratory Society statement: Key concepts and advances in pulmonary rehabilitation. *Am J Respir Crit Care Med.* 2013;188:e13-64.

17. Bauldoff GS, Carlin BW, eds. *Guidelines for Pulmonary Rehabilitation Programs.* 5th ed. Champaign, IL: Human Kinetics; 2019.

18. Palermo P, Corra U. Exercise prescription for training and rehabilitation in patients with heart and lung disease. *Ann Am Thor Soc.* 2017;14(suppl1):S59-S66.

19. Nakazawa A, Cox NS, Holland AE. Current best practice in rehabilitation in interstitial lung disease. *Ther Adv Respir Dis.* 2017;11(2):115-128

20. Arena R. Exercise testing and training in chronic lung disease and pulmonary arterial hypertension. *Prog Cardiovasc Dis.* 2011;53:454-463.

21. Vitacca M, Paneroni. Rehabilitation of patients with coexisting COPD and heart failure. *J COPD.* 2018;15(3):231-237.

22. Vogelmeier CF, Criner GJ, Martinez, FJ, et al. Global strategy for the diagnosis, management, and prevention of chronic obstructive pulmonary disease. 2017 report. GOLD executive summary. *Am J Respir Crit Care Med.* 2017;195(5):557-582.

Chapter 11: Younger Adults Section

1. Audelin MC, Savage PD, Ades PA. Changing clinical profile of patients entering cardiac rehabilitation/secondary prevention programs: 1996 to 2006. *J Cardiopulm Rehabil Prev.* 2008;28(5):299-306.

2. Opotowsky AR, Rhodes J, Landzberg MJ, et al. A Randomized Trial Comparing Cardiac Rehabilitation to Standard of Care for Adults With Congenital Heart Disease. *World J PediatrCongenit Heart Surg.* 2018;9(2):185-193.

3. De S, Searles G, Haddad H. The prevalence of cardiac risk factors in women 45 years of age or younger undergoing angiography for evaluation of undiagnosed chest pain. *Can JCardiol.* 2002;18(9):945-948.

4. Madala MC, Franklin BA, Chen AY, et al. Obesity and age of first non-ST-segment elevation myocardial infarction. *J Am Coll Cardiol.* 2008;52(12):979-985.

5. Dunlay SM, Pack QR, Thomas RJ, Killian JM, Roger VL. Participation in cardiac rehabilitation, readmissions, and death after acute myocardial infarction. *Am J Med.* 2014;127(6):538-546.

6. Ribeiro PA, Boidin M, Juneau M, Nigam A, Gayda M. High-intensity interval training in patients with coronary heart disease: Prescription models and perspectives. *Ann Phys Rehabil Med.* 2017;60(1):50-57.

7. Ellingsen O, Halle M, Conraads V, et al. High-intensity interval training in patients with heart failure with reduced ejection fraction. *Circulation.* 2017;135(9):839-849.

8. Pfaeffli L, Maddison R, Whittaker R, et al. A mHealth cardiac rehabilitation exercise intervention: Findings from content development studies. *BMC Cardiovasc Disord.* 2012;12:36.

9. Varnfield M, Karunanithi M, Lee CK, et al. Smartphone-based home care model improved use of cardiac rehabilitation in postmyocardial infarction patients: Results from a randomised controlled trial. *Heart.* 2014;100(22):1770-1779.

10. Daniels KM, Arena R, Lavie CJ, Forman DE. Cardiac rehabilitation for women across the lifespan. *Am J Med.* 2012;125(9):937 e931-937.

11. Beckie TM, Fletcher G, Groer MW, Kip KE, Ji M. Biopsychosocial health disparities among young women enrolled in cardiac rehabilitation. *J Cardiopulm Rehabil Prev.* 2015;35(2):103-113.

12. Milani RV, Lavie CJ. prevalence and profile of metabolic syndrome in patients following acute coronary events and effects of therapeutic lifestyle change with cardiac rehabilitation. Am J Cardiol. 2003;92:50-54.

13. Lavie CJ, Milani RV. Adverse psychological and coronary risk profiles in young patients with coronary artery disease and benefits of formal cardiac rehabilitation. *Arch Intern Med.* 2006;166(17):1878-1883.

Chapter 11: Older Adults Section

1. Forman DE, Rich MW, Alexander KP, et al. Cardiac care for older adults. Time for a new paradigm. *J Am Coll Cardiol.* 2011;57(18):1801-1810.

2. Heidenreich PA, Trogdon JG, Khavjou OA, et al. Forecasting the future of cardiovascular disease in the United States: A policy statement from the American Heart Association. *Circulation.* 2011;123(8):933-944.

3. Benjamin EJ, Blaha MJ, Chiuve SE, et al. Heart disease and stroke statistics-2017 Update: A report from the American Heart Association. *Circulation.* 2017;135(10):e146-e603.

4. Richardson LA, Buckenmeyer PJ, Bauman BD, et al. Contemporary cardiac rehabilitation: Patient characteristics and temporal trends over the past decade. *J Cardiopulm Rehabil.* 2000;20(1):57-64.

5. Audelin MC, Savage PD, Ades PA. Changing clinical profile of patients entering cardiac rehabilitation/secondary prevention programs: 1996 to 2006. *J Cardiopulm Rehabil Prev.* 2008;28(5):299-306.

6. Suaya JA, Shepard DS, Normand SL, et al. Use of cardiac rehabilitation by Medicare beneficiaries after myocardial infarction or coronary bypass surgery. *Circulation.* 2007;116(15):1653-1662.

7. Forman DE, Sanderson BK, Josephson RA, et al. Heart Failure as a Newly Approved Diagnosis for Cardiac Rehabilitation: Challenges and Opportunities. *J Am Coll Cardiol.* 2015;65(24):2652-2659.

8. Schopfer DW, Forman DE. Cardiac rehabilitation in older adults. *Can J Cardiol.* 2016;32(9):1088-1096.

9. Menezes AR, Lavie CJ, Forman DE, et al. Cardiac rehabilitation in the elderly. *Prog Cardiovasc Dis.* 2014;57(2):152-159.

10. Doll JA, Hellkamp A, Ho PM, et al. Participation in Cardiac Rehabilitation Programs Among Older Patients After Acute Myocardial Infarction. *JAMA Intern Med.* 2015;175(10):1700-1702.

11. Gurewich D, Prottas J, Bhalotra S, et al. System-level factors and use of cardiac rehabilitation. *J Cardiopulm Rehabil Prev.* 2008;28(6):380-385.

12. Ruano-Ravina A, Pena-Gil C, Abu-Assi E, et al. Participation and adherence to cardiac rehabilitation programs. A systematic review. *Int J Cardiol.* 2016;223:436-443.

13. Bell SP, Orr NM, Dodson JA, et al. What to expect from the evolving field of Geriatric Cardiology. *J Am Coll Cardiol.* 2015;66(11):1286-1299.

14. Forman DE, Maurer MS, Boyd C, et al. Multimorbidity in Older Adults With Cardiovascular Disease. *J Am Coll Cardiol.* 2018;71(19):2149-2161.

15. Tinetti ME, Fried TR, Boyd CM. Designing health care for the most common chronic condition—Multimorbidity. *JAMA.* 2012;307(23):2493-2494.

16. Kanaan AO, Donovan JL, Duchin NP, et al. Adverse drug events after hospital discharge in older adults: Types, severity, and involvement of Beers Criteria Medications. *J Am Geriatr Soc.* 2013;61(11):1894-1899.

17. Rossello X, Pocock SJ, Julian DG. Long-Term Use of Cardiovascular Drugs: Challenges for Research and for Patient Care. *J Am Coll Cardiol.* 2015;66(11):1273-1285.

18. Afilalo J, Alexander KP, Mack MJ, et al. Frailty assessment in the cardiovascular care of older adults. *J Am Coll Cardiol.* 2014;63(8):747-762.

19. Bibas L, Levi M, Bendayan M, et al. Therapeutic interventions for frail elderly patients: Part I. Published randomized trials. *Prog Cardiovasc Dis.* 2014;57(2):134-143.

20. Marzetti E, Calvani R, Tosato M, et al. Physical activity and exercise as countermeasures to physical frailty and sarcopenia. *Aging Clin Exp Res.* 2017;29(1):35-42.

21. Molino-Lova R, Pasquini G, Vannetti F, et al. Effects of a structured physical activity intervention on measures of physical performance in frail elderly patients after cardiac rehabilitation: A pilot study with 1-year follow-up. *Intern Emerg Med.* 2013;8(7):581-589.

22. McGlory C, van Vliet S, Stokes T, et al. The impact of exercise and nutrition in the regulation of skeletal muscle mass. *J Physiol.* 2018.

23. Forman DE, Santanasto AJ, Boudreau R, et al. Impact of incident heart failure on body composition over time in the health, aging, and body composition study population. *Circ Heart Fail.* 2017;10(9).

24. Fried LP, Tangen CM, Walston J, et al. Frailty in older adults: Evidence for a phenotype. *J Gerontol A Biol Sci Med Sci.* 2001;56(3):M146-156.

25. Rockwood K, Song X, MacKnight C, et al. A global clinical measure of fitness and frailty in elderly people. *CMAJ.* 2005;173(5):489-495.

26. Forman DE, Alexander KP. Frailty: A Vital Sign for Older Adults With Cardiovascular Disease. *Can J Cardiol.* 2016;32(9):1082-1087.

27. Agarwal KS, Kazim R, Xu J, et al. Unrecognized Cognitive Impairment and Its Effect on Heart Failure Readmissions of Elderly Adults. *J Am Geriatr Soc.* 2016;64(11):2296-2301.

28. Forman DE, Arena R, Boxer R, et al. Prioritizing functional capacity as a principal end point for therapies oriented to older adults with cardiovascular disease: A scientific statement for healthcare professionals from the American Heart Association. *Circulation.* 2017;135(16):e894-e918.

29. Krumholz HM. Post-hospital syndrome—An acquired, transient condition of generalized risk. *N Engl J Med.* 2013;368(2):100-102.

30. Baldasseroni S, Pratesi A, Francini S, et al. Cardiac rehabilitation in very old adults: Effect of baseline functional capacity on treatment effectiveness. *J Am Geriatr Soc.* 2016;64(8):1640-1645.

31. Freedman VA, Martin LG, Schoeni RF. Recent trends in disability and functioning among older adults in the United States: A systematic review. *JAMA.* 2002;288(24):3137-3146.

32. Daniels KM, Arena R, Lavie CJ, et al. Cardiac rehabilitation for women across the lifespan. *Am J Med.* 2012;125(9):937.e931-937.

33. Benton MJ, Silva-Smith AL. Accuracy of body mass index versus lean mass index for prediction of sarcopenia in older women. *J Frailty Aging.* 2018;7(2):104-107.

34. Gaalema DE, Savage PD, Rengo JL, et al. Financial incentives to promote cardiac rehabilitation participation and adherence among Medicaid patients. *Prev Med.* 2016;92:47-50.

35. Tinetti ME, Esterson J, Ferris R, et al. Patient priority-directed decision making and care for older adults with multiple chronic conditions. *Clin Geriatr Med.* 2016;32(2):261-275.

36. Kritchevsky SB, Forman DE, Callahan K, et al. Pathways, contributors, and correlates of functional limitation across specialties: Workshop summary. *J Gerontol A Biol Sci Med Sci.* 2018.

37. Reeves GR, Gupta S, Forman DE. Evolving role of exercise testing in contemporary cardiac rehabilitation. *J Cardiopulm Rehabil Prev.* 2016;36(5):309-319.

38. Riebe D, Ehrman JK, Liguori G, Maier M. *ACSM's Guidelines for Exercise Testing and Prescription.* 10th ed. Philadelphia: Lippincott Williams & Wilkins; 2018.

39. Chodzko-Zajko WJ, Proctor DN, Fiatarone Singh MA, et al. American College of Sports Medicine position stand. Exercise and physical activity for older adults. *Med Sci Sports Exerc.* 2009;41(7):1510-1530.

40. Syed FA, Ng AC. The pathophysiology of the aging skeleton. *Curr Osteoporosis Rep.* 2010;8(4):235-240.

41. Fielding RA, LeBrasseur NK, Cuoco A, et al. High-velocity resistance training increases skeletal muscle peak power in older women. *J Am Geriatr Soc.* 2002;50(4):655-662.

42. Clemson L, Fiatarone Singh MA, Bundy A, et al. Integration of balance and strength training into daily life activity to reduce rate of falls in older people (the LiFE study): Randomised parallel trial. *BMJ.* 2012;345:e4547.

43. Guralnik JM, Simonsick EM, Ferrucci L, et al. A short physical performance battery assessing lower extremity function: Association with self-reported disability and prediction of mortality and nursing home admission. *J Gerontol.* 1994;49(2):M85-94.

44. Joshua AM, D'Souza V, Unnikrishnan B, et al. Effectiveness of progressive resistance strength training versus traditional balance exercise in improving balance among the elderly - A randomised controlled trial. *J Clin Diagn Res.* 2014;8(3):98-102.

45. Sattelmair JR, Pertman JH, Forman DE. Effects of physical activity on cardiovascular and noncardiovascular outcomes in older adults. *Clin Geriatr Med.* 2009;25(4):677-702, viii-ix.

46. Wisloff U, Stoylen A, Loennechen JP, et al. Superior cardiovascular effect of aerobic interval training versus moderate continuous training in heart failure patients: A randomized study. *Circulation.* 2007;115(24):3086-3094.

47. Arena R, Myers J, Forman DE, et al. Should high-intensity-aerobic interval training become the clinical standard in heart failure? *Heart Fail Rev.* 2013;18(1):95-105.

48. Rutledge T, Redwine LS, Linke SE, et al. A meta-analysis of mental health treatments and cardiac rehabilitation for improving clinical outcomes and depression among patients with coronary heart disease. *Psychosom Med.* 2013;75(4):335-349.

49. Mortensen MB, Falk E. Primary prevention with statins in the elderly. *J Am Coll Cardiol.* 2018;71(1):85-94.

50. Fleg JL, Forman DE, Berra K, et al. Secondary prevention of atherosclerotic cardiovascular disease in older adults: A scientific statement from the American Heart Association. *Circulation.* 2013;128(22):2422-2446.

51. Savarese G, Gotto AM, Jr., Paolillo S, et al. Benefits of statins in elderly subjects without established cardiovascular disease: A meta-analysis. *J Am Coll Cardiol.* 2013;62(22):2090-2099.

52. Baigent C, Blackwell L, Emberson J, et al. Efficacy and safety of more intensive lowering of LDL cholesterol: A meta-analysis of data from 170,000 participants in 26 randomised trials. *Lancet.* 2010;376(9753):1670-1681.

53. Baigent C, Keech A, Kearney PM, et al. Efficacy and safety of cholesterol-lowering treatment: Prospective meta-analysis of data from 90,056 participants in 14 randomised trials of statins. *Lancet.* 2005;366(9493):1267-1278.

54. Cannon CP, Braunwald E, McCabe CH, et al. Intensive versus moderate lipid lowering with statins after acute coronary syndromes. *N Engl J Med.* 2004;350(15):1495-1504.

55. Rodriguez F, Maron DJ, Knowles JW, et al. Association between intensity of statin therapy and mortality in patients with atherosclerotic cardiovascular disease. *JAMA Cardiol.* 2017;2(1):47-54.

56. Cannon CP, Blazing MA, Giugliano RP, et al. Ezetimibe added to statin therapy after acute coronary syndromes. *N Engl J Med.* 2015;372(25):2387-2397.

57. Lloyd-Jones DM, Evans JC, Levy D. Hypertension in adults across the age spectrum: current outcomes and control in the community. *JAMA.* 2005;294(4):466-472.

58. Williamson JD, Supiano MA, Applegate WB, et al. Intensive vs standard blood pressure control and cardiovascular disease outcomes in adults aged ≥75 Years: A randomized clinical trial. *JAMA.* 2016;315(24):2673-2682.

59. Fleg JL, Aronow WS, Frishman WH. Cardiovascular drug therapy in the elderly: Benefits and challenges. *Nat Rev Cardiol.* 2011;8(1):13-28.

60. Whelton PK, Carey RM, Aronow WS, et al. 2017 ACC/AHA/AAPA/ABC/ACPM/AGS/APhA/ASH/ASPC/NMA/PCNA guideline for the prevention, detection, evaluation, and management of high blood pressure in adults: A report of the American College of Cardiology/American Heart Association Task Force on Clinical Practice Guidelines. *J Am Coll Cardiol.* 2018;71(19):e127-e248.

61. Wright JT, Jr., Williamson JD, Whelton PK, et al. A randomized trial of intensive versus standard blood-pressure control. *N Engl J Med.* 2015;373(22):2103-2116.

62. Saneei P, Salehi-Abargouei A, Esmaillzadeh A, et al. Influence of dietary approaches to stop hypertension (DASH) diet on blood pressure: A systematic review and meta-analysis on randomized controlled trials. *Nutr Metab Cardiovasc Dis.* 2014;24(12):1253-1261.

63. Savage PD, Banzer JA, Balady GJ, et al. Prevalence of metabolic syndrome in cardiac rehabilitation/secondary prevention programs. *Am Heart J.* 2005;149(4):627-631.

64. Kirkman MS, Briscoe VJ, Clark N, et al. Diabetes in older adults. *Diabetes Care.* 2012;35(12):2650-2664.

65. Harvey-Berino J. Weight loss in the clinical setting: Applications for cardiac rehabilitation. *Coron Artery Dis.* 1998;9(12):795-798.

66. Lee SJ, Boscardin WJ, Stijacic Cenzer I, et al. The risks and benefits of implementing glycemic control guidelines in frail older adults with diabetes mellitus. *J Am Geriatr Soc.* 2011;59(4):666-672.

67. Zinman B, Wanner C, Lachin JM, et al. Empagliflozin, cardiovascular outcomes, and mortality in type 2 diabetes. *N Engl J Med.* 2015;373(22):2117-2128.

68. Ades PA, Savage PD, Brawner CA, et al. Aerobic capacity in patients entering cardiac rehabilitation. *Circulation*. 2006;113(23):2706-2712.

69. Mallik S, Krumholz HM, Lin ZQ, Kasl SV, Mattera JA, Roumains SA, Vaccarino V. Patients with depression have lower health status benefits after coronary artery bypass surgery. *Circulation*. 2005(111):271-277.

70. Swardfager W, Herrmann N, Dowlati Y, et al. Relationship between cardiopulmonary fitness and depressive symptoms in cardiac rehabilitation patients with coronary artery disease. *J Rehabil Med*. 2008;40(3):213-218.

71. Rutledge T, Linke SE, Krantz DS, et al. Comorbid depression and anxiety symptoms as predictors of cardiovascular events: Results from the NHLBI-sponsored Women's Ischemia Syndrome Evaluation (WISE) study. *Psychosom Med*. 2009;71(9):958-964.

72. Sheikh JI, Yesavage JA. Geriatric Depression Scale (GDS): recent findings and development of a shorter version. *Clinical Gerontology*. 1986;5:165-173.

73. Kroenke K, Spitzer RL, Williams JB. The PHQ-9: validity of a brief depression severity measure. *J Gen Intern Med*. 2001;16(9):606-613.

74. Heffner JE, Barbieri C. End-of-life care preferences of patients enrolled in cardiovascular rehabilitation programs. *Chest*. 2000;117(5):1474-1481.

75. Gellert C, Schottker B, Brenner H. Smoking and all-cause mortality in older people: Systematic review and meta-analysis. *Arch Intern Med*. 2012;172(11):837-844.

76. Reid RD, Mullen KA, Pipe AL. Systematic approaches to smoking cessation in the cardiac setting. *Curr Opin Cardiol*. 2011;26(5):443-448.

77. Zullo MD, Dolansky MA, Josephson RA, et al. Older Adult Attendance in Cardiac Rehabilitation: Impact of functional status and postacute care after acute myocardial infarction in 63 092 Medicare beneficiaries. *J Cardiopulm Rehabil Prev*. 2018;38(1):17-23.

78. Oerkild B, Frederiksen M, Hansen JF, et al. Home-based cardiac rehabilitation is as effective as centre-based cardiac rehabilitation among elderly with coronary heart disease: Results from a randomised clinical trial. *Age Ageing*. 2011;40(1):78-85.

79. Varnfield M, Karunanithi M, Lee CK, et al. Smartphone-based home care model improved use of cardiac rehabilitation in postmyocardial infarction patients: Results from a randomised controlled trial. *Heart*. 2014;100(22):1770-1779.

Chapter 11: Women and Men Section

1. Heart Disease Facts. CDC website. www.cdc.gov/heartdisease/facts.htm. Published November 28, 2017. Accessed October 28, 2019.

2. Garcia M, Mulvagh SL, Merz CNB, Buring JE, Manson JE. Cardiovascular disease in women: Clinical perspectives. *Circ Res*. 2016;118(8):1273-1293. doi:10.1161/CIRCRESAHA.116.307547

3. Shaw LJ, Bairey Merz CN, Pepine CJ, et al. Insights from the NHLBI-sponsored Women's Ischemia Syndrome Evaluation (WISE) Study: Part I: Gender differences in traditional and novel risk factors, symptom evaluation, and gender-optimized diagnostic strategies. *J Am Coll Cardiol*. 2006;47(3 Suppl S):4S-20S. doi:10.1016/j.jacc.2005.01.072

4. Shaw LJ, Shaw RE, Merz CNB, et al. Impact of ethnicity and gender differences on angiographic coronary artery disease prevalence and in-hospital mortality in the American College of Cardiology-National Cardiovascular Data Registry. *Circulation*. 2008;117(14):1787-1801. doi:10.1161/CIRCULATIONAHA.107.726562

5. Anand SS, Islam S, Rosengren A, et al. Risk factors for myocardial infarction in women and men: Insights from the INTERHEART study. *Eur Heart J*. 2008;29(7):932-940. doi:10.1093/eurheartj/ehn018

6. Canto JG, Rogers WJ, Goldberg RJ, et al. Association of age and sex with myocardial infarction symptom presentation and in-hospital mortality. *JAMA*. 2012;307(8):813-822. doi:10.1001/jama.2012.199

7. Mosca L, Barrett-Connor E, Wenger NK. Sex/gender differences in cardiovascular disease prevention: What a difference a decade makes. *Circulation*. 2011;124(19):2145-2154. doi:10.1161/CIRCULATIONAHA.110.968792

8. Gu Q, Burt VL, Paulose-Ram R, Dillon CF. Gender differences in hypertension treatment, drug utilization patterns, and blood pressure control among US adults with hypertension: Data from the National Health and Nutrition Examination Survey 1999-2004. *Am J Hypertens*. 2008;21(7):789-798. doi:10.1038/ajh.2008.185

9. Bird CE, Fremont AM, Bierman AS, et al. Does quality of care for cardiovascular disease and diabetes differ by gender for enrollees in managed care plans? *Womens Health Issues*. 2007;17(3):131-138.

10. Chou AF, Scholle SH, Weisman CS, Bierman AS, Correa-de-Araujo R, Mosca L. Gender disparities in the quality of cardiovascular disease care in private managed care plans. *Womens Health Issues*. 2007;17(3):120-130. doi:10.1016/j.whi.2007.03.002

11. Lloyd-Jones DM, Huffman MD, Karmali KN, et al. Estimating longitudinal risks and benefits from cardiovascular preventive therapies among Medicare patients: The Million Hearts Longitudinal ASCVD Risk Assessment Tool: A special report from the American Heart Association and American College of Cardiology. *J Am Coll Cardiol*. 2017;69(12):1617-1636. doi:10.1016/j.jacc.2016.10.018

12. Dale CM, Angus JE, Seto Nielsen L, et al. "I'm no superman": Understanding diabetic men, masculinity, and cardiac rehabilitation. *Qual Health Res*. 2015;25(12):1648-1661. doi:10.1177/1049732314566323

13. Appelman Y, van Rijn BB, Ten Haaf ME, Boersma E, Peters SAE. Sex differences in cardiovascular risk factors and disease prevention. *Atherosclerosis*. 2015;241(1):211-218. doi:10.1016/j.atherosclerosis.2015.01.027

14. Huxley R, Barzi F, Woodward M. Excess risk of fatal coronary heart disease associated with diabetes in men and women: Meta-analysis of 37 prospective cohort studies. *BMJ*. 2006;332(7533):73-78. doi:10.1136/bmj.38678.389583.7C

15. Flegal KM, Carroll MD, Ogden CL, Curtin LR. Prevalence and trends in obesity among US adults, 1999-2008. *JAMA*. 2010;303(3):235-241. doi:10.1001/jama.2009.2014

16. Fitzgerald KR. Review of article: Prevalence of obesity and trends in the distribution of body mass index among US adults, 1999-2010 by Katherine M. Flegal, PhD; Margaret D. Carroll, MSPH; Brian K. Kit, MD; Cynthia L. Ogden, PhD (*JAMA* 2012;307:491-7). *J Vasc Nurs Off Publ Soc Peripher Vasc Nurs*. 2013;31(3):131-132. doi:10.1016/j.jvn.2013.06.004

17. Schiller JS, Lucas JW, Peregoy JA. Summary Health Statistics for U.S. Adults: National Health Interview Survey, 2011. Hyattsville; 2011.

18. Sattelmair J, Pertman J, Ding EL, Kohl HW 3rd, Haskell W, Lee I-M. Dose response between physical activity and risk of coronary heart disease: a meta-analysis. *Circulation*. 2011;124(7):789-795. doi:10.1161/CIRCULATIONAHA.110.010710

19. Regitz-Zagrosek V, Oertelt-Prigione S, Prescott E, et al. Gender in cardiovascular diseases: impact on clinical manifestations, management, and outcomes. *Eur Heart J*. 2016;37(1):24-34. doi:10.1093/eurheartj/ehv598

20. Goff DC, Lloyd-Jones DM, Bennett G, et al. 2013 ACC/AHA guideline on the assessment of cardiovascular risk: a report of the American College of Cardiology/American Heart Association Task Force on Practice Guidelines. *J Am Coll Cardiol*. 2014;63(25 Pt B):2935-2959. doi:10.1016/j.jacc.2013.11.005

21. Shufelt CL, Pacheco C, Tweet MS, Miller VM. Sex-Specific Physiology and Cardiovascular Disease. *Adv Exp Med Biol*. 2018;1065:433-454. doi:10.1007/978-3-319-77932-4_27

22. Kramer MCA, Rittersma SZH, de Winter RJ, et al. Relationship of thrombus healing to underlying plaque morphology in sudden coronary death. *J Am Coll Cardiol*. 2010;55(2):122-132. doi:10.1016/j.jacc.2009.09.007

23. Mead H, Andres E, Katch H, Siegel B, Regenstein M. Gender differences in psychosocial issues affecting low-income, underserved patients' ability to manage cardiovascular disease. *Womens Health Issues*. 2010;20(5):308-315. doi:10.1016/j.whi.2010.05.006

24. Szerencsi K, van Amelsvoort LGPM, Viechtbauer W, Mohren DCL, Prins MH, Kant I. The association between study characteristics and outcome in the relation between job stress and cardiovascular disease - a multilevel meta-regression analysis. *Scand J Work Environ Health*. 2012;38(6):489-502. doi:10.5271/sjweh.3283

25. Beckie TM, Fletcher GF, Beckstead JW, Schocken DD, Evans ME. Adverse baseline physiological and psychosocial profiles of women enrolled in a cardiac rehabilitation clinical trial. *J Cardiopulm Rehabil Prev*. 2008;28(1):52-60.

26. Goodman H, Firouzi A, Banya W, Lau-Walker M, Cowie MR. Illness perception, self-care behaviour and quality of life of heart failure patients: A longitudinal questionnaire survey. *Int J Nurs Stud*. 2013;50(7):945-953. doi:10.1016/j.ijnurstu.2012.11.007

27. Xiang X, An R. Depression and onset of cardiovascular disease in the US middle-aged and older adults. *Aging Ment Health*. 2015;19(12):1084-1092. doi:10.1080/13607863.2014.1003281

28. Mendes de Leon CF, Krumholz HM, Seeman TS, et al. Depression and risk of coronary heart disease in elderly men and women: New Haven EPESE, 1982-1991. Established Populations for the Epidemiologic Studies of the Elderly. *Arch Intern Med*. 1998;158(21):2341-2348.

29. Caulin-Glaser T, Maciejewski PK, Snow R, LaLonde M, Mazure C. Depressive symptoms and sex affect completion rates and clinical outcomes in cardiac rehabilitation. *Prev Cardiol.* 2007;10(1):15-21.

30. Komorovsky R, Desideri A, Rozbowsky P, Sabbadin D, Celegon L, Gregori D. Quality of life and behavioral compliance in cardiac rehabilitation patients: A longitudinal survey. *Int J Nurs Stud.* 2008;45(7):979-985. doi:https://dx.doi.org/10.1016/j.ijnurstu.2007.06.008

31. Lichtman JH, Bigger TJ, Blumenthal JA, et al. Depression and coronary heart disease: recommendations for screening, referral, and treatment: A science advisory from the American Heart Association Prevention Committee of the Council on Cardiovascular Nursing, Council on Clinical Cardiology. *Circulation.* 2008;118(17):1768-1775. doi:10.1161/CIRCULATIONAHA.108.190769.

32. Arroll B, Goodyear-Smith F, Crengle S, Gunn J, Kerse N, Fishman T, Falloon K, Hatcher S. Validation of PHQ-2 and PHQ-9 for major depression in the primary care population. *Ann Fam Med.* 2010;8(4):348-353.

33. Hamm LF, Sanderson BK, Ades PA, et al. Core competencies for cardiac rehabilitation/secondary prevention professionals: 2010 update: Position statement of the American Association of Cardiovascular and Pulmonary Rehabilitation. *J Cardiopulm Rehabil Prev.* 2011;31(1):2-10. doi:10.1097/HCR.0b013e318203999d

34. World Heart Federation: Go Red for Women. WHF website. https://www.world-heart-federation.org/programmes/go-red-women/. Accessed October 28, 2019.

35. Mosca L, Mochari H, Christian A, et al. National study of women's awareness, preventive action, and barriers to cardiovascular health. *Circulation.* 2006;113(4):525-534.

36. Heran BS, Chen JM, Ebrahim S, et al. Exercise-based cardiac rehabilitation for coronary heart disease. *Cochrane Database Syst Rev.* 2011;(7):CD001800. doi:10.1002/14651858.CD001800.pub2

37. Wenger NK. Current status of cardiac rehabilitation. *J Am Coll Cardiol.* 2008;51(17):1619-1631. doi:10.1016/j.jacc.2008.01.030

38. Balady GJ, Williams MA, Ades PA, et al. Core components of cardiac rehabilitation/secondary prevention programs: 2007 update: A Scientific Statement From the American Heart Association Exercise, Cardiac Rehabilitation, and Prevention Committee, the Council on Clinical Cardiology; the Councils on Cardiovascular Nursing, Epidemiology and Prevention, and Nutrition, Physical Activity, and Metabolism; and the American Association of Cardiovascular and Pulmonary Rehabilitation . *J Cardiopulm Rehabil Prev.* 2007;27(3):121-129. doi:10.1097/01.HCR.0000270696.01635.aa

39. Balady GJ, Ades PA, Bittner VA, et al. Referral, enrollment, and delivery of cardiac rehabilitation/secondary prevention programs at clinical centers and beyond: a presidential advisory from the American Heart Association. *Circulation.* 2011;124(25):2951-2960. doi:10.1161/CIR.0b013e31823b21e2.

40. Piepoli MF, Hoes AW, Agewall S, et al. 2016 European Guidelines on cardiovascular disease prevention in clinical practice. *Eur Heart J.* 2016;37(29):2315-2381. doi:10.1093/eurheartj/ehw106.

41. Aragam KG, Moscucci M, Smith DE, et al. Trends and disparities in referral to cardiac rehabilitation after percutaneous coronary intervention. *Am Heart J.* 2011;161(3):544-551.e2. doi:10.1016/j.ahj.2010.11.016.

42. Suaya JA, Shepard DS, Normand S-LLT, Ades PA, Prottas J, Stason WB. Use of cardiac rehabilitation by Medicare beneficiaries after myocardial infarction or coronary bypass surgery. *Circulation.* 2007;116(15):1653-1662. doi:10.1161/CIRCULATIONAHA.107.701466

43. Samayoa L, Grace SL, Gravely S, et al. Sex differences in cardiac rehabilitation enrollment: A meta-analysis. *Can J Cardiol.* 2014;30(7):793-800. doi:10.1016/j.cjca.2013.11.007.

44. Colella TJF, Gravely S, Marzolini S, et al. Sex bias in referral of women to outpatient cardiac rehabilitation? A meta-analysis. *Eur J Prev Cardiol.* 2015. doi:10.1177/2047487314520783

45. Scott LAB, Ben-Or K, Allen JK, Benz Scott LA. Why are women missing from outpatient cardiac rehabilitation programs? A review of multilevel factors affecting referral, enrollment, and completion. *J Womens Health.* 2002;11(9):773-791.

46. Grace SL, Gravely-Witte S, Kayaniyil S, Brual J, Suskin N, Stewart DE. A multisite examination of sex differences in cardiac rehabilitation barriers by participation status. *J Women's Heal.* 2009;18(2). doi:10.1089/jwh.2007.0753

47. Shanmugasegaram S, Oh P, Reid RD, McCumber T, Grace SL. Cardiac rehabilitation barriers by rurality and socioeconomic status: A cross-sectional study. *Int J Equity Health.* 2013;12(1):72. doi:http://dx.doi.org/10.1186/1475-9276-12-72

48. Resurreccion DM, Motrico E, Rigabert A, et al. Barriers for nonparticipation and dropout of women in cardiac rehabilitation programs: A systematic review. *J Womens Health.* 2017;07:7. doi:https://dx.doi.org/10.1089/jwh.2016.6249

49. Supervía M, Medina-Inojosa JR, Yeung C, et al. Cardiac rehabilitation for women: A systematic review of barriers and solutions. *Mayo Clin Proc.* 2017;92(4):565-577. doi:10.1016/j.mayocp.2017.01.002

50. Grace SL, Shanmugasegaram S, Gravely-Witte S, Brual J, Suskin N, Stewart DE. Barriers to cardiac rehabilitation: Does age make a difference? *J Cardiopulm Rehabil Prev.* 2009;29(3):183-187. doi:10.1097/HCR.0b013e3181a3333c

51. Berger JS, Elliott L, Gallup D, et al. Sex differences in mortality following acute coronary syndromes. *JAMA.* 2009;302(8):874-882. doi:10.1001/jama.2009.1227

52. Whooley MA, de Jonge P, Vittinghoff E, et al. Depressive symptoms, health behaviors, and risk of cardiovascular events in patients with coronary heart disease. *JAMA.* 2008;300(20):2379-2388. doi:10.1001/jama.2008.711

Chapter 11: Race and Culture Section

1. Benjamin EJ, Virani SS, Callaway CW, Chamberlain AM, Chang AR, Cheng S, et al. Heart disease and stroke statistics—2018 update. A report from the American Heart Association. *Circulation.* 2018; 137:e67-e492.

2. Graham G. Disparities in cardiovascular disease risk in the United States. *Curr Cardiol Rev.* 2015;11:238-245.

3. Annual estimates of the resident population by sex, race, and Hispanic origin for the United States, states, and counties: April 1, 2010 to July 1, 2017. U.S. Census Bureau, Population Division. https://factfinder.census.gov/faces/tableservices/jsf/pages/productview.xhtml?src=bkmk#Release date: June 2018. Accessed October 28, 2019.

4. 2010 Census summary file 1—Technical documentation prepared by the U.S. Census. Bureau. https://www.census.gov/prod/cen2010/doc/sf1.pdf. Published September 2012. Accessed October 28, 2019.

5. Chasteen, JC. *Born in Blood and Fire: A Concise History of Latin America. 1.* New York: Norton; 2001.

6. Lloyd-Jones DM, Hong Y, Labarthe D, et al. Defining and setting national goals for cardiovascular health promotion and disease reduction: The American Heart Association's strategic impact goal through 2020 and beyond. *Circulation.* 2010; 121:586-613.

7. Smedley BD, Stith AY, Nelson AR, editors. Unequal treatment: Confronting racial and ethnic disparities in health care (2003). Committee on Understanding and Eliminating Racial and Ethnic Disparities in Health Care, Board on Health Policy, Institute of Medicine. Washington, DC: National Academy Press; 2002.

8. Egede LE. Race, ethnicity, culture, and disparities in health care. Gen Intern Med. 2006; 21: 667-669.

9. Howard G, Prineas R, Moy C, et al. Racial and geographic differences in awareness, treatment, and control of hypertension: the reasons for geographic and racial differences in stroke study. *Stroke.* 2006;37:1171-1178.

10. Sorlie PD, Backlund E, Johnson NJ, et al. Mortality by Hispanic status in the United States. *JAMA.* 1993;270:2464-2468.

11. Borrell LN, Lancet EA. Race/ethnicity and all-cause mortality in U.S. adults: Revisiting the Hispanic paradox. *Am J Public Health.* 2012; 102:836-843.

12. Rodriguez CJ, Allison M, Daviglus ML, et al. Status of cardiovascular disease and stroke in Hispanics/Latinos in the United States: A science advisory from the American Heart Association. *Circulation.* 2014;130:593-625M.

13. Ye J, Rust G, Baltrus P, et al. Cardiovascular risk factors among Asian Americans: Results from a national health survey. *Ann Epidemiol.* 2009;19:718-23.

14. Pleis JR, Lucas JW, Ward BW. Summary health statistics for U.S. Adults: National Health Interview Survey, 2008. *Vital Health Stat 10.* 2009;242:1-157.

15. Denny CH, Coolidge JN, Williams GI, et al. *Atlas of Heart Disease and Stroke Among American Indians and Alaska Natives* Atlanta, GA: U.S. Department of Health and Human Services, Centers for Disease Control and Prevention and Indian Health Service; 2005.

16. Health, United States, 2015: With special feature on racial and ethnic health disparities. CDC, National Center for Health Statistics website. www.cdc.gov/nchs/data/hus/hus15.pdf. Published May, 2016. Accessed October 4, 2018.

17. Li S, Fonarow GC, Mukamal K, et al. Sex and racial disparities in cardiac rehabilitation referral at hospital discharge and gaps in long-term mortality. *Heart Assoc.* 2018;7:e008088.

18. Sun EY, Jadotte Y, Halperin W. Disparities in cardiac rehabilitation participation in the United States: a systematic review and meta-analysis. *J Cardiopulm Rehabil Prev.* 2017; 37:2-10.

19. Supervía M, Medina-Inojosa JR, Yeung C, et al. Cardiac rehabilitation for women: A systematic review of barriers and solutions. *Mayo Clin Proc.* 2017;*92:*565-577.

20. Castellanos LR, Viramontes O, Bains NK, et al. Disparities in cardiac rehabilitation among individuals from racial and ethnic groups and rural communities. A systematic review. *J Racial Ethn Health Disparities.* 2018; 5:1-11.

21. Mensah GA, Cooper RS, Siega-Riz AM, et al. Reducing cardiovascular disparities through community-engaged implementation research. A National Heart, Lung, and Blood Institute Workshop Report. *Circ Res.* 2018;122:213-230.

22. Roth GA, Dwyer-Lindgren L, Bertozzi-Villa A, et al. Trends and patterns of geographic variation in cardiovascular mortality among U.S. counties, 1980-2014. *JAMA.* 2017;317:1976-1992.

23. Leigh JA, Alvarez M, Rodriguez CJ. Ethnic minorities and coronary heart disease: An update and future directions. *Curr Atheroscler Rep.* 2016;18:9.

24. Goff DC, Bertoni AG, Kramer H, et al. Dyslipidemia prevalence, treatment, and control in the multi-ethnic study of atherosclerosis (MESA) gender, ethnicity, and coronary artery calcium. *Circulation.* 2006;113:647-656.

25. Mathews R, Wang TY, Honeycutt E, et al. Persistence with secondary prevention medications after acute myocardial infarction: Insights from the TRANSLATE-ACS study. *Am Heart J.* 2015;170:62-9J.

26. Pollock B, Hamman BL, Sass DM, et al. Effect of gender and race on operative mortality after isolated coronary artery bypass grafting. *Am J Cardiol.* 2015;115:614-618.

27. Popescu I, Cram P, Vaughan-Sarrazin MS. Differences in admitting hospital characteristics for black and white Medicare beneficiaries with acute myocardial infarction. *Circulation.* 2011;123(23):2710-2716.

28. U.S. Department of Health and Human Services Office of Minority Health. Assuring Cultural Competence in Health Care: Recommendations for National Standards and Outcomes-Focused Research Agenda. Washington, DC: U.S. Government Printing Office; 2000.

29. CAHPS cultural competence item set. Agency for Healthcare Research and Quality website. https://cahps.ahrq.gov/surveys-guidance/item-sets/cultural/index.html. Accessed September 20, 2018.

30. AHA/HRET Guides: Becoming a culturally competent health care organization. HPOE website. www.hpoe.org/resources/ahahret-guides/1395. Published June 18, 2013. Accessed October 28, 2019.

31. U.S. Department of Health and Human Services: Office of Minority Health. *The National CLAS Standards.* Washington, DC: U.S. Department of Health and Human Services; 2013.

32. Scrimshaw SC, Fullilove MT, Fielding JE. Culturally competent healthcare systems: A systematic review. *Am J Prev Med.* 2003;24:68-79.

33. Midence L, Mola A, Terzic CM, Thomas RJ, Grace SL. Ethnocultural diversity in cardiac rehabilitation. *J. Cardiopulm Rehabil Prev.* 2014;34:437-444.

34. Yeager KA, Bauer-Wu S. Cultural humility: Essential foundation for clinical researchers. *Appl Nurs Res.* 2013;4:251-256.

Chapter 11: Socioeconomic Considerations Section

1. Üskül AeK, Oishi S. *Socio-Economic Environment and Human Psychology: Social, Ecological, and Cultural Perspectives.* New York: Oxford University Press; 2018.

2. Institute of Medicine (U.S.). Committee on Health and Behavior: Research Practice and Policy. *Health and Behavior: The Interplay of Biological, Behavioral, and Societal Influences.* Washington, DC: National Academy Press; 2001.

3. Clark AM, DesMeules M, Luo W, Duncan AS, Wielgosz A. Socioeconomic status and cardiovascular disease: risks and implications for care. *Nat Rev Cardiol.* 2009;6(11):712-722.

4. Galobardes B, Shaw M, Lawlor DA, Lynch JW, Davey Smith G. Indicators of socioeconomic position (part 1). *J Epidemiol Community Health.* 2006;60(1):7-12.

5. Galobardes B, Shaw M, Lawlor DA, Lynch JW, Davey Smith G. Indicators of socioeconomic position (part 2). *J Epidemiol Community Health.* 2006;60(2):95-101.

6. Galobardes B, Morabia A, Bernstein MS. Diet and socioeconomic position: Does the use of different indicators matter? *Int J Epidemiol.* 2001;30(2):334-340.

7. Messer LC, Laraia BA, Kaufman JS, et al. The development of a standardized neighborhood deprivation index. *J Urban Health.* 2006;83(6):1041-1062.

8. Williams DR, Mohammed SA, Leavell J, Collins C. Race, socioeconomic status, and health: Complexities, ongoing challenges, and research opportunities. *Ann N Y Acad Sci.* 2010;1186:69-101.

9. Eisner MD, Blanc PD, Omachi TA, et al. Socioeconomic status, race and COPD health outcomes. *J Epidemiol Community Health.* 2011;65(1):26-34.

10. Guralnik JM, Leveille SG. Race, ethnicity, and health outcomes—Unraveling the mediating role of socioeconomic status. *Am J Public Health.* 1997;87(5):728-730.

11. Wister AV. The effects of socioeconomic status on exercise and smoking: Age-related differences. *J Aging Health.* 1996;8(4):467-488.

12. Levinson AH. Where the U.S. tobacco epidemic still rages: Most remaining smokers have lower socioeconomic status. *J Health Care Poor Underserved.* 2017;28(1):100-107.

13. Brown-Johnson CG, England LJ, Glantz SA, Ling PM. Tobacco industry marketing to low socioeconomic status women in the U.S.A. *Tob Control.* 2014;23(e2):e139-146.

14. Leng B, Jin Y, Li G, Chen L, Jin N. Socioeconomic status and hypertension: A meta-analysis. *J Hypertens.* 2015;33(2):221-229.

15. Pechey R, Monsivais P. Socioeconomic inequalities in the healthiness of food choices: Exploring the contributions of food expenditures. *Prev Med.* 2016;88:203-209.

16. Sobal J, Stunkard AJ. Socioeconomic status and obesity: A review of the literature. *Psychol Bull.* 1989;105(2):260-275.

17. Shohaimi S, Boekholdt MS, Luben R, Wareham NJ, Khaw KT. Distribution of lipid parameters according to different socio-economic indicators—The EPIC-Norfolk prospective population study. *BMC Public Health.* 2014;14:782.

18. Connolly V, Unwin N, Sherriff P, Bilous R, Kelly W. Diabetes prevalence and socioeconomic status: A population based study showing increased prevalence of type 2 diabetes mellitus in deprived areas. *J Epidemiol Community Health.* 2000;54(3):173-177.

19. Lorant V, Deliege D, Eaton W, Robert A, Philippot P, Ansseau M. Socioeconomic inequalities in depression: a meta-analysis. *Am J Epidemiol.* 2003;157(2):98-112.

20. Hare DL, Toukhsati SR, Johansson P, Jaarsma T. Depression and cardiovascular disease: A clinical review. *Eur Heart J.* 2014;35(21):1365-1372.

21. Whooley MA, Wong JM. Depression and cardiovascular disorders. *Annu Rev Clin Psychol.* 2013;9:327-354.

22. Gaalema DE, Elliott RJ, Morford ZH, Higgins ST, Ades PA. Effect of socioeconomic status on propensity to change risk behaviors following myocardial infarction: Implications for healthy lifestyle medicine. *Prog Cardiovasc Dis.* 2017;60(1):159-168.

23. Albert MA, Glynn RJ, Buring J, Ridker PM. Impact of traditional and novel risk factors on the relationship between socioeconomic status and incident cardiovascular events. *Circulation.* 2006;114(24):2619-2626.

24. Avendano M, Kunst AE, Huisman M, et al. Socioeconomic status and ischaemic heart disease mortality in 10 western European populations during the 1990s. *Heart.* 2006;92(4):461-467.

25. Rawshani A, Svensson AM, Zethelius B, Eliasson B, Rosengren A, Gudbjornsdottir S. Association between socioeconomic status and mortality, cardiovascular disease, and cancer in patients with type 2 diabetes. *JAMA Intern Med.* 2016;176(8):1146-1154.

26. Amarasingham R, Moore BJ, Tabak YP, et al. An automated model to identify heart failure patients at risk for 30-day readmission or death using electronic medical record data. *Med Care.* 2010;48(11):981-988.

27. Alter DA, Naylor CD, Austin P, Tu JV. Effects of socioeconomic status on access to invasive cardiac procedures and on mortality after acute myocardial infarction. *N Engl J Med.* 1999;341(18):1359-1367.

28. Rao SV, Schulman KA, Curtis LH, Gersh BJ, Jollis JG. Socioeconomic status and outcome following acute myocardial infarction in elderly patients. *Arch Intern Med.* 2004;164(10):1128-1133.

29. Harlan WR, 3rd, Sandler SA, Lee KL, Lam LC, Mark DB. Importance of baseline functional and socioeconomic factors for participation in cardiac rehabilitation. *Am J Cardiol.* 1995;76(1):36-39.

30. Valencia HE, Savage PD, Ades PA. Cardiac rehabilitation participation in underserved populations. Minorities, low socioeconomic, and rural residents. *J Cardiopulm Rehabil Prev.* 2011;31(4):203-210.

31. Nielsen KM, Faergeman O, Foldspang A, Larsen ML. Cardiac rehabilitation: health characteristics and socio-economic status among those who do not attend. *Eur J Public Health.* 2008;18(5):479-483.

32. Cooper AF, Jackson G, Weinman J, Horne R. Factors associated with cardiac rehabilitation attendance: a systematic review of the literature. *Clin Rehabil.* 2002;16(5):541-552.

33. Bachmann JM, Mayberry LS, Wallston KA, et al. Relation of Perceived Health Competence to Physical Activity in Patients With Coronary Heart Disease. *Am J Cardiol.* 2018;121(9):1032-1038.

34. Bachmann JM, Shah AS, Duncan MS, et al. Cardiac rehabilitation and readmissions after heart transplantation. *J Heart Lung Transplant.* 2017.

35. Suaya JA, Stason WB, Ades PA, Normand SL, Shepard DS. Cardiac rehabilitation and survival in older coronary patients. *J Am Coll Cardiol.* 2009;54(1):25-33.

36. Suaya JA, Shepard DS, Normand SL, Ades PA, Prottas J, Stason WB. Use of cardiac rehabilitation by Medicare beneficiaries after myocardial infarction or coronary bypass surgery. *Circulation.* 2007;116(15):1653-1662.

37. Hammill BG, Curtis LH, Schulman KA, Whellan DJ. Relationship between cardiac rehabilitation and long-term risks of death and myocardial infarction among elderly Medicare beneficiaries. *Circulation.* 2010;121(1):63-70.

38. Gaalema DE, Savage PD, Rengo JL, et al. Patient characteristics predictive of cardiac rehabilitation adherence. *J Cardiopulm Rehabil Prev.* 2017;37(2):103-110.

39. Bachmann JM, Huang S, Gupta DK, et al. Association of neighborhood socioeconomic context with participation in cardiac rehabilitation. *J Am Heart Assoc.* 2017;6(10).

40. Neubeck L, Freedman SB, Clark AM, Briffa T, Bauman A, Redfern J. Participating in cardiac rehabilitation: A systematic review and meta-synthesis of qualitative data. *Eur J Prev Cardiol.* 2012;19(3):494-503.

41. Health Policy & Reimbursement Update: Proposed 2019 Medicare Regulations. American Association of Cardiovascular and Pulmonary Rehabilitation website. www.aacvpr.org/Advocacy/Reimbursement-Updates. Published July 31, 2018. Accessed October 24, 2019.

42. Karmali KN, Davies P, Taylor F, Beswick A, Martin N, Ebrahim S. Promoting patient uptake and adherence in cardiac rehabilitation. *Cochrane Database Syst Rev.* 2014(6):CD007131.

43. Gaalema DE, Savage PD, Rengo JL, Cutler AY, Higgins ST, Ades PA. Financial incentives to promote cardiac rehabilitation participation and adherence among Medicaid patients. *Prev Med.* 2016;92:47-50.

44. Jansen T, Rademakers J, Waverijn G, Verheij R, Osborne R, Heijmans M. The role of health literacy in explaining the association between educational attainment and the use of out-of-hours primary care services in chronically ill people: A survey study. *BMC Health Serv Res.* 2018;18(1):394.

45. Friis K, Lasgaard M, Rowlands G, Osborne RH, Maindal HT. Health literacy mediates the relationship Between educational attainment and health behavior: A Danish population-based study. *J Health Commun.* 2016;21(sup2):54-60.

46. AACVPR Outpatient Cardiac Rehabilitation Registry Selected Data Elements. American Association of Cardiovascular and Pulmonary Rehabilitation website. www.aacvpr.org//Portals/0/Registry/AACVPR%20CR%20Registry%20Data%20Elements.pdf. Published November 2013. Accessed October 24, 2019.

47. Cooper AF, Weinman J, Hankins M, Jackson G, Horne R. Assessing patients' beliefs about cardiac rehabilitation as a basis for predicting attendance after acute myocardial infarction. *Heart.* 2007;93(1):53-58.

48. Shanmugasegaram S, Gagliese L, Oh P, et al. Psychometric validation of the cardiac rehabilitation barriers scale. *Clin Rehabil.* 2012;26(2):152-164.

49. Mattson CC, Rawson K, Hughes JW, Waechter D, Rosneck J. Health literacy predicts cardiac knowledge gains in cardiac rehabilitation participants. *Health Education Journal.* 2015;74(1):96-102.

50. Kripalani S, Weiss BD. Teaching about health literacy and clear communication. *J Gen Intern Med.* 2006;21(8):888-890.

51. Bandura A. Self-efficacy: Toward a unifying theory of behavioral change. *Psychol Rev.* 1977;84(2):191-215.

52. Slovinec D'Angelo ME, Pelletier LG, Reid RD, Huta V. The roles of self-efficacy and motivation in the prediction of short- and long-term adherence to exercise among patients with coronary heart disease. *Health Psychol.* 2014;33(11):1344-1353.

53. Clark DO, Patrick DL, Grembowski D, Durham ML. Socioeconomic status and exercise self-efficacy in late life. *J Behav Med.* 1995;18(4):355-376.

54. Woodgate J, Brawley LR. Self-efficacy for exercise in cardiac rehabilitation: Review and recommendations. *J Health Psychol.* 2008;13(3):366-387.

55. Miller WR, Rollnick S. *Motivational interviewing: preparing people to change addictive behavior.* New York: Guilford Press; 1991.

56. Miller WR, Rollnick S. *Motivational Interviewing: Preparing People for Change.* 2nd ed. New York: Guilford Press; 2002.

57. Rollnick S, Butler CC, Kinnersley P, Gregory J, Mash B. Motivational interviewing. *BMJ.* 2010;340:c1900.

58. Edwards EJ, Stapleton P, Williams K, Ball L. Building skills, knowledge and confidence in eating and exercise behavior change: Brief motivational interviewing training for healthcare providers. *Patient Educ Couns.* 2015;98(5):674-676.

Chapter 12

1. Hamm LF, Sanderson BK, Ades PA, et al. Core competencies for cardiac rehabilitation/secondary prevention professionals: 2010 update. *J Cardiopulm Rehabil Prev.* 2011;31:2-10.

2. Balady GJ, Williams MA, Ades PA, et al. Core components of cardiac rehabilitation/secondary prevention programs: 2007 update: A scientific statement from the American Heart Association and the American Association of Cardiovascular and Pulmonary Rehabilitation. *Circulation.* 2007;115:2675-2682.

3. Suaya JA, Shepard DS, Normand ST, et al. Use of cardiac rehabilitation by Medicare beneficiaries after myocardial infarction or coronary bypass surgery. *Circulation.* 2007;116:1653-1662.

4. Arena R, Williams, M, Forman DE, Cahalin LP, et al. Increasing referral and participation rates to outpatient cardiac rehabilitation: The valuable role of healthcare professionals in the inpatient and home health settings. *Circulation.* 2012;125:1321-1329.

5. Thomas RJ, Balady G, Banka G, et al. 2018 ACC/AHA clinical performance and quality measures for cardiac rehabilitation: A report of the American College of Cardiology/American Heart Association Task Force on Performance Measures. J Am Coll Cardiol. 2018 Apr 24;71(16):1814-1837. doi: 10.1016/j.jacc.2018.01.004.

6. LaBresh KA, Fonarow GC, Smith SC, et al. Improved treatment of hospitalized coronary artery disease patients with the Get With the Guidelines program. *Crit Pathw Cardiol.* 2007;6:98-105.

7. Gurewich D, Prottas J, Bhalotra S, et al. System-level factors and use of cardiac rehabilitation. *J Cardiopulm Rehabil Prev.* 2008;28:380-385.

8. Grace SL, Russell KL, Reid RD, et al. Effect of cardiac rehabilitation referral strategies on utilization rates. *Arch Intern Med.* 2011;171:235-241.

9. Pub 100-03 Medicare National Coverage Determination, Transmittal 125, Change Request 7113, September 24, 2010. Intensive Cardiac Rehabilitation (ICR) Programs (20.31). Centers for Medicare & Medicaid Services website. https://www.cms.gov/Medicare/Medicare-General-Information/MedicareApprovedFacilitie/ICR.html Published 8/18/15.. Accessed October 1, 2019.

10. National Coverage Determination (NCD) for Pritikin Program (20.31.1). Centers for Medicare & Medicaid website. www.cms.gov/Medicare. Issued September 24, 2010. Accessed July 8, 2018.

11. National Coverage Determination (NCD) for Ornish Program for Reversing Heart Disease (20.31.2). Centers for Medicare & Medicaid Services website. https://www.cms.gov/medicare-coverage-database/details/nca-tracking-sheet.aspx?NCAId=240&NcaName=Intensive+Cardiac+Rehabilitation+. Issued September 24, 2010. Accessed July 8, 2018.

12. National Coverage Determination (NCD) for Benson-Henry Institute Cardiac Wellness Program (20.31.3). Centers for Medicare & Medicaid Services website. https://www.cms.gov/medicare-coverage-database/details/nca-decision-memo.aspx?MCDIndexType=1&mcdtypename=Guidance+Documents&NCAId=271&NcaName=Intensive+Cardiac+Rehabilitation+(ICR)+Program+-+Benson-Henry+Institute+Cardiac+Wellness+Program&ExpandComments=n&type=lcd&page=results.asp&lmrp_id=26765&lmrp_version=31&basket=lcd*3a%2426765*-3a%2431*3a%24b%253E+Botulinum+Toxin+Types+A+and+B+-+4I-84AB-R5%252Fb%253E*3a%24MAC+-+Part+B*3a%24TrailBlazer+Health+Enterprises%257C%257C+LLC+(04402)*3a%24&bc=gAAAAAAAAAAA%3D%3D&. Accessed July 8, 2018.

13. Gaalema DE, Savage PD, Leadholm K, et al. Clinical and demographic trends in cardiac rehabilitation: 1996-2015. *J Cardiopulm Rehabil Prev.* 2019 Jul;39(4):266-273. doi:10.1097/HCR.0000000000000390

14. National Coverage Determination (NCD) for Cardiac Rehabilitation Programs for Chronic Heart Failure (20.10.1). Centers for Medicare & Medicaid Services website. https://www.cms.gov/medicare-coverage-database/details/nca-decision-memo.aspx?NCAId=270&NcaName=Cardiac+Rehabilitation+(CR)+Programs+-+Chronic+Heart+Failure&DocID=CAG-00437N&bc=gAAAAAgAQCAA&. Issued February 18, 2014. Accessed August 30, 2018.

15. Ades PA, Savage PD, Toth MJ, et al. High-calorie-expenditure exercise. A new approach to cardiac rehabilitation for overweight coronary patients. *Circulation.* 2009;119:2671-2678.

16. Donnelly JE, Blair SN, Jakicic JM, et al. ACSM position stand. Appropriate physical activity intervention strategies for weight loss and prevention of weight regain for adults. *Med Sci Sports Exerc.* 2009;41(2):459-471.

17. Savage PD, Ades PA. Pedometer step counts predict cardiac risk factors at entry to cardiac rehabilitation. *J Cardiopulm Rehabil Prev.* 2008;28:370-377.

18. Ayabe M, Brubaker PH, Dobrosielski D, et al. The physical activity patterns of cardiac rehabilitation program participants. *J Cardiopulm Rehabil Prev.* 2004;24:80-86.

19. Jones NL, Schneider PL, Kaminsky LA, et al. An assessment of the total amount of physical activity of patients participating in a phase III cardiac rehabilitation program. *J Cardiopulm Rehabil Prev.* 2007;27:81-85.

20. Leon AS, Franklin BA, Costa F, et al. Cardiac rehabilitation and secondary prevention of coronary heart disease: An American Heart Association scientific statement in collaboration with the American Association of Cardiovascular and Pulmonary Rehabilitation. *Circulation.* 2005;111:369-376.

21. Squires RW, Kaminsky LA, Porcari JP, et al. Progression of exercise training in early outpatient cardiac rehabilitation: An official statement from the AACVPR. *J Cardiopulm Rehabil Prev.* 2018;38:139-146.

22. Savage PD, Antkowiak ME, Ades PA. Failure to improve cardiopulmonary fitness in cardiac rehabilitation. *J Cardiopulm Rehabil Prev.* 2009;29:284-291.

23. Department of Health and Human Services, Centers for Medicare and Medicaid Services. Publication No. 100-06. Change request 6850. https://www.cms.gov/Regulations-and-Guidance/Guidance/Transmittals/downloads/R170FM.pdf. Published May 21, 2010. Accessed October 11, 2019.

24. *Federal Register,* Vol. 74, No. 226, Section 410.49. https://www.govinfo.gov/content/pkg/FR-2009-11-25/html/E9-26502.htm. Published November 25, 2009:62004-62005. \Accessed October 11, 2019.

25. Ades PA, Keteyian SJ, Wright JS, et al. Increasing cardiac rehabilitation participation from 20% to 70%: A road map from the Million Hearts Cardiac Rehabilitation Collaborative. *Mayo Clin Proc.* 2017;92(2):234-242.

26. Hammill BG, Curtis LH, Schulman KA, Whellan DJ. Relationship between cardiac rehabilitation and long-term risks of death and myocardial infarction among elderly Medicare beneficiaries. *Circulation.* 2010;121:63-70.

27. Dunlay SM, Pack QR, Thomas RJ, et al. Participation in cardiac rehabilitation, readmissions, and death after acute myocardial infarction. *Am J. Med.* 2014;127(6):538-546.

28. Jolliffe J, Rees K, Taylor R, et al. Exercise-based rehabilitation for coronary heart disease. *Cochrane Database Syst Rev.* 2001;1:CD001800.

29. Taylor R, Brown A, Jolliffe J, et al. Exercise-based rehabilitation for patients with coronary heart disease: Systematic review and meta-analysis of randomized controlled trials. *Am J Med.* 2004;116:682-692.

30. Tharrett KJ, Peterson JA. *ACSM's Health/Fitness Facility Standards and Guidelines.* 4th ed. Champaign, IL: Human Kinetics. 2012;63-79,97.

31. Title 42 Code of Federal Regulations: 42 CFR, Section 482.56. Conditions of participation: Outpatient services. U.S. Government Publishing Office website. https://www.govinfo.gov/app/details/CFR-2011-title42-vol5/CFR-2011-title42-vol5-sec482-56. Issued October 1, 2011. Accessed October 11, 2019.

32. Title 42 Code of Federal Regulations: 42 CFR, Section 410.49. Cardiac rehabilitation program and intensive cardiac rehabilitation program: Conditions of coverage. Centers for Medicare & Medicaid Services website. https://www.cms.gov/Regulations-and-Guidance/Guidance/Transmittals/Downloads/R126BP.pdf.Published May 21, 2010. Accessed October 11, 2019.

33. King ML, Williams MA, Fletcher GF, et al. Medical director responsibilities for outpatient cardiac rehabilitation/secondary prevention programs. *J Cardiopulm Rehabil.* 2005;25:315-320.

34. Fletcher SM, McBurney H. Strategic moments: Identifying opportunities to engage clients in attending cardiac rehabilitation and maintaining lifestyle changes. *J Cardiopulm Rehabil Prev.* 2016;36:346-351.

35. Sanderson BK, Shewchuk RM, Bittner V. Cardiac rehabilitation and women: What keeps them away? *J Cardiopulm Rehabil Prev.* 2010;30:12-21.

Chapter 13

1. Outcome tools resource guide. American Association of Cardiovascular and Pulmonary Rehabilitation (AACVPR) website. www.aacvpr.org/Resources/Resources-for-Professionals. 2002. Accessed May 3, 2018.

2. Verrill D, Graham H, Vitcenda M, Peno-Green L, Kramer V, Corbisiero T. Measuring behavioral outcomes in cardiopulmonary rehabilitation. *J Cardiopulm Rehabil Prev.* 2009;29(3):193-203. doi:10.1097/HCR.0b013e3181927843

3. Buckley J, Doherty P, Furze G, et al. *Standards and Core Components for Cardiovascular Disease Prevention and Rehabilitation.* Heart. 2019 Apr;105(7):510-515.

4. Grace SL, Turk-Adawi KI, Contractor A, et al. Cardiac rehabilitation delivery model for low-resource settings: An international council of cardiovascular prevention and rehabilitation consensus statement. *Prog Cardiovasc Dis.* 2016;59(3):303-322. doi:10.1016/j.pcad.2016.08.004

5. Grace SL, Turk-Adawi KI, Contractor A, et al. Cardiac rehabilitation delivery model for low-resource settings. *Heart.* 2016;102(18):1449-1455. doi:10.1136/heartjnl-2015-309209

6. Woodruffe S, Neubeck L, Clark RA, et al. Australian Cardiovascular Health and Rehabilitation Association (ACRA) Core Components of Cardiovascular Disease Secondary Prevention and Cardiac Rehabilitation 2014. *Hear Lung Circ.* 2015;24(5):430-441. doi:10.1016/j.hlc.2014.12.008

7. Porter ME. What is value in health care? *N Engl J Med.* 2010;363(26):2477-2481. doi:10.1056/NEJMp1011024

8. Anderson L, Oldridge N, Thompson DR, et al. Exercise-based cardiac rehabilitation for coronary heart disease. *J Am Coll Cardiol.* 2016;67(1):1-12. doi:10.1016/j.jacc.2015.10.044

9. Santiago De Araujo Pio C, Marzolini S, Pakosh M, Grace SL. Effect of cardiac rehabilitation dose on mortality and morbidity: A systematic review and meta-regression analysis. *Mayo Clin Proc.* 2017;92(11):1644-1659. doi:10.1016/j.mayocp.2017.07.019

10. How to improve. Institute for Healthcare Improvement website. www.ihi.org/resources/Pages/HowtoImprove/ScienceofImprovement HowtoImprove.aspx. Accessed June 7, 2018.

11. AACVPR outpatient cardiac rehabilitation data registry. American Association for Cardiovascular and Pulmonary Rehabilitation (AACVPR) website. www.aacvpr.org/Registry/Cardiac-Rehab-Registry. Accessed June 7, 2018.

12. Balady GJ, Williams MA, Ades PA, et al. Core components of cardiac rehabilitation/secondary prevention programs: 2007 update. *Circulation.* 2007;115(20):2675-2682. doi:10.1161/CIRCULATIONAHA.106.180945

13. Green L, Kreuter M. *Health Program Planning: An Educational and Ecological Approach.* 4th ed. New York: McGraw-Hill Higher Education; 2005.

14. Zullo MD, Jackson LW, Whalen CC, Dolansky MA. Evaluation of the recommended core components of cardiac rehabilitation practice: An opportunity for quality improvement. *J Cardiopulm Rehabil Prev.* 2012;32(1):32-40. doi:10.1097/HCR.0b013e31823be0e2

15. Piepoli MF, Hoes AW, Agewall S, et al. 2016 European guidelines on cardiovascular disease prevention in clinical practice: The Sixth Joint Task Force of the European Society of Cardiology and Other Societies on Cardiovascular Disease Prevention in Clinical Practice (constituted by representatives of 10 societies and by invited experts). *Eur Heart J.* 2016;37(29):2315-2381. doi:10.1093/eurheartj/ehw106

16. American College of Sports Medicine. *Guidelines for Exercise Testing and Prescription.* 7th ed. Philadelphia: Lippincott Williams & Wilkins; 2006.

17. Pogosova N, Saner H, Pedersen SS, et al. Psychosocial aspects in cardiac rehabilitation: From theory to practice. A position paper from the Cardiac Rehabilitation Section of the European Association of Cardiovascular Prevention and Rehabilitation of the European Society of Cardiology. *Eur J Prev Cardiol.* 2015;22(10):1290-1306. doi:https://dx.doi.org/10.1177/2047487314543075

18. American Thoracic Society statement: Guidelines for the six minute walk test. *Am J Respir Crit Care Med.* 2002;166(1):111-117. doi:10.1164/ajrccm.166.1.at1102

19. Podsiadlo D, Richardson S. The timed "Up and Go": A test of basic functional mobility for frail elderly persons. *J Am Geriatr Soc.* 1991;39(2):142-148.

20. Hlatky MA, Boineau RE, Higginbotham MB, et al. A brief self-administered questionnaire to determine functional capacity (the Duke Activity Status Index). *Am J Cardiol.* 1989;64(10):651-654.

21. Beck AT, Steer RA, Brown GK. *BDI-II - Beck Depression Inventory: Manual.* San Antonio, Texas: Psychological Corporation; 1996.

22. Radloff LS. The CES-D Scale. *Appl Psychol Meas.* 1977;1(3):385-401. doi:10.1177/014662167700100306

23. Zigmond AS, Snaith RP. The hospital anxiety and depression scale. *Acta Psychiatr Scand.* 1983;67(6):361-370.

24. Spitzer RL, Kroenke K, Williams JB. Validation and utility of a self-report version of PRIME-MD: The PHQ primary care study. *JAMA.* 1999;282(18):1737-1744. doi:10.1001/jama.282.18.1737

25. Eichenauer K, Feltz G, Wilson J, Brookings J. Measuring psychosocial risk factors in cardiac rehabilitation. *J Cardiopulm Rehabil Prev.* 2010;30(5):309-318. doi:10.1097/HCR.0b013e3181d6f937

26. Craig CL, Marshall AL, Sjöström M, et al. International physical activity questionnaire: 12-country reliability and validity. *Med Sci Sports Exerc.* 2003;35(8):1381-1395. doi:10.1249/01.MSS.0000078924.61453.FB

27. Morisky DE, DiMatteo MR. Improving the measurement of self-reported medication nonadherence: Response to authors. *J Clin Epidemiol.* 2011;64(3):255-263.

28. Connor SL, Gustafson JR, Sexton G, Becker N, Artaud-Wild S, Connor WE. The diet habit Survey: A new method of dietary assessment that relates to plasma cholesterol changes. *J Am Diet Assoc.* 1992;92(1):41-47.

29. Kris-Etherton P, Eissenstat B, Jaax S, et al. Validation for MEDFICTS, a dietary assessment instrument for evaluating adherence to total and saturated fat recommendations of the National Cholesterol Education Program Step 1 and Step 2 diets. *J Am Diet Assoc.* 2001;101(1):81-86. doi:10.1016/S0002-8223(01)00020-7

30. Taylor AJ, Wong H, Wish K, et al. Validation of the MEDFICTS dietary questionnaire: A clinical tool to assess adherence to American Heart Association dietary fat intake guidelines. *Nutr J.* 2003;2(1):4. doi:10.1186/1475-2891-2-4

31. Ghisi GL de M, Grace SL, Thomas S, Evans MF, Oh P. Development and psychometric validation of the second version of the Coronary Artery Disease Education Questionnaire (CADE-Q II). *Patient Educ Couns.* 2015;98(3):378-383. doi:10.1016/j.pec.2014.11.019

32. Oldridge NB. Outcome assessment in cardiac rehabilitation: Health-related quality of life and economic evaluation. *J Cardiopulm Rehabil.* 1997;17(3):179-194.

33. Kane R. *Understanding Health Care Outcome Research.* Gaithersburg, MD: Aspen Publishers; 1997.

34. Kempen GI, van Sonderen E, Sanderman R. Measuring health status with the Dartmouth COOP charts in low-functioning elderly. Do the illustrations affect the outcomes? *Qual Life Res.* 1997;6(4):323-328.

35. Ware JE, Sherbourne CD. The MOS 36-item short-form health survey (SF-36). I. Conceptual framework and item selection. *Med Care.* 1992;30(6):473-483.

36. Wiklund I. The Nottingham Health Profile-A measure of health-related quality of life. *Scand J Prim Health Care.* 1990;1(Supplement):15-18.

37. Donabedian A. The Quality of Care. *JAMA.* 1988;260(12):1743. doi:10.1001/jama.1988.03410120089033

38. Taherzadeh G, Filippo DE, Kelly S, et al. Patient-Reported Outcomes in Cardiac Rehabilitation. *J Cardiopulm Rehabil Prev.* 2016;36:230-239. doi:10.1097/HCR.0000000000000142

39. Moore SM, Kramer FM. Women's and men's preferences for cardiac rehabilitation program features. *J Cardiopulm Rehabil.* 1996;16(3):163-168.

40. Glasgow RE, Wagner EH, Schaefer J, Mahoney LD, Reid RJ, Greene SM. Development and validation of the Patient Assessment of Chronic Illness Care (PACIC). *Med Care.* 2005;43(5):436-444.

41. Thomas RJ, King M, Lui K, Oldridge N, Piña IL, Spertus J. AACVPR/ACCF/AHA 2007 performance measures on cardiac rehabilitation for referral to and delivery of cardiac rehabilitation/secondary prevention services. *J Cardiopulm Rehabil Prev.* 2007;27:260-290.

42. Thomas RJ, King M, Lui K, Oldridge N, Piña IL, Spertus J. AACVPR/ACCF/AHA 2010 Update: Performance measures on cardiac rehabilitation for referral to cardiac rehabilitation/secondary prevention services: A report of the American Association of Cardiovascular and Pulmonary Rehabilitation and the American College. *J Cardiopulm Rehabil Prev.* 2010;56(5):279-288. doi:10.1016/j.jacc.2010.06.006

43. Thomas RJ, Balady G, Banka G, et al. 2018 ACC/AHA Clinical performance and quality measures for cardiac rehabilitation. A Report of the American College of Cardiology/American Heart Association Task Force on Performance Measures. *Circ Cardiovasc Qual Outcomes.* 2018;11(4).

44. Grace SL, Poirier P, Norris CM, Oakes GH, Somanader DS, Suskin N. Pan-Canadian development of cardiac rehabilitation and secondary prevention quality indicators. *Can J Cardiol.* 2014;30(8):945-948.

45. Doherty P, Salman A, Furze G, Dalal HM, Harrison AS. Does cardiac rehabilitation meet minimum standards: An observational study using UK national audit? *Open Hear.* 2017;4(1):1-5. doi:10.1136/openhrt-2016-000519

46. Piepoli MF, Corra U, Adamopoulos S, et al. Secondary prevention in the clinical management of patients with cardiovascular diseases. Core components, standards and outcome measures for referral and delivery: A policy statement from the cardiac rehabilitation section of the European Association for Cardiovascular Prevention & Rehabilitation. *Eur J Prev Cardiol.* 2014;21(6):664-681. doi:10.1177/2047487312449597

47. Moghei M, Oh P, Chessex C, Grace S. Cardiac rehabilitation quality improvement. *J Cardiopulm Rehabiliation Prev.* 2018; (Under Revision).

48. Gude WT, van Engen-Verheul MM, van der Veer SN, de Keizer NF, Peek N. How does audit and feedback influence intentions of health professionals to improve practice? A laboratory experiment and field study in cardiac rehab. *BMJ Qual Saf.* 2016:1-9.

49. Grace SL, Chessex C, Arthur H, et al. Systematizing inpatient referral to cardiac rehabilitation 2010: Canadian Association of Cardiac Rehabilitation and Canadian Cardiovascular Society joint position paper. *Can J Cardiol.* 2011;27(2):192-199. doi:10.1016/j.cjca.2010.12.007

50. Midence L, Mola A, Terzic CM, Thomas RJ, Grace SL. Ethnocultural diversity in cardiac rehabilitation. *J Cardiopulm Rehabil Prev.* 2014;34(6):437-444. doi:10.1097/HCR.0000000000000089

51. Thomas RJ, Chiu JS, Goff DC, et al. Reliability of abstracting performance measures: Results of the cardiac rehabilitation referral and reliability (CR3) project. *J Cardiopulm Rehabil Prev.* 2014;34(3):172-179. doi:10.1097/HCR.0000000000000048

52. King M, Bittner V, Josephson R, Lui K, Thomas RJ, Williams MA. Medical director responsibilities for outpatient cardiac rehabilitation/secondary prevention programs: 2012 Update: A Statement for health care professionals from the American Association of Cardiovascular and Pulmonary Rehabilitation and the American Heart Association. *Circulation.* 2012;126(21):2535-2543. doi:10.1161/CIR.0b013e318277728c

53. Ghisi GL de M, Chaves GS da S, Britto RR, Oh P. Health literacy and coronary artery disease: A systematic review. *Patient Educ Couns.* 2018;101(2):177-184. doi:10.1016/j.pec.2017.09.002

54. Berwick DM. A primer on leading the improvement of systems. *BMJ.* 1996;312(7031):619-622.

55. Poffley A, Thomas E, Grace SL, et al. A systematic review of cardiac rehabilitation registries. *Eur J Prev Cardiol.* 2017;24(15):1596-1609. doi:10.1177/2047487317724576

56. Pack QR, Johnson LL, Barr LM, et al. Improving cardiac rehabilitation attendance and completion through quality improvement activities and a motivational program. *J Cardiopulm Rehabil Prev.* 2013;33(3):153-159. doi:10.1097/HCR.0b013e31828db386

57. Pack QR, Squires RW, Lopez-Jimenez F, et al. Participation rates, process monitoring, and quality improvement among cardiac rehabilitation programs in the United States: A National Survey. *J Cardiopulm Rehabil Prev.* 2015;35(3):173-180. doi:10.1097/HCR.0000000000000108

58. Straus S, Tetroe J, Graham ID, eds. *Knowledge Translation in Health Care: Moving from Evidence to Practice.* Vol 1. Oxford, Chichester, Hoboken: Blackwell; 2009.

59. Santiago de Araujo Pio C, Chaves GSS, Davies P, Taylor RS, Grace SL. Promoting patient uptake and adherence in cardiac rehabilitation. *Cochrane Database Syst Rev.* 2018;(Under revision).

60. Santiago, C.S.P., Beckie, T., Sarrafzadegan, N., et al. Promoting patient utilization of outpatient cardiac rehabilitation: A joint International Council and Canadian Association of Cardiovascular Prevention and Rehabilitation Position Statement. *Int J Cardiol.* 2019 Jul 4. pii: S0167-5273(19)31295-1.

61. The Deming cycle: or PDSA and PDCA. www.quality-improvement-matters.com/deming-cycle.html. Accessed June 4, 2018.

62. Grace SL, Parsons TL, Duhamel TA, Somanader D, Suskin N. The quality of cardiac rehabilitation in canada: A report of the Canadian Cardiac Rehab Registry. *Can J Cardiol.* 2014;30(11):1452-1455. doi:10.1016/j.cjca.2014.06.016

63. Benzer W, Rauch B, Schmid JP, et al. Exercise-based cardiac rehabilitation in twelve European countries results of the European cardiac rehabilitation registry. *Int J Cardiol.* 2017;228:58-67. doi:10.1016/j.ijcard.2016.11.059

Chapter 14

1. Thompson PD, Franklin BA, Balady GJ, et al. Exercise and acute cardiovascular events: Placing the risks into perspective: A scientific statement from the American Heart Association. *Circulation.* 2007;115:2358-2368.

2. Gaalema et al. Clinical and demographic trends in cardiac rehabilitation: 1996-2015. *JCRP.* J Cardiopulm Rehabil Prev. 2017 Mar;37(2):103-110.

3. Hospital accreditation. The Joint Commission website. www.jointcommission.org/accreditation/hospitals.aspx. Accessed June 27, 2018.

4. Critical access hospital accreditation. The Joint Commission website. www.jointcommission.org/accreditation/critical_access_hospital.aspx. Accessed June 27, 2018.

5. Ambulatory health care accreditation. The Joint Commission website. www.jointcommission.org/accreditation/ambulatory_healthcare.aspx. Accessed June 27, 2018.

6. Seeking home care accreditation. The Joint Commission website. www.jointcommission.org/accreditation/home_care.aspx. Accessed June 27, 2018.

7. Gerald LB, Sanderson B, Fish L, et al. Advance directives in cardiac and pulmonary rehabilitation patients. *J Cardiopulm Rehabil Prev.* 2000;20:340-345.

8. Heffner JE, Barbieri C. End-of-life care preferences of patients enrolled in cardiovascular rehabilitation programs. *Chest.* 2000;117:1474-1481.

9. Peterson JA, Tharrett SJ. *ACSM's Health/Fitness Facility Standards and Guidelines.* Champaign, IL: Human Kinetics; 2012.

10. Pina IL, Apstein CS, Balady GJ, et al. Exercise and heart failure. *Circulation.* 2003;107:1210-1225.

11. O'Connor CM, Whellan DJ, Lee KL, et al. Efficacy and Safety of Exercise Training in Patients With Chronic Heart Failure: HF-ACTION Randomized Controlled Trial. *JAMA : the journal of the American Medical Association.* 2009;301(14):1439-1450.

12. Lopez-Jimenez F, Kramer VC, Masters B, et al. Recommendations for managing patients with diabetes mellitus in cardiopulmonary rehabilitation. *J Cardiopulm Rehabil Prev.* 2012;32:101-112.

13. Lichtman JH, Bigger JT, Blumenthal JA, et al. Depression and coronary heart disease. Recommendations for screening referral, and treatment. *Circulation.* 2008;118:1768-1775.

14. Lichtman JH, Froelicher ES, Blumenthal JA, et al. Depression as a risk factor for poor prognosis among patients with acute coronary syndrome: Systematic review and recommendations: A scientific statement from the American Heart Association. *Circulation.* 2014;129(12):1350-1369.

15. American Heart Association. *BLS for Healthcare Providers Student Manual.* Dallas: American Heart Association; 2016.

16. American Heart Association. *ACLS Provider Manual.* Dallas: American Heart Association: 2016

17. Perkins GD, Jacobs IG, Nadkarni VM, et al. Cardiac arrest and cardiopulmonary resuscitation outcome reports: Update of the Utstein Resuscitation Registry templates for out-of-hospital cardiac arrest: A statement for healthcare professionals from a Task Force of the International Liaison Committee on Resuscitation (American Heart Association, European Resuscitation Council, Australian and New Zealand Council on Resuscitation, Heart and Stroke Foundation of Canada, InterAmerican Heart Foundation, Resuscitation Council of Southern Africa, Resuscitation Council of Asia);

and the American Heart Association Emergency Cardiovascular Care Committee and the Council on Cardiopulmonary, Critical Care, Perioperative and Resuscitation. *Resuscitation.* 2015;96: 328-340.

18. Kronick SL, Kurz MC, Lin S, et al. Part 4: Systems of care and continuous quality improvement: 2015 American Heart Association guidelines update for cardiopulmonary resuscitation and emergency cardiovascular care. *Circulation.* 2015;132(18 Suppl 2):S397-413.

19. Balady GJ, Chaitman B, Driscoll D, et al. Recommendations for cardiovascular screening, staffing and emergency policies at health/fitness facilities. *Circulation.* 1998;97:2283-2293.

20. Balady GJ, Chaitman B, Foster C, et al. Automated external defibrillators in health/fitness facilities. *Circulation.* 2002;105:1147-1150.

21. Neumar RW, Shuster M, Callaway CW, et al. Part 1: Executive Summary: 2015 American Heart Association guidelines update for cardiopulmonary resuscitation and emergency cardiovascular care. *Circulation.* 2015;132(18 Suppl 2):S315-367.

22. Arena R, Williams M, Forman DE, et al. Increasing referral and participation rates to outpatient cardiac rehabilitation: The valuable role of healthcare professionals in the inpatient and home health settings. *Circulation.* 2012;125:1321-1329.

23. Smith KM, McKelvie RS, Thorpe KE, et al. Six-year follow-up of a randomized controlled trial examining hospital versus home-based exercise training after coronary artery bypass graft surgery. *Heart.* 2011;97:1169-1174.

24. Anderson L, Sharp GA, Norton RJ, et al. Home-based versus centre-based cardiac rehabilitation. *Cochrane Database Syst Rev.* 2017;6:Cd007130.

25. Harris DE, Record NB. Cardiac rehabilitation in community settings. *J Cardiopulm Rehabil.* 2003;23:250-259.

26. Ades PA, Pashkow FJ, Fletcher G, et al. A controlled trial of cardiac rehabilitation in the home setting using electrocardiographic and voice transtelephonic monitoring. *Am Heart J.* 2000;139:543-548.

27. Sparks KE, Shaw DK, Eddy D, et al. Alternatives for cardiac rehabilitation patients unable to return to a hospital-based program. *Heart Lung.* 1993;22:298-303.

28. Piotrowicz E, Baranowski R, Bilinska M, et al. A new model of home-based telemonitored cardiac rehabilitation in patients with heart failure: Effectiveness, quality of life, and adherence. *Eur J Heart Fail.* 2010;12(2):164-17.

29. Aufderheide T, Hazinski MF, Nichel G, et al. Community lay rescuer automated external defibrillator programs: Key state legislative components and implementation strategies. *Circulation.* 2006;113:1260-1270.

30. Pashkow FJ. Issues in contemporary cardiac rehabilitation: A historical perspective. *J Am Coll Cardiol.* 1993;21(3):822-834.

31. Haskell WL. Cardiovascular complications during exercise training of cardiac patients. *Circulation.* 1978;57(5):920-924.

32. Van Camp SP, Peterson RA. Cardiovascular complications of outpatient cardiac rehabilitation programs. *JAMA.* 1986;256(9):1160-1163.

33. Giallauria F, Lucci R, D'Agostino M, , et al. Two-year multicomprehensive secondary prevention program: Favorable effects on cardiovascular functional capacity and coronary risk profile after acute myocardial infarction. *J Cardiovasc Med (Hagerstown).* 2009;10(10):772-780.

34. Giannuzzi P, Temporelli PL, Marchioli R, , et al. Global secondary prevention strategies to limit event recurrence after myocardial infarction: Results of the GOSPEL study, a multicenter, randomized controlled trial from the Italian Cardiac Rehabilitation Network. *Arch Intern Med.* 2008;168(20):2194-2204.

35. Lear SA, Spinelli JJ, Linden W, et al. The Extensive Lifestyle Management Intervention (ELMI) after cardiac rehabilitation: A 4-year randomized controlled trial. *Am Heart J.* 2006;152(2):333-339.

Index

Note: The italicized *f* and *t* following page numbers refer to figures and tables, respectively.

A

AACVPR. *See* American Association of Cardiovascular and Pulmonary Rehabilitation (AACVPR)

AAPM (Advanced Alternative Payment Model) 8

ABI (ankle–brachial index) 187, 187*t*

ACC. *See* American College of Cardiology (ACC)

accelerometers 101, 102*f*, 103*f*

acceptance and commitment therapy (ACT) 88

accreditation of facilities 234

ACLS (advanced cardiac life support) medications 260, 261, 264

ACS (acute coronary syndrome) 8, 16, 150-151

ACSM. *See* American College of Sports Medicine (ACSM)

ACSM's Guidelines for Exercise Testing and Prescription 151, 154, 188*t*

ACT (acceptance and commitment therapy) 88

action stage 92

activities of daily living (ADLs)
  assessment of 16, 19, 39, 46, 167
  exercise and 65, 154, 195, 203
  flexibility training and 68
  in outcomes assessment 245
  rehabilitation and 16-17, 23, 156
  in transitional settings 23, 27

acute coronary syndrome (ACS) 8, 16, 150-151

ADA (Americans with Disabilities Act) 232

adherence, gaps in 9-10, 9*f*, 131

ADLs. *See* activities of daily living (ADLs)

admission criteria, for IPCR programs 27-28, 27*f*

Advanced Alternative Payment Model (AAPM) 8

advanced cardiac life support (ACLS) medications 260, 261, 264

advance directives 256

AEDs (automatic external defibrillators) 260, 261, 263

aerobic exercise training 113, 183-184, 204-205. *See also* cardiorespiratory endurance training

African Americans 111, 129, 214-217, 214*f*, 216*t*

AHA. *See* American Heart Association (AHA)

air pollution 143-148, 144*t*, 148*t*

alcohol use 72, 77, 121, 129*t*

American Association of Cardiovascular and Pulmonary Rehabilitation (AACVPR)
  continuum of care 10, 11*t*, 242
  core competencies 25, 224, 226*t*-230*t*, 231, 240-241
  core components 224-225, 245*t*-246*f*, 246-247
  CR Outcomes Matrix 244-249, 245*t*-246*t*
  facilities and equipment 232
  performance measures 22-23, 51
  program certification 224-225, 231, 244
  registry of outcome data 244, 247, 249-250, 252, 254

American College of Cardiology (ACC)
  ASCVD risk calculator 108
  on CR patients with CVD 150
  on depression screening 139
  on dyslipidemia 105, 107, 108, 109
  on exercise testing 37-38, 40
  exercise testing certification 39, 150
  on heart failure 78, 167, 168*t*
  after heart valve surgery 158
  on hypertension 76-77, 124-129, 125*t*, 130
  on hypoglycemia and hyperglycemia 119*t*
  on lifestyle modification 129*t*
  on nutrition 75*t*, 76-77
  on PAD 187, 189, 192
  performance measures of 3, 10-12, 11*t*, 250
  on psychosocial concerns 139, 211

American College of Sports Medicine (ACSM) 39-40, 60, 68*t*, 103, 127, 168*t*

American Heart Association (AHA)
  on behavior change 89
  on cardiorespiratory fitness 98, 103
  on communication with patient 23
  on CPR and ECC 261
  on CR after heart valve surgery 158
  on CR for patients with CVD 150
  on CVD and stroke reduction 2

on dyslipidemia and nutrition 105, 107, 108-109

on emergency planning 260, 261, 263

on exercise testing supervision 39

on exercise with PAD 187, 187*t*, 189, 192

on heart failure 78, 167, 168*t*

on hypertension 76-77, 124-125, 125*t*, 127-130, 129*t*

on nutrition 73, 75*t*

on patient education 91

performance measures of 3, 10-12, 11*t*, 50

on psychosocial concerns 138, 139

on tobacco cessation 123, 124

on weight loss 134

American Indians and American Natives 214*f*, 215, 216*t*

anger, evaluation of 51, 137, 139, 198, 210-211

angina
  atypical 44-45
  CR for patients with 150, 153, 157, 182, 237
  diagnosis of 44
  endurance exercise and 63
  exercise and 19, 37-38, 40, 54, 58, 62
  patient screening for 35, 157, 256-257
  in Phase 3 262
  rating scale 42-43, 234
  standing orders 267

ankle–brachial index (ABI) 187, 187*t*

antioxidants 72, 73

anxiety 9, 138, 140-141, 159-160

aortic regurgitation (AR) 157-158

aortic stenosis 157, 160

arrhythmias. *See* dysrhythmias

arsenic pollution 147

ASCVD (atherosclerotic cardiovascular disease) 105, 107, 108-110

Asian Americans 214, 214*f*, 215, 216*t*

assessment, patient
  of activities of daily living 16, 19, 39, 46, 167
  in behavior modification 89-91
  of cardiorespiratory fitness 103, 105
  core competencies 29, 226*t*
  daily 19, 55
  in diabetes 112-113
  discharge readiness 23

assessment, patient *(continued)*
    guideline on 17
    of initial mobilization 20
    inpatient 16-21, 18*f*, 20*f*
    of inpatient activity program 18
    interviewing 17, 46
    of muscular strength 67
    patient-reported 188-189
    psychosocial 139-140
    risk factor checklist 18*f*
    of tobacco use 120-121
    walking tests 187-188
assist devices 205
asthma 194, 194*t*
atherosclerotic cardiovascular disease (ASCVD) 105, 107, 108-110
atherosclerotic disease. *See also* peripheral artery disease
    cholesterol levels and 106, 108, 228*t*
    environmental factors in 145, 146, 147
    PAD and 186, 191
    process of 103
    revascularization and 150-151
    risk factors for 35, 36, 105
    risk stratification for 50, 53
    secondary prevention of 153
atrial fibrillation 157, 161-162. *See also* dysrhythmias
audits, program 251-252
automatic external defibrillators (AEDs) 260, 261, 263

B
balance training 113-114, 204
basic life support (BLS) training 240-241, 259, 261, 262-264
behavior modification 87-96. *See also* tobacco cessation
    barriers to engagement 52, 89, 93, 94
    as collaboration 89, 94
    educating the patient 22, 90-91
    emotions in 88
    environment in 89, 93, 94
    feedback in 95
    goal setting 80-82, 81*t*, 93-94
    initial assessment 89-90
    lapses and relapses 96, 122
    maximizing participation in 88
    in nutrition 80-82, 81*t*
    outcomes domain 247
    plan development 88, 90, 93-94
    rewards in 95-96
    self-efficacy and 222
    stages of change in 90, 91-93
    in weight loss 134, 134*t*
benchmarking outcomes 253, 259
beta-blockers 45, 107, 130-131, 151

Black Americans 111, 129, 214-217, 214*f*, 216*t*
blood glucose monitoring 115-119, 116*t*, 117*t*, 118*t*, 119*t*, 258
blood pressure. *See also* hypertension
    air pollution and 145-146
    core competencies in 227*t*
    in exercise 41, 54, 63*t*, 68*t*
    after heart transplantation 179
    measurement 125-126, 125*t*, 174
    in metabolic syndrome 133*t*
    therapeutic goals 128
    white coat effect 126-127
BLS (basic life support) training 240-241, 259, 261, 262-264
body composition 18, 51, 64, 132, 202
body mass index (BMI) 132-133, 133*t*, 146
bradycardia 268
Bruce Protocol 39-40, 41*t*, 42
Bundled Payment Care Initiative (BPCI) 4, 8

C
CABG (coronary artery bypass graft) 35, 51, 150, 154-157
CAD (coronary artery disease) 45, 135, 151, 153, 216*t*
cadmium pollution 147
caffeine, hypertension and 77
carbohydrates 70-71, 77, 114
cardiac allograft vasculopathy (CAV) 175, 176*t*, 177
cardiac arrest 258-259
cardiac rehabilitation/secondary prevention (CR/SP) programs. *See also* inpatient cardiac rehabilitation; outpatient cardiac rehabilitation/secondary prevention
    AACVPR certification of 224-225, 231, 244
    benefits of 2, 3, 12
    bundled payment 4, 8
    care coordination strategies 4-5
    continuum of care 8-12, 9*f*, 11*t*, 242
    costs of 221
    dropout rates 64
    exercise capacity and timing 152
    home-based 4-5, 209
    Medicare provision for 4
    for myocardial infarction 150
    nutrition education 82-85
    for older adults 202-203
    performance measures in 2-3
    Phase 3 programs 262-263
    population health and 2-3
    reduction goals 50, 53
    tobacco use in 120-121

    underutilization of 2, 3, 4-5, 12
    value-based care 3
cardiac reinnervation 179, 182, 182*f*
cardiac resynchronization therapy (CRT) 164
cardiopulmonary arrest emergency standing orders 266-267
cardiopulmonary exercise testing 44. *See also* exercise testing
cardiorespiratory endurance training 62-65, 63*t*, 99, 168-170, 170*t*, 183-184. *See also* exercise training
cardiorespiratory fitness (CRF) 62, 98-99, 100, 103, 105
cardiovascular disease (CVD)
    air pollution and 144-147
    alcohol and 72, 121
    atherosclerotic 105, 107, 108-110
    CR enrollment timing 152
    exercise prescription 151
    gender and 202, 209-213, 210*t*, 216*t*
    nicotine replacement and 124
    nutrition and 70, 70*f*, 71, 73-74
    physical activity risks 53-54, 56
    prevalence of 2, 150
    in racial and ethnic groups 214-215, 214*f*, 216*t*
    reduction goals 2
    revascularization in 150-151, 152-153
    risk factors 18*f*, 50, 52-54, 56, 206-207
    secondary prevention 153
    socioeconomic status 220-222
care coordination 4-5
case management approach 50, 52-58
CAV (cardiac allograft vasculopathy) 175, 176*t*, 177
Centers for Medicare and Medicaid Services (CMS) 189-191, 224, 234, 235-236, 238, 244. *See also* Medicare
cerebrovascular accident (CVA) 108, 112, 216*t*, 258, 269
certification. *See also* accreditation
    Medicare 234
    personnel 25, 39, 137, 225, 240-242
    program 224, 231, 244
Certified Diabetes Educator (CDE) 112
CHD. *See* coronary heart disease (CHD)
cholesterol 72-73, 84, 105-106, 107-110, 109*t*. *See also* dyslipidemia; high-density lipoprotein cholesterol; lipid management; low-density lipoprotein cholesterol
chronic heart failure 53-54
chronic lung disease 193-195, 194*t*
chronic obstructive pulmonary disease (COPD) 193-195, 194*t*
chronic renal insufficiency 178

CLAS Standards, National 219
claudication
    intermittent 43
    PAD and 186-188
    pharmacologic treatment 192
    rating scale 42, 43, 188t
    supervised exercise therapy 189-191, 192-193
    symptoms of 186
clinical exercise physiologists 241
clinical pathways 23-26, 24t, 26t
CMS (Centers for Medicare and Medicaid Services) 189-191, 224, 234, 235-236, 238, 244. *See also* Medicare
cognitive decline 201
community-site programs 189, 191, 263-264
complete revascularization 152
confidentiality 233, 235
congestive heart failure 165, 167t. *See also* heart failure
contemplation stage 91-92
Continuous Quality Improvement (CQI) 231, 253-254
continuum of care 7-13
    in CR/SP 8-12, 9f, 11t, 242
    in discharge planning 22-23
    program administration and 242
    reducing gaps in 10-13, 11t
    skilled nursing facilities and 208
COPD (chronic obstructive pulmonary disease) 193-195, 194t
Core Competencies 25, 224, 226t-230t, 231, 240-241
core components 224-225, 245t-246t, 246-247
coronary artery bypass graft (CABG) 35, 51, 150, 154-157
coronary artery disease (CAD) 45, 135, 151, 153, 216t
coronary heart disease (CHD)
    age and 198, 206
    asymptomatic 112-113
    depression in 208, 211
    interventions in 123
    obesity and 131-132, 135
    in racial and ethnic groups 214
    smoking and 119
counseling
    behavior modification 93, 95-96
    daily exercise 114, 135
    mental health 142
    nutritional 76, 79, 85, 130, 132, 226t
    psychosocial 140, 141, 171t, 208
    spiritual needs 142
    substance abuse 142
    tobacco 122-123, 208, 220

CQI (Continuous Quality Improvement) 231, 253-254
CRE (cardiorespiratory endurance training) 62-65, 63t, 99, 168-170, 170t, 183-184
C-reactive protein (CRP) 210t
CRF (cardiorespiratory fitness) 62, 98-99, 100, 103, 105
CR/SP. *See* cardiac rehabilitation/secondary prevention (CR/SP) programs
CR specialists 25, 26t
CRT (cardiac resynchronization therapy) 164
cultural competence 217-218
cultural diversity. *See* racial and ethnic groups
CVA (cerebrovascular accident) 108, 112, 216t, 258, 269
CVD. *See* cardiovascular disease (CVD)
cycle ergometers 40, 42, 42t

D
Daily Emergency Cart Checklist 272-273
dairy foods 71, 74
DASH (Dietary Approaches to Stop Hypertension) 73, 74, 75t, 76, 77-78, 129-130, 129t
data management 250-252
DBN (discharge before noon) 16
delivery models 225, 231
depression
    adherence and 9, 137-138
    in heart disease patients 136-138, 139, 159-160
    after heart transplant 178
    interventions for 140-141
    physical activity and 140
    risk stratification and 54
    screening for 139, 258
    social support and 137
    symptoms of 138
    in women 210-211, 211t
diabetes 110-119. *See also* insulin resistance; Type 2 diabetes
    air pollution and 146
    blood glucose monitoring with exercise 115-118, 116t, 117t, 118t, 119t
    comorbid conditions in 110-111
    core competencies in 228t
    exercise prescription in 113-114
    foot care in 112, 114-115
    after heart transplant 178
    lipids and 107, 108
    nutrition and 71, 77
    in older adults 207-208
    in outcomes matrix 245t
    PAD and 186-187

preexercise testing in 112-113, 116t, 117t, 118t
    in racial and ethnic groups 214-215, 216t
    statistics on 110
    Type 1 diabetes 110-111, 113, 117t
diet. *See* nutrition
Dietary Approaches to Stop Hypertension (DASH) 73, 74, 75t, 76, 77-78, 129-130, 129t
dietitians 79, 80t, 85-86
disabilities, patients with 28, 232
discharge before noon (DBN) 16
discharge planning 16, 22-23, 22f, 24, 24t, 30
disparities in health and health care
    cultural competency 217-218
    national CLAS standards on 219
    racial, ethnic, and geographical 215-217, 216t
    socioeconomic 202, 210-211, 218-222, 220t
dobutamine stress echocardiography (DSE) 46
documentation
    of emergencies 259
    emergency standing orders 261, 266-269
    individualized treatment plans 82, 83f
    informed consent for exercise testing 38, 41
    intervention summaries 258-262
    for outcome analysis 251-252
    physician notification 270-271
    smoking history 121-123
dose–response relationship 63-64, 99
drug therapy. *See* medications
DSE (dobutamine stress echocardiography) 46
DSM-5 138
dyslipidemia 103-110. *See also* cholesterol; lipid management
    demographics and 198, 206-207, 209, 216t
    after heart transplant 175, 178
    as risk factor 18t, 35, 51, 103, 105-106, 216t
    treatment of 107-110, 109t
dyspnea
    assessment and screening 258
    in chronic lung disease 193-194
    emergency standing orders 269
    with exercise 40, 44, 160, 171t
    in heart failure 165, 167, 168t
    rating scale 42-43
dysrhythmias 146, 157, 160-165, 166t, 257

E

early ambulation 16, 19

ECGs. *See* electrocardiograms (ECGs)

echocardiography 45, 158-159

education. *See also* behavior modification

  for behavior change 22, 90-91

  classroom methodologies 84

  in clinical pathways 24, 24*t*

  of diabetes patients 114

  for emergencies 256, 261-264

  on equipment and supplies 27

  on the exercise floor 84-85

  of heart failure patients 171*t*

  inpatient 20-22, 27, 30

  in-service 25-26

  iPEEP format 84

  nutritional 82-85

  of older adults 206

  outcomes review in 252-253

  outpatient 55, 56, 60

  on psychosocial issues 141

  safety-related information 19

  for supervision during exercise 55

  written materials for 85, 90-91

egg consumption 73

electrocardiograms (ECGs)

  during exercise 56-58, 65, 185

  in exercise testing 44, 54-55

  in physical examination 34, 51

  remote monitoring 263

  risk stratification and 58

electronic cigarettes 21, 124

Emergency Equipment Maintenance Log 277

emergency planning

  advance directives 256

  for at-home services 263

  for community-site facilities 263-264

  documentation 259-260

  emergency plans 56, 261-262

  equipment 259, 260, 261, 272-277

  home health personnel 263, 264

  intervention summaries 258-262

  in Phase 3 CR programs 262-263

  physician notification 270-271

  potential risks in programs 256-258

  training 256, 261-262, 263, 264

  transportation to hospitals 262, 292

emergency standing orders 261, 266-269

emotions 88

energy balance–weight equation 64, 133

environment, health and 143-148, 144*t*, 148*t*, 210-211

equipment

  for community sites 264

  for emergencies 259, 260, 261, 272-277

for home health personnel 264

for inpatient rehabilitation 26-27, 232

maintenance of 39, 260

for outpatient rehabilitation 232-234

ethnic diversity. *See* racial and ethnic groups

exercise. *See also* exercise testing; exercise training; physical activity

  adverse responses to 262

  air pollution and 147-148

  blood pressure during 126, 127

  clinical supervision of 55, 56, 58

  contraindications 36-38, 39, 160

  diabetes and 111-119

  after heart transplant 179

  remote supervision 263

  risk stratification for 38, 50-55, 58

  in weight loss 58-59, 64, 135-136

exercise capacity 152

exercise echocardiography 45

exercise intolerance 157, 167, 174, 230*t*-231*t*, 258, 262

exercise nuclear imaging 45-46

exercise physiologists 241

exercise prescription

  cardiorespiratory endurance training 63*t*, 65*t*

  in cardiovascular disease 151

  in chronic lung disease 195

  in diabetes 113-114

  in dysrhythmias 161, 162

  in heart failure 169-170, 170*t*

  in heart transplantation 185-186

  in LVAD support 173-174

  program delivery models 225

  in valvular heart disease 159

exercise specialists 241

exercise testing 33-47

  cardiopulmonary 44

  in cardiovascular disease 151

  contraindications to 36-38

  diabetes and 113

  dysrhythmias and 36, 39, 40, 162

  for exercise tolerance 262

  facilities and equipment 39, 232-233, 234

  heart failure and 38, 39

  heart transplantation and 182-183

  with imaging modalities 45-46

  informed consent in 38, 41

  interpretation of 44-45

  interviews and questionnaires 46, 101-102, 104-105

  in ischemia detection 44

  job simulation 37, 46-47

  medications and 39

  modality and protocols 39-42, 41*t*, 42*t*

in older adults 44

in outcomes matrix 245*t*

personnel in 39

pharmacologic stress testing 46

repeating 34

revascularization and 151

risk stratification 36-37, 38, 50-55, 58

safety in 37-39

6-minute walk test 34, 46

symptom rating scales for 42-43

termination of 39-42

valve replacement and 51

exercise training. *See also* resistance training

  blood pressure measurement in 126, 127

  after CABG 154-157

  cardiorespiratory endurance 62-65, 63*t*, 99, 168-170, 170*t*, 183-184

  chronic lung disease and 194, 195

  contraindications for 36-38

  core competencies 230*t*

  dose–response relationship 63-64, 99

  dysrhythmias and 162

  flexibility training 67-68, 68*t*, 113, 204, 245*t*

  heart failure and 168-170, 170*t*

  heart transplantation and 183, 184-185

  in home settings 189, 191, 263

  hypertension and 129

  informed consent in 38, 41

  LVAD and 172

  for older adults 44, 203-205

  in outcomes matrix 245*t*

  PAD and 189-191, 192-193

  revascularization and 151-152

  valve replacement and 51

F

facilities 231-234. *See also* equipment

fats, dietary 71

FFQs (food frequency questionnaires) 79

fiber, dietary 71

fiscal accountability 231

fish consumption 73

flexibility training 67-68, 68*t*, 113, 204, 245*t*

food frequency questionnaires (FFQs) 79

foot care 112, 114-115

frailty 200-201

fruits, consumption of 73

functional decline 201-202

G

games, education through 85

gay patients 214

glucose monitoring 115-119, 116*t*, 117*t*, 118*t*, 119*t*, 258

goals
  in behavior modification 80-82, 81*t*, 93-94
  in cardiac rehabilitation 17, 50, 53
  in CVD reduction 2

H

HDL-C. *See* high-density lipoprotein cholesterol (HDL-C)
health educators 241
health insurance companies 235
Health Insurance Portability and Accountability Act of 1996 (HIPAA) 235
health outcomes domain 248-249, 250
heart failure (HF) 165-175
  air pollution and 146
  assessment and screening 257
  cardiorespiratory training in 168-170, 170*t*
  chronic 53-54
  clinical manifestations of 165, 167-168, 168*t*, 169*t*
  congestive 165, 167*t*
  diabetes and 216*t*
  disability evaluation 167
  left ventricular assist devices 171-175, 172*f*
  non-ischemic 108
  nutrition and 78, 84
  practice considerations in 170-171, 171*t*
  in racial and ethnic groups 216*t*
  secondary prevention after 170-171
  statistics on 165
heart rate (HR) 56-58, 65, 162-163, 179, 180*f*, 263
heart rate reserve (HRR) 62, 179
heart transplantation 175-186
  graded exercise testing 182-183
  graft dysfunction 176
  immunosuppression and 184
  medical conditions after 176*t*
  medications in 177, 177*t*, 184
  nonrejection medical problems 177-178
  orthotopic technique in 175-176, 176*f*
  psychological factors in 178-179
  rejection of 176-177, 185
  responses to exercise after 179-182, 180*f*, 181*f*
  statistics on 175
heart valve replacement and repair 51, 108, 157-160
HF. *See* heart failure (HF)
high-density lipoprotein cholesterol (HDL-C)
  medications for 107, 108-110
  in metabolic syndrome 133

nutrition and 70-71, 72, 77
recommended levels of 106
screening for 18, 51, 106
tobacco use and 120
high-intensity interval training (HIIT) 152, 157, 168, 185, 205
HIPAA (Health Insurance Portability and Accountability Act of 1996) 235
Hispanic Americans 214-215, 214*f*, 216*t*, 217
home-based secondary prevention 4-5, 209
home health care 27*f*, 28-29
HR (heart rate) 56-58, 65, 162-163, 179, 180*f*, 263
HRR (heart rate reserve) 62, 179
HTN. *See* hypertension (HTN)
hyperglycemia. *See also* diabetes
  assessment and screening 257-258
  blood glucose monitoring 115-119, 116*t*, 117*t*, 118*t*, 119*t*
  care in 117*t*, 118*t*
  diagnosis 124-125, 124*t*
  emergency standing orders for 267-268
  signs and symptoms of 119*t*
hyperlipidemia. *See* lipid management
hypertension (HTN) 124-131
  classification of 124-128, 124*t*, 125*t*
  in CVD 18*f*, 19, 207
  diabetes and 112, 216*t*
  emergency standing orders for 268
  after heart transplant 178
  intervention 76-77, 128-130, 129*t*
  masked 126-127
  nutrition and 74, 76-77, 84
  in outcomes matrix 245*t*-246*t*
  performance measure 131
  pharmacologic treatment 130-131
  pulmonary 176, 195
  in racial and ethnic groups 216*t*
  resistant 127
  white coat effect 126-127
hypoglycemia 115-119, 116*t*, 117*t*, 118*t*, 119*t*, 257-258, 267
hypotension 112, 258, 268

I

ICD (implantable cardioverter-defibrillators) 163-164, 174
ICR (Intensive Cardiac Rehabilitation) 224, 236, 238
imaging, in exercise testing 45-46
implantable cardioverter-defibrillators (ICD) 163-164, 174
inactivity 18*t*, 51, 98-103, 102*f*, 103*f*, 208
individualized treatment plans (ITP) 82, 83*f*, 237, 238-239, 247, 252

infection 152, 177-178
inflammation
  age and 200
  atherosclerosis and 103
  chronic lung disease and 193
  diabetes and 110, 114, 207
  exercise and 204
  heart disease and 137
  nutrition and 71-74
  obesity and 131, 207
  pollution and 144, 145-147
information management 235
informed consent 38, 41
inpatient cardiac rehabilitation (IPCR) 15-31. *See also* cardiac rehabilitation/secondary prevention programs
  abnormal responses to 19
  activities of daily living and 16, 19
  admission criteria 27-28, 27*f*
  ambulation safety assessment 19
  clinical pathways 23-26, 24*t*, 26*t*
  common activities in 19-20, 20*t*
  components of 16
  continuity in 31
  daily assessment 19
  decreasing length of stay 16, 22
  discharge planning in 22-23, 22*f*
  early family involvement 22
  early mobilization 16, 19
  heart transplantation and 184-185
  initial assessment in 16-19, 18*f*, 20*f*
  patient education 20-22, 27, 30
  physician referral to 16, 17, 18*f*, 19
  progression of activities in 19
  space and equipment 26-28, 27*f*, 232
  staffing in 25-26, 26*t*, 31
  tobacco cessation 21, 122
  transitional programming in 23
insulin resistance. *See also* diabetes
  air pollution and 146
  in CVD risk 50, 52
  exercise and 111, 114
  metabolic syndrome and 132-133
  nutrition and 70-71, 206
  obesity and 131, 207-208
  in older adults 207
insurance and reimbursement 235-238
Intensive Cardiac Rehabilitation (ICR) 224, 236, 238
International Physical Activity Questionnaire (IPAQ) 101-102, 104-105
interventions
  for air pollution effects 147-148, 148*t*
  follow-up checklist 22*f*
  for hypertension 76-77, 128-130, 129*t*

interventions *(continued)*
    intervention summaries 258-262
    for psychosocial concerns 140-141
    for revascularization of valve patients 150-157
    for tobacco cessation 21, 120-121, 122-123
    in valvular heart disease 158-160
    for weight management 132, 133-136, 134*t*
interviews of patients 17, 46
intravenous line placement 269
intuitive eating (IE) 80
IPAQ (International Physical Activity Questionnaire) 101-102, 104-105
IPCR. *See* inpatient cardiac rehabilitation (IPCR)
iPEEP format 84
ischemia
    air pollution and 146
    critical limb 186
    dysrhythmias and 164
    during exercise 54, 63, 65, 112
    exercise testing and 36, 37, 40, 44, 113, 162
    heart transplantation and 176-177, 182
    imaging modalities and 45-46
    pharmacologic tests 45
    revascularization and 152-153
    risk stratification and 36, 54, 65
    screening and 256-257
ischemic threshold 151
ITP. *See* individualized treatment plans (ITP)

L
LDL-C. *See* low-density lipoprotein cholesterol (LDL-C)
lead pollution 143, 147
learning assessment tools 21-22
left bundle branch block 45, 55
left ventricular assist devices (LVAD) 28, 171-175, 172*f*
length of stay 16, 22
LGBT populations 214
lifestyle intervention 128-130, 129*t*
lipid management. *See also* dyslipidemia
    clinical evaluation 106-107
    core competencies in 228*t*
    dietary guidelines for 107
    long-term follow-up in 110
    in older patients 206-207
    in outcomes matrix 245*t*
    pharmacologic treatment 107-110, 109*t*
    programming on 84
    in racial and ethnic groups 214-215
    recommended levels 106

    therapeutic lifestyle changes for 107
    tobacco and 120
lipoproteins 106. *See also* high-density lipoprotein cholesterol; low-density lipoprotein cholesterol
low-density lipoprotein cholesterol (LDL-C)
    as CVD risk factor 52, 206-207
    glycemic control and 77
    nutrition and 70-71, 72, 73, 76
    in older patients 206-207
    recommended levels of 106
    reduction of 107-109, 109*t*
    tobacco use and 120
LVAD. *See* left ventricular assist devices (LVAD)

M
macronutrients 70-72
maintenance stage 59-60, 92, 262-263
masked hypertension 126-127
maximal exercise tests 105
ME (mindful eating) 80
meat consumption 73
Medicaid 221
medical directors 34, 39, 57, 237, 239, 240
medical evaluation 16-17, 34-36, 51. *See also* exercise testing
medical history 17, 34-35, 39, 51, 127
medical nutrition therapy (MNT) 77, 85
Medicare
    advance directives and 256
    care coordination in 4
    CR provisions 150, 157-158, 165, 170, 235-238
    documentation for 237, 238-239
    on exercise in PAD 189-191
    on health care providers 234, 236
    home and transitional care 28-29
    on Intensive CR 224, 236, 238
    on measuring outcomes 143
    on nutritional consults 85
    on outpatient CR 236-238
    program certification 234
    psychosocial screening and 139
    reimbursement by 221, 231, 235-236
medications
    automatic refills 94
    in diabetes 207-208
    exercise testing and 39
    in heart failure 165
    in heart transplantation 177, 177*t*
    in hypertension 130-131
    in lipid management 107, 108-110
    in PAD 192
    polypharmacy 200
    psychotropic 140

    in tobacco cessation 122, 123-124
Mediterranean (MEDIT) diet 73, 75, 75*t*, 77, 78, 135
men
    CR participation by 211-213, 212*t*
    CVD rates in 209, 210*t*, 216*t*
    psychosocial considerations in 210-211, 211*t*
    younger 198
mental health professionals 142, 241
metabolic equivalents (METs) 42, 42*t*, 64, 100, 105
metabolic syndrome
    in CR programs 132
    as CVD risk factor 50, 52, 216*t*
    diabetes and 216*t*, 228
    diagnosis of 132-133, 133*t*
    in older patients 207
    in racial and ethnic groups 216*t*
    treatment of 58, 132
metal pollutants 147
micronutrients 72
mindful eating (ME) 80
minerals 72
minorities. *See* racial and ethnic groups
mitral regurgitation (MR) 157-158, 160
MNT (medical nutrition therapy) 77, 85
Monthly Emergency Cart Checklist 274-276
motivational interviews 80, 88, 121, 222
MR (mitral regurgitation) 157-158, 160
multimorbidity 200
myalgias 108
myocardial infarction (MI) 150, 220

N
National Standards for Culturally and Linguistically Appropriate Services (CLAS) 219
Native Americans 214*f*, 215, 216*t*
negative predictive value 45
neuropathy, peripheral 112, 114
nicotine replacement therapy 123-124
non-Hispanic whites (NHW) 214, 214*f*, 215-217, 216*t*
nuclear imaging, in exercise testing 45-46
nutrition 69-86
    AHA on 73, 75*t*, 76-78
    assessment tools 79, 80*t*
    behavioral change for 80-82, 81*t*
    counseling 76, 79, 85, 130, 132, 226*t*
    CR care plan 79-82
    Dietary Guidelines for Americans 76
    dietitian–CR partnership 85-86
    education on 82-85
    food plans 74-76, 75*t*, 82-83, 83*f*, 135
    glycemic control 77
    in ITPs 82, 83*f*, 237, 238-239

macronutrients 70-72, 77
micronutrients 72
in obesity 64, 78-79
for older adults 206
in outcomes matrix 245*t*
specific categories of foods 73-74
nuts, consumption of 73

O
obesity and overweight. *See also* weight management
    classification of 132-133, 133*t*
    in current CR programs 132
    demographics of 131, 131*f*, 207-208, 216*t*
    diabetes in 110, 131-132, 216*t*
    energy balance–weight loss equation 64, 133
    health effects of 131-132, 161, 162
    lipid management and 107
    metabolic syndrome and 132-133, 133*t*
    nutrition guidelines in 78-79
obesity paradox 133
occupational therapists 241
older adults
    CR tailored to 200-203
    exercise training 44, 203-205
    facility- versus home-based CR 208-209
    participation 199-200, 202, 211-213
    program success with 205-206
    risk factor control in 44, 206-208
    secondary prevention in 199
    skilled nursing facilities 27, 27*f*, 208
    sociocultural issues and 210-211
omega-3 fatty acids 110
osteoporosis 178
outcomes assessment and utilization 243-254
    assessment of 51, 237, 244
    behavioral outcomes domain 247-248
    benchmarking 253, 259
    clinical outcomes domain 247-248
    CR Outcomes Matrix 244-249, 245*t*-246*t*
    data collection and management 250-251, 252
    health outcomes domain 248-249, 250
    national registries 221-222, 244, 247, 249-250, 252
    psychosocial 143
    Quality Improvement using 253-254
    reporting and interpreting 252-253
    resources 254
    service outcomes domain 249-250
    socioeconomic status and 220-222
outcomes-based programming 224

Outpatient Cardiac Rehabilitation Registry 221-222
outpatient cardiac rehabilitation/secondary prevention (CR/SP) 49-60. *See also* cardiac rehabilitation/secondary prevention programs; exercise testing
    barriers to participation 60, 211-213, 213*t*, 220-221
    case management 50, 52-58
    clinical supervision during exercise 39, 55, 56, 58
    early outpatient exercise program 55-56
    ECG monitoring in 56-58
    emergency plans 56, 60
    enrollment systems 10, 51
    exercise testing 36-47, 41*t*, 42*t*
    exercise training 50-55, 58
    facilities and equipment for 232-234
    future directions of 60
    in heart failure 168-171, 170*t*, 171*t*
    in heart transplantation 185-186
    innovation in 58-59, 242
    maintenance phase 59-60, 262-263
    medical evaluation 16, 17, 34-36, 51
    Medicare on 236-238
    nutritional care plan 79-85, 80*t*, 81*t*
    patient assessment and screening 256-258
    practice guidelines for 50-58
    program delivery models 225, 231
    standing orders to initiate 265
    tobacco cessation in 122-123
    weight loss programs 133-136, 134*t*
outpatient education 55, 56, 60
overweight 132-133, 133*t*. *See also* obesity

P
pacemakers 162-163, 164
PAD. *See* peripheral artery disease (PAD)
particulate matter (PM) 143-146, 144*t*
patient navigators 28-29
PDSA (Plan-Do-Study-Act) model 253-254
peak oxygen uptake 44, 172-173, 180-182, 181*f*
performance measures
    in discharge planning 22-23, 50
    documenting 252
    goals of 3, 4, 10-12, 11*t*
    on hypertension 124, 126, 130-131
    outcomes and 143
    for program priorities 224
    psychosocial 139, 142, 258
    referral for nutritional consult 85-86
    referral from inpatient setting 22-23
    referral to outpatient setting 50, 150, 157, 158

on tobacco use 119-120, 122
peripheral artery disease (PAD) 186-193, 187*t*, 188*t*
personnel
    burnout of 7
    certification of 25, 39, 86, 137, 240-242
    in exercise testing 55, 56
    in freestanding centers 261
    home health 263-264
    in maintenance phase 60, 262-263
    medical director 34, 39, 57, 237, 239, 240
    performance review 242
    program director 65, 225, 231, 239, 240-241, 264
    program staff 240-242
    training and skills of 239-240, 261
pharmacologic therapy. *See* medications
Phase 3 CR programs 262-263
physical activity 98-103. *See also* exercise
    assessment of 46-47, 100-103, 102*f*, 103*f*, 104-105
    cardiorespiratory fitness 98-99, 100
    components of 100
    counseling 230*t*
    dose–response relationship 63-64, 99
    hypertension and 129, 129*t*
    inactivity as risk factor 98-100, 99*f*
    in inpatient CR 26, 30
    monitoring 101
    outside of CR 64, 65-66
    recommendations for 53, 100
    safety factors 62
    in weight loss 58-59, 64, 135-136
physical examination 16, 17, 34-36, 51
physical inactivity 18*t*, 51, 98-103, 102*f*, 103*f*, 208
physical therapists 241
physician notification of untoward event 270-271
phytosterols 72
Plan-Do-Study-Act (PDSA) model 253-254
plant-based diets 86. *See also* nutrition
PM (particulate matter) 143-146, 144*t*
policies and procedures 234-235. *See also* program administration
polypharmacy 200
polyphenols 72, 73
positive predictive value 45
posthospitalization syndrome 201-202
potassium 76, 129*t*, 130
precontemplation stage 91
premature ventricular contractions (PVCs) 268
preparation stage 92

program administration 223-242. *See also* performance measures; personnel
    contemporary delivery models 225, 231
    Continuous Quality Improvement 231, 253-254
    continuum of care 242
    core competencies 25, 225, 226*t*-230*t*, 240-241
    core function 240
    documentation 238-239
    facilities and equipment 231-234
    fiscal accountability 231
    insurance and reimbursement 235-238
    maximizing utilization 224
    outcomes-based programming 224
    in outcomes matrix 245*t*
    performance and quality 224
    personnel 239-242
    policies and procedures 234-235
    program comprehensiveness 225
    program director 65, 225, 231, 239, 240-241, 264
    program priorities 224-231
    staff education and review 242
program director 65, 225, 231, 239, 240-241, 264
protein, dietary 71-72, 77
psychosocial concerns 136-143. *See also* counseling; education; interventions
    anxiety 9, 138
    assessments in 139-140, 237
    core competencies 137, 139, 229*t*
    counseling in 140, 141, 142
    depression 9, 54, 136-138, 139
    diagnoses 137
    exercise and 140
    guidelines 139, 141, 142
    interventions 140-142
    medical history 35
    medications in 140
    in older adults 208, 210-211
    outcomes measurement 143, 246*t*
    referral to other providers 142-143
    social support 138, 141
    stress management in 141-142
pulmonary HTN 176, 194, 195
PVCs (premature ventricular contractions) 268

Q

Quality Improvement (QI) 13, 231, 253-254
quality measures 10-12, 11*t*
quality of life 59, 139, 142, 167, 249-250

R

racial and ethnic groups 111, 129, 214-218, 214*t*, 216*t*, 220*t*
range of motion 67-68, 68*t*, 185
rate-responsive pacing 163
rating scales 42-43, 234, 288*t*
readiness to change 52, 79, 91
referral
    assessment of 231, 250-251
    automatic 10, 51, 86
    in continuum of care 4-5, 10-12, 16-17
    CVD and 150, 154, 158
    to dietitians 79, 80*t*, 85-86
    in discharge planning 11*t*, 12, 22-23, 26*f*
    disparities in 215, 217
    hypertension and 130
    impacts of increased 58-59
    Medicare on 237
    to mental health specialists 137, 139-143, 208, 211, 258
    older adults 189, 192, 199
    PAD and 189, 192
    in performance measures 11*t*, 12, 50, 224
    strategies to increase 2-3, 56, 213, 213*t*, 224, 232
    tobacco use and 120, 122
    underutilization of CR and 2, 4, 12, 137, 202, 224
    of women 202, 211, 213*t*
registered dietitians 134-135, 241
registered nurses 241
registries, participation in 244, 247, 249-250, 252
relaxation training 141-142
religious needs 137, 139, 142
resistance training
    benefits of 66-67, 68*t*
    in diabetes 113
    in heart failure 170, 170*t*
    in heart transplantation 184, 185-186
    in LVAD patients 174
    in older adults 203-204
    in outcomes matrix 245*t*
    in PAD 191
    after revascularization 156
respiratory therapists 241
restrictive lung diseases 194, 194*t*
revascularization 150-157, 192
risk factors. *See also* diabetes; dyslipidemia; hypertension; interventions; obesity; tobacco use
    in air pollution 143-147, 144*f*
    assessment and management of 18*f*, 20, 22, 50-52
    inactivity as 98-100, 99*f*
    multiple 52
    in older adults 44, 206-208
risk reduction. *See* behavior modification
risk stratification
    for atherosclerotic disease 50, 53
    for cardiac or respiratory arrest 53-54
    for depression 54
    for exercise 38, 50-55, 58
    exercise testing and 36-47, 41*t*, 42*t*, 50-55, 58
    for ischemia 36, 54, 65

S

safety. *See also* emergency planning
    in ambulation 19
    in exercise 56-58, 62, 67, 151, 162-163
    in exercise testing 37-39
    facilities and equipment and 233-234
    of medications 108
    for older adults 205
    in resistance training 67
    supervision during exercise 39, 55, 56, 58
saturated fatty acids (SFAs) 71, 73-74, 107
secondary prevention. *See also* outpatient cardiac rehabilitation/secondary prevention
    in continuum of care 9, 9*f*, 153
    in home settings 189, 191, 263
    importance of 153
    initiation of 9, 9*f*
    remote ECG monitoring 263
sensitivity of exercise testing 44-45
service outcomes domain 249-250
SES (socioeconomic status) 202, 210-211, 218-222, 220*t*
SET (supervised exercise therapy) 189-191, 192
sexual concerns 137
SFAs (saturated fatty acids) 71, 73-74, 107
simulated job tests 37, 46-47
sitting time 98, 101
6-minute walk test (6MWT) 34, 46, 65, 105, 203
skilled nursing facilities (SNFs) 27, 27*f*, 208
smoking. *See* tobacco cessation; tobacco use
social isolation 93, 138
social support 138, 141
socioeconomic status (SES) 202, 210-211, 218-222, 220*t*
sodium 72, 74, 75*t*, 76-78, 129-130, 129*t*
space requirements 26-27
specificity of exercise testing 45

spiritual needs and counseling 137, 139, 142

staff training for emergencies 256, 261-262

standing orders. *See* emergency standing orders

Standing Orders to Initiate Outpatient Cardiac Rehabilitation 264

statins 106, 107-108, 109*t*, 177, 206-207

stationary cycling 40, 42, 42*t*

stenosis 158

sternal healing 35, 51, 155-157

strength training. *See* resistance training

stress management 2, 141-142, 251

stress testing. *See* exercise testing

stroke 108, 112, 216*t*, 258, 269

sugar intake 70-71

supervised exercise therapy (SET) 189-191, 192

supervising physicians 57, 237

symptom rating scales 42-43

syncope or near-syncope 128, 160, 258

T

tachycardia 269

TG (triglycerides) 70, 72-73, 77, 106-107, 110, 133

Timed Up-and-Go (TUG) test 188

tobacco cessation 21, 92, 120-123, 229*t*, 245*t*

tobacco use 50, 119-121, 208, 216*t*

traffic pollution 144-146

trans fats 71, 107

transitional planning 23

transitional settings 19, 27-29, 27*f*, 30-31

transplantation. *See* heart transplantation

transportation to hospitals 262, 269

treadmill ergometers 39-40, 41*t*, 187-188

triglycerides (TG) 70, 72-73, 77, 106-107, 110, 133

Triple Aim framework 2, 3, 7

TUG (Timed Up-and-Go) test 188

Type 1 diabetes (T1DM) 110-111, 113, 117*t*. *See also* diabetes

Type 2 diabetes (T2DM). *See also* diabetes
air pollution and 146-147
controlling 84, 85, 110-111, 118*t*
demographics and 198, 207-208, 209
diet programming on 84
exercise and 99-100, 111, 113, 118*t*
glycemic control 77
nutrition and 71-72, 74, 75*t*, 77
obesity and 207-208
prevalence of 110

V

value-based care 3, 12

valvular heart disease (VHD) 157-160

vegetarian diets 75*t*, 76, 135

very low-density lipoprotein cholesterol (VLDL-C) 106

vitamins 72

vocational rehabilitation counselors 241-242

W

waist circumference measurements 132

walking 187-188, 189, 191

warm-ups, for older adults 203

weight management. *See also* obesity and overweight
in arrhythmias 162
behavioral modification in 89-90, 93-94, 129, 129*t*, 247
core competencies in 227*t*
in CR/SP programs 132, 133-136, 134*t*
in diabetes 77, 111, 207
diet in 64, 78-79, 84, 134-135
in dyslipidemia 107
energy balance–weight loss equation 64, 133
exercise in 58-59, 64, 111, 135-136, 225
guidelines on 78-79, 132
hypertension and 76, 129
identifying overweight patients 132-133
in older adults 207
in outcomes matrix 245*t*
in younger patients 198

white coat effect 126-127

women
CVD in 202, 209-210, 210*t*, 216*t*
program participation by 211-213, 213*t*
psychosocial considerations for 210-211, 211*t*
referral of 202, 211, 213*t*
younger 198

Y

younger adults 198, 200, 208-211

About the AACVPR

Founded in 1985, the **American Association of Cardiovascular and Pulmonary Rehabilitation (AACVPR)** is a multidisciplinary professional association comprised of health professionals who serve in the field of cardiac and pulmonary rehabilitation. AACVPR is dedicated to improving the quality of life for patients and their families by reducing morbidity, mortality, and disability from cardiovascular and pulmonary disease through education, prevention, rehabilitation, research, and disease management. AACVPR provides educational, networking, and professional development opportunities such as live webcasts and online modules, an annual conference and affiliate meetings, professional and program certifications, outpatient data registries, legislative advocacy, leadership opportunities, and more. AACVPR membership is comprised of cardiovascular and pulmonary physicians, nurses, exercise physiologists, physical therapists, behavioral scientists, respiratory therapists, dieticians, and nutritionists. For more information, visit www.aacvpr.org.

Contributors

EDITORS

Patrick D. Savage, MS, FAACVPR
Associate Director of Cardiac Rehabilitation
University of Vermont Medical Center
Burlington, Vermont

Jonathan K. Ehrman, PhD, FACSM, FAACVPR
Associate Director of Preventive Cardiology and
Director of Clinical Weight Management Program
Henry Ford Medical Group
Detroit, Michigan

CONTRIBUTORS

Philip A. Ades, MD, FACC, MAACVPR
Professor of Medicine and Director of Preventive
Cardiology
University of Vermont Medical Center
Burlington, Vermont

Justin M. Bachmann, MD, MPH, FACC
Cardiologist and Assistant Professor of Medicine
Vanderbilt University Medical Center
Nashville, Tennessee

Alison L. Bailey, MD, FACC
Director of Preventive Cardiology and Cardiac
Rehabilitation
Erlanger Heart and Lung Institute
Chattanooga, Tennessee

Alexis L. Beatty, MD, MAS
Cardiologist and Health Services Researcher
VA Palo Alto Health Care System
Palo Alto, California

Cathie Biga, MSN, FACC
President/CEO
Cardiovascular Management of Illinois
Chairman Board of Managers, MedAxiom
Darien, Illinois

Brian Carlin, MD, FCCP, MAACVPR, FAARC
Senior Staff Physician
Pittsburgh Critical Care Associates
Pittsburgh, Pennsylvania

Sheri R. Colberg, PhD, FACSM
Professor Emerita of Exercise Science
Old Dominion University
Norfolk, Virginia

Mary Dolansky, PhD, RN, FAAN
Associate Professor at Frances Payne Bolton School
of Nursing; Assistant Professor in the Department
of Population and Quantitative Health Sciences,
School of Medicine; Director of the QSEN
Institute; and Senior Faculty Scholar for the VA
Quality Scholars Program
Case Western University
Cleveland, Ohio

Emma Fletcher, MS, MVB
Research and Teaching Assistant
Baylor University
Waco, Texas

Daniel Forman, MD
Chair of Geriatric Cardiology
University of Pittsburgh Department of Medicine
Pittsburgh, Pennsylvania

Diann Galeema, PhD
Assistant Professor of Psychiatry and Psychology
Vermont Center on Behavior and Health, University
of Vermont
Burlington, Vermont

Naomi Gauthier, MD
Director, Cardiac Fitness Program
Instructor of Pediatrics, Harvard Medical School
Boston, Massachusetts

Carly Goldstein, PhD
Assistant Professor (Research), The Warren Alpert
Medical School
Brown University
Research Scientist, The Miriam Hospital
Providence, Rhode Island

Paul M. Gordon, PhD, MPH, FACSM
Professor and Chair of the Department of Health,
Human Performances, and Recreation
Baylor University School of Education
Waco, Texas

Sherry L. Grace, PhD, FCCS, FAACVPR, CRFC
Professor in the Faculty of Health at York
University, University Health Network,
University of Toronto; Senior Scientist in
Toronto Rehabilitation Institute's Cardiovascular
Rehabilitation and Prevention Program; and
Director of Cardiac Rehabilitation Research for
Peter Munk Cardiac Centre
Toronto, Canada

(continued)

CONTRIBUTORS *(CONTINUED)*

Joel Hughes, PhD, FAACVPR
Professor and Director of Clinical Training
Kent State University Department of Psychological Sciences
Kent, Ohio

Dennis J. Kerrigan, PhD, FACSM
Director of Outpatient Exercise Programs at Edith and Benson Ford Heart and Vascular Institute, and Preventive Cardiology Specialist for Henry Ford Hospital

Steven J. Keteyian, PhD
Director of Preventive Cardiology at Henry Ford Medical Group and Adjunct Professor in Wayne State University Department of Physiology
Detroit, Michigan

Sherrie Khadanga, MD
Assistant Professor of Medicine
University of Vermont Medical Center
Burlington, Vermont

Kirstine Laerum Sibilitz, MD, PhD
Department of Cardiology
The Heart Centre, Rigshospitalet, Copenhagen University Hospital
Copenhagen, Denmark

Karen Lui, RN, MS, MAACVPR
Associate
GRQ Consultants
Sarasota, Florida

Ryan Mays, PhD, MPH
Assistant Professor, Adult and Gerontological Health Cooperative
School of Nursing, University of Minnesota
Minneapolis, Minnesota

Ana Mola, PhD, ANP-BC
Clinical Assistant Professor of Rehabilitation Medicine, Care Transition and Population Management
NYU Langone Medical Center
New York, New York

Jonathan Myers, PhD
Health Research Scientist and Director of the Exercise Research Laboratory
Palo Alto Veterans Affairs Health Care System
Palo Alto, California

Alexander Opotowsky, MD, MPH, MMsc
Codirector of Boston Adult Congenital Heart (BACH) Research and Associate Professor of Pediatrics
Harvard Medical School
Boston, Massachusetts

Quinn R. Pack, MD, MsC, FAACVPR
Cardiologist and Medical Director
Cardiac Rehabilitation and Wellness Baystate
Springfield, Massachusetts

Jonathan Powell, MD
Cardiovascular Disease Fellow
University of Tennessee Health and Science Center College of Medicine
Chattanooga, Tennessee

Jason L. Rengo, MS, FAACVPR
Senior Clinical Exercise Physiologist, Cardiac Rehabilitation
University of Vermont Medical Center
South Burlington, Vermont

Killian Robinson, MD, FAHA, FACC, FACP
Cardiologist Consultant
Sligo University Hospital
Sligo, Ireland

Ellen Schaaf Aberegg, MA, LD, RD, FAACVPR
Nutritional and Cardiac Rehabilitation Consultant
Westerville, Ohio

Ray W. Squires, PhD
Professor of Medicine
Program Director, Cardiovascular Health and Rehabilitation
Mayo Clinic Department of Cardiovascular Medicine
Rochester, Minnesota

Marta Supervia, MD, MSc, CCRP
Physical Medicine and Rehabilitation Physician, Coordinator of Cardiac Rehabilitation Program for Adults and Children, Head of Physical and Medicine Rehabilitation Research Group at Gregorio Marañón General University Hospital, Gregorio Marañón Health Research Institute; and Research Collaborator in the Mayo Clinic Department of Cardiovascular Medicine
Madrid, Spain

Carmen Terzic, MD, PhD
Chair of the Department of Physical Medicine and Rehabilitation, Professor of Physical Medicine and Rehabilitation, and Associate Professor of Medicine
Mayo Graduate School of Medicine, Mayo Clinic College of Medicine
Rochester, Minnesota

Diane J. Treat-Jacobson, PhD, RN, FAAN
Professor, Associate Dean for Research, and Cora Meidl Siehl Chair in Nursing Research for Improved Care
University of Minnesota School of Nursing
Minneapolis, Minnesota

REVIEWERS

Philip A. Ades, MD, FACC, MAACVPR
Professor of Medicine, University of Vermont College of Medicine
Director of Preventive Cardiology, University of Vermont Medical Center
Burlington, Vermont

Gerene S. Bauldoff, PhD, RN, FCCP, MAACVPR, FAAN
Professor of Clinical Nursing
Ohio State University School of Nursing
Columbus, Ohio

Theresa M. Beckie, PhD, MN, RN, FAHA, FAAN
Associate Dean of the College of Nursing, Professor in the College of Medicine Cardiology, and Associate Dean of the PhD Program
University of South Florida
Tampa, Florida

Vera Bittner, MD, MSPH MAACVPR
Professor of Medicine and Section Head of General Cardiology, Prevention, and Imaging in the Division of Cardiovascular Disease; and Medical Director of the Coronary Care Unit and the University Hospital Cardiac Rehabilitation Program
University of Alabama at Birmingham
Birmingham, Alabama

Eileen G. Collins, PhD, RN, FAACVPR, FAAN
Professor in the Department of Biobehavioral Health Science
University of Illinois at Chicago College of Nursing
Chicago, Illinois

Pat Comoss, RN, BS, MAACVPR
Nurse Consultant
Cardiac Rehabilitation Nursing Enrichment Consultants, Inc.
Harrisburg, Pennsylvania

Kent A. Eichenauer, PsyD, FAACVPR
Clinical Psychologist
Urbana, Ohio

Anne M. Gavic-Ott, MPA, RCEP, MAACVPR
Manager of Cardiopulmonary Rehabilitation
Northwest Community Hospital
Arlington Heights, Illinois

Richard A. Josephson, MS, MD, FACC, FACP, FAHA, FAACVPR
Professor of Medicine at Case Western Reserve University, and Director of Cardiac Cardiovascular and Pulmonary Rehabilitation for University Hospitals
Cleveland, Ohio

Leonard A. Kaminsky, PhD, FACSM, FAACVPR, FAHA
Professor of Clinical Exercise Physiology, Director of the Fisher Institute for Health and Well Being, and John and Janice Fisher Distinguished Professor of Wellness
Ball State University
Muncie, Indiana

Selena Lauren Baker, MS, RDN, LD
Clinical Nutrition Manager
Indiana University Health, West Central Region
Lafayette, Indiana

Carl "Chip" J. Lavie, MD, FACC, FACP, FCCP, FESPM
Medical Director of Cardiac Rehabilitation and Preventive Cardiology at John Ochsner Heart and Vascular Institute, and Professor of Medicine in the Ochsner Clinical School
University of Queensland
New Orleans, Louisiana

Lauretta Quinn, PhD, RN, CDE, FAHA, FAAN
Clinical Professor in the Department of Biobehavioral Health Science
University of Illinois at Chicago
Chicago, Illinois

Jason L. Rengo, MS, FAACVPR
Senior Clinical Exercise Physiologist, Cardiac Rehabilitation
University of Vermont Medical Center
Burlington, Vermont

Charlotte Teneback, MD
Pulmonologist and Associate Professor
University of Vermont Medical Center, Larner College of Medicine at University of Vermont
Burlington, Vermont

Karam Turk-Adawi, MPH, MSSc, PhD
Assistant Professor of Public Health
Qatar University
Doha, Qatar

Mark A. Williams, PhD, MAACVPR
Professor of Medicine,
Creighton University School of Medicine
Omaha, Nebraska

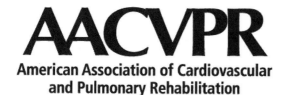

Promoting Health & Preventing Disease

Love the *AACVPR Guidelines for Cardiac Rehabilitation Programs, Sixth Edition*, but not sure what else AACVPR has to offer? See below for more information about AACVPR initiatives.

Membership

Membership with AACVPR offers ways to grow your knowledge, advance your career, and shape the field of cardiovascular and pulmonary rehabilitation to save and improve lives. AACVPR members have access to the *Journal of Cardiopulmonary Rehabilitation and Prevention*, the ability to earn continuing education credits through AACVPR's Live Webcast series, regular updates on reimbursement, the opportunity to serve on national committees, discounted registration to AACVPR Annual Meetings and other events, and much more.

Program Certification

AACVPR offers the Cardiac and Pulmonary Rehabilitation Program Certification process, the only peer-reviewed accreditation process designed to review individual facilities for adherence to standards and guidelines developed and published by the AACVPR and other professional societies. AACVPR-certified programs are leaders in cardiac and pulmonary rehabilitation because they offer the most advanced practices available and have proven track records of high quality patient care.

Professional Certifications & Certificates

The Certified Cardiac Rehabilitation Professional (CCRP), is the only certification aligned with the published CR competencies. In 2018, AACVPR and the American Association for Respiratory Care launched the Pulmonary Rehabilitation Certificate, a program that provides PR professionals the knowledge necessary to be an effective member of the pulmonary rehabilitation team.

Education

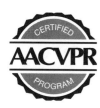

AACVPR offers a number of high-quality educational opportunities, including the in-person AACVPR Annual Meeting, printed resources like the *AACVPR Guidelines for Cardiac Rehabilitation Programs*, Live Webcast series, online courses like the *Essentials of Cardiac Rehabilitation* and the *Essentials of Pulmonary Rehabilitation*, *Staff Competencies for Core Components*, and much more.

Outpatient Data Registries

The AACVPR Outpatient Cardiac & Pulmonary Rehabilitation Registries are unique and powerful tools for tracking patient outcomes and program performance in meeting evidence-based guidelines for secondary prevention of cardiac and pulmonary diseases. AACVPR is now developing a Data Analytic Center, which will allow researchers to access data from the Registries while maintaining registry security and quality.

Legislation and Advocacy Work

AACVPR is a leading advocate for the practice of cardiac and pulmonary rehabilitation, and has a long history of challenging legislation and regulation that negatively impacts the care of patients. Our advocacy efforts are varied to ensure that the interests of our members are made known to a wide array of decision makers. From AACVPR's Annual Day on the Hill to the numerous reimbursement resources available on the website, AACVPR works to gain recognition and support for the live-saving work of cardiopulmonary professionals.

For more information, visit www.aacvpr.org